Pharmacology of Ocular Therapeutics

Thirumurthy Velpandian
Editor

Pharmacology of Ocular Therapeutics

Adis

Editor
Thirumurthy Velpandian
Ocular Pharmacology and Pharmacy
Dr. RP Centre for Ophthalmic Sciences
New Delhi
India

ISBN 978-3-319-25496-8   ISBN 978-3-319-25498-2 (eBook)
DOI 10.1007/978-3-319-25498-2

Library of Congress Control Number: 2015960760

Springer Cham Heidelberg New York Dordrecht London

Printed on acid-free paper

Adis is a brand of Springer
Springer International Publishing AG Switzerland is part of Springer Science+Business Media (www.springer.com)

अज्ञानतिमिरान्धस्य ज्ञानाञ्जनशालाकया ।
चक्षुरुन्मीलितं येन तस्मै श्रीगुरवे नमः ॥३॥

Salutations to the Guru, who with the poultice of knowledge opens the eyes of one who is blinded by the darkness of ignorance

Sage Vyasa (Vedic Age)

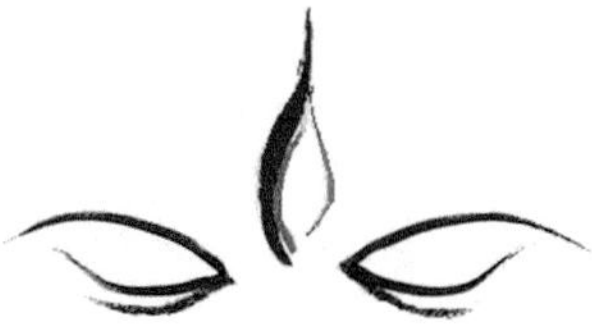

Dedicated to
All my respected gurus

Preface

Archaeological evidence now supports that drugs and various surgeries were used in the treatment of eye diseases by ancient Greeks and Mesopotamians, as well as Indus Valley civilisations during the Vedic age. Bits and pieces of this information can be seen now in recent transcripts deciphered from epigraphs, palm leaf scripts and tablets. Superstitious believes of people in such times also played a major role in eye medications not only for the eye but also for healing various ailments of the body. Priests and monks demonstrated their magical remedies by touching or adding a collyrium on eyes of people affected by various diseases. Psychedelic plants causing visual hallucinations were used in various tribes to transcend into a supernatural world according to his good or bad deeds. Altogether, it is very interesting to understand how the beliefs of societies around the world influenced the remedies on the eye or their effect on vision.

Though the use of herbal and mineral medicines for eye diseases was known to many earlier civilisations of the world, the rationale of treatment started with the systematic understanding about the molecular aspects of the internal structures of the eye along with conditions affecting their function. In the middle of the twentieth century, drugs developed or used for systemic diseases were commonly tested for ocular diseases. Therefore, ocular drug development after considering the constraints exerted by the eye was not adopted as a popular strategy. Although, the first edition of Goodman Gillman's *Pharmacological Basis of Therapeutics* was published in 1941, until its ninth edition in 1996, ocular pharmacology was not dealt as a separate chapter, indicating the slow development of understanding and drug development for ocular conditions.

The prime aim of this book is to deal with such key aspects which are not usually covered by other books and authors. To make a centreline understanding towards the pharmacology of drugs in ocular perspective, invited experts have contributed their wisdom as chapters pertaining to various aspects. Extemporaneously prepared drug formulations, as miscellaneously prepared agents, do not fall under any particular chapter and are considered as an extension of dispensing pharmacy. This book specifically deals with such formulations which are of immense importance in day-to-day ophthalmic practice along with newer dimensions in ocular biochemistry, pharmacogenomics, blood ocular barriers affecting ocular pharmacokinetics, mucoadhesive polymers, tear substitutes, contact lens solutions, drugs acting through ANS, ocular diagnostic agents, therapy for ocular tumours, systemic and ocular toxicity of drugs, etc.

It gives me an immense pleasure to edit the key aspects of this book *Pharmacology of Ocular Therapeutics*. I thank all the authors who have accepted my invitation and contributed their provincial expertise in their own engaging manner.

I hope this book will be a stimulus for research scholars and postgraduates in ophthalmology, optometry, pharmacy, pharmacology and nursing to think about expanding their domain understanding and to broaden their exploratory thoughts. I thank all my research scholars for their help in compiling the chapters of this book. I also thank Springer for coming forward to provide the much needed public access of its contents by publishing the same. I must acknowledge my family for their understanding and support whenever I have taken the liberty of using their time for my academic pursuits.

தாமின் புறுவது உலகின் புறக் கண்டு காமுறுவர் கற்றறிந் தார்	"The learned foster learning more On seeing the world enjoy their lore"
Kural 399 by Thiruvalluvar (1–3 Century BC)	

New Delhi, India Thirumurthy Velpandian

Contents

Contributors

Tushar Agarwal, MD Cornea Services, Dr. Rajendra Prasad Center for Ophthalmic Sciences, All India Institute of Medical Sciences, New Delhi, India

Narayanasamy Angayarkanni, PhD Biochemistry and Cell Biology Department, Sankara Nethralaya, Vision Research Foundation, Chennai, India

Renu Agarwal, PhD Faculty of Medicine, Universiti Teknologi MARA, Sungai Buloh, Selangor Darul Ehsan, Malaysia

Carlos Alves, PhD School of Pharmacy, University of Coimbra, Coimbra, Portugal

Neelima Aron, MD Cornea Services, Dr. Rajendra Prasad Center for Ophthalmic Sciences, All India Institute of Medical Sciences, New Delhi, India

Rajinder K. Bhardwaj, MS, PhD d3 Medicine, Parsippany, NJ, USA

Subramaniam Rajesh Bharathi Devi RS Mehta Jain Department of Biochemistry and Cell Biology, Vision Research Foundation, Sankara Nethralaya, Chennai, India

Alain Bron, MD University Hospital, Dijon, France

Monica Chaudhry, M. Optom Department of Optometry and Vision Science, Amity University, Haryana, India

Bhavna Chawla, MS (Ophthalmol) Ocular Oncology & Pediatric Ophthalmology Service, Dr. Rajendra Prasad Center for Ophthalmic Sciences, All India Institute of Medical Sciences, New Delhi, India

Karunakaran Coral RS Mehta Jain Department of Biochemistry and Cell Biology, Vision Research Foundation, Sankara Nethralaya, Chennai, India

Jose Cunha-Vaz, MD, PhD, FAAO Department of Ophthalmology, Coimbra University Hospital, Coimbra, Portugal

Tanuj Dada, MD Dr. Rajendra Prasad Center for Ophthalmic Sciences, All India Institute of Medical Sciences, New Delhi, India

Ujjalkumar S. Das, MPharm Ocular Pharmacology and Pharmacy, Dr. Rajendra Prasad Center for Ophthalmic Sciences, All India Institute of Medical Sciences, New Delhi, India

Kavitha Duraipandi, MD, FICO, DNB Department of Ophthalmology, Dr. Rajendra Prasad Center for Ophthalmic Sciences, All India Institute of Medical Sciences, New Delhi, India

Rosa Fernandes, PhD Laboratório de Farmacologia e Terapêutica Experimental, IBILI – Faculdade de Medicina da Universidade de Coimbra, Coimbra, Portugal

Suresh Kumar Gupta, PhD, DSc, FIPS, FIACS Pharmacology/Clinical Research, Delhi Institute of Pharmaceutical Sciences and Research (DIPSAR), University of Delhi, New Delhi, India

Nabanita Halder, PhD Ocular Pharmacology and Pharmacy, Dr. Rajendra Prasad Center for Ophthalmic Sciences, All India Institute of Medical Sciences, New Delhi, India

Parul Ichhpujani, MD Glaucoma and Neuro-ophthalmology Services, Department of Ophthalmology, Government Medical College and Hospital, Chandigarh, India

Gaurav K. Jain, PhD Department of Pharmaceutics, Faculty of Pharmacy, Jamia Hamdard (Hamdard University), New Delhi, India

Jayabalan Nirmal, PhD School of Materials Science and Engineering, NTU-Northwestern Nanomedicine Institute@NTU, Nanyang Technological University, Singapore

Rama Jayasundar, PhD Department of NMR, All India Institute of Medical Sciences, New Delhi, India

Atul Kumar, MD, FAMS Vitreous-Retina Service, Dr. Rajendra Prasad Center for Ophthalmic Sciences, All India Institute of Medical Sciences, New Delhi, India

Govindasamy Kumaramanickavel, MD Narayana Nethralaya, Bangalore, India Aditya Jyot Eye Hospital, Mumbai, India

Francisco Batel Marques, PhD Centre for Heath Technology Assessment and Drug Research (CHAD), AIBILI Association for Innovation and Biomedical Research on Light and Image (AIBILI), Coimbra, Portugal

Rajani Mathur, PhD Department of Pharmacology, Delhi Institute of Pharmaceutical Sciences and Research (DIPSAR), New Delhi, India

Kanuj Mishra, MBiotech Department of Biotechnology, All India Institute of Medical Sciences, New Delhi, India

S.N. Mohanraj, MD Nethradhama Superspeciality Eye Hospital, Bangalore, India

Sujata Mohanty, PhD Stem Cell Facility, DBT-Centre for Excellence of Stem Cell Research, All India Institute of Medical Sciences, New Delhi, India

Laxmi Moksha, MPharm Ocular Pharmacology and Pharmacy, Dr. Rajendra Prasad Center for Ophthalmic Sciences, All India Institute of Medical Sciences, New Delhi, India

Madhu Nath, RN (H), MSc (Clin Res) Department of Ophthalmology, Dr. Rajendra Prasad Center for Ophthalmic Sciences, All India Institute of Medical Sciences, New Delhi, India

Anuradha V. Pai, PhD Ocular Pharmacology and Pharmacy, Dr. Rajendra Prasad Center for Ophthalmic Sciences, All India Institute of Medical Sciences, New Delhi, India

Santosh Patnaik, MPharm Ocular Pharmacology and Pharmacy, Dr. Rajendra Prasad Center for Ophthalmic Sciences, All India Institute of Medical Sciences, New Delhi, India

Swati Phuljhele Ophthalmology, Dr. Rajendra Prasad Center for Ophthalmic Sciences, All India Institute of Medical Sciences, New Delhi, India

Ramalingam Kalainesan Rajeshkumar, MS BioTech, MPhil, PhD Ocular Pharmacology and Pharmacy, Dr. Rajendra Prasad Center for Ophthalmic Sciences, All India Institute of Medical Sciences, New Delhi, India

Manu Saini, MD Cornea Services, Dr. Rajendra Prasad Center for Ophthalmic Sciences, All India Institute of Medical Sciences, New Delhi, India

Aluru Venkata Saijyothi RS Mehta Jain Department of Biochemistry and Cell Biology, Vision Research Foundation, Sankara Nethralaya, Chennai, India

Rohit Saxena, MD Ophthalmology, Dr. Rajendra Prasad Center for Ophthalmic Sciences, All India Institute of Medical Sciences, New Delhi, India

Srinivasan Senthilkumari, PhD Scientist II, Department of Ocular Pharmacology, Aravind Medical Research Foundation (AMRF), Madurai, Tamil Nadu, India

Rachna Seth, MD Division of Pediatric Oncology, Department of Pediatrics, All India Institute of Medical Sciences, New Delhi, India

Charu Sharma, PhD Department of Internal Medicine, College of Medicine and Health Sciences, UAE University, Al-Ain, UAE

Hanuman Prasad Sharma, MPharm Ocular Pharmacology and Pharmacy, Dr. Rajendra Prasad Center for Ophthalmic Sciences, All India Institute of Medical Sciences, New Delhi, India

Namrata Sharma, MD Cornea Services, Dr. Rajendra Prasad Center for Ophthalmic Sciences, All India Institute of Medical Sciences, New Delhi, India

Aruna Singh, MPharm Department of NMR, All India Institute of Medical Sciences, New Delhi, India

Murugesan Vanathi, MD Cornea Services, Dr. Rajendra Prasad Center for Ophthalmic Sciences, All India Institute of Medical Sciences, New Delhi, India

Thirumurthy Velpandian, BPharm, MS(Pharmacol), PhD Ocular Pharmacology and Pharmacy, Dr. Rajendra Prasad Centre for Ophthalmic Sciences, All India Institute of Medical Sciences, New Delhi, India

Sharmilee Vetrivel, MBiotech Department of Biotechnology, All India Institute of Medical Sciences, New Delhi, India

Arumugam Ramamoorthy Vijayakumar, PhD Ophthalmic Pharmaceutical Division, Appasamy Associates, Arumbakkam, Chennai, India

Manu Saini, MD Cornea Services, Dr. Rajendra Prasad Center for Ophthalmic Sciences, All India Institute of Medical Sciences, New Delhi, India

Chapter 1
Ocular Pharmacology and Therapeutics: Origin, Principle, Challenges, and Practices

Thirumurthy Velpandian and Suresh Kumar Gupta

Abstract Recent revelations on the origin of eye specific applications bring out the fascinating history from various civilizations. Use of black kohl eyeliner and the possible science behind it has been explored through contemporary technology. Chemical analysis of the contents of the pyxis recovered from the Roman vessel that was shipwrecked off the coast of Tuscany more than 2000 years ago, showed the presence of higher amounts of zinc which might have been used to treat eye infections. Literatures available from ancient civilizations indicate the use of many INTERESTING drug formulations for the eye. This chapter narrates the history for such usage attributing to the development of medications for ocular therapeutics, principles of ocular therapy and challenges in applying ocular pharmacology to therapeutics.

1.1 Origin of Eye Medications in the Human History

Almost in all ancient civilizations, the eye and vision had a special place in their evolution. Eye paint was used as a remedy to strive against evil spirits entering through nine vulnerable openings in the body in ancient Mesopotamia. The importance of ophthalmic ointments and eye paint was particularly signified in the Egyptian culture. The importance of the eye was immortalized through the myth of the Eye of Horus which says that one eye represents the moonlight while the other

T. Velpandian, BPharm, MS(Pharmacol), PhD (✉)
Ocular Pharmacology and Pharmacy, Dr. Rajendra Prasad Centre for Ophthalmic Sciences, All India Institute of Medical Sciences, New Delhi 110 029, India
e-mail: tvelpandian@hotmail.com

S.K. Gupta, PhD, DSc, FIPS, FIACS
Pharmacology/Clinical Research, Delhi Institute of Pharmaceutical Sciences and Research (DIPSAR), University of Delhi, New Delhi, India

Research (DIPSAR), University of Delhi, New Delhi, India

T. Velpandian (ed.), *Pharmacology of Ocular Therapeutics*,
DOI 10.1007/978-3-319-25498-2_1

eye represents the sunshine. The two eyes altogether thus represent the power of human intellect. Blindness, in turn, was seen as a divine punishment. To protect the eyes from blindness, Egyptians used to apply drops and ointments, to chase away insects and demons that were associated with a variety of eye infections.

The Egyptian physicians for eye diseases carried a special kit that contained a black kohl make up and green chrysocolla. Kohl served multiple roles in the Egyptian culture. Moreover, the Egyptian of all social classes smeared their eyelids with black kohl eyeliner in veneration of the deities. Kohl also signified one's status in the society with the glossiest, highest-quality kohl denoting one's upper class status in society while the less wealthy applied kohl of fire soot. Kohl applied liberally around the eyes helped to reduce the sun's glare, to repel flies, and to provide cooling relief from the heat. It also trapped errant dust and dirt common in the desert.

The typical composition of kohl which was used in Egypt in the recent past has been reported to contain crushed stibnite, burnt almonds, lead, oxidized copper, ochre, ash, malachite, and chrysocolla (Murube 2013), whereas the original composition of kohl used in ancient Egypt is now known from the work of French researchers reported in 2010. They have analyzed 52 kohl samples from the Egyptian make up containers residing at the Louvre museum in Paris. The research of their study reported the presence of trace amounts of four uncommon lead species: galena (PbS), cerussite (PbCO3), phosgenite (Pb2Cl2CO3), and laurionite (Pb(OH)Cl) in the cosmetics (Tapsoba et al. 2010).

Kohl was predominantly composed of the mineral galena, a dark, metallic lead-based product that is also known by the chemical name lead sulfide (PbS). The minerals were further reported to be crushed and mixed with several other ingredients such as ground pearls, rubies and emeralds, silver and gold leaves, frankincense, coral, and medicinal herbs such as saffron, fennel, and neem . The resulting formulation was then diluted in liquids such as oil, gum, animal fats, milk, or water to solubilize the lead and assist in its eventual facial smearing. Thus the composition of kohl made authors of the study to quote that "it is clear that such intentional production remains the first known example of a large scale chemical process" (BMJ 1909).

When researchers exposed skin cells to the lead sulfates found in kohl, they discovered that the lead ions elicited a profound immunological response. The cultured cells released one of the most important messenger molecule in the immune system, nitric oxide gas (NO); this gaseous molecule serves as an activating messenger to bacteria-eating macrophage cells and stimulates blood flow by increasing the diameter of capillaries, encouraging rapid immune cell movement within the bloodstream. The abovementioned molecular interaction of kohl illustrates its role not only as a beautifying cosmetic but also an antibacterial ointment. As eye infections would have been a common problem in tropical marshy places such as Nile area, application of kohl must have played a prominent role in the Egyptian custom (Tapsoba et al. 2010).

In death, pouches containing kohl were buried alongside the departed, illustrating its indispensable role in the Egyptian traditions. Kohl also observes a mention in the Egyptian manuscript – Ebers papyrus, the oldest known medical texts in existence. In the hieroglyphic manuscript dating from 1550 BC, Egyptians mention detailed herbal preparations for eyedrops, salves, and ointments. However, an old Babylonian tablet (16–20 century BC) from Nippur showing medication for various parts of the body is the oldest known prescription of an ointment for eyes (BAM IV

393). Neo-Babylonian tablets (5–6 century BC) dealing exclusively with eye diseases have been discovered. These contain prescriptions of ointments for eyes. The individual instructions begin with a list of ingredients and end with the conditions for which the ointment has to be used (BAM IV 383, Attia and Buisson 2006).

Apart from the ores of lead in the kohl, the use of zinc in ocular medication was well documented in one of Galen's treatises, Medicines according to Places.

> Cleaned Cadmia (zinc oxide), 28 drams; hematite stone, burnt and washed, 24 drams; Cyprian ash (i.e. copper), 24 drams; myrrh, 48 drams; saffron, 4 drams; Spanish opium-poppy, 8 drams; white pepper, 30 grains; gum, 6 drams; dilute with Italian wine. Use with an egg **(Galen, Compositions of medicines according to places 4.8, 12.774 Khun)**

This timeless application of zinc in ocular medication came from a breaking finding in the history of medicine which came to light in the year 2013 with the findings from the analysis of the contents of a shipwreck Relitto del Pozzino dated 140–130 BCE. The vessel was laying about 18 m underwater in the Baratti Gulf, not far from the remains of the important Etruscan city of Populonia, a key port along trade routes across the Mediterranean. It was thought to be a trading ship sailing from the Asia Minor and Greece areas, carrying wine, glass cup, and lamps off the coast of Tuscany near Etruscan town of Populonia in Italy (Fig. 1.1).

The boat was found to have various pharmacological preparations along with a surgery hook, a mortar 136 wooden drug vials, and in particular several tin boxes (pyxides) (Fig. 1.2). X-ray examination of the tin boxes revealed the presence of well-preserved circular tablets in dry form even after resting in the seafloor for such a long time of 2000 years. Interestingly, five grey disc-shaped tablets enclosed in the watertight tin pyxis lying on the seabed of the Baratti Gulf wrapped in dense marine flora revealed a rare archaeological finding about the medicine used 2120 years before (Fig. 1.3).

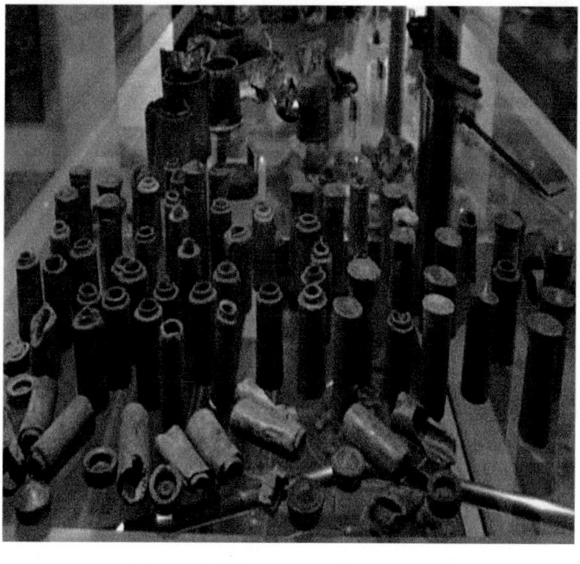

Fig. 1.1 Picture showing boxwoods recovered from the shipwrecked Relitto del Pozzino can be seen on display at the Archaeological Museum of Populonia in Piombino, Italy

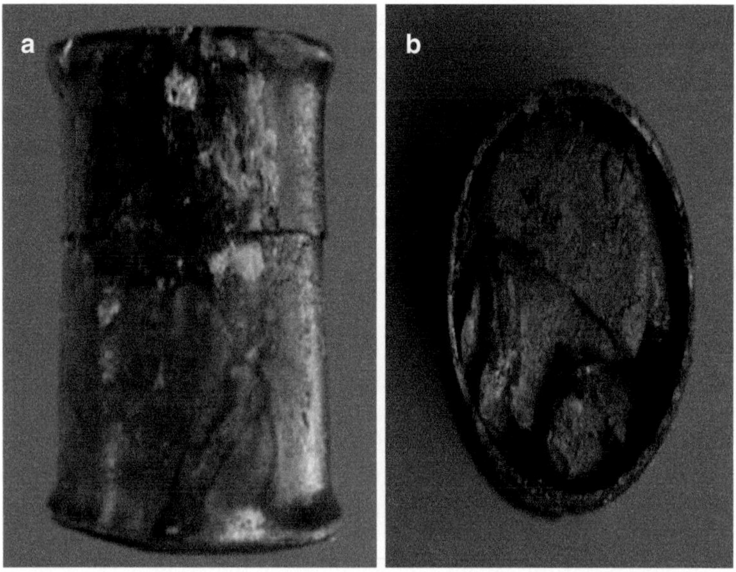

Fig. 1.2 Airtight tin container kept in a boxwood stored aboard of a Roman vessel that was shipwrecked off the coast of Tuscany more than 2,000 year ago. The A/6 pyxis before it was opened (**a**) and the pyxis showing it content (**b**) (Gianna et al. 2013; reproduced with permission)

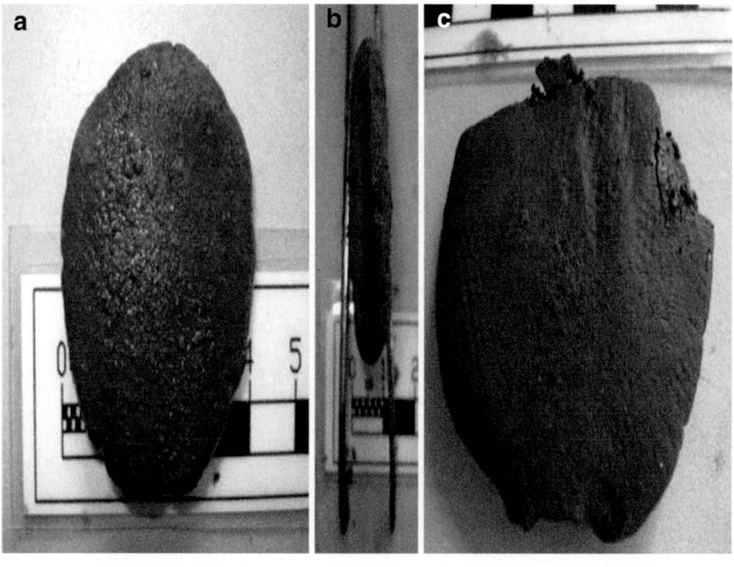

Fig. 1.3 Picture showing grey tablets, each about the shape of a circular makeup sponge, inside an airtight tin container stored aboard a Roman vessel that was shipwrecked off the coast of Tuscany more than 2,000 year ago. (**a**) The Front (**b**) side & (**c**) back view profile of tablet found in the A/6 pyxis (Giachi et al. 2013 reproduced with permission). *Note*: chemical analyses revealed the presence of starch, pine resin, beeswax, and fats in the ancient drugs, with higher amount of zinc compounds indicating that it might have been used to treat eye infections

Subjecting them for chemical analysis using advanced analytical instruments revealed extraordinary information on the composition of the tablets and on their possible therapeutic use. Hydrozincite (zinc hydroxycarbonate) and smithsonite (zinc carbonate) were two of the most abundant ingredients of the Pozzino tablets, along with starch, animal and plant lipids, and pine resin. From the composition, the authors reached a conclusion that the Pozzino tablets were used for ophthalmic purposes.

Concurrently Roman oculist stamps demonstrate a classification of ocular disease, a system of treatment, and reveal the names of practitioners (Marmion 1995). Roman oculist stamps were associated with collyria, and collyrium stamps are parallelepipedic stones that were used in the Roman world, between the second part of the first century and the fourth century A.D., to stamp eye medicine (Perez-Cambrodi et al. 2013). The Latin expression collyrium (eyewash) comes from the Greek name κο λλυ′ ρα, which means "small round loaves" (Giachi et al. 2013). These seals specifically those of Roman eye medicine were inscribed according to the Greek medical tradition indicating the name of the patient, therapeutic instructions, method of administration, etc. Thus, the Greek medical texts reveal the influence of the Greek ophthalmology on Roman eye medicine (Pardon-Labonnelie 2014). Collyrium also refers to the composition of powders brought to a pasty consistence with a liquid and formed into tentlike structure for insertion into (Murube J, 2007a).

Another usage of the vocabulary of collyrium refers to Keshanjana (collyrium), an Ayurvedic formulation prepared out of Keshamasi (ash prepared by scalp hairs) mixed with Goghrita (cow ghee). This particular preparation is indicated for treating Chushkashipaka (dry eye syndrome) in Vagbhatta Samhitas and classical Ayurvedic treatises (Kartar et al. 2014). Ayurvedic and Siddha medical systems originated from different parts of India reported several medicines for ocular use (Subbarayappa 1997; Ven Murthy et al. 2010). Ayurveda dates back to the Vedic period of the Indus Valley Civilization (about 3000 BC) and has been passed on through generations of oral tradition, like the other four sacred texts (Rigveda, Yajurveda, Samaveda, and Atharvanaveda) which were composed between the twelfth and seventh century BC (Ven Murthy et al. 2010).

In the ancient Indian Ayurvedic texts, Shalakya tantra is referred as one among Ashtang Ayurveda (eight super specialities) specifically for the diagnosis, treatment, and prevention of all the diseases occurring above the neck such as eyes, nose, ear, mouth, and head. According to the Vedic scripts, the father of Shalakya tantra was referred as King Nimi (king of Videha). Among the eight super speciality disciplines, Netra Chikitsa is considered as referring to the treatment for ocular diseases.

Anjanam is an ancient Ayurvedic eyeliner and paint explained for cleansing and therapeutic purposes (Fig. 1.4). Although it has been known to exist in the ancient Ayurvedic literature, its relevance to the origin of its use has not been studied systematically. Although the effects of plants with psychoactive substances have been manifested in many ways, one account in Indian Ayurvedic literature details about the use of Datura. "Harita Samhita" explains, Datura root is crushed in water and strained liquid is used in instilling in sore eyes (conjunctivitis). Cannabis extract was used for sore eyes by the Egyptians around 2000 BC (Webley K 2010). They have also used squill for dropsy under the mystic name of the "Eye of Typhon."

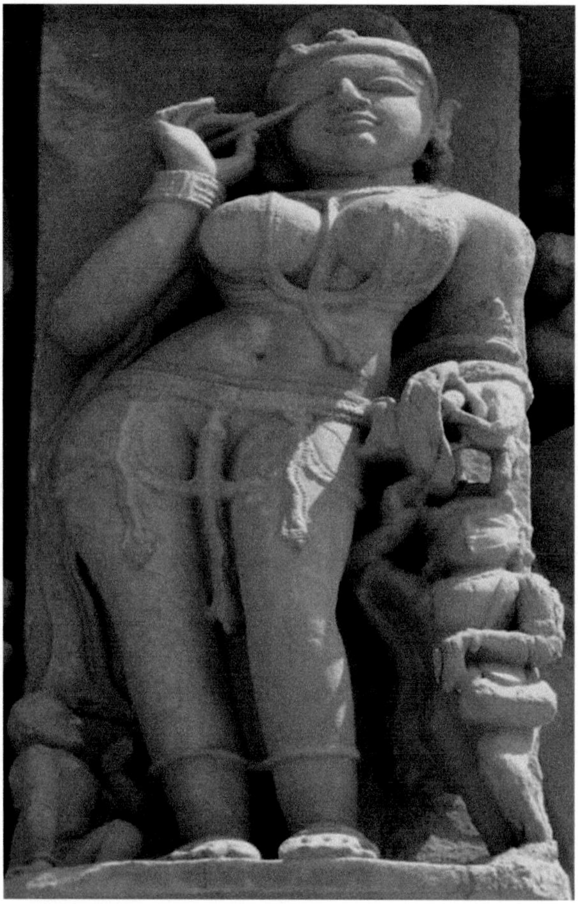

Fig. 1.4 The tenth century carving on stone at Parshvanath temple, Madhya Pradesh, India, showing an *Apsaras* (angel) applying kajal (collyrium)

Chinese philosopher Mo-Zi (fifth to fourth century BC), recorded the effects of pharmaceutical substances on the quality of eyes "there is a drug for this. if one eats it, the eye will become sharp and the eye will be clear.". However, the Wan wu text among the Fu-yang bamboo manuscripts found in the tomb of Xiahou Zao, the Lord of Ruyin who died in 165 BC, quotes the recommendation "Ox gall brightens the eye so that one may climb on high on slip thirty-five" (Shaughnessy 2014).

In a Celtic leech-book preserved in the University of Leyden (nineteenth century), shows the treatment for the dimness for eyes. One of the formulations contained pound fennel roots, mixed with honey and boiled over slow fire, with cistern water or woman's milk and smearing eyes with the fat of a fox (Adipe vulpis). Another remedy claims a mixture of a child's urine (lotium infantis) with the best honey; add a decoction of fennel roots (Thompson 1897).

An excellent recipe for sore eyes was the juice of the calyx of the red honeysuckle prescribed in 1553. The flowers had to have been gathered kneeling and repeating nine Paternosters in honor of the Trinity, nine more "to greet our Ladye," and a creed. The abovementioned My Ladye Falkenbrydge's recipe for eyewater was thus much esteemed and ran as: "Corne-flowers gathered with their cuppes and bruyse them; macerate them in snow or snow water for twenty-four hours, then dystyl in a moderate sandebath and applye it night and morning" (Thompson 1897).

Interestingly the old apothecary's prescriptions in 1685 were composed of strange ingredients, including crab's eyes and boar's teeth, or powdered pearls, and viper broth (Thompson 1897).

At the same time, eyedrops were also used miraculously to cure dental pain. A writer of the Time states that the itinerant dentist was also a well-known figure at the street corner. For 100 marks, he would put out both your eyes and quite cure your inflammation with one drop of his aqua mirabilis, at 12 pence a drop (fifteenth century).

Over a period of centuries, eye diseases were not classified; especially the two major problems were not clearly differentiated. It is somewhere in 1820 that a clear differentiation between glaucoma and cataract was seen in the history. The earliest understanding towards the usage of any substance having a meaningful ocular use come from the observations of the Greek women. The Greek women used the juice of the berries of *Atropa belladonna* to enlarge their pupils for cosmetic reasons. In Italy belladonna refers to "beautiful lady." The alluring beauty of Queen Cleopatra of the last century BCE has been attributed to her dilated pupils by using the extracts from the Egyptian henbane (*Hyoscyamus niger*). Friedlieb Ferdinand Runge, a German chemist, demonstrated the mydriatic effect of the extract of the deadly nightshade in 1819. Atropine in its crystalline form was isolated in 1831 by the German pharmacist Heinrich F. G. Mein. However, atropine has been used for more than a century now by ophthalmologists throughout the world for dilating iris.

It is interesting to know that the knowledge about the dilation property of belladonna was existing for long among the Greek women for making themselves attractive. The same practice has been continued even today when modern photographers use the same technique to make female portraits with attractive eyes. Discovery of contact lenses make this practice in modern times more comfortable by largely using cosmetic contact lenses to give the illusion of dilated eyes. The rationale for the hypothesis came from the investigations of Tombs and Silverma (2004) that the reproductive strategies of males are best served by unequivocal female sexual interest and arousal indicated by dilated pupils (Tombs and and Silverma 2004).

Pilocarpine preparations have been used since 1870s with their first record starting in the mid-nineteenth century. During that time, European visitors to Old Calabar, an eastern province of Nigeria and Africa, came to know about the native belief in the power of the seeds of a local plant to determine whether individuals were innocent or guilty of misdemeanor. Missionaries who arrived in Calabar in 1846 realized that the particular bean was responsible for more than 120 deaths annually. This information rapidly reached Scotland, the home of the missionaries' parent church for evaluation. Slowly, exploration of the bean started and reached a stage when Balfour's comprehensive botanical description of the bean plant appeared as *Physostigma venenosum*. In 1863 a young Edinburgh ophthalmologist, Argyll Robertson, published a paper announcing the arrival of the first agent that constricted the pupil of the eye (Proudfoot 2006).

The drug was an extract of Calabar beans, and Argyll Robertson openly admitted that he had been alerted to its unusual property by his physician friend, Thomas Fraser. Later Fraser extensively studied the action of Calabar bean on the eye and noted down its opposing action to atropine. However, in 1864, an ophthalmologist, Niemetschek, working in Prague in 1864 recommended Calabar bean extract to his friend Kleinwächter who was treating a young man with atropine intoxication (Nickalls and Rudorfer 1980). This rendered the patient to survive atropine toxicity and incidence establishing the beans antagonism of atropine. In 1870 Fraser reported his firm belief that physostigmine and atropine were mutually antagonistic at a physiological level and opened a new era in cholinergic system for further careful interpretations (Proudfoot 2006). The modern understanding about glaucoma pharmacology began in 1862 along with the isolation of physostigmine from the Calabar bean. The discovery of epinephrine's intraocular pressure-lowering capacity came along some 40 years later (Realini 2011). In the twentieth century, ocular drug development took an advanced pace along with the rapid development of drugs for cardiovascular and central nervous system disorders (Table 1.1).

The need to administer pilocarpine frequently everyday has been unfavorable for many glaucoma patients. In the 1980s, beta-blockers were developed, reducing the administration frequency to twice a day. In 1999, prostaglandin-type ophthalmic preparations that require a once-a-day administration appeared on the market, easing the burden of frequent administration. During the process of the development of these new ophthalmic agents, Ocusert, a sustained-release pilocarpine preparation that is inserted into pre-corneal area only once a week, was designed and applied clinically (Komatsu 2007).

In modern ocular therapeutics, several plant-derived products like *Atropa belladonna* (Atropine), Datura specs (tropane alkaloids), *Physostigma venenosum* (physostigmine), *Pilocarpus jaborandi* (pilocarpine), *Ephedra* (ephedrine), and *Cannabis sativa* (cannabis) were identified and reported to have some relevance directly or indirectly to various ocular conditions. Interestingly, they are being used in its original form; their semisynthetic derivatives are having a strong holding in the modern ophthalmic practice for either therapeutic or diagnostic purposes.

Table 1.1 Significant milestones in the development of drugs for ocular therapeutics

1831	Atropine isolated in crystalline form
1870	Physostigmine isolated
1875	Pilocarpine isolated
1885	Effect of pilocarpine on IOP recorded
1920	Nonselective sympathomimetics (epinephrine and dipivefrin)
1950	Oral carbonic anhydrase inhibitors (acetazolamide)
1970	Beta-blockers (timolol, levobunolol)
1990	Topical carbonic anhydrase inhibitors, fluoroquinolones antibacterial photodynamic therapy
2000	Intraocular antiangiogenic agents (ranibizumab, bevacizumab, pegaptanib)

1.2 Principles of Ocular Therapy

After the Second World War, sterility of drug for eye has been recognized as a mandate for topical eyedrops. Usage of preservatives came into picture to avoid bacterial contamination or growth in the multi-dose eyedrop vial for their use up to 30 days after opening. However, few fundamental aspects need emphasis while administering them to the patients or self-administration. One need to remember the appropriate way of application of an eyedrop (Table. 1.2). Most of the eyedrops are clear-colored or colorless solutions with or without preservatives, iso-osmotic and buffered to have neutral pH, with exception in suspensions like prednisolone acetate, dexamethasone, basifloxacin, etc. Application of eyedrops with lesser volume (drop size) or single drop is known to have better ocular bioavailability as compared to larger volume or multiple drops.

Cornea is a specialized tissue, devoid of blood vessels having hydrophobic epithelium followed by hydrophilic stroma thereby restricting the entry of both hydrophobic and hydrophilic compounds for gaining access to aqueous humor. Cornea is highly sensitive for pH of the ingredients, osmolarity (hypo and hyper), nonspecific irritants, and pH of the formulations. The pH and nonspecific irritation can induce reflux tearing which in turn washes away the pre-corneal drugs. Predominately, drugs applied topically take transcellular diffusion pathway as corneal epithelium is reported to have tight intracellular junctions (zona occludens); therefore, less than 5 % of the topically applied drug dosage reaches aqueous humor. As less amount of drug reaches into aqueous humor, conventionally, drug concentrations are increased considerably in the applied drops to reach adequate levels for the pharmacological activity.

However, the modern understanding for the transfer of drugs across cornea is explained much better by the presence of drug transporter proteins in corneal epithelium and endothelium. These transporters are physiologically responsible for the

Table 1.2 How to apply eyedrops

Clean hands with soap solution and dry it
Open the dropper cap
Do not touch the tip of the dropper
Slightly tilt the head backwards
Gently pull the lower eyelid with one hand
Place only one drop of the drug solution into the lower fornix (do not apply two drops)
Close the eyes and sit quietly for 1 min
If possible apply a gentle pressure on the tear duct by pressing near medical canthus with index finger for a while – this will avoid the immediate entry of drug solution into the lacrimal drainage system
If two different drops need to administered, it should be done by with the interval of at least 15 min between them
Close the eyedropper without touching the dropper tip and store it in a cool and dry place
Unpreserved eyedrops must be kept in refrigerator at 2–6 °C

uptake of nutrients for the survival of cornea and to maintain its transparency by regulating its homeostasis. Systemically, administered drug seldom reaches adequate concentration into the tissues of the eye with the considerable concentration for expected pharmacological action. Most of the systemically administered antibiotics were reported to fail to reach adequate concentration due to the presence of blood-ocular barriers (Velpandian 2009).

Therefore, selecting appropriate route of drug administration to the eye is expected to having better pharmacodynamic profiles. Based on requirement, subtenon, retrobulbar, subconjunctival, intracameral, intravitreal, and peribulbar routes are preferred to comply required drug concentration at a particular site in the eye.

1.3 Challenges in Ocular Therapeutics

Ocular therapeutics is the only area in which the drugs used more than 100 years ago are still having its presence in clinical practice. Despite the multidimensional drug development approaches of the contemporary period, it is rare to see any specific agent being developed for ocular use considering the penetration constraints exerted by the eye after topical or systemic administration. Most of the drugs, approved for systemic use, are often exploited for ocular use without rationalizing the penetration characteristics in the drug development stage. Lack of considerable market size for drugs other than for glaucoma and retinal neovascular conditions could have been the major limiting factor for not getting much of industrial emphasis for ocular-specific drug discovery. Due to the application of modern techniques on traditional knowledge, ocular applications of herbal drugs are continuously increasing. However, in most of the cases, there are isolated publications on animal models or human studies which are not having any big impact for their wider use in ocular therapeutics. Therefore, developing drug specific for the eye with the consideration of its constraints would be beneficial for the further development of ocular pharmacology and its application to therapeutics.

1.4 Ocular Pharmacology and Its Practice

Ocular applications of many drugs are due to their mutual borrowings from several fields of medicine. However, all of them may not been approved for its ocular use due to the lack of initiation for the application to the regulatory authorities for their use in ophthalmology. Off-label use of drugs is commonly evident in ophthalmology; therefore, requirement of a compounding pharmacy in the final translation of drugs approved for other systemic use for ocular therapeutics. One of the chapters in this book deals with extensively about this aspect in detail. Along with the increasing knowledge about the pathology of ocular disease, we are sure that usage of extemporaneously prepared drugs might increase further in the future. During such attempts, a rational approach is expected to justify their appropriate usage in ocular therapeutics.

References

BMJ. The ophthalmology of the pharaohs. BMJ. 1909;2(2543):902.

Giachi G, et al. Ingredients of a 2,000-y-old medicine revealed by chemical, mineralogical, and botanical investigations. Proc Natl Acad Sci U S A. 2013;110(4):v1193–6.

Jeanette CF. Cuneiform tablets on eye diseases. In: Attia A, Buisson G, editors, Mesopotamian medicine from hammurabi to hippocrates. Proceedings of the International Conference "Oeil malade et mauvais oeil," Collège de France, Paris, 23rd June 2006 published by Brill, Boston; 2009.

Kartar SD, Kartar JS, Nayan RB, Vinay RS. Quality control evaluation of Keshamasi, Keshanjana and Keshamasi eye ointment. Ayu. 2014;35(1):58–62.

Komatsu Y. A history of the development of eye drops used to treat glaucoma. Yakushigaku Zasshi. 2007;42(1):7–16. Japanese. PubMed.

Marmion VJ. The Roman oculist stamps. Bull Soc Belge Ophtalmol. 1995;259:215–7.

Murube J. Collyrium: where does this word come from? Ocul Surf. 2007a;5(4):264–8. PubMed.

Murube J. Hunain's eye: the oldest preserved scientific image of the ocular surface. Ocul Surf. 2007b;5(3):207–12. PubMed.

Murube J. Ocular cosmetics in ancient times. Ocul Surf. 2013;11(1):2–7.

Nickalls RWD and Rudorfer MV. Physostigmine for anticholinergic drug poisoning. 1980; 316 (8194):589–90.

Pardon-Labonnelie M. Collyrium names attested on stone tablets: the example of the Helvetian corpus. Stud Anc Med. 2014;42:240–55. PubMed.

Perez-Cambrodi RJ, Pinero DP, Mavrou A, Cervino A, Brautaset R, Murube del Castillo J. Collyria seals in the Roman Empire. Acta Med Hist Adriat. 2013;11(1):89–100.

Proudfoot A. The early toxicology of physostigmine: a tale of beans, great men and egos. Toxicol Rev. 2006;25(2):99–138.

Realini T. A history of glaucoma pharmacology. Optom Vis Sci. 2011;88(1):36–8.

Shaughnessy EL. Recently discovered manuscripts of the Yi Jing (I Ching) and related texts. New York: Columbia University Press; 2014.

Subbarayappa BV. Siddha medicine: an overview. Lancet. 1997;350(20/27):1843–4.

Tapsoba I, Arbault S, Walter P, Amatore C. Finding out egyptian gods' secret using analytical chemistry: biomedical properties of egyptian black makeup revealed by amperometry at single cells. Anal Chem. 2010;82(2):457–60.

Thompson CJS. The mystery and romance of alchemy and pharmacy. London: The Scientific Press Ltd. 1897, XIX. p. 97.

Tombs S, Silverma I. Pupillometry: a sexual selection approach. Evol Hum Behav. 2004; 25(4):221–8.

Ven Murthy MR, Ranjekar PK, Ramassamy C, Deshpande M. Scientific basis for the use of Indian ayurvedic medicinal plants in the treatment of neurodegenerative disorders: ashwagandha. Cent Nerv Syst Agents Med Chem. 2010;10(3):238–46.

Velpandian T. Intraocular penetration of antimicrobial agents in ophthalmic infections and drug delivery strategies. Expert Opin Drug Deliv. 2009 Mar;6(3):255–70.

Webley K. Brief history: medical marijuana. Time, 21 June 2010.

Zeitschrift für celtische Philologie (ZcP). 1(1): Pages 17–25, ISSN (Online) 1865-889X, ISSN (Print) 0084-5302, DOI: 10.1515/zcph.1897.1.1.17, October 2009.

Chapter 2
Opportunities for the Development of Newer Drugs for Ocular Use

Rajinder K. Bhardwaj

Abstract Both anatomically and physiologically, eye is a unique organ containing several widely varied structures with independent physiological functions. Eye has a number of distinct features in contrast to other organs as it is isolated from systemic access by the blood-retinal, blood-aqueous, and blood-vitreous barriers. Topically administered drugs as instillations on eye face a hydrodynamic surface wherein the physio-chemical properties of the drug determine its penetration across the cornea. Therefore, drug development for eye requires extensive developmental considerations to overcome these barriers. This chapter reveals the novel targets for ocular drug research in the areas of neovascularization, glaucoma, AMD, pharmacological vitreolysis, genomic studies and drug delivery.

2.1 Introduction

Compromised visual functions or any disruption to the delicate and complex anatomy of eye can result into ocular discomfort or loss of vision, which can substantially deteriorate quality of life. The visual impairment is a serious public health problem, and the condition will get worse in the next 30 years due to (a) aging population, (b) increase in chronic diseases affecting eyes, and (c) changing demographics of the global population (Alward 2003). The ocular diseases such as cataract, diabetic retinopathy, age-related macular degeneration (AMD), and glaucoma are common among aging population (Akpek and Smith 2013). In addition, there are other diseases such as idiopathic intracranial hypertension, retinoblastoma, usher syndrome, and uveal coloboma that can affect the eye and could result into ocular discomfort (Alward 2003; Akpek and Smith 2013). Both anatomically and

R.K. Bhardwaj, MS, PhD
Clinical Pharmacology, d3 Medicine, Parsippany, NJ, USA
e-mail: rajinder.bhardwaj@gmail.com

T. Velpandian (ed.), *Pharmacology of Ocular Therapeutics*,
DOI 10.1007/978 3 319 25498 2_2

physiologically, eye is a unique organ containing several widely varied structures with independent physiological functions. Eye has a number of unique features when compared to the other organs as it is isolated from systemic access by the blood-retinal, blood-aqueous, and blood-vitreous barriers. Therefore, research in ocular pharmacology provides both benefits and challenges for drug discovery and delivery in developing new medicines for eye diseases. Moreover, wide variation of ocular sizes and physiology among animal models add another challenge in translation of results from one species of animal to another and eventually to humans (Alward 2003).

As per the published reports, the patient burden related to ocular blindness and visual impairment represents a substantial amount (Rein et al. 2006). The total economic burden related to eye diseases report submitted to the National Eye Institute (NEI) of the National Institutes of Health (NIH) in 1981 was $14.1 billion, whereas later it was reported that the approximate economic impact of major visual disorders among patients aged 40 years has been estimated at US$35.4 billion in the USA (Rein et al. 2006). The centers for disease control and prevention are actively involved in identifying steps and priorities to strengthen global surveillance systems to help assess and monitor disparities in eye health and vision loss. The market size for drugs used in eye diseases is estimated to be $12 billion (US); however, there appears to be a lack of enough new drug molecules (Rein et al. 2006). Despite advances in ophthalmic medicine in recent decades and large market potential, there remains significant opportunity to improve ocular patient care with lower cost of services. As life expectancy increases, so does the incidence of ophthalmic disease; therefore, high prevalence of ocular diseases has created significant opportunities for companies to develop innovative medicines and new technologies. Moreover recent advances in the molecular understanding of ophthalmic disease biology have added an unprecedented opportunity to develop new treatments. In the present chapter, we discuss the current opportunities and challenges for the development of newer drugs for ocular diseases.

2.2 Novel Targets in Ocular Research

To foster the translation of ideas into innovation, this section describes current understanding and novel drug targets in ocular research as a basis for the discovery and development of new therapeutic approaches (Fig. 2.1).

2.3 Anti-VEGF Therapy

Vascular endothelial growth factor (VEGF) has been associated with retinal diseases such as AMD, diabetic retinopathy, retinopathy of prematurity, sickle cell retinopathy, retinal vascular occlusion, and inherited retinal dystrophies (Bock et al. 2007;

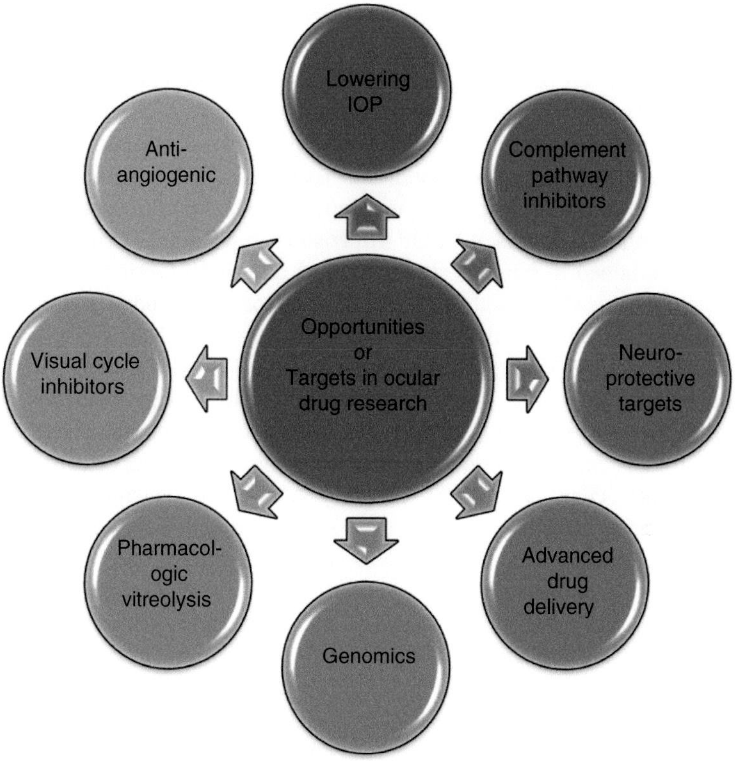

Fig. 2.1 Schematic of target areas in ocular research

Shams and Ianchulev 2006). The VEGF is a dimeric glycoprotein (approximately 40 kDa), a potent endothelial cell mitogen that stimulates proliferation, migration, and tube formation leading to angiogenic growth of new blood vessels (Bock et al. 2007; Shams and Ianchulev 2006). The VEGF family consists of seven members in mammals, which are VEGF-A (also known as VEGF), VEGF-B to VEGF-F, and PlGF (placental growth factor) (Bock et al. 2007; Shams and Ianchulev 2006). The VEGF receptors belong to the receptor tyrosine kinase family and named as VEGFR-1/Flt-1, VEGFR-2/KDR/Flk-1, Flt-3/Flk-2, and VEGFR-3/Flt-4 receptors (Yancopoulos et al. 2000). The first two receptors, i.e., VEGFR-1/Flt-1 and VEGFR-2/KDR/Flk-1, are primarily involved in angiogenesis, and the latter two VEGF receptors are involved in hematopoiesis and lymphangiogenesis (Yancopoulos et al. 2000).

VEGF expressions were seen in astrocytes of the neuroblastic layer near the optic disc and in Müller cells of the inner nuclear layer (Stone et al. 1995). The expression of VEGF advances towards the periphery with a gradual downregulation in the central retina (Stone et al. 1995). The retinal cells that are involved in the production of VEGF are retinal pigmented epithelium (RPE), astrocytes, Müller cells, vascular endothelium, and ganglion cells (Provis et al. 1997). The gene expression of VEGF is regulated by oxygen tension that helps tissues adjust vascular supply to oxygen demand (Goldberg and Schneider 1994). Animal models involving rats and mice demonstrated that retinal cells produce adequate levels of VEGF, and its expression was decreased in response to hyperoxia thus playing an important role in retinopathy under hypoxic conditions (Alon et al. 1995; Pierce et al. 1996). Additionally, studies under hypoxic conditions have shown Müller cells and astrocytes produce higher amounts of VEGF (Morrison and Aschner 2007). Furthermore, clinical data obtained in humans also suggested role of VEGF in retinopathy and other ocular diseases (Penn et al. 2008). This is supported by studies where levels of VEGF were increased in ocular fluid from patients with diabetic retinopathy and other retinal neovascularizing diseases (Adamis et al. 1994; Pe'er et al. 1995).

Ocular anti-VEGF therapy approach represents one of the significant advances in ocular drug therapy (Penn et al. 2008). Multiple studies in patients have demonstrated the role of antiangiogenic therapies targeting VEGF as an effective therapy in treating AMD (Penn et al. 2008). Globally, AMD is the leading cause of legal blindness, affecting 10–13 % of adults over 65 years of age based on increased life expectancy (Friedman et al. 2004). Additionally, the growing negative impact of environmental risk factors such as arteriosclerosis, obesity, and smoking is expected to double the AMD by 2020 (Friedman et al. 2004). Patients affected by AMD have shown improvements with anti-VEGF treatments (Penn et al. 2008). In addition, the improvement in their vision was enhanced due to increased understanding of the mechanisms of ocular angiogenesis (Schmidt-Erfurth et al. 2014).

Bevacizumab is a recombinant humanized monoclonal antibody that blocks angiogenesis by inhibiting VEGF. It was the first clinically available angiogenesis inhibitor (Rosenfeld et al. 2005). Bevacizumab was approved by the Food and Drug Administration (FDA) in 2004 as anti-VEGF therapy for AMD (Rosenfeld et al. 2005). Moshfeghi et al. studied the effect of systemic bevacizumab therapy on patients with AMD in a 24-week uncontrolled open-label clinical study. The results showed improvement in visual acuity within the first 2 weeks and by 24 weeks (Moshfeghi et al. 2006). Overall, the bevacizumab therapy was well tolerated and effective in patients (Moshfeghi et al. 2006). Another monoclonal antibody fragment (Fab) is ranibizumab, which was created from the same parent mouse antibody as bevacizumab, and the effectiveness is similar to that of bevacizumab (Schmucker et al. 2012). Heier et al. assessed the safety of ranibizumab in treating AMD in a multidose study. Sixty-four patients with subfoveal predominantly or minimally classic AMD-related choroidal neovascularization were enrolled in the study (Heier et al. 2006). The results demonstrated improvement in visual acuity from baseline and decease in areas of leakage and subretinal fluid (Heier et al. 2006). Additionally, repeated intravitreal injections of ranibizumab had a good safety profile in subjects with neovascular AMD (Heier et al. 2006).

Aflibercept is another example that inhibits receptor binding by trapping VEGF in the extracellular space (Stewart 2013). It inhibits the activity of the vascular endothelial growth factor subtypes VEGF-A and VEGF-B thus inhibiting the growth of new blood vessels (Stewart 2013). Zehetner et al. studied the systemic levels of vascular endothelial growth factor before and after intravitreal injection of aflibercept in patients with exudative AMD (Zehetner et al. 2015). Seven days after intravitreal injection of aflibercept, plasma levels were significantly reduced to values below the minimum detectable dose (MDD) in 17 of 19 patients (89.5 %) resulting in a median VEGF concentration of <9 pg/ml ($p<0.001$) (Zehetner et al. 2015). The reduction persisted throughout 1 month with values below the MDD in 5 of 19 patients (26.3 %) and a median measurement of 17.0 pg/ml ($p<0.001$) (Zehetner et al. 2015). Thus the results demonstrated significant reduction of VEGF levels throughout the observational period of 4 weeks suggesting role of anti-VEGF therapy and effectiveness against AMD (Zehetner et al. 2015). In a recent study, Kawashima et al. looked at the visual and anatomic outcomes in response to the changing treatment to aflibercept in patients with neovascular AMD and polypoidal choroidal vasculopathy (PCV) refractory to previous treatment with ranibizumab. The results suggested switching to aflibercept is generally effective regardless of patient genotype (Kawashima et al. 2014). Comparing between the ocular diseases, PCV patients showed benefit more significantly than AMD patients (Kawashima et al. 2014). In an another study, Michalewski et al. studied efficacy of single dose of aflibercept in bevacizumab nonresponders patients with persistent intraretinal or subretinal fluid treated with 6 or more monthly bevacizumab (Michalewski et al. 2014). After switching to aflibercept, the visual acuity was significantly improved ($p=0.01$) and was stable for the remaining 6 months of the study suggesting aflibercept improves visual outcome in bevacizumab nonresponders (Michalewski et al. 2014). Moreover, Peden et al. reported the long-term outcomes in eyes receiving fixed-interval dosing of anti-VEGF therapy in the form of ranibizumab, bevacizumab, or aflibercept administration for at least 5 years in 109 eyes with exudative AMD. The results showed greatest visual gains at 5 and 7 years in those patients with AMD with vision stabilizing or improving in 93.2 % of eyes with anti-VEGF therapy (Peden et al. 2015). Additionally, 43.2 % of patients maintained driving vision in the treatment eye at 7 years compared with 10.1 % at baseline suggesting better outcomes with continuous therapy over sporadic therapy (Peden et al. 2015).

In addition to AMD, other indications such as diabetic macular edema (DME) and proliferative diabetic retinopathy have also been explored to be treated by anti-VEGF therapy (Penn et al. 2008). Diabetic macular edema (DME) is one of the primary causes of visual impairment due to diabetic retinopathy (Penn et al. 2008). The traditional standard treatment of DME is photocoagulation, but with the advent of anti-VEGF therapies, the role of anti-VEGF agents has become increasingly explored (Penn et al. 2008). Adelman et al. compared the efficacy of different ocular drug therapies in the treatment of DME using clinical information provided on 2603 patients with macular edema including 870 patients with DME. The administration of anti-VEGF therapy resulted in significant improvement in visual functions in DME patients (Adelman et al. 2015). The use of anti-VEGF therapy also produced an inhibition of vascular proliferation which resulted into improvement of vision of people with proliferative diabetic retinopathy (Martinez-Zapata et al. 2014). The proliferative diabetic retinopathy is a complication of diabetic retinopathy where panretinal photocoagulation (PRP) is the treatment of choice (Martinez-Zapata et al. 2014). In a study reported by Kambhampati et al., dendrimer triamcinolone acetonide conjugates used as antiangiogenic agent in proliferative diabetic retinopathy showed efficacy by suppressing VEGF production in hypoxic retinal pigment epithelial cells (Kambhampati et al. 2015).

There are various other alternative approaches to inhibit ocular angiogenesis that can be explored during ocular drug discovery and development to improve vision loss related to neovascularization and diabetic retinopathy (Penn et al. 2008; Jacot and Sherris 2011). The PI3K/AKT/MTOR pathway is an intracellular signaling pathway important in regulating the cell cycle. The inhibition of PI3K/AKT/MTOR pathway presents a unique opportunity for the management of ocular neovascularization and diabetic retinopathy (Penn et al. 2008; Jacot and Sherris 2011). The PI3K/AKT/MTOR inhibitors work by suppressing HIF-1α, VEGF, leakage, and breakdown of the blood-retinal barrier thus imparting a pronounced inhibitory effect on inflammation (Penn et al. 2008; Jacot and Sherris 2011). Eventually, the inhibitors also suppress IkappaB kinase (IKK) and nuclear factor kappa-light-chain-enhancer of activated B cells (NF-κB) along with downstream inflammatory cytokines, chemokines, and adhesion molecules (Penn et al. 2008). Jacot et al. and Sasore et al. have studied deciphering combinations of PI3K/AKT/mTOR pathway drugs which could result into augmenting antiangiogenic efficacy in vivo (Jacot et al. 2011; Sasore et al. 2014). Using both the zebra fish intersegmental vessel and hyaloid vessel assays to measure the in vivo antiangiogenic efficacy of PI3K/Akt/mTOR pathway inhibitors, the results highlighted the potential of combinations of PI3K/AKT/mTOR pathway inhibitors to safely and effectively treat ocular neovascularization (Sasore et al. 2014). Additionally, some other examples of PI3K/AKT/MTOR inhibitors are everolimus and palomid drugs which are under clinical development in patients with wet AMD (Sasore et al. 2014).

Another potential approach in ocular drug discovery is sphingosine-1-phosphate (S1P), a signaling sphingolipid, also known as lysosphingolipid (Maines et al. 2006). It is an extracellular ligand for S1P receptor 1 and involved in the regulation of a variety of cellular processes. Skoura et al. in the murine model of oxygen-induced retinopathy demonstrated a knockout of S1P2 receptors has been shown to mitigate vascular growth and permeability (Skoura et al. 2007). Preclinical studies have shown intravitreous anti-S1P monoclonal antibody inhibited CNV formation and subretinal collagen deposition (Xie et al. 2009). The mechanism of action of S1P appears to be independent from those of anti-VEGF agents, indicating the potential of S1P antibodies to serve as a monotherapy, or it could be an adjunct therapy to anti-VEGF agents for the treatment of neovascular AMD (Xie et al. 2009).

2.4 Lowering Intraocular Pressure (IOP)

Glaucoma is a progressive optic neuropathy which results into loss of vision caused by impairment of trabecular meshwork, optic nerve head, and retinal ganglion cells (Sommer et al. 1991). It is also described as a group of eye disorders that result in optic nerve damage, often associated with IOP (Sommer et al. 1991). Glaucoma can be categorized into (a) open-angle and (b) closed-angle glaucoma (Sommer et al. 1991). The open-angle glaucoma is developed slowly over time, is painless, and often has no symptoms until the disease has progressed significantly (Sommer et al. 1991). The treatment of open-angle glaucoma is to lower the pressure or utilize pressure-reducing glaucoma surgeries (Sommer et al. 1991). The other form as closed-angle glaucoma resulting from a sudden spike in intraocular pressure is associated with sudden eye pain, redness, nausea, and vomiting, and it is treated as a medical emergency (Sommer et al. 1991). These two forms of glaucoma have affected 60.5 million people worldwide in 2010, and this number would increase to 79.6 million by 2020 (Resnikoff et al. 2004). Epidemiological studies have shown that African-American with ages 60 and older and people with a family history of glaucoma are susceptible to glaucoma (Resnikoff et al. 2004). Significant advances are being made by pharmaceutical companies and academia for the successful management of glaucoma that include discovery of novel molecular entities and delivery systems to improve medical therapy. Thus, discovering new drugs to lower IOP is another potential area in ocular research.

Intraocular pressure is a condition when the rate of aqueous inflow is the same as the rate of aqueous outflow (Liu and Weinreb 2011). The aqueous humor is drained by trabecular meshwork and the uveoscleral pathway, whereas it is secreted into the eye by the ciliary body (Weinreb 2011). The IOP shows diurnal variation for normal eyes, ranging from 3 to 6 mmHg, and the variation may increase in glaucomatous eyes (Sena and Lindsley 2013). Ocular hypertension is the most important risk factor for glaucoma, and it has been observed that increase in IOP is associated with certain types of glaucoma, as well as iritis or retinal detachment. The IOP can be elevated due to anatomic problems, increasing age, inflammation of the eye, genetic factors, and side effect from coadministered medication (Sena and Lindsley 2013).

Multiple classes of medications are used to treat glaucoma, with several different drugs in each class (Sommer et al. 1991; Resnikoff et al. 2004; Liu et al. 2011). Among the multiple therapeutic agents for lowering IOP in glaucoma, cholinergic agents have been extensively used as they act on muscarinic receptors located on the ciliary muscle to increase outflow through the trabecular meshwork (Migdal 2000). The most common drug that is used under cholinergic agent is pilocarpine; however, its use is limited by the ocular side effect such as miosis, myopia, browache, and dimming of vision (Migdal 2000). Another category of medication is carbonic anhydrase inhibitors that act through suppressing the activity of carbonic anhydrase enzyme (Scozzafava and Supuran 2014). The primary function of carbonic anhydrase enzyme is to interconvert carbon dioxide and bicarbonate to maintain acid-base balance in blood and other tissues and to help transport carbon dioxide out of tissues (Scozzafava and Supuran 2014). The dorzolamide and brinzolamide are the most commonly utilized carbonic anhydrase inhibitors to lower intraocular pressure in patients with open-angle glaucoma or ocular hypertension (Scozzafava and Supuran 2014; Pinard et al. 2013). Another target to lower IOP is the use of beta-adrenergic receptor blockers (Nathanson 1981). Beta-blockers are a class of drugs that are developed earlier for the management of cardiac arrhythmias; however, they have shown to reduce IOP by reducing aqueous humor formation (Nathanson 1981). They act by blocking adrenergic β-receptor from activation of adenylyl cyclase and cAMP formation to regulate aqueous humor formation in the ciliary process (Nathanson 1981). Timolol, a beta-blocker, has been used to treat open-angle and occasionally secondary glaucoma acts by reducing aqueous humor production through blockage of the beta-receptors on the ciliary epithelium (Daka and Trkulja 2014). Inoue et al. evaluated dorzolamide and timolol fixed-combination eyedrops versus the separate use of both drugs in 34 patients with either primary open-angle glaucoma or ocular hypertension. The replacement of concomitant treatment with dorzolamide or timolol maleate eyedrops with dorzolamide/timolol maleate combination eyedrops improved protocol adherence and preserved the IOP (Inoue et al. 2012).

The alpha-adrenergic receptor, a G protein-coupled receptor (GPCR) agonist, is used in the treatment of glaucoma by decreasing the production of aqueous fluid by the ciliary bodies of the eye and also by increasing uveoscleral outflow (Arthur and Cantor 2011). The most common alpha-adrenergic receptors used clinically are apraclonidine, brimonidine, and dipivefrin (Arthur and Cantor 2011). Fan et al. studied daytime and nighttime effects of brimonidine on IOP and aqueous humor dynamics in thirty participants with ocular hypertension. The results in subjects with ocular hypertension showed brimonidine treatment for 6 weeks significantly reduced seated IOP during the day by increasing uveoscleral outflow (Fan et al. 2014). Chen et al. evaluated the comparison of efficacy and safety of brimonidine with those of apraclonidine in preventing IOP elevations after anterior segment laser surgery in 80 patients (Chen 2005). The results demonstrated a single preoperative drop of brimonidine had similar efficacy and safety as apraclonidine in preventing IOP elevations immediately after anterior segment laser surgery (Chen 2005). Developing prostaglandin F receptor (PTGFR) analogs is another area as these agents have shown to increase aqueous outflow by altering the composition of the extracellular matrix in the ciliary muscle and trabecular meshwork (Lindén and Alm 1999). The analogs for PTGFR have been reported to be the most effective of the IOP-lowering agents; however, adverse effects such as lengthening and thickening of eyelashes have been observed suggesting the need of developing safer PTGFR analogs (Lindén and Alm 1999). The most common analogs are latanoprost, travoprost, bimatoprost, and unoprostone (Lindén and Alm 1999). The PF04217329 is another selective agonist of prostaglandin E receptor 2 in clinical development with studies showing significant reduction of IOP in patients with primary open-angle glaucoma and ocular hypertension (Schachar et al. 2011).

Another potential target in the treatment of glaucoma is developing drugs targeting Rho/ROCK pathway (Wang et al. 2013). It plays an important role in the synthesis of extracellular matrix components in the aqueous humor outflow tissue and the permeability of Schlemm's canal endothelial cells (Wang et al. 2013). The activation of the Rho/ROCK pathway results in trabecular meshwork (TM) contraction (Wang et al. 2013). In addition, the inhibition of this pathway would provoke relaxation of TM with subsequent increase in outflow facility resulting in decrease of IOP (Wang et al. 2013). The RhoA/ROCK pathway is also involved in optic nerve neuroprotection, improves retinal ganglion cell (RGC) survival, and promotes RGC axon regeneration (Wang et al. 2013). Overall, ROCK inhibitors have the ability to lower IOP in patients with primary open-angle glaucoma and/or ocular hypertension by increasing the outflow through the trabecular meshwork (Wang et al. 2013). Another class of drugs used in glaucoma are macrolides (El Sayed et al. 2006; Rasmussen et al. 2014). These are a group of drugs whose activity stems from the presence of a macrolide ring. The latrunculins are novel marine compounds isolated from the sponge *Latrunculia magnifica* that have the ability to inhibit actin polymerization thus resulting in increased outflow (El Sayed et al. 2006). Rasmussen et al. evaluated the safety, tolerability, and IOP-lowering effect of latrunculin in patients with ocular hypertension or early primary open-angle glaucoma. In a randomized, placebo-controlled, ascending-dose study in patients, twice daily latrunculin significantly lowered IOP compared with contralateral, placebo-treated eyes, with few and mild ocular adverse events (Rasmussen et al. 2014).

Recently, endothelin system has also been reported to be involved in the processes that lead to vascular dysregulation in glaucoma (Good and Kahook 2010). Endothelin, a vasoconstrictive agent, has shown to be elevated in aqueous humor of patients with glaucoma thus capable of inducing the contraction of both trabecular meshwork cells and the cellular matrix (Good and Kahook 2010). The endothelin receptor would be another target to lower IOP and could constitute a potential new treatment modality to manage glaucoma through IOP reduction. Resch et al. studied the effect of dual endothelin receptor blockade on ocular blood flow in patients with glaucoma and healthy subjects. Bosentan 500 mg daily for 8 days was administered in fourteen patients with primary open-angle glaucoma (Resch et al. 2009). Retinal arteries and veins showed a significant dilatation after administration of bosentan with increased choroidal and optic nerve head blood flow.

Connective tissue growth factor (CTGF) has also been involved in the pathogenesis of glaucoma (Su et al. 2013). The CTGF induces extracellular matrix (ECM) synthesis and contractility in human trabecular meshwork (HTM) cells (Su et al. 2013). Su et al. studied adenovirus-carried connective tissue growth factor on extracellular matrix in trabecular meshwork and its role on aqueous humor outflow facility. The results of the study suggested transfection with adenovirus-CTGF significantly affects the aqueous humor outflow pattern thus demonstrating CTGF is one of the novel targets for treatment of primary open-angle glaucoma (Su et al. 2013). Overall, better knowledge about trabecular outflow pathway, cytoskeletal reorganization, and cell adhesion may be needed in discovering new drug molecules for glaucoma.

2.5 Complement Pathway Inhibitors

The complement system, an innate immunity system of the body, consists of a number of small proteins found in the blood that supports the ability of antibodies and phagocytic cells to clear pathogens from an organism (Jha et al. 2007). Additionally, these plasma and membrane bound proteins play an important role in the defense against infection and in the modulation of immune and inflammatory responses (Jha et al. 2007). Various studies have reported the complement system pathway in the eye (cornea, aqueous humor, tears, and retina) (Jha et al. 2007). In addition, different proteins which are present in ocular tissues that regulate the activation of the complement system are C1 esterase inhibitor (C1 inhibitor), decay-accelerating factor (DAF), membrane cofactor protein (MCP), MAC-inhibitory protein (MAC-IP), factor I, and factor H (Jha et al. 2007). Sohn et al. have reported that complement system works at the level of C3 convertase to prevent the intraocular inflammation (Sohn et al. 2007). The complement system is involved in protecting cornea from pathogenic microorganisms and inflammatory antigens in response to bacterial infection (Mondino et al. 1996).

Both humans and preclinical animal models have shown the involvement of complement pathway in the pathogenesis of a large number of diseases, including ocular diseases (Thurman and Holers 2006). The ocular disease include corneal diseases, autoimmune uveitis, AMD, and diabetic retinopathy. Sivaprasad et al. determined the role of systemic complement activation in the pathogenesis of AMD (Sivaprasad et al. 2007). In 42 subjects each with early age-related maculopathy and neovascular (wet) age-related macular degeneration, plasma complement C3adesArg levels and a single nucleotide polymorphism at position 402 of the complement factor H gene (CFH) were determined (Sivaprasad et al. 2007). The results demonstrated increase in the complement C3adesArg concentration compared to the age-matched controls suggesting C3adesArg is an indicator of complement activation in AMD (Sivaprasad et al. 2007). The complement pathway has also been involved in non-exudative AMD as studies conducted by Johnson et al. have shown the accumulation of abnormal extracellular deposits, called drusen, adjacent to the basal surface of the retinal-pigmented epithelium cells (Johnson et al. 2011). Joachim et al. evaluated the incidence, progression, and associated risk factors of medium drusen in AMD patients. Among 1317 participants at risk, the 15-year cumulative incidence of medium drusen was 13.9 %, and the increasing age and the presence of at least-risk alleles of the CFH were associated with a higher incidence (Joachim et al. 2015). Additionally, the progression rate to late AMD in the eyes with both medium drusen and retinal pigmentary abnormalities was fourfold higher than that in the eyes with medium drusen alone (Joachim et al. 2015).

Under the complement activation family, factor H is another member of the regulators and also called as complement control protein (Józsi and Zipfel 2008). It is a soluble glycoprotein with 155 kDa structure which is involved in the regulation of alternative pathway of the complement system (Józsi and Zipfel 2008). It helps the complement system in directing towards pathogens or other dangerous material and does not damage host tissue (Józsi and Zipfel 2008). In ocular pharmacology, factor H-like proteins regulate the complement system by acting as a cofactor for factor H-mediated inactivation of C3b (Zipfel et al. 2002). In addition, factor H-like proteins are present in vitreous fluid of the eyes and expressed by retinal pigment epithelium cells (Zipfel et al. 2002). A variation in factor H gene is associated with a significant risk in humans with AMD (Hageman et al. 2005). Khandhadia et al. investigated whether modification of liver complement factor H (CFH) production, by alteration of liver CFH Y402H genotype through liver transplantation, influences the development of AMD in patients greater than 55 years (Khandhadia et al. 2013). The results showed AMD was associated with recipient CFH Y402H genotype and local intraocular complement activity is important in AMD pathogenesis (Khandhadia et al. 2013). The involvement of complement system plays an important role in the pathogenesis of diabetic retinopathy (Kastelan et al. 2007). Gerl et al. evaluated the presence of activated complement components in eyes affected by diabetic retinopathy in the eyes of 50 deceased donors with diabetic retinopathy and of 10 nondiabetic subjects with uveal melanoma (Gerl et al. 2002). Utilizing immunohistochemical studies, extensive deposits of complement C5b-9 complexes were detected in the choriocapillaris in diabetic retinopathy (Gerl et al. 2002). The presence of C3d, C5b-9, and vitronectin suggested that complement activation occurs to completion in the eyes affected by diabetic retinopathy.

Complement system has also been involved in uveitis, a disease associated with inflammation of the uvea (Mondino et al. 1984). Under uveitis, anterior uveitis (AU) is the most prevalent form of uveitis, and complement activation products such as C3b and C4b have been demonstrated to be present in the eyes of patients with AU (Mondino et al. 1984). Jha et al. reported complement system plays a critical role in the development of experimental autoimmune anterior uveitis. In an animal model, autoimmune anterior uveitis was induced by immunization with bovine melanin-associated antigen (Jha et al. 2007). The results demonstrated a correlation between ocular complement activation and disease progression in autoimmune anterior uveitis (Jha et al. 2007). Moreover, the incidence and severity of disease were dramatically reduced after active immunization in complement-depleted rats thus suggesting presence of complement was critical for local production of cytokines, chemokines, and adhesion molecules (Jha et al. 2007). The finding suggested complement activation plays a central role in the pathogenesis of ocular autoimmunity and may serve as a potential target for therapeutic intervention (Jha et al. 2007). The complement system has also been involved in protecting cornea from insults due to pathogenic microorganisms and inflammatory antigens (Cleveland et al. 1983). Depletion of complement system protein C3 may result into corneal infection (Cleveland et al. 1983). Therefore, suggesting the functions associated with C3, such as opsonization and regulation of phagocytosis, may be critical in protection of the cornea from bacterial infection. In summary, various strategies in drug discovery can be explored to modulate complement system for discovering new medicine in ocular diseases.

2.6 Visual Cycle Inhibitors

Visual cycle inhibitors act by reducing the accumulation of fluorophores in retinal pigment epithelium cells (Mata et al. 2000; Sparrow et al. 2000). The visual cycle is involved in regenerating 11-cis-retinal by sequence of enzymatic reactions through a pathway located in both retinal pigment epithelium and photoreceptor cells (Mata et al. 2000; Sparrow et al. 2000). This pathway serves as a substrate for the uptake of retinol by the retinal pigment epithelium cells within the eye, whereas aberrant accumulation of cellular debris or lipofuscin results into ocular disease (Mata et al. 2000; Sparrow et al. 2000). The ACU-4429 is a first in class small-molecule visual cycle modulator that inhibits the isomerase complex (Kubota et al. 2012). In mouse model of retinal degeneration, after 45-min dark adaptation, electroretinographic findings demonstrated dose-related slowing of the rate of recovery after administration of ACU-4429 (Kubota et al. 2012). In another study, Moiseyev et al. studied inhibition of visual cycle by A2E through direct interaction with retinal pigment epithelium 65 isomerohydrolase and implications in stargardt disease (Moiseyev et al. 2010). Pyridinium bis-retinoid A2E is a major component of lipofuscin which accumulates in retinal pigment epithelium cells in stargardt disease and contributes to the disease pathogenesis (Moiseyev et al. 2010). The study demonstrated A2E efficiently inhibits with retinal pigment epithelium 65 isomerohydrolase enzyme (Moiseyev et al. 2010). Furthermore, the experiments demonstrated the fluorescence of retinal pigment epithelium 65 isomerohydrolase decreased upon incubation with A2E suggesting A2E inhibits the regeneration of 11-cis retinal, a mechanism by which A2E may impair vision in stargardt disease (Moiseyev et al. 2010).

Other visual cycle inhibitor that is under clinical development is fenretinide, an oral synthetic retinoid derivative (Berni and Formelli 1992). Under physiological conditions, the retinol necessary for the regeneration of 11-cis-retinal is delivered to the retinal pigment cells in a complex formed by retinol-binding protein (RBP), retinol, and transthyretin (TTR) (Berni and Formelli 1992). Fenretinide works through binding to the RBP in the circulation and prevents the association with retinol thus inhibiting the transport of retinol to the RPE and decreasing its presence in the visual cycle (Berni and Formelli 1992). Additionally, RBP-fenretinide complex is removed by the kidneys through urine, thus reducing the circulating quantity of RBP (Berni and Formelli 1992; Mata et al. 2013). Samuel et al. studied the effect of fenretinide in inducing ubiquitin-dependent proteasomal degradation of stearoyl-CoA desaturase in human retinal pigment epithelial cells (Samuel et al. 2014). The study demonstrated fenretinide decreased stearoyl-CoA desaturase protein and enzymatic activity suggesting role of fenretinide against retinal diseases (Samuel et al. 2014). In a study with 246 patients for treatment of geographic atrophy in AMD, the efficacy of fenretinide was studied after oral administration of 100 and 300 mg dosing for 2 years (Mata et al. 2013). The results demonstrated dose-dependent reversible reductions in serum RBP-retinol, reduced lesion growth rates, and reduced rate of choroidal neovascularization (Mata et al. 2013). In summary, discovering compounds to be visual cycle inhibitors is a promising area in ocular research, and the discovery of novel compounds can benefit various ocular diseases.

2.7 Pharmacologic Vitreolysis

With increasing knowledge of vitreoretinal disorders and the role of anomalous posterior vitreous detachment in vitreomaculopathies, pharmacologic vitreolysis has emerged as a new treatment modality (Sebag 1998). Pharmacologic vitreolysis is a nonsurgical approach to release tractional forces at the vitreoretinal interface by injecting an enzyme with proteolytic activity against fibronectin and laminin into the vitreous cavity (Sebag 1998). Sebag firstly defined pharmacologic vitreolytic compounds as agents that alter the molecular organization of vitreous in an effort to reduce or eliminate its role in disease (Sebag 1998). The agents used as pharmacologic vitreolysis can be classified by their mechanism of action, whether they induce liquefaction of the vitreous (liquefactant) or vitreous separation from the retina (interfactant) (Bandello et al. 2013). The tissue plasminogen activator (tPA), plasmin, microplasmin, nattokinase, and vitreosolve are believed to be both liquefactants and interfactants, whereas hyaluronidase is used as liquefactant. The majority of agents used for pharmacologic vitreolysis are enzymes (tPA, microplasmin, nattokinase, chondroitinase, dispase, and hyaluronidase), whereas the nonenzymatic agents used are urea/vitreosolve and arginine-glycine-aspartate peptides (Bandello et al. 2013).

Plasmin, a nonspecific serine protease, acts by degrading fibrin and other extracellular matrix components, including laminin and fibronectin (Liotta et al. 1981). Plasmin may also indirectly generate increased levels of other nonspecific proteases such as matrix metalloproteinases and elastase (Baramova et al. 1997). Both preclinical and clinical studies have shown ability of plasmin to achieve a complete vitreoretinal separation (Liotta et al. 1981). In addition, strong correlation was observed between plasmin concentration, exposure time, and the resultant extent of vitreoretinal separation (Liotta et al. 1981). Plasmin as autologous plasmin enzyme (APE) was used in the surgical treatment of pediatric traumatic macular holes (Margherio et al. 1998), stage 5 retinopathy of prematurity (Wu et al. 2008), and complicated X-linked retinoschisis showing improved anatomic outcomes. Ocriplasmin (microplasmin) is a recombinant product which has proteolytic activity of targeting vitreoretinal interface such as fibronectin and laminin (Tsui et al. 2012). The mechanism of ocriplasmin involves two steps, i.e., it is involved in vitreoretinal separation and vitreous liquefaction (Tsui et al. 2012). Ocriplasmin has shown greater penetration of vitreous and epiretinal tissues as compared to plasmin with reduced risk of microbial contamination associated with blood derivatives (Tsui et al. 2012). Multiple studies in animal models have shown its activity using porcine, rat, and rabbit eyes (Tsui et al. 2012). Ocriplasmin demonstrated efficacy and safety for the treatment of patients with symptomatic vitreomacular adhesion or vitreomacular traction, including patients with macular holes (Khoshnevis and Sebag 2015). The patients treated with ocriplasmin were more likely not to require vitrectomy surgery (Khoshnevis and Sebag 2015). In a clinical trial with 125 patients who underwent pars plana vitrectomy for the treatment of either vitreomacular traction or macular hole, the results suggested ocriplasmin injection at a dose of 125 μg led to a greater likelihood of induction and progression of posterior vitreous detachment than placebo injection (Khoshnevis and Sebag 2015). The other pharmacologic vitreolysis agent chondroitinase acts by degrading chondroitin sulfate, whereas nattokinase has a strong fibrinolytic affect (Bandello et al. 2013). Dispase is a protease which cleaves fibronectin, collagen IV, and, to a lesser extent, collagen I, and hyaluronidase acts by dissolving the glycosaminoglycan network of the vitreous gel thus electively considered a liquefactant (Bandello et al. 2013).

Pharmacologic vitreolysis is an emerging form of drug therapy that is based upon recent advances in our understanding of vitreous biochemistry and the role of anomalous posterior vitreous detachment in the pathophysiology of vitreoretinopathies. The role of enzymatic vitreolytic agents have been studied; however, additional studies are needed to develop more effective drugs. Studies involving nonenzymatic agents could also be explored as a potential agents for vitreolysis without collateral damage to adjacent structures. Additionally, combining an anti-VEGF with a vitreolytic agent to counteract the pathogenesis of neovascularization is another area to be explored. Moreover, extensive in vitro testing of present and new agents should be carried out in appropriate animal model studies before treating patients with evidence of efficacy.

2.8 Neuroprotective Targets

Discovery of neuroprotective compounds is another therapeutic target for diseases related to the eye. Multiple retinal diseases such as glaucoma, diabetic retinopathy, and AMD are associated with neurodegenerative disorders in which neurodegeneration happens in retinal ganglion cells (Schmidt et al. 2008). Cascade of cellular signaling events can be triggered by the stimulation of interleukin one receptors, JUN receptors, glutamate receptors, and tumor necrosis factor receptors (TNFRs) which results retinal neurons to undergo apoptosis (Schmidt et al. 2008). This could also result into activation of the proapoptotic proteins such as BCL-2 antagonist of cell death (BAD), BH3-interacting domain death agonist (BID), and BCL-2-associated X protein (BAX), which further releases cytochrome c and activates the caspase pathways (Schmidt et al. 2008). New drug molecules can be discovered as neuroprotective agents as they should (a) have specific and relevant receptor on the target tissue, (b) have adequate penetration to reach the target tissue in pharmacologically effective concentrations, (c) increase the neuronal survival or decrease neuronal damage in animal models, and (d) show efficacy in clinical trials.

The N-methyl-D-aspartate receptor (NMDA) is a glutamate receptor and ion channel protein found in nerve cells (Yucel et al. 2003). The activation of the NMDA receptor signaling pathway could lead to excitotoxicity wherein intracellular calcium overloads retinal ganglion cells causing cell death through apoptosis (Yucel et al. 2003). Kim et al. studied the relationship between the NMDA receptors and retinal ganglion cells in a rat model of chronic ocular hypertension using memantine (10 mg/kg), a NMDA antagonist, administered orally once daily for up to 5 weeks (Kim et al. 2007). Administration of memantine showed significant reduction in retinal ganglion cells and NMDA receptor expression in the eyes of rats suggesting that excessive expression of NMDA receptors are involved in retinal ganglion cell death in glaucoma (Kim et al. 2007).

Ciliary neurotrophic factor (CNTF), originally discovered in chicken embryo, has shown neuroprotection of rod photoreceptors in multiple retinal degeneration models across several species (Chen and Li 2011). Pease et al. studied the neuroprotective effect of CNTF after laser-induced glaucoma in Wistar rats (Pease et al. 2009). The administration CNTF had a significant protective effect, with 15 % less retinal ganglionic axon cell death. Additionally, there was a quantitative increase in CNTF expression in retinas exposed to single viral vectors carrying each gene thus confirming that CNTF can exert a protective effect in experimental glaucoma (Pease et al. 2009).

The use α2-adrenergic agonists have been another promising approach as they have shown neuroprotective effects by increasing the retinal ganglionic cells and axonal function in models utilizing both ocular hypertension and other optic nerve injuries (Wen et al. 1996). The well-known α2-adrenergic agonists used in ocular therapy are brimonidine and apraclonidine. Lindsey et al. studied differential protection of injured retinal ganglion cell dendrites by brimonidine (Lindsey et al. 2015). The results demonstrated brimonidine treatment significantly slowed the complete loss of retinal ganglionic cell dendrites and significantly slowed the reduction of total dendrite length and branching complexity. In addition to α2-adrenergic agonists, β-blockers are likely to exert a secondary neuroprotective effect. The neuroprotective effect of β-blockers is primarily via regulation of sodium and calcium channels, which are linked to the release of glutamate and subsequent activation of NMDA receptors.

Carbonic anhydrase (CA) isoenzyme as discussed before has been involved in the aqueous humor production in the human anterior segment (Vasudevan et al. 2011; Kniep et al. 2006). The carbonic anhydrase inhibitor dorzolamide has been involved in reducing the apoptotic pathways (Kniep et al. 2006). Another approach is developing 5-HT1A agonists as they have shown to have neuroprotective effects against excitotoxic neuronal damage in animal models (Schmidt et al. 2008). Collier et al. evaluated the efficacy of 5-HT (1A) agonists to protect the retina from severe blue light-induced photooxidative damage (Collier et al. 2011). Administrating AL-8309A in rats provided potent and structural protection suggesting the mechanism of protection is rapidly activated and protection persists for longer period (Collier et al. 2011). The use of neuroprotectant agents in ocular diseases is undoubtedly appealing; however, additional studies (both preclinical and clinical) are needed to extrapolate mechanisms of such agents to human patients.

2.9 Genomics

Genomic studies have gained attention for the past couple of decades because ocular complication have shown strong genetic component in the disease progression. There have been reports on different degrees of primary open-angle glaucoma observed in different population suggesting role of genetic variation (Cooke Bailey et al. 2013). It has been observed that prevalence of primary open-angle glaucoma in individuals of African ancestry is several-fold higher than in those of European ancestry (Cooke Bailey et al. 2013). Similarly, genetic abnormality has also been associated with diabetic retinopathy where frequency of diabetic retinopathy varies among different ethnicities and its prevalence is higher in individuals with a positive family history (Cooke Bailey et al. 2013). Drug discovery efforts could be targeted to the disease-related gene-encoding proteins. The International Age-related Macular Degeneration Genomics Consortium (IAMDGC) is involved in designing dataset which could help in understanding disease susceptibility loci and genomic regions contributing to disease susceptibility for the common blinding ocular disorders (Cooke Bailey et al. 2013).

Stem cell therapy is another area that has gained interest in order to achieve ocular tissue repair and/or regeneration (Eveleth 2013). The retinal pigment cells can be derived from patients with geographic atrophy who have a high-genetic-risk genotype, and these cells can be subjected to an in vitro high-throughput screen to identify small molecules that can prevent their death or enhance survival (Eveleth 2013). A considerable progress has been made in the genomic research to develop clinically useful gene-based tests and therapeutic strategies targeted to the diseases. Advances in novel gene-based tests and therapies in ocular diseases can help in reducing the global burden of visual impairment.

2.10 Ocular Drug Delivery

Bioavailability of ocular drugs administered to the anterior segment of the eye is limited by the corneal and conjunctival epithelial barriers of the eye (Morrison and Khutoryanskiy 2014). The eyedrops are rapidly drained from the ocular surface thus resulting into low bioavailability (Morrison and Khutoryanskiy 2014). The topical absorption can be increased by increasing the dosage forms, but they have not gained wide acceptance in the patients as administration of topical ocular medications does not reach the posterior segment drug targets. Currently there is an enormous growing interest in the posterior segment drug delivery (Morrison and Khutoryanskiy 2014) as multiple posterior segment diseases cannot be treated effectively with current methods. Intraocular or periocular injections could be associated with significant complications and often need to be repeated at regular intervals. Posterior segment delivery of both small and large molecules is challenging thus suggesting a need of ocular delivery system (Morrison and Khutoryanskiy 2014).

Due to the anatomic location of the eye, blood-ocular barriers, and an array of efflux transporters, the delivery of drug to the ocular targets becomes more challenging. Increasing number of sustained release drug delivery devices using different mechanisms are being studied. Other methods on ocular drug delivery that can be explored in drug discovery are using viscosity enhancers, mucoadhesives, and penetration enhancers to promote drug transport into the eye. Another area of active research and development is ocular insert as this method has a drug-loaded device that resides in the cul-de-sac under the eyelids or fits directly on the cornea like a contact lens where these devices are often designed to control release of drug molecules. Utilization of nanoparticles into ocular diseases is another area due to their unique capability of enhancing drug efficacy through preferential targeting to disease sites (Morrison and Khutoryanskiy 2014).

Gillies et al. studied head-to-head comparison of a dexamethasone implant (Ozurdex) versus bevacizumab (Avastin) for center-involving diabetic macular edema (DME) in 88 eyes of 61 patients (Gillies et al. 2014). The clinical study results demonstrated dexamethasone implant achieved similar rates of visual acuity improvement compared with bevacizumab (Gillies et al. 2014). Cunha-Vaz et al. showed sustained delivery fluocinolone acetonide vitreous implants on long-term benefits in patients with chronic diabetic macular edema (Cunha-Vaz et al. 2014). The results demonstrated that sustained delivery fluocinolone acetonide vitreous implants provide substantial visual benefit for up to 3 years who do not respond to other therapy (Cunha-Vaz et al. 2014).

Among various approaches to optimize drug delivery, applications of nanomedicine can have essential roles. Nanoparticles have offered numerous exciting possibilities in health care, and there are clinically approved nanoparticles therapies for treating ophthalmic diseases. The pegaptanib, an anti-VEGF aptamer conjugated with branched polyethylene glycol, has been approved for the treatment of AMD (Trujillo et al. 2007). Additionally, combining synthetic chemistry with a basic understanding of protein-polymer interactions has led to the efficient encapsulation and controlled delivery of proteins. Kalita et al. studied in vivo intraocular distribution and safety of periocular nanoparticle carboplatin for treatment of advanced retinoblastoma in humans (Kalita et al. 2014). The study was designed to determine the intraocular distribution and safety of polymethyl methacrylate nanoparticles loaded with carboplatin after posterior subtenon injection in six patients scheduled to undergo planned uniocular enucleation (Kalita et al. 2014). The highest level of carboplatin was detected in retina indicating an increased facilitated trans-scleral transport of nanoparticle carboplatin.

Encapsulated cell technology (ECT) is another technique where desired therapeutic proteins overexpressed through genetically engineered cells are encapsulated into semipermeable capsules (Tao 2006). The ECT facilitates the diffusion of nutrients and proteins with the advantage of preventing attack by the host immune system (Tao 2006). These technologies are particularly promising as the therapeutic potential of proteins and monoclonal antibodies is increasingly becoming realized in ophthalmology, particularly for halting retinal angiogenesis (Tao 2006). Zhang et al. studied ciliary neurotrophic factor delivered by encapsulated cell intraocular implants for treatment of geographic atrophy in AMD (Zhang et al. 2011). In a pilot, proof of concept phase 2 study, Zhang et al. evaluated ciliary neurotrophic factor (CNTF) delivered via an intraocular encapsulated cell technology implant for the treatment of geographic atrophy in a multicenter, double-masked, sham-controlled dose-ranging study (Zhang et al. 2011). Both the implant and the implant procedure were well tolerated (Zhang et al. 2011). The findings suggested that CNTF delivered by the encapsulated cell technology implant appeared to slow the progression of vision loss in geographic atrophy (Zhang et al. 2011).

Many successes in prolonging retention time and reducing administration frequency have been achieved in ocular drug delivery approaches using biodegradable or nonbiodegradable polymers. Various other approaches such as novel therapeutic molecules such as an antisense oligonucleotide or a small interfering RNA might be applicable in the ophthalmic field. Additional studies are needed in this field that might help in improving patient's and doctor's compliance.

2.11 Conclusions

Pharmaceutical industry spends billion US dollars on research and development each year on new drug discovery and development; however, right selection of drug target is one of the challenges which needs considerable attention. There have been multiple targets reported in literature as a potential to discover new ocular drugs; however, more knowledge may be required to better understand the characteristics and biological diversity of targets. Presently, therapies targeting VEGF have shown efficacy against eye diseases such as AMD, diabetic macular edema, and retinal vein-occlusive diseases; however, new agents targeting with higher efficacy for these diseases can be discovered. Additionally, several other blinding disorders, such as geographic atrophy, for which no effective therapies are currently available, can be explored for drug targets in ocular research. Similarly, new drug molecules targeting other areas such as lowering IOP, visual cycle inhibitors, protein vitrolysis, and neuroprotective agents can be explored. In addition, use of genomics and ocular drug release platforms to deliver either small or large molecule drugs is an important focus of future research. Finally, we need to develop suitable in vitro models and translational research where animal models can accurately recapitulate ophthalmic diseases in humans in order to validate new therapeutic agents before embarking on expensive clinical trials. In conclusion, discovering new drug molecules and preventing the loss of vision will present both great opportunities and challenges in the coming years.

References

Adamis AP, Miller JW, Bernal MT, D'Amico DJ, Folkman J, Yeo TK, Yeo KT. Increased vascular endothelial growth factor levels in the vitreous of eyes with proliferative diabetic retinopathy. Am J Ophthalmol. 1994;118(4):445–50.

Adelman R, Parnes A, Michalewska Z, Parolini B, Boscher C, Ducournau D. Strategy for the management of diabetic macular edema: the European vitreo-retinal society macular edema study. Biomed Res Int. 2015;2015:352487.

Akpek EK, Smith RA. Overview of age-related ocular conditions. Am J Manag Care. 2013;19(5 Suppl):S67–75.

Alon T, Hemo I, Itin A, Pe'er J, Stone J, Keshet E. Vascular endothelial growth factor acts as a survival factor for newly formed retinal vessels and has implications for retinopathy of prematurity. Nat Med. 1995;1:1024–8.

Alward WL. Biomedicine. A new angle on ocular development. Science. 2003;299:1527–8.
Arthur S, Cantor LB. Update on the role of alpha-agonists in glaucoma management. Exp Eye Res. 2011;93(3):271–83.
Bandello F, La Spina C, Iuliano L, Fogliato G, Parodi MB. Review and perspectives on pharmacological vitreolysis. Ophthalmologica. 2013;230(4):179–85.
Baramova EN, Bajou K, Remacle A, L'Hoir C, Krell HW, Weidle UH, Noel A, Foidart JM. Involvement of PA/plasmin system in the processing of pro-MMP-9 and in the second step of pro-MMP-2 activation. FEBS Lett. 1997;405:157–62.
Berni R, Formelli F. In vitro interaction of fenretinide with plasma retinol-binding protein and its functional consequences. FEBS Lett. 1992;308:43–5.
Bock F, König Y, Dietrich T, Zimmermann P, Baier M, Cursiefen C. Inhibition of angiogenesis in the anterior chamber of the eye. Ophthalmologe. 2007;104:336–44.
Chen TC. Brimonidine 0.15% versus apraclonidine 0.5% for prevention of intraocular pressure elevation after anterior segment laser surgery. J Cataract Refract Surg. 2005;31(9):1707–12.
Chen R, Li GL. Neuroprotection of retinal degenerative disease by ciliary neurotrophic factor. Zhonghua Yan Ke Za Zhi. 2011;47(6):568–72.
Cleveland RP, Hazlett LD, Leon MA, Berk RS. Role of complement in murine corneal infection caused by Pseudomonas aeruginosa. Invest Ophthalmol Vis Sci. 1983;24(2):237–42.
Collier RJ, Patel Y, Martin EA, Dembinska O, Hellberg M, Krueger DS, Kapin MA, Romano C. Agonists at the serotonin receptor (5-HT(1A)) protect the retina from severe photo-oxidative stress. Invest Ophthalmol Vis Sci. 2011;52(5):2118–26.
Cooke Bailey JN, Sobrin L, Pericak-Vance MA, Haines JL, Hammond CJ, Wiggs JL. Advances in the genomics of common eye diseases. Hum Mol Genet. 2013;22(R1):R59–65.
Cunha-Vaz J, Ashton P, Iezzi R, Campochiaro P, Dugel PU, Holz FG, Weber M, Danis RP, Kuppermann BD, Bailey C, Billman K, Kapik B, Kane F, Green K, FAME Study Group. Sustained delivery fluocinolone acetonide vitreous implants: long-term benefit in patients with chronic diabetic macular edema. Ophthalmology. 2014;121(10):1892–903.
Daka Q, Trkulja V. Efficacy and tolerability of mono-compound topical treatments for reduction of intraocular pressure in patients with primary open angle glaucoma or ocular hypertension: an overview of reviews. Croat Med J. 2014;55(5):468–80.
El Sayed KA, Youssef DT, Marchetti D. Bioactive natural and semisynthetic latrunculins. J Nat Prod. 2006;69(2):219–23.
Eveleth DD. Cell-based therapies for ocular disease. J Ocul Pharmacol Ther. 2013;29(10):844–54.
Fan S, Agrawal A, Gulati V, Neely DG, Toris CB. Daytime and nighttime effects of brimonidine on IOP and aqueous humor dynamics in participants with ocular hypertension. J Glaucoma. 2014; 23(5):276–81.
Friedman DS, O'Colmain BJ, Muñoz B, Tomany SC, McCarty C, de Jong PT, Nemesure B, Mitchell P, Kempen J. Prevalence of age-related macular degeneration in the United States. Arch Ophthalmol. 2004;122:564–72.
Gerl VB, Bohl J, Pitz S, Stoffelns B, Pfeiffer N, Bhakdi S. Extensive deposits of complement C3d and C5b-9 in the choriocapillaris of eyes of patients with diabetic retinopathy. Invest Ophthalmol Vis Sci. 2002;43(4):1104–8.
Gillies MC, Lim LL, Campain A, Quin GJ, Salem W, Li J, Goodwin S, Aroney C, McAllister IL, Fraser-Bell S. A randomized clinical trial of intravitreal bevacizumab versus intravitreal dexamethasone for diabetic macular edema: the BEVORDEX study. Ophthalmology. 2014;121(12): 2473–81.
Goldberg MA, Schneider TJ. Similarities between the oxygen-sensing mechanisms regulating the expression of vascular endothelial growth factor and erythropoietin. J Biol Chem. 1994;269: 4355–9.
Good TJ, Kahook MY. The role of endothelin in the pathophysiology of glaucoma. Expert Opin Ther Targets. 2010;14(6):647–54.
Hageman GS, Anderson DH, Johnson LV, Hancox LS, et al. A common haplotype in the complement regulatory gene factor H (HF1/CFH) predisposes individuals to age-related macular degeneration. Proc Natl Acad Sci U S A. 2005;102(20):7227–32.

Heier JS, Antoszyk AN, Pavan PR, Leff SR, Rosenfeld PJ, Ciulla TA, Dreyer RF, Gentile RC, Sy JP, Hantsbarger G, Shams N. Ranibizumab for treatment of neovascular age-related macular degeneration: a phase I/II multicenter, controlled, multidose study. Ophthalmology. 2006;113(4): 633.e1–4.

Inoue K, Shiokawa M, Sugahara M, Wakakura M, Soeda S, Tomita G. Three-month evaluation of dorzolamide hydrochloride/timolol maleate fixed-combination eye drops versus the separate use of both drugs. Jpn J Ophthalmol. 2012;56(6):559–63.

Jacot JL, Sherris D. Potential therapeutic roles for inhibition of the PI3K/Akt/mTOR pathway in the pathophysiology of diabetic retinopathy. J Ophthalmol. 2011;2011:589813.

Jha P, Bora PS, Bora NS. The role of complement system in ocular diseases including uveitis and macular degeneration. Mol Immunol. 2007;44(16):3901–8.

Joachim ND, Mitchell P, Kifley A, Wang JJ. Incidence, Progression, and Associated Risk Factors of Medium Drusen in Age-Related Macular Degeneration: Findings from the 15-Year Follow-up of an Australian Cohort. JAMA Ophthalmol. 2015;133(6):698–705.

Johnson LV, Forest DL, Banna CD, Radeke CM, Maloney MA, Hu J, Spencer CN, Walker AM, Tsie MS, Bok D, Radeke MJ, Anderson DH. Cell culture model that mimics drusen formation and triggers complement activation associated with age-related macular degeneration. Proc Natl Acad Sci U S A. 2011;108(45):18277–82.

Józsi M, Zipfel PF. Factor H family proteins and human diseases. Trends Immunol. 2008;29(8): 380–7.

Kalita D, Shome D, Jain VG, Chadha K, Bellare JR. In vivo intraocular distribution and safety of periocular nanoparticle carboplatin for treatment of advanced retinoblastoma in humans. Am J Ophthalmol. 2014;157(5):1109–15.

Kambhampati SP, Mishra MK, Mastorakos P, Oh Y, Lutty GA, Kannan RM. Intracellular delivery of dendrimer triamcinolone acetonide conjugates into microglial and human retinal pigment epithelial cells. Eur J Pharm Biopharm. 2015;pii: S0939 -6411(15):00095–8.

Kastelan S, Zjacić-Rotkvić V, Kastelan Z. Could diabetic retinopathy be an autoimmune disease? Med Hypotheses. 2007;68(5):1016–8.

Kawashima Y, Oishi A, Tsujikawa A, Yamashiro K, Miyake M, Ueda-Arakawa N, Yoshikawa M, Takahashi A, Yoshimura N. Effects of aflibercept for ranibizumab-resistant neovascular age-related macular degeneration and polypoidal choroidal vasculopathy. Graefes Arch Clin Exp Ophthalmol. 2015;253(9):1471–7.

Khandhadia S, Hakobyan S, Heng LZ, et al. Age-related macular degeneration and modification of systemic complement factor H production through liver transplantation. Ophthalmology. 2013;120(8):1612–8.

Khoshnevis M1, Sebag J. Pharmacologic vitreolysis with ocriplasmin: rationale for use and therapeutic potential in vitreo-retinal disorders. BioDrugs. 2015;29(2):103–12.

Kim JH, Lee NY, Jung SW, Park CK. Expression of N-methyl-d-aspartate receptor 1 in rats with chronic ocular hypertension. Neuroscience. 2007;149(4):908–16.

Kniep EM, Roehlecke C, Ozkucur N, Steinberg A, Reber F, Knels L, Funk RH. Inhibition of apoptosis and reduction of intracellular PH decrease in retinal neural cell cultures by a blocker of carbonic anhydrase. Invest Ophthalmol Vis Sci. 2006;47(3):1185–11892.

Kubota R, Boman NL, David R, Mallikaarjun S, Patil S, Birch D. Safety and effect on rod function of ACU-4429, a novel small-molecule visual cycle modulator. Retina. 2012;32(1):183–8.

Lindén C, Alm A. Prostaglandin analogues in the treatment of glaucoma. Drugs Aging. 1999;14(5):387–98.

Lindsey JD, Duong-Polk KX, Hammond D, Chindasub P, Leung CK, Weinreb RN. Differential protection of injured retinal ganglion cell dendrites by brimonidine. Invest Ophthalmol Vis Sci. 2015;56(3):1789–804.

Liotta LA, Goldfarb RH, Brundage R, Siegal GP, Terranova V, Garbisa S. Effect of plasminogen activator (urokinase), plasmin, and thrombin on glycoprotein and collagenous components of basement membrane. Cancer Res. 1981;41:4629–36.

Liu JHK, Weinreb RN. Monitoring intraocular pressure for 24 h. Br J Ophthalmol. 2011;95(5): 599–600.

Maines LW, French KJ, Wolpert EB, Antonetti DA, Smith CD. Pharmacologic manipulation of sphingosine kinase in retinal endothelial cells: implications for angiogenic ocular diseases. Invest Ophthalmol Vis Sci. 2006;47(11):5022–31.

Margherio AR, Margherio RR, Hartzer M, Trese MT, Williams GA, Ferrone PJ. Plasmin enzyme-assisted vitrectomy in traumatic pediatric macular holes. Ophthalmology. 1998;105:1617–20.

Martinez-Zapata MJ, Martí-Carvajal AJ, Solà I, Pijoán JI, Buil-Calvo JA, Cordero JA, Evans JR. Anti-vascular endothelial growth factor for proliferative diabetic retinopathy. Cochrane Database Syst Rev. 2014;11:D008721.

Mata NL, Weng J, Travis GH. Biosynthesis of a major lipofuscin fluorophore in mice and humans with ABCR-mediated retinal and macular degeneration. Proc Natl Acad Sci U S A. 2000;97:7154–9.

Mata NL, Lichter JB, Vogel R, Han Y, Bui TV, Singerman LJ. Investigation of oral fenretinide for treatment of geographic atrophy in age-related macular degeneration. Retina. 2013;33(3):498–507.

Michalewski J, Nawrocki J, Trębińska M, Michalewska Z. Switch to a single dose of aflibercept in bevacizumab nonresponders with AMD. Can J Ophthalmol. 2014;49(5):431–5.

Migdal C. Glaucoma medical treatment: philosophy, principles and practice. Eye (Lond). 2000;14:515–8.

Moiseyev G, Nikolaeva O, Chen Y, Farjo K, Takahashi Y, Ma JX. Inhibition of the visual cycle by A2E through direct interaction with RPE65 and implications in Stargardt disease. Proc Natl Acad Sci U S A. 2010;107(41):17551–6.

Mondino BJ, Glovsky MM, Ghekiere L. Activated complement in inflamed aqueous humor. Invest Ophthalmol Vis Sci. 1984;25(7):871–3.

Mondino BJ, Chou HJ, Sumner HL. Generation of complement membrane attack complex in normal human corneas. Invest Ophthalmol Vis Sci. 1996;37(8):1576–81.

Morrison DG, Aschner M. Vascular endothelial growth factor response to insulin-like growth factor in normoxic and hypoxic cell culture. Invest Ophthalmol Vis Sci. 2007;48:E-Abstract 1735.

Morrison PW, Khutoryanskiy VV. Advances in ophthalmic drug delivery. Ther Deliv. 2014;5(12):1297–315.

Moshfeghi AA, Rosenfeld PJ, Puliafito CA, Michels S, Marcus EN, Lenchus JD, Venkatraman AS. Systemic bevacizumab (Avastin) therapy for neovascular age-related macular degeneration: twenty-four-week results of an uncontrolled open-label clinical study. Ophthalmology. 2006;113(11):2002.e1–12.

Nathanson JA. Human ciliary process adrenergic receptor: pharmacological characterization. Invest Ophthalmol Vis Sci. 1981;21:798–804.

Pease ME, Zack DJ, Berlinicke C, Bloom K, Cone F, Wang Y, Klein RL, Hauswirth WW, Quigley HA. Effect of CNTF on retinal ganglion cell survival in experimental glaucoma. Invest Ophthalmol Vis Sci. 2009;50(5):2194–200.

Peden MC, Suñer IJ, Hammer ME, Grizzard WS. Long-term outcomes in eyes receiving fixed-interval dosing of anti-vascular endothelial growth factor agents for wet age-related macular degeneration. Ophthalmology. 2015;122(4):803–8.

Pe'er J, Shweiki D, Itin A, Hemo I, Gnessin H, Keshet E. Hypoxia-induced expression of vascular endothelial growth factor by retinal cells is a common factor in neovascularizing ocular diseases. Lab Invest. 1995;72(6):638–45.

Penn JS, Madan A, Caldwell RB, Bartoli M, Caldwell RW, Hartnett ME. Vascular endothelial growth factor in eye disease. Prog Retin Eye Res. 2008;27(4):331–71.

Pierce EA, Foley ED, Smith LE. Regulation of vascular endothelial growth factor by oxygen in a model of retinopathy of prematurity. Arch Ophthalmol. 1996;114(10):1219–28.

Pinard MA, Boone CD, Rife BD, Supuran CT, McKenna R. Structural study of interaction between brinzolamide and dorzolamide inhibition of human carbonic anhydrases. Bioorg Med Chem. 2013;21(22):7210–5.

Provis JM, Leech J, Diaz CM, Penfold PL, Stone J, Keshet E. Development of the human retinal vasculature: cellular relations and VEGF expression. Exp Eye Res. 1997;65:555–68.

Rasmussen CA, Kaufman PL, Ritch R, Haque R, Brazzell RK, Vittitow JL. Latrunculin B Reduces Intraocular Pressure in Human Ocular Hypertension and Primary Open-Angle Glaucoma. Transl Vis Sci Technol. 2014;3(5):1.

Rein DB, Zhang P, Wirth KE, Lee PP, Hoerger TJ, McCall N, Klein R, Tielsch JM, Vijan S, Saaddine J. The economic burden of major adult visual disorders in the United States. Arch Ophthalmol. 2006;124:1754–60.

Resch H, Karl K, Weigert G, Wolzt M, Hommer A, Schmetterer L, Garhöfer G. Effect of dual endothelin receptor blockade on ocular blood flow in patients with glaucoma and healthy subjects. Invest Ophthalmol Vis Sci. 2009;50(1):358–63.

Resnikoff S, Pascolini D, Etya'ale D, Kocur I, Pararajasegaram R, Pokharel GP, Mariotti SP. Global data on visual impairment in the year 2002. Bull World Health Organ. 2004;82:844–51.

Rosenfeld PJ, Moshfeghi AA, Puliafito CA. Optical coherence tomography findings after an intravitreal injection of bevacizumab (avastin) for neovascular age-related macular degeneration. Ophthalmic Surg Lasers Imaging. 2005;36:331–5.

Samuel W1, Kutty RK, Duncan T, Vijayasarathy C, Kuo BC, Chapa KM, Redmond TM. Fenretinide induces ubiquitin-dependent proteasomal degradation of stearoyl-CoA desaturase in human retinal pigment epithelial cells. J Cell Physiol. 2014;229(8):1028–38.

Sasore T, Reynolds AL, Kennedy BN. Targeting the PI3K/Akt/mTOR pathway in ocular neovascularization. Adv Exp Med Biol. 2014;801:805–11.

Schachar RA, Raber S, Courtney R, Zhang M. A phase 2, randomized, dose–response trial of taprenepag isopropyl (PF-04217329) versus latanoprost 0.005% in open-angle glaucoma and ocular hypertension. Curr Eye Res. 2011;36(9):809–17.

Schmidt KG, Bergert H, Funk RH. Neurodegenerative diseases of the retina and potential for protection and recovery. Curr Neuropharmacol. 2008;6(2):164–78.

Schmidt-Erfurth U, Chong V, Loewenstein A, Larsen M, Souied E, Schlingemann R, Eldem B, Monés J, Richard G, Bandello F, European Society of Retina Specialists. Guidelines for the management of neovascular age-related macular degeneration by the European Society of Retina Specialists (EURETINA). Br J Ophthalmol. 2014;98(9):1144–67.

Schmucker C, Ehlken C, Agostini HT, Antes G, Ruecker G, Lelgemann M, Loke YK. A safety review and meta-analyses of bevacizumab and ranibizumab: off-label versus gold standard. PLoS One. 2012;7(8):e42701.

Scozzafava A, Supuran CT. Glaucoma and the applications of carbonic anhydrase inhibitors. Subcell Biochem. 2014;75:349–59.

Sebag J. Pharmacologic vitreolysis. Retina. 1998;18(1):1–3.

Sena DF, Lindsley K. Neuroprotection for treatment of glaucoma in adults. Cochrane Database Syst Rev. 2013;2, CD006539.

Shams N, Ianchulev T. Role of vascular endothelial growth factor in ocular angiogenesis. Ophthalmol Clin North Am. 2006;19(3):335–44.

Sivaprasad S, Adewoyin T, Bailey TA, Dandekar SS, Jenkins S, Webster AR, Chong NV. Estimation of systemic complement C3 activity in age-related macular degeneration. Arch Ophthalmol. 2007;125(4):515–9.

Skoura A, Sanchez T, Claffey K, Mandala SM, Proia RL, Hla T. Essential role of sphingosine 1-phosphate receptor 2 in pathological angiogenesis of the mouse retina. J Clin Invest. 2007;117(9):2506–16.

Sohn JH, Bora PS, Jha P, Tezel TH, Kaplan HJ, Bora NS. Complement, innate immunity and ocular disease. Chem Immunol Allergy. 2007;92:105–14.

Sommer A, Tielsch JM, Katz J, Quigley HA, Gottsch JD, Javitt J, Singh K. Relationship between intraocular pressure and primary open angle glaucoma among white and black Americans: the Baltimore eye survey. Arch Ophthalmol. 1991;109(8):1090–5.

Sparrow JR, Nakanishi K, Parish CA. The lipofuscin fluorophore A2E mediates blue light induced damage to retinal pigmented epithelial cells. Invest Ophthalmol Vis Sci. 2000;41:1981–9.

Stewart MW. Aflibercept (VEGF Trap-Eye) for the treatment of exudative age-related macular degeneration. Expert Rev Clin Pharmacol. 2013;6(2):103–13.

Stone J, Itin A, Alon T, Pe'er J, Gnessin H, Chan-Ling T, Keshet E. Development of retinal vasculature is mediated by hypoxia-induced vascular endothelial growth factor (VEGF) expression by neuroglia. J Neurosci. 1995;15:4738–47.

Su Y, Cheng J, Liu H, Wang F, Zhao S. Adenovirus conducted connective tissue growth factor on extracellular matrix in trabecular meshwork and its role on aqueous humor outflow facility. Mol Biol Rep. 2013;40(11):6091–6.

Tao W. Application of encapsulated cell technology for retinal degenerative diseases. Expert Opin Biol Ther. 2006;6(7):717–26.

Thurman JM, Holers VM. The central role of the alternative complement pathway in human disease. J Immunol. 2006;176(3):1305–10.

Trujillo CA, Nery AA, Alves JM, Martins AH, Ulrich H. Development of the anti-VEGF aptamer to a therapeutic agent for clinical ophthalmology. Clin Ophthalmol. 2007;1(4):393–402.

Tsui I, Pan CK, Rahimy E, Schwartz SD. Ocriplasmin for vitreoretinal diseases. J Biomed Biotechnol. 2012;2012:354979.

Vasudevan SK, Gupta V, Crowston JG. Neuroprotection in glaucoma. Indian J Ophthalmol. 2011;59(Suppl):S102–13.

Wang J, Liu X, Zhong Y. Rho/Rho-associated kinase pathway in glaucoma (Review). Int J Oncol. 2013;43(5):1357–67.

Wen R, Cheng T, Li Y, Cao W, Steinberg RH. α2-adrenergic agonists induce basic fibroblast growth factor expression in photoreceptors in vivo and ameliorate light damage. J Neurosci. 1996;16:5986–92(1).

Wu WC, Drenser KA, Lai M, Capone A, Trese MT. Plasmin enzyme-assisted vitrectomy for primary and reoperated eyes with stage 5 retinopathy of prematurity. Retina. 2008;28 suppl 3:S75–80.

Xie B, Shen J, Dong A, Rashid A, Stoller G, Campochiaro PA. Blockade of sphingosine-1-phosphate reduces macrophage influx and retinal and choroidal neovascularization. J Cell Physiol. 2009;218(1):192–8.

Yancopoulos GD, Davis S, Gale NW, Rudge JS, Wiegand SJ, Holash J. Vascular-specific growth factors and blood vessel formation. Nature. 2000;407:242–8.

Yucel YH, Zhang Q, Weinreb RN, Kaufman PL, Gupta N. Effects of retinal ganglion cell loss on magno-, parvo-, koniocellular pathways in the lateral geniculate nucleus and visual cortex in glaucoma. Prog Retin Eye Res. 2003;22:465–81.

Zehetner C, Kralinger MT, Modi YS, Waltl I, Ulmer H, Kirchmair R, Bechrakis NE, Kieselbach GF. Systemic levels of vascular endothelial growth factor before and after intravitreal injection of aflibercept or ranibizumab in patients with age-related macular degeneration: a randomised, prospective trial. Acta Ophthalmol. 2015;93(2):e154–9.

Zhang K, Hopkins JJ, Heier JS, Birch DG, Halperin LS, Albini TA, Brown DM, Jaffe GJ, Tao W, Williams GA. Ciliary neurotrophic factor delivered by encapsulated cell intraocular implants for treatment of geographic atrophy in age-related macular degeneration. Proc Natl Acad Sci U S A. 2011;108(15):6241–5.

Zipfel PF, Skerka C, Hellwage J, Jokiranta ST, Meri S, Brade V, Kraiczy P, Noris M, Remuzzi G. Factor H family proteins: on complement, microbes and human diseases. Biochem Soc Trans. 2002;30(Pt 6):971–8.

Chapter 3
Drug Transport Across Blood-Ocular Barriers and Pharmacokinetics

Jose Cunha-Vaz, Francisco Batel Marques, Rosa Fernandes, Carlos Alves, and Thirumurthy Velpandian

Abstract Systemically administered drugs do not reach or have limited diffusion into the eye due to the presence of various ocular barriers. Therefore, intravitreal, intracameral, subconjunctival and sub-tenon routes are the preferred options for directly injecting drugs to into the eyes or ocular structures. Presence of drug transporters in the ocular or retinal barriers play a vital role in the ocular pharmacokinetics of the drugs administered by systemic or direct injection routes. This chapter discusses the involvement of various transporters in providing barrier functions for the transport of drugs in and out of eye. It also discusses about the general principles regarding ocular pharmacokinetics of drugs applied systemically and topically. Studies revealing the functional importance of transporters in barriers and models developed to predict the ocular kinetics of drugs, pharmaceutical factors, ocular drug metabolism and elimination are discussed to give further understanding while selecting a suitable drug for ocular therapy.

J. Cunha-Vaz, MD, PhD, FAAO (✉)
Department of Ophthalmology, Coimbra University Hospital, Coimbra, Portugal
e-mail: cunhavaz@aibili.p

F.B. Marques, PhD
Centre for Heath Technology Assessment and Drug Research (CHAD),
AIBILI Association for Innovation and Biomedical Research on Light and Image (AIBILI),
Azinhaga de Santa Comba, Celas 3000-548, Coimbra, Portugal

R. Fernandes, PhD
Laboratório de Farmacologia e Terapêutica Experimental,
IBILI – Faculdade de Medicina da Universidade de Coimbra,
Azinhaga de Santa Comba, Celas 3000-548, Coimbra, Portugal

C. Alves, PhD
School of Pharmacy, University of Coimbra,
Azinhaga de Santa Comba, Celas 3000-548, Coimbra, Portugal

T. Velpandian, BPharm, MS(Pharmacol), PhD
Ocular Pharmacology and Pharmacy, Dr. RP Centre for Ophthalmic Sciences,
All India Institute of Medical Sciences, New Delhi 110 029, India
e-mail: tvelpandian@hotmail.com

T. Velpandian (ed.), *Pharmacology of Ocular Therapeutics*,
DOI 10.1007/978-3-319-25498-2_3

3.1 Blood-Ocular Barriers

Jose Cunha-Vaz, MD, PhD, FAAO, Francisco Batel Marques, PhD,
Rosa Fernandes, PhD, and Carlos Alves, PhD

3.1.1 Introduction

The objective of medical therapy is to achieve the best favorable effects of drugs and to avoid their undesirable, unwanted side effects. The principles of pharmacokinetics – absorption, distribution, metabolism or biotransformation, and elimination – constitute a key knowledge for the appropriate choice and clinical success of therapeutic drug regimens (Buxton and Benet 2011). Unlike the vast majority of human organs, the eye is relatively excluded from the access of systemic circulating blood by several barriers (Jordan and Jordán and Ruíz-Moreno 2013). Therefore, direct administration of drugs in the eye, either topically or by ocular injection, is considered as specific routes of drug administration (Jordán and Ruíz-Moreno 2013). In order to have pharmacological activity, a drug must be present at the local site of action, which, in turn, requires its absorption and distribution. Absorption refers to the extent of drug reaching the systemic blood circulation or the central compartment (Buxton and Benet 2011). For oral administered drugs, several variables influence the absorption, such as the physical state of the drug, the blood flow at the local absorption, and the presence of ionized/nonionized forms (Buxton and Benet 2011). However, bioavailability is the concept reflecting the amount of drug reaching the local action after the absorption process and constitutes the most clinically meaningful pharmacokinetic concept (Buxton and Benet 2011).

During their passage through the body, drugs have to cross several cell membranes. This process may occur by passive transport (paracellular transport or diffusion) or by active transport (facilitated diffusion or drug transporters) (Buxton and Benet 2011). The later involves the active participation of molecular cell structures (Buxton and Benet 2011). It usually occurs as a movement against a concentration gradient and is an energy-consuming process (Buxton and Benet 2011).

The treatment of several eye diseases is based on the topical administration of drugs. They may act at the ocular surface or may need to cross epithelial cells (cornea, conjunctiva, or both) to reach local action (Attar et al. 2005). Transporters, particularly of peptide nature, are present in those tissues and regulate the action of several drugs (Attar et al. 2005). Drug-metabolizing enzymes have also been characterized in ocular tissues, with drug metabolism induction and inhibition properties as well as polymorphisms, particularly in cytochrome P450 expressions (Attar et al. 2005).

However, systemic administered drugs do not reach or have limited diffusion in the eye, due to the presence of ocular barriers, giving place to the need of directly inject drugs (intravitreous administration) (Jordán and Ruíz-Moreno 2013).

3.1.2 Ocular Barriers to the Penetration of Systemically Administered Drugs

The situation in the blood-ocular barriers is better understood if we consider two main barrier systems in the eye. One, regulating exchanges between blood and the intraocular fluids and involving a variety of structures, concerns the primary and ciliary body and is called the blood-aqueous barrier. Here, inward movements from the blood into the eye predominate. The aqueous humor is secreted into the posterior chamber by the ciliary processes from where it flows through the pupil into the anterior chamber and leaves the eye by bulk flow at the chamber angle by the trabecular or uveoscleral routes. There are diffusional solute exchanges between the aqueous humor and the surrounding tissues, the posterior chamber, and the vitreous compartment (Adler 1962; Bito 1977; Cunha-Vaz and Maurice 1967).

The other barrier, particularly tight, where outward movement from the eye into the blood appears to predominate and where the penetration into the eye of only a few important metabolic products in allowed, is called the blood-retinal barrier. It is responsible for homeostasis of the neuroretina.

3.1.3 Ocular Barriers to the Penetration of Topically Instilled Drugs

3.1.3.1 The Blood-Aqueous Barrier (BAB)

The blood-aqueous barrier is formed by the nonpigmented epithelium of the ciliary body, the posterior iris epithelium, the endothelium of the iris vessels with junctions of the leaky type, and the endothelium of Schlemm's canal (Chen et al. 2008). The BAB excludes aqueous and vitreous humors from blood plasma proteins to avoid compromising the transparency of intraocular fluids and to maintain their osmotic and chemical equilibrium (Butler et al. 1988). The aqueous, which is the fluid in the anterior and posterior chambers, is produced by the nonpigmented ciliary epithelium of the ciliary body (Chen et al. 2008). The aqueous humor maintains a normal homeostatic environment and is essential to the proper functioning of anterior chamber tissues (Chowdhury et al. 2010). The reason for a different composition of the aqueous humor comparing to the plasma resides in two physiological characteristics of the anterior segment: the blood-aqueous barrier and the active transport of various organic and inorganic substances by the ciliary epithelium. The greatest differences are the low protein and high ascorbate concentrations in the aqueous relative to plasma (200 times less and 20 times greater, respectively) (Gabelt and Kaufman 2011).

The BAB supports the nutrition and function of the cornea and lens (Chen et al. 2008). Ocular inflammation, intraocular surgery, trauma, or vascular diseases may cause alterations in the BAB (Chen et al. 2008). The aqueous becomes cloudy due to leakage of plasma proteins into the posterior and anterior chambers. The presence of fibrinogen and other proteins may turn the aqueous plasmoid (Hosoya and Tomi 2005). When the breakdown of the BAB occurs, inflammatory cells may be present in the aqueous. However, for BAB the expression of drug transporters and metabolizing enzymes has not been characterized; therefore, its role on ocular drug kinetics lacks elucidation (Chen et al. 2008; Urtti 2006).

The BAB is not as able as the BRB in respect to limiting molecular diffusion (Occhiutto et al. 2012). It was identified that after intravenous injection, substances such as inulin, chloride, sucrose, phosphate, potassium, sodium, urea, proteins, and some antibiotics could be found on the anterior side of the vitreous humor resulting from the ciliary circulation. However, these substances could not reach the retina directly due to the blood-retinal barrier (Occhiutto et al. 2012).

3.1.3.2 The Blood-Retinal Barrier (BRB)

The BRB is a physiological barrier that regulates ion, protein, and water flux into and out of the retina and prevents leakage into the retina of macromolecules and other harmful agents (Cunha-Vaz 1979, 2004). This barrier, which has many similarities to the blood-brain barrier, is essential to the integrity of the retina, and once BRB damage occurs, vision may become impaired (Cunha-Vaz 1997, 1979, 2010).

The BRB consists of inner and outer components (inner BRB [iBRB] and outer BRB [oBRB]) (Cunha-Vaz 2010). It provides metabolic support to the neural and glial cells through a unique vascular structure while minimizing interference with light sensing (Runkle and Antonetti 2011). The oBRB is constituted by the retinal pigment epithelium and is located at the posterior of the eye, controlling exchange of nutrients with the choroidal vessels (Runkle and Antonetti 2011). The vascular and epithelial components of the blood-retinal barrier maintain the specialized environment of the neural retina (Runkle and Antonetti 2011).

3.1.3.3 The Inner Blood-Retinal Barrier (iBRB)

The iBRB is established by the tight junctions (zonulae occludentes) between retinal endothelial cells (Cunha-Vaz 2010). The retinal endothelial layer functions as an epithelium and is directly associated with its differentiation and with the polarization of BRB function (Cunha-Vaz 2010). This continuous endothelial cell layer, which forms the main structure of the iBRB, rests on a basal lamina that is covered by the processes of astrocytes and Müller glia cells (Cunha-Vaz 2010). Pericytes are also present in the iBRB, encased in the basal lamina, in contact with the endothelial cells, but they do not form a continuous layer and therefore do not contribute to the diffusional barriers (Jordán and Ruíz-Moreno 2013). Astrocytes, Müller cells, and pericytes are considered to affect maturation and maintenance of the

BRB by transmitting regulatory signals to endothelial cells indicating changes in the microenvironment of the retinal neuronal circuitry (Cunha-Vaz 2010; Schlosshauer 2007).

The vascular endothelium found in the adult retina and the brain shows similar structural characteristics, though some differences have been identified, such as a higher density of interendothelial junctions and the lack of g-glutamyl transpeptidase (gGT) in the retinal endothelium (Schlosshauer 2007; Vinores 1995). The development of the endothelial network and the formation of the iBRB are characterized by a primary construction phase followed by a secondary destruction period until the adult layout is sculptured (Schlosshauer 2007). Furthermore, the initial vascular network is leaky. The expression of barrier characteristics appears to be one of the latest steps during maturation (Schlosshauer 2007).

Retinal Vascular Endothelial Cells

The retinal vascular endothelial capillaries are composed by non-fenestrated cells which have a paucity of vesicles (Cunha-Vaz 2010). Such vesicles promote receptor-mediated processes of endocytosis or transcytosis. Other mechanism for diffusion of substances across the BRB is the channel-facilitated transport using transmembrane proteins, such as the glucose transporter GLUT1 which supplies glucose to the neuronal tissue (Cunha-Vaz 2010). The disruption of the iBRB in pathological conditions is associated with increased vesicle formation and disrupted endothelial membranes and may develop before opening of the tight junctions being detected (Cunha-Vaz 2010).

Retinal Vascular Endothelial Tight Junctions

The main function of the tight junctions, TJs, is the ion, water, and nutrient flow regulation between the retina and blood vessels, as well as the protection of the neural retina from inflammatory cells and their toxic products found in the systemic circulation (Vinores 1995; Gardner et al. 2002; Kaur et al. 2008). Tight junctions may also serve as regulatory centers that can help to coordinate several cell processes, such as the regulation of cell morphology, proliferation, and establishment and maintenance of apico-basal polarity (Kaur et al. 2008).

The TJs of the retinal vascular endothelium are formed by fusion of the outer leaflets of adjacent endothelial cell membranes (Fernandes et al. 2012). The TJ complex contains at least 40 transmembrane proteins and internal adapter proteins that regulate paracellular flux (Fernandes et al. 2012). Transmembrane proteins constituting the TJ are occludins, claudins, and junctional adhesion molecules. Adapter proteins are localized below the membrane and act as TJ organizers and cytoskeleton anchors (Fernandes et al. 2012). The TJs are regulated by signal transduction through cyclic AMP levels, or tyrosine kinases, for example (Fernandes et al. 2012).

Müller Glia Cells, Astrocytes, and Pericytes

The close spatial relationship between Müller glia cells and blood vessels in the retinal suggests that these cells have a critical role in the formation and maintenance of the BRB by regulating the functions of the barrier cells in the uptake of nutrients and in the disposal of metabolites under normal conditions (Cunha-Vaz 2010). Muller cells have matrix metaloproteinases that promote proteolytic degradation of TJ proteins occludins.

Astrocytes in the iBRB play a critical role during normal inner retinal vascularization (Dorrell et al. 2002; Fruttiger et al. 1996; Provis et al. 2000), and degeneration of retinal astrocytes in ischemic tissues is associated with failure of the blood-retinal barrier in oxygen-induced retinopathies (Chan-Ling and Stone 1992; Dorrell et al. 2010). These cells are originated from the optic nerve and migrate to the retinal nerve fiber layer during retinal vascular development, to closely associate with the retinal vessels helping to maintain their integrity (Cunha-Vaz 2010). Astrocytes enhance the expression of the TJ protein Z0.1 which has a role in moderate TJ integrity (Cunha-Vaz 2010).

Pericytes support endothelial cells by secreting angiopoietin 1, which induces the protein expression of occlud and other proteins integrating TJ. These cells help in the regulation of vascular tone, secretion of extracellular materials and in the process of phagocytosis (Cunha-Vaz 2010).

3.1.3.4 The Outer Blood-Retinal Barrier (oBRB)

The outer blood-retinal barrier is formed by a single layer of retinal pigment epithelial (RPE) cells that are interconnected in their apical side by TJs (zona occludens) (Fernandes et al. 2012). The permeable Bruch's membrane separates the RPE from the overlying fenestrated choriocapillaris (Fernandes et al. 2012). The RPE is fundamental to regulate the access of nutrients from the blood to the photoreceptors and in the elimination of waste products and maintenance of retinal adhesion (Cunha-Vaz 2010). Besides these features that serve the (outer) retina in general, the metabolic relationship between the RPE villi and the photoreceptors is considered critical for the maintenance of visual function.

RPE Cells

RPE cells regulate water content and lactic acid removal generated by the characteristic high metabolic rates in the retina (Jordán and Ruíz-Moreno 2013). The adhesion of the retina to the RPE is based on the interphotoreceptor matrix, which is synthesized by the RPE (Steinberg and Wood 1979). The viscosity and bonding properties of the matrix are dependent on its hydration and ionic composition, both of which are controlled by vectorial flux of water and selected ions. The net effect of several RPE pump systems is a movement of water across the RPE in the apical-to-basal, i.e., retina-choroid, direction (Zauberman 1979). The water transport is linked with ion transport, organic anion transport, and other drainage mechanisms (Cunha-Vaz 2010).

The RPE is further involved in photoreceptor outer segment renewal (Fernandes 2012). RPE cells also transport glucose and retinol from blood to the photoreceptors (Cunha-Vaz 2010).

RPE Tight Junctions

The TJs of the RPE cells are anchored to the actin cytoskeleton of RPE cells, interact with signaling molecules, and are important for the establishment of cell polarity (Cunha-Vaz 2010). These junctions restrict the paracellular movement of larger molecules between neighboring RPE cells (Cunha-Vaz 2010). As the retinal vascular endothelium TJs, occludins, claudins, and adapter proteins have been detected in the RPE TJs (Cunha-Vaz 2010). The TJ complexes of the iBRB and oBRB allow the establishment of the polarities of the BRB, restricting paracellular diffusion of blood-barrier compounds in the neuronal tissues (Cunha-Vaz 2010).

3.1.3.5 BRB and Ocular Immune Privilege

The immune response has developed and evolved to protect the organism from invasion and damage by a wide range of pathogens. With time, the immune system has developed destructive responses that are specific for pathogens as well as tissues. However, such tissue injury may have a devastating effect on the function of an organ such as the eye, which needs to maintain optical stability (Cunha-Vaz 2009).

The existence of ocular immune privilege is dependent on multiple factors such as immunomodulatory factors and ligands, regulation of the complement system within the eye, tolerance-promoting antigen-presenting cells (APCs), unconventional drainage pathways, and, with particular relevance, the existence of the blood-ocular barriers (Cunha-Vaz 2009).

The blood-ocular barriers provide a relative sequestration of the anterior chamber, vitreous humor, and neurosensory retina from the immune system and create the necessary environment for the existence of ocular immune privilege (Fernandes 2012). The evolution of immune privilege as a protective mechanism for preserving the function of vital and delicate organs such as the eye has resulted in a complex system with multiple regulatory safeguards for the control of both innate and adaptive immunity (Cunha-Vaz 2009). The consequences of inadvertent bystander tissue destruction by antigen-nonspecific inflammation can be so catastrophic to the organ or host that a finely tuned regulatory system is needed to ensure the integrity of the ocular tissues and maintain optical relationships (Fernandes 2012; Cunha-Vaz 2009).

There are also several lines of evidence that point to immunosuppressive functions in BRB cells, RPE cells, and retinal endothelial cells. These immunosuppressive effects are apparently due to the secretion of a variety of soluble factors, such as cytokines and growth factors (Cunha-Vaz 2009).

3.1.3.6 Regulation of the Microenvironment of the Retina: BRB Transport Systems

The presence of TJ in the BRB prevents free diffusion of polar nutrients essential for the metabolism of the retina, and therefore, the BRB must contain specific transport proteins that are expressed at the plasma membranes of the retinal epithelial and endothelial cells. Epithelial (oBRB) and endothelial (iBRB) cells exhibit a polarized expression of transport carriers in the apical/luminal and basolateral/abluminal plasma membranes (Fernandes 2012). The orientation of these carriers results in preferential blood-to-retina influx or retina-to-blood efflux transport of substrates or in facilitated transport in either direction depending on the concentration gradient of the solutes across the BRB (Fernandes 2012).

Potential routes for facilitated transport across the BRB are the blood-to-retina influx transport system that acts as an energy supply system for the retina, since the iBRB supplies metabolic substrates from the circulating blood, such as glucose, amino acids, vitamins, and nucleosides, to the retina (Fernandes 2012). The other is the retina-to-blood efflux transport system that acts to get rid of hydrophobic xenobiotics and neurotransmitter metabolites (Fernandes 2012).

3.1.3.7 Energy Transport System

The blood-to-retina influx transporters operating at the iBRB supply hydrophilic substrates to the retina. The retina, one of the most metabolically active tissues in the body, uses glucose as its main energy source. Being a hydrophilic molecule, glucose does not freely cross the barrier and its transport from blood into retina is mediated by facilitative glucose transporters, named GLUT1 (Takata et al. 1992; Fernandes et al. 2003). The distribution of GLUT1 at the iBRB is asymmetric, being its expression at the abluminal membrane approximately two- and threefold greater than that at the luminal membrane in humans and rats, respectively (Takata et al. 1992; Fernandes et al. 2003). The higher density of GLUT1 on the abluminal membrane of the retinal endothelial cells suggests that glucose transport is limited at the blood-luminal rather than the abluminal-interstitial interface. In experimental animal models of type 1 and type 2 diabetes, as well as in vitro studies where endothelial cells were exposed to elevated glucose, it has been shown that there is a downregulation of GLUT1 in retinal endothelial cells (Badr et al. 2000; Fernandes et al. 2004).

Besides glucose, dehydroascorbic acid (DHA), which is an oxidized form of vitamin C, is rapidly transported across the BRB via GLUT1 and accumulates as ascorbic acid in the retina. DHA uptake by GLUT1 is competitively inhibited by D-glucose (Minamizono et al. 2006). DHA transport from the blood to the retina decreases with increasing blood D-glucose concentration under diabetic conditions due to the inhibition of DHA uptake by GLUT1 at the BRB (Minamizono et al. 2006). This can lead to the increased oxidative stress observed in diabetic retinas.

In addition to D-glucose, L-lactic acid appears to be required as an energy source in photoreceptors (Poitry-Yamate et al. 1995), and the transport of this solute between retina and blood seems to be mediated by the monocarboxylate transporter 1 (MCT1). Immunoreactivity for this transporter was found both in luminal and abluminal membranes of rat endothelial cells (Gerhart et al. 1999). It has been shown that the uptake of labeled L-lactic acid is inhibited by protonophores, MCT inhibitors, and a number of other monocarboxylates and monocarboxylic drugs, such as salicylic and valproic acids (Alm and Törnquist 1985; Hosoya et al. 2001). These results suggest that these transports are an attractive route for monocarboxylate drug delivery to the posterior segment of the eye.

Creatine, which plays an essential role in supporting ATP homeostasis in the retina, is transported by creatine transporter (CRT) (Nakashima et al. 2004). The storage and administration of phosphate-bound energy is mediated by the conversion of creatine to phosphocreatine. It has been found to be an asymmetrical distribution of CRT at luminal and abluminal membranes of rat retinal endothelial cells (Nakashima et al. 2004).

In glycolysis, glucose is oxidized to either lactate or pyruvate. Both glycolysis and the tricarboxylic acid cycle generate energy in the form of ATP. Therefore, GLUT1, MCT1, and CRT transporters may act in synergy to maintain energy homeostasis in the retina.

3.1.3.8 Nucleoside Transport System

Adenosine is an important intracellular signaling molecule that is involved in retinal neurotransmission, blood flow, vascular development, and response to ischemia trough cell surface adenosine receptors (Ghiardi et al. 1999; Lutty and McLeod 2003).

The expression at the mRNA level of several equilibrative nucleoside transporters ENT1, ENT2, CNT1, and CNT2 has been detected in retinal endothelial cells (Nagase et al. 2006). By regulating the concentration of adenosine available to cell surface receptors, these transporters influence the retinal physiological processes mentioned above. ENT2 is also responsible for the uptake of some antiviral and anticancer nucleoside drugs (Yao et al. 2001; Baldwin et al. 2004). This has led to the hypothesis that ENT2 at the iBRB could be a potential route for delivering nucleoside drugs from the circulating blood to the retina.

3.1.3.9 Organic Anion Transport System

In order to maintain a constant milieu in the neural retinal, the BRB also carries out the efflux transport of harmful substances like neurotransmitter metabolites, toxins, and xenobiotics (Cunha-Vaz and Maurice 1967).

Members of the family of organic anion-transporting polypeptides (OATP) mediate the Na + -independent transport of a wide range of amphipathic organic compounds, including bile salts, organic dyes, steroid conjugates, thyroid hormones, anionic oligopeptides, numerous drugs, and other xenobiotic substances (Hagenbuch and Meier 2003). Transporters of the family of OATP (OATP2 and OATP14) have been identified in the rat inner and outer BRB (Gao et al. 2002).

3.1.3.10 ABC Transporters

ABC transporters (ATP-binding cassette) are a superfamily of membrane proteins that play a major role in restricting the bioavailability of many drugs in various tissues by pumping agents (with consumption of ATP) from the lipid bilayer or cytoplasm back into the extracellular fluid (Mannermaa et al. 2006). In the ocular tissues, the ABC transporters of greatest significance for efflux transport are P-glycoprotein (P-gp), multidrug resistance-associated proteins (MRP), and breast cancer protein (BCRP) (Mannermaa et al. 2006).

The ABC superfamily is subdivided into seven subfamilies based on similarities in domain structure, nucleotide-binding folds, and transmembrane domains (Dean et al. 2001). The general structure of ABC transporters is composed of 12 transmembrane regions, split into two halves, each with a nucleotide-binding domain (NBD) (Altenberg 2004).

P-gp (MDR1) mediates the efflux of a wide range of drugs from the intracellular to the extracellular space (Fojo et al. 1987). The list of its substrates/inhibitors is continually growing and includes anticancer agents, antibiotics, antivirals, calcium channel blockers, and immunosuppressive agents (Altenberg 2004). P-gp has been shown to be expressed in rat retinal capillaries and cultures of rat retinal endothelial cells (Greenwood 1992; Shen et al. 2003; Hosoya and Tomi 2005). The P-gp-mediated drug efflux pump on the apical plasma membrane of the conjunctiva plays a role in restricting the conjunctival absorption of some lipophilic drugs and xenobiotics.

BCRP (ABCG2) has only one ABC and six putative transmembrane domains, being referred to as a half-ABC transporter, most likely functioning as a homodimer (Krishnamurthy and Schuetz 2006) ABCG2 shows great affinity not only for drugs but also for phototoxic compounds that can cause light-induced damage to the retina (Boulton et al. 2001). BCRP was found to be present in the luminal membrane of mouse capillary endothelial cells by immunolabeling and was shown to be expressed in mouse and rat retinas (Asashima et al. 2006).

These drug efflux pumps at the BRB could act by restricting the distribution of xenobiotics, including drugs and phototoxins, in the retina. Modulation of such efflux mechanisms in conjunction with the treatment of ocular tissues in retinal diseases remains a major challenge.

3.1.3.11 Relevance of the Blood-Retinal Barrier in the Treatment of Retinal Diseases

When administered systemically, drugs must pass the BRB in order to reach therapeutic levels in the retina. Drug entrance into the retina depends on a number of factors, including the plasma concentration profile of the drug, the volume of its distribution, plasma protein binding, and the relative permeability of the BRB (Cunha-Vaz 1979). To obtain therapeutic concentrations within the retina, new strategies must be considered such as delivery of nanoparticles, chemical modification of drugs to enhance BRB transport, coupling of drugs to vectors, etc. (Cunha-Vaz 2010; Fernandes et al. 2012). The BRB must be considered as a dynamic interface that has the physiological function of specific and selective membrane transport from blood to retina and active efflux from retina to blood for many compounds, as well as degradative enzymatic activities (Cunha-Vaz 2009). Better understanding of the transports systems at the BRB will be extremely useful for drug design. Efflux pumps must be effectively circumvented to enhance drug absorption across the retina (Cunha-Vaz 2010). Modulating a drug substrate targeting an influx transporter offers great potential. In this strategy, drugs must be designed such that the modified compounds become substrates of nutrient transporters, leading to enhanced absorption across the ocular barriers. In addition, efflux is effectively circumvented due to diminished or no affinity of the drug molecule toward efflux pumps due to structural modification and binding to the influx transporter (Cunha-Vaz 2010).

Eyedrops are now being developed for the treatment of posterior segment diseases. However, they are generally considered to be of limited benefit. Newer prodrug formulations that achieve high concentrations of the drug in the posterior segment may have a role in the future. Meanwhile, periocular injection is one modality that has offered mixed results (Cunha-Vaz 2010; Fernandes et al. 2012).

Finally, recent years have seen a generalized and surprisingly safe utilization of intravitreal injections, a form of administration that circumvents the BRB. Steroids and a variety of anti-vascular endothelial growth factor (anti-VEGF) drugs have been administered through intravitreal injections to a large number of patients without significant side effects and demonstrating good acceptance by the patients. Intravitreal injections can achieve high drug concentrations in the vitreous humor and retina, preserving BRB integrity and its crucial protective function (Cunha-Vaz 2010). At present, the major challenge appears to be the need to decrease the number of intravitreal injections, which, in the case of anti-VEGF treatments, are given every 6 weeks to maintain efficacy. The search for safe slow-delivery devices or implantable biomaterials is ongoing, but the invasive approach to retinal disease treatment appears to be an effective way of rapidly reaching therapeutic levels in the retina in the presence of a functioning BRB (Cunha-Vaz 2010; Fernandes et al. 2012).

3.1.4 Conclusion

It has been shown to be particularly difficult to reach therapeutic drug concentrations in the retina using traditional routes of administration, other than the exception of intravitreal injections. Topical treatments generally present favorable benefit/risk ratios but have been limited to ocular anterior segment pathologies. The BRB is an obstacle to drug penetration and circulation within the retina, since transporters expressed by this barrier play a decisive role on drug bioavailability to this tissue.

3.2 Ocular Pharmacokinetics and Factors Affecting Ocular Disposition of Drugs

Thirumurthy Velpandian

Drug transfer across the ocular barriers is expected to govern the pharmacokinetics of drugs which in turn affect their dynamic properties. Drug entry into the ocular structures is conventionally enabled by systemic, intraocular (intracameral and intravitreal), periocular (sub-tenon and subconjunctival), and topical administrations. Except direct injection into the ocular compartments such as intravitreal or intracameral, all other routes for ocular drug administration would be governed by their systemic pharmacokinetics where they behave as sites for drug absorption.

Systemic drugs seldom reach effective concentration (above ED50 or MIC 90) into normal ocular tissues. Therefore, systemic drug routes are not preferred for most of the ocular diseases. Failure to reach adequate drug level into ocular structures can be attributed to their therapeutic failure at many instances. Typically, eye has been reported to have two predominant pathways of drug elimination. After direct injection some drugs are eliminated from vitreous through retinal pathway (Posterior) and some of them are reported to be eliminated through anterior pathway. Hence, ocular disposition of drugs can play an independent role unlike other places where they are not guarded by blood organ barriers.

3.2.1 Pharmacokinetics of the Topically Applied Drugs

Pre-corneal factors are the key determinants of the absorption of the topically administered drugs into the eye. Based on the port of entry, pharmacokinetics of the drugs into anterior and posterior segments of the eye can be classified. If absorption takes place through the cornea or conjunctiva after topical instillation of drugs such as eyedrops, the levels reaching aqueous humor are suggestive of the extent of its

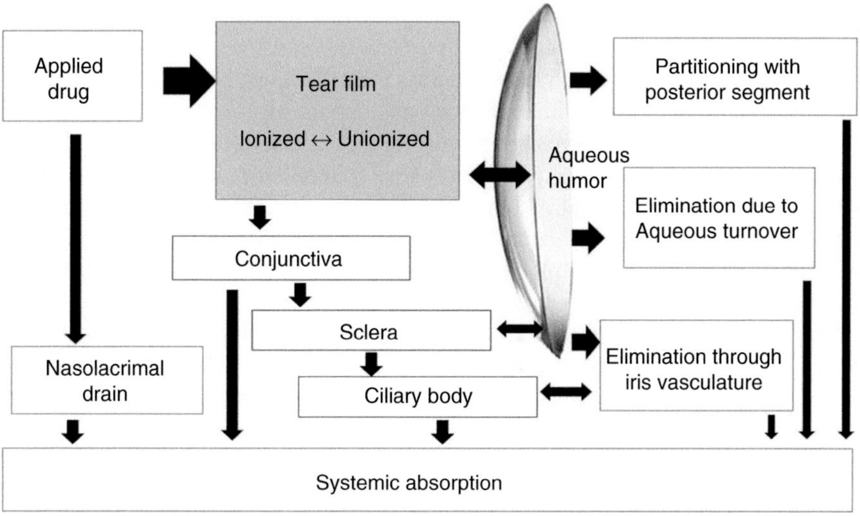

Fig. 3.1 Schematic representation of the fate of topically applied drugs on the eye and their disposition

penetration. The elimination kinetics of the drug from the aqueous humor is favored through anterior pathways of elimination including aqueous drainage, absorption into iris vasculature, re-equilibration with corneal tissues, and reverse draining to the posterior segment through retinal blood vessels (Fig. 3.1). In most of the cases, the former route is favored than the later. Effect of coadministered drugs are also reported to influence ocular absorption of drugs. Topically instilled anesthetic agents significantly suppressed the rate of tear turnover and thereby increased pre-corneal drug residence time (Patton and Robinson 1975).

3.2.2 Pre-corneal Factors Affecting Ocular Penetration of Drugs after Topical Application

In the air-corneal interface, one would see several layers of physiological importance involved in the maintenance of corneal integrity and transparency very efficiently. The outer most layer is a mono lipid layer floating on the tear film having hydrophobic lipids toward air and amphiphilic lipids in the lipid-water interface thereby giving integrity. These lipids are secreted by meibomian glands, which are embedded in the tarsal plate of the upper and lower eyelids giving protection against aqueous evaporation. The cornea produces a small proportion of the aqueous layer as well as mucins in the glycocalyx. The conjunctiva secretes substantial electrolytes and water into the aqueous layer and mucins into the mucous layer. At the same time, the conjunctiva can also absorb electrolytes, water, and applied drugs from the tear film thereby modifying their pharmacokinetics. Although five layers of the cornea are very distinct, the corneal epithelium, stroma, and endothelium are the layers that gain pharmacological importance as far as drug penetration is concerned. In these layers, drug transport across the cornea can be modulated by drug transporters present in the epithelium and endothelium. However, the resistance for the transport of the drug across these membranes is also affected by the physiochemical nature of the molecule. The corneal epithelium is hydrophobic and the stroma is hydrophilic; thereby both water-soluble and lipid-soluble drugs cannot penetrate freely. The cornea behaves as a typical biological membrane in which most of the drugs cross this structure either by intracellular or transcellular diffusion (Lee and Robinson 1986).

Topically applied eyedrops exceeding the volume of 20 μl would be drained from the cul-de-sac via nasolacrimal duct or removed externally by blinking. Application of low volumes of eyedrop would be beneficial for getting better bioavailability. Volume of solution delivered by commercial eye droppers can be between 25–50 μl and if the subject is not blinking, eye can hold upto 30 μl if instilled carefully. However, reflex blinking may increase both solution drainage and overflow from the conjunctival sac. Decreasing the volume of instillation is expected to improve risk-to-benefit ratio of the potent compounds known to have systemic toxicity (Lynch et al. 1987).

Most of the topically applied drugs are the salts of acids or bases like ciprofloxacin HCl, timolol maleate, prednisolone acetate, pilocarpine trinitrate, atropine sulfate, bromfenac sodium, etc. Drug molecules in the tear film can be influenced or get influenced by the tear film pH depending on their concentration and property. Therefore, the extent of their ocular bioavailability would depend upon their ionization constant (pKa) under the given pH of the pre-corneal tear film. The unionized compounds show higher lipophilicity enabling them to cross the outer epithelium. Apart from pKa, molecular weight, preservatives, presence of surfactants, vehicle, and osmolarity of the formulation are the other factors that determine the ocular pharmacokinetics of the drugs. Certain topical drug preservatives like benzalkonium chloride are reported to increase the ocular bioavailability of the topically applied drugs by disrupting the corneal membrane.

Most of the topically instilled drugs reach their Cmax in aqueous humor between 15 min to 2 hrs. Based on the frequency of drug administration hourly or 2 hourly, the levels can substantially be increased to reach pharmacologically accepted concentration in the cornea, conjunctiva, and aqueous humor. Pre-corneal drug residence time is largely dependent upon the bidirectional equilibration of drug levels reaching in between the cornea and tear film which slowly decrease along with time. This aspect gains much importance when trying to reach adequate antimicrobial drug levels after repeated drug instillation in case of corneal or conjunctival bacterial infections. Corneal nerves are very sensitive to non-specific stimulation, pH and osmolarity, the pre-corneal elimination of drugs which is in equilibrium with tissues can be accelerated in case if the lacrimal secretion is increased by the stimulation of sensory nerves of the cornea due to the nature of the drug component or formulation factors. Composition of topical formulation (drug vehicle) has also been reported to influence the topical penetration of drugs (Hardberger et al. 1975; McCarthy 1975).

3.2.3 Compartment Models Used to Predict Ocular Kinetics of Drugs

Compartment models are mathematical equations used to predict the drug disposition beyond the tissues/fluids in which the drug concentration is quantified. This information is required to understand the movement of drugs across various tissues and organs along with the elimination of drugs from the primary compartment. Usually for systemic pharmacokinetics, blood would serve as a central compartment from where the drug elimination predominately happens. In eye, anterior chamber administration of amikacin and chloramphenicol followed one compartmental model (Mayers et al. 1991). Following bolus administration of the hydrophobic immune-suppressant drug cyclosporine into the anterior chamber, its clearance from the aqueous humor was predicted by one-compartment model with the terminal half-life of 30–40 h, where as for the aqueous to tissue distribution into the cornea, a two-compartment model was employed (Oh et al. 1995).

Typically, when the analysis of drug partition into systemic and ocular tissues needs to be done, two-compartment model best suited the purpose considering that the multiple sites of tissue distribution is involved. Two-compartment modeling was successfully used by several investigators to predict the drug partitioning from tear film to ocular tissues for their effect as well as systemic absorption causing side effects. The advantage of timolol with thickening agent (gel) was compared with simple topical solution of timolol in rabbits. A two-compartment pharmacokinetic model was used to fit the aqueous humor level for determining the drainage (kd) and absorption rate constants (ka) in the pre-corneal area as well as the elimination rate constant (ke) of timolol in the aqueous humor. This study reported that gel has a longer retention time in eyes to improve ocular bioavailability and lesser systemic side effects (Chiang et al. 1996). Sasaki and coworkers (2000) predicted concentrations of tilisolol in the aqueous humor after instillation with CMC vehicle from the tear concentrations. Its ocular and systemic absorption was analyzed by a mathematical model including a diffusion process and a two-compartment model with first-order absorption, respectively. Similarly, a two-compartment model was successfully used for topically instilled gentamicin (Eljarrat-Binstock et al. 2004) and chlorhexidine gluconate (Xuguang et al. 2006). Presence of drug transporters is well recognized in the blood-ocular barriers; therefore, systemically administered drugs partitioning into the humors or tissues are subjected to their susceptibility for drug influx/efflux mechanisms. Systemically administered P-gp substrate (Rho-123) was best fitted with a three-compartment model and shifted to a two-compartment model upon its blocker administration in rabbits. This shift has increased intraocular penetration of compounds across blood-ocular barriers (Senthilkumari et al. 2008a, b). A three-compartment physiological-based pharmacokinetic (PK) model with a bidirectional transfer between the cornea and aqueous humor and a unidirectional transfer between the aqueous humor and iris-ciliary body was used to describe an antiglaucoma agent 1-ethyl-6-fluoro,1,2,3,4-tetrahydroquinoline in rabbits. Using its ED50 values derived from pressure-lowering activity (pharmacody-

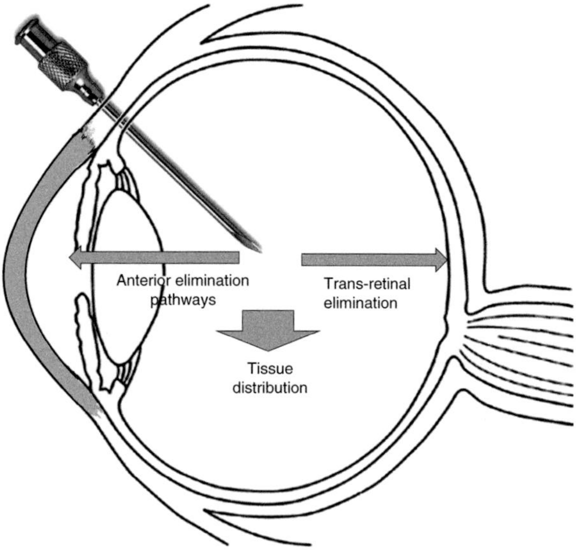

Fig. 3.2 Elimination pathways of intravitreally injected drugs

namic property), the PK-PD model was derived to explain pharmacodynamics of iris-ciliary body concentration time data (Pamulapati and Schoenwald 2012).

Intravitreally administered drugs reaching the systemic circulation is of concern for their toxicity (Fig. 3.2). Systemic pharmacokinetics of intravitreally administered ranibizumab in patients with retinal vein occlusion (RVO) or diabetic macular edema (DME) was predicted using one-compartment pharmacokinetics model with first-order absorption and elimination rate constants. This population kinetic study found that there is no difference among conditions like AMD, RVO, and DME as far as the systemic exposure of VEGF antibody is concerned (Zhang et al. 2014).

Subconjunctival injection of gentamicin was fitted into one compartmental model (van Rooyen et al. 1991). Antibacterial agents such as ciprofloxacin and fleroxacin (Miller et al. 1992) were also predicted with single-compartment model after direct intravitreal administration. A population pharmacokinetic metabolism model was used to describe the concentrations of ciprofloxacin in serum, aqueous and vitreous humor by a four-compartment PK linear model after oral administration.

Single-dose administration as eyedrop raises aqueous humor levels within a period of 30–60 min and mostly the levels fall within 4 h. Being underprivileged organ, eye lacks first-line immune defense mechanisms in the humors, antimicrobial drug levels above the MIC of microbe is required for their activity. Therefore, during corneal infections, hourly or 2 hourly instillations of antimicrobial agents are preferred. To estimate the appropriate drug schedule, pharmacokinetic simulations are helpful. Aqueous humor kinetics of single and multiple doses of topical, non-preserved voriconazole (VZ) were studied in human eyes comparing hourly versus 2 hourly instillations (Senthilkumari et al. 2010). Single-dose ocular kinetics of 1 % VZ resulted in a maximum mean aqueous concentration of 3.333 ± 1.61 μg/ml in

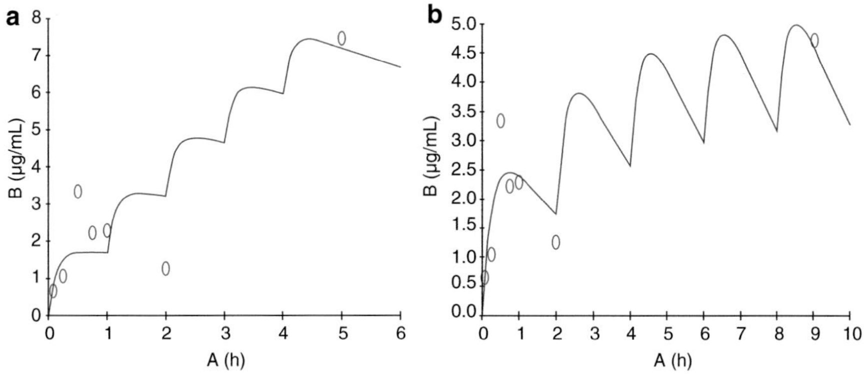

Fig. 3.3 PK simulation from our laboratory showing the predicted concentration of voriconazole in aqueous humor achieved hourly (A), 2 hourly (5 doses) instillation of voriconazole topical application in patients undergoing cataract surgery (*o* observed, -- predicted) (Senthilkumari et al. 2010)

30 min; multidose kinetic study revealed that hourly and bihourly dosing resulted in mean aqueous concentrations of 7.47 ± 2.14 µg/ml and 4.69 ± 2.7 µg/ml, respectively (Fig. 3.3).

Serial sampling of the humors of the eye is not a feasible task in human or animals while conducting ocular pharmacokinetic studies. Therefore, the model of collecting samples at various time points after the administration of drug is followed in all the studies except few studies indicating the worth of microdialysis for serial sampling in animals. Many of the ocular drugs were investigated in the literature for their intraocular penetration, but only few of them were interpreted with the help of pharmacokinetic models to explain their ocular disposition.

After a single topical instillation of tritiated clonidine HCl solution (0.2 %) at the volume of 30 µl into rabbit eyes, Chiang and Schoenwald (1986) evaluated clonidine ocular pharmacokinetics. Seven different tissues and plasma were excised and assayed for drug concentration over 180 min. They have also generated data at steady state levels of drug in cornea using an infusion assembly. The data were analysed by fitting them into physiological and a classical diffusion pharmacokinetic models. This study reported that the physiological model parameters were fit to the topical infusion data and showed good agreement between the predicted and experimental data.

3.2.4 *Drug Interaction in Topically Applied Drugs*

More than one eyedrops are often required to be administered together at times. In such conditions, chemical incompatibility has been observed which is causing one of them to precipitate in the lower fornix. This is a potential cause for the reduction of pre-corneal drug availability of the topically applied drugs. Ciprofloxacin hydrochloride deposition on the lower fornix of the eye due to its pH incompatibility has been claimed as the advantage of pre-corneal deposits as drug depots "ciprofloxacin HCl precipitates." However, redistribution or dissolution of these deposits back to increase tear film concentrations have not been proved. Ocular pharmacokinetics of the topically applied drug also gets altered by coadministered drugs when they are competing for the same transport mechanism (Nirmal et al. 2013a). Coadministration of local anesthetics and antimuscarinic agents might increase ocular bioavailability of the drugs by decreasing tear film secretion. This interaction so far is attributed to the decrease in tear film secretion; however, other interactions on the corneal transport mechanism require further studies.

3.2.5 Ocular Drug Levels after Systemic Administration

Ocular pharmacokinetics of 1,3-bis(2-chloroethyl)-1-nitrosourea (BCNU) was investigated using its levels in vitreous and aqueous humors after its systemic administration in rabbits. This study compared systemic, topical, and subconjunctival administrations and suggested that topical application of BCNU is the best and subconjunctival injection the second best route for treating an iris tumor and that intravenous injection is the best route for choroidal and retinal tumors (Ueno et al. 1982).

Aqueous humor penetration of amikacin was assessed in the anterior chamber of the human eyes using radioimmunoassay. This study reported that bactericidal concentrations of amikacin were not achieved by topical or intravenous administration. Subconjunctival injection also did not produce consistent bactericidal concentration of amikacin in the aqueous humor. This study has also reported that iris pigment binding as one of the factor responsible for the poor levels reached (Eiferman and Stagner 1982). Several clinical studies showed that inadequate penetration of antimicrobial agents into the eye after their systemic administration as a limitation for ocular infections (Velpandian 2009). Only after multiple doses orally administered fluoroquinolones like ciprofloxacin reached significant levels in the vitreous above the MIC for most of the ocular pathogenic organisms (Keren et al. 1991). Inadequate penetration of different classes of drugs into non-inflammed eyes after systemic administration has been well documented by many investigations.

3.2.6 Factors Affecting Ocular Penetration of Drugs

Aqueous ophthalmic drug solutions typically exhibit low bioavailability due to various loss processes such as drainage, tear turnover, nonproductive absorption, and protein binding. Suspensions may improve bioavailability, but because of a short residence time and a low corneal permeability rate constant, the dissolution rate of the drug and its intrinsic solubility must be considered.

Topically applied hydrophobic compounds like amphotericin B showed undetectable levels of drug after single application; however, after repeated application, therapeutic levels reached the cornea in the normal eyes of rabbits. In inflamed eyes the levels reached high quickly but fell rapidly (O'Day et al. 1986). Corneal inflammation that induced increased drug penetration across the cornea is not well documented in the literature due to the difficulties encountered in sampling aqueous humor from patients undergoing ocular surgeries.

3.2.7 Ocular Drug Metabolism

Although the liver is still the major organ involved in the biotransformation of drugs, drug metabolism in the eye is often pursued as a avenue for the development of designer drugs. The corneal epithelium is the source of amidases and esterases which favors the optimization of dosage forms using the concept of prodrugs. Latanoprost and dipivefrin are the best examples for the prodrugs to get into their active form after the metabolism in the cornea. In the cornea, the presence of aminopeptidases and other peptidases has also been reported, and their involvements in the metabolism of drugs are confirmed (Lee et al. 1986). While studying the ocular pharmacokinetics of topically applied phenylephrine, Antoine et al. (1984) reported that the corneal epithelium is responsible for the metabolic degradation of phenylephrine which occurred following its topical instillation. While working with levobunolol for topical antiglaucoma treatment, Tang-Liu and coworkers (1987) demonstrated that the major sites of ocular metabolism were the corneal epithelium and the iris-ciliary body. On passage across the cornea, 4.7 % of topically applied levobunolol dose was biotransformed to an active metabolite dihydrolevobunolol and subsequently became bioavailable to intraocular tissues. Another 12 % of the topical levobunolol dose entered the systemic circulation as metabolite after presystemic biotransformation. Nakamura et al. (2005) examined the expression levels of the different conjugation enzymes, sulfotransferases, UDP-glucuronosyl transferases (UGTs), and glutathione S-transferases (GSTs), in ocular tissues. In 5-week-old animals, the CYP genes, CYP2B2 and CYP3A1, were abundantly expressed in the lens, with higher CYP1A1 expression detectable in the extra-lenticular tissues, of both genders. They have also reported that in general, the expression levels of the CYPs and sulfotransferases declined with age, whereas the levels of the UGTs and GSTs increased. These results demonstrate that the expression profiles of drug-metabolizing enymes show both region- and age-specific patterns in rat ocular tissues. Presence of various metabolizing enzymes and their physiological function has been targeted for ocular drug delivery (Duvvuri et al. 2004).

3.2.8 Elimination Pathways of the Drugs

A major pathway for systemic absorption of topically applied drug has been reported to be through the walls of the gastrointestinal tract (Anderson 1980). Schmitt et al. (1980) evaluated the penetration of radiolabeled timolol into the rabbit eye after topical instillation and after intravenous injection in animals. This study reported that the levels of radioactivity were considerably greater in ocular tissues after instillation as compared with intravenous injection, whereas in extraocular tissues, the levels were similar after both routes of administration. This study has also reported that in ocular instillation, only unchanged timolol was present in the aqueous humor, whereas both timolol and metabolites were present in the serum. After intravenous administration, timolol was rapidly metabolized and metabolites appeared in the serum and aqueous humor. Pharmacokinetic studies conducted after the intravitreal injection of drugs revealed that two predominating pathways are involved in the clearance of drugs. Most of the drugs are cleared through posterior elimination pathway through retinal blood vessels Drugs like aminoglycoside antibiotics follow anterior pathway through aqueous humor and iris (Barza et al. 1983; Gupta et al. 2000; Nirmal et al. 2012).

3.2.9 Functional Importance of Blood-Ocular Barriers Affecting Pharmacokinetics

Drug penetration across blood-ocular barriers is now well recognized; therefore, beyond pharmaceutical parameters, their susceptibility for various transporters is expected to govern their pharmacokinetics. Probenecid (Benemid) was the agent first explored to elevate serum penicillin concentrations (Burnell and Kirby 1951). The interest to evaluate the impact on the concentration of penicillin derivatives in ocular fluids (Barza et al. 1973; Salminen 1978). However, these studies showed that administration of probenecid had an enhancing effect on ocular cloxacillin concentration allowing improved drug diffusion into the eye by means of an elevated plasma concentration and had no specific ocular effect. In the subsequent studies after the intravitreal administration of carbenicillin, concomitant intraperitoneal dosing of probenecid prolonged the vitreal half-life of carbenicillin and showed that beta-lactam antibiotics are eliminated via the retinal route. Ever since, observations and curiosities among the researchers led to better fundamental understanding regarding the involvement of drug transporters in blood-ocular barriers. Using retinal capillary endothelial cell lines presence and function of various transporters were explored (Hosoya and Tomi 2005; Mannermaa et al. 2006). Subsequently, functional importance of such transporters for the penetration of xenobiotics reported in animals (Senthilkumari et al. 2009; Nirmal et al 2012; Gunda et al. 2006)

Although, the presence of transporter proteins in the blood-ocular barriers has been well documented, their extent and role affecting pharmacological action have come to light after the systematic explorations in the last decade. In these controlled experiments, probes were used as a substrate and their pharmacokinetic modulation was assessed after blocking the functions of transporters with respective agents.

Functional role of P-gp and ocular tissue distribution of intravitreally injected rhodamine 123 (Rho-123) was evaluated in the presence of P-gp-specific blocker (GF 120918) in normal as well as rifampicin-fed rabbits using microdialysis and

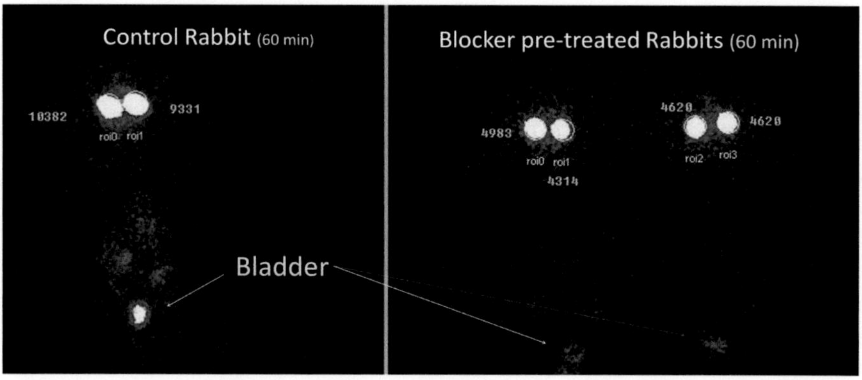

Fig. 3.4 Static planar gamma camera image of rabbits following intravitreal injection of ^{99m}Tc-ofloxacin in rabbits. Note: Control rabbit bladder showing higher radioactivity

direct sampling technique. This study revealed that intravenously injected blocker significantly altered the ocular disposition of intravitreally injected P-gp substrate. Rifampicin pretreatment did not upregulate P-gp transporters of the retina to the extent to affect the intravitreal kinetics of Rho-123 significantly (Senthilkumari et al. 2008a). The impact of P-glycoprotein (P-gp) blockade on the intravenous (i.v.) pharmacokinetics of Rho-123 and the subsequent effect on its disposition in ocular and non-ocular tissues were studied using rabbits. This study concluded that increasing the ocular concentration of systemically given drugs may not be possible with the degree of P-gp blockade achieved when using GF120918 (P-gp blocker) at the studied concentration after intravenous administration (Senthilkumari et al. 2008b). The effect of P-glycoprotein modulation at blood-ocular barriers using gamma scintigraphy in rabbits is shown in Fig. 3.4. This confirmed the involvement of P-glycoprotein in the intraocular disposition of susceptible drugs (Senthilkumari et al. 2009).

Although aminoglycoside antibiotics were reported to be cleared through the anterior route (Barza et al. 1983), while studying OCT transporters, Nirmal et al. (2013b) concluded that the clearance of organic cation transporter (OCT) substrates favors the anterior elimination pathway. The functional importance of (OCT) on the ocular disposition of intravitreally injected substrate tetraethyl ammonium (TEA) was assessed in rabbits (Nirmal et al. 2013b); this study concluded that intravitreally injected OCT substrates may follow an anterior elimination pathway and prolonged residence time in the vitreous humor. This study showed that OCT may not be active from vitreous to blood route in the blood-retinal barrier.

The potential pharmacokinetic role of organic cation transporters in modulating the trans-corneal penetration of its substrates administered topically has been studied in rabbits. This study concluded that OCT is functionally active in the cornea causing uptake of their substrates from tear to the aqueous humor. When administering their substrates/blockers topically, both may be competing for OCT for their uptake across the cornea, thereby decreasing the corneal penetration. Hence, OCT can have a potential pharmacokinetic role in modulating the ocular bioavailability of their substrates which are used topically for ocular therapeutics (Nirmal et al. 2013b). The role of organic cation transporters was studied in the ocular disposition of its intravenously injected substrate in rabbits by quantifying the levels of its substrate in the presence and absence of blockers. This study revealed that in most of the tissues, OCTs are functionally present from apical to basolateral. The gene expression studies also showed the presence of OCT1, OCTN1, and OCTN2 in various ocular tissues studied. This study suggested that OCTs are functionally active in blood-ocular barriers and involved in the transport of its substrate from blood to vitreous humor (Nirmal et al. 2013a). Moreover, this study also revealed the precorneal availability of OCT substrate through lacrimal secretion indicating the possibility of utilizing them for the delivery of drug to the tear film through systemic route (Nirmal et al. 2010). Apart from OCT, OAT, and P-gp transporters, PEPT transporters have been used for the delivery of stable dipeptide prodrugs for improved absorption of acyclovir (Talluri et al. 2008).

Most of the drugs used in ophthalmic therapeutics are developed for systemic diseases, which are subsequently included for ocular use after toxicity studies. Developing any drug with the understanding of the constraints of the eye was not a popular strategy followed. Much of the emphasis was made on pharmaceutical solutions rather than relevant molecular parameters. The cornea is a live tissue that behaves much beyond simple biomatrix; therefore, in vitro studies may not be having much relevance in the in vivo scenario. To enable in silico screening of drugs, techniques like cassette dosing are being developed to assess the possibility of enhanced topical penetration with less number of animals (Sharma et al. 2011). Along with the increasing knowledge about the barrier functions, it is clear that the in-depth knowledge of the molecular properties like drug transport susceptibility, and interaction of drugs with their physiological/pathological targets are expected to govern ocular pharmacokinetics and toxicity of drugs in the future.

3.3 Conclusion

In the current state of knowledge, it is evident that developing ocular specific drug to meet the target site concentration with reduced systemic exposure is a possible reality. Screening drugs with better ocular pharmacokinetics for their projected use in ophthalmic therapeutics is the rationalized approach for ocular drug development.

References

Adler FH. Textbook of physiology of the eye. St. Louis: CV Mosby; 1962.

Alm A, Törnquist P. Lactate transport through the blood-retinal and the blood-brain barrier in rats. Ophthalmic Res. 1985;17(3):181–4.

Altenberg GA. Structure of multidrug-resistance proteins of the ATP-binding cassette (ABC) superfamily. Curr Med Chem Anticancer Agents. 2004;4(1):53–62.
Anderson JA. Systemic absorption of topical ocularly applied epinephrine and dipivefrin. Arch Ophthalmol. 1980;98(2):350–3.
Antoine ME, Edelhauser HF, O'Brien WJ. Pharmacokinetics of topical ocular phenylephrine HCl. Invest Ophthalmol Vis Sci. 1984;25(1):48–54.
Asashima T, Hori S, Ohtsuki S, Tachikawa M, Watanabe M, Mukai C, Kitagaki S, Miyakoshi N, Terasaki T. ATP-binding cassette transporter G2 mediates the efflux of phototoxins on the luminal membrane of retinal capillary endothelial cells. Pharm Res. 2006;23(6): 1235–42.
Attar M, Shen J, Ling KH, Tang-Liu D. Ophthalmic drug delivery considerations at the cellular level: drug-metabolising enzymes and transporters. Expert Opin Drug Deliv. 2005;2(5): 891–908.
Badr GA, Tang J, Ismail-Beigi F, Kern TS. Diabetes downregulates GLUT1 expression in the retina and its microvessels but not in the cerebral cortex or its microvessels. Diabetes. 2000; 49(6):1016–21.
Baldwin SA, Beal PR, Yao SY, King AE, Cass CE, Young JD. The equilibrative nucleoside transporter family, SLC29. Pflugers Arch. 2004;447(5):735–43.
Barza M, Baum J, Birkby B, Weinstein L. Intraocular penetration of carbenicillin in the rabbit. Am J Ophthalmol. 1973;75(2):307–13.
Barza M, Kane A, Baum J. Pharmacokinetics of intravitreal carbenicillin, cefazolin, and gentamicin in rhesus monkeys. Invest Ophthalmol Vis Sci. 1983;24(12):1602–6.
Bito LZ. The physiology and pathophysiology of intraocular fluids. Exp Eye Res. 1977; 25(Suppl):273–90.
Boulton M, Rózanowska M, Rózanowski B. Retinal photodamage. J Photochem Photobiol B. 2001;64(2–3):144–61.
Burnell JM, Kirby WM. Effectiveness of a new compound, benemid, in elevating serum penicillin concentrations. J Clin Invest. 1951;30(7):697–700.
Butler JM, Unger WG, Grierson I. Recent experimental studies on the blood-aqueous barrier: the anatomical basis of the response to injury. Eye (Lond). 1988;2(Suppl):S213–20.
Buxton ILO, Benet LZ. Section I, Chapter 2: Pharmacokinetics: the dynamics of drug absorption, distribution, metabolism, and elimination. In: The pharmacological basis of therapeutics. 12th ed. New York: The McGraw-Hill Companies, Inc.; 2011. p. 17–39.
Chan-Ling T, Stone J. Degeneration of astrocytes in feline retinopathy of prematurity causes failure of the blood-retinal barrier. Invest Ophthalmol Vis Sci. 1992;33(7):2148–59.
Chen MS, Hou PK, Tai TY, Lin BJ. Blood-ocular barriers. Tzu Chi Med J. 2008;20(1):25–34.
Chiang CH, Ho JI, Chen JL. Pharmacokinetics and intraocular pressure lowering effect of timolol preparations in rabbit eyes. J Ocul Pharmacol Ther. 1996;12(4):471–80.
Chiang CH, Schoenwald RD. Ocular pharmacokinetic models of clonidine-3H hydrochloride. J Pharmacokinet Biopharm. 1986;14(2):175–211.
Chowdhury UR, Madden BJ, Charlesworth MC, Fautsch MP. Proteome analysis of human aqueous humor. Invest Ophthalmol Vis Sci. 2010;51(10):4921–31.
Cunha-Vaz J. The blood-ocular barriers. Surv Ophthalmol. 1979;23(5):279–96.
Cunha-Vaz JG. The blood-ocular barriers: past, present, and future. Doc Ophthalmol. 1997;93(1–2): 149–57.
Cunha-Vaz JG. The blood-retinal barriers system. Basic concepts and clinical evaluation. Exp Eye Res. 2004;78(3):715–21.
Cunha-Vaz J. The blood-retinal barrier in retinal disease. Eur Ophthal Rev. 2009;3(2):105–8.
Cunha-Vaz J. Blood-retinal barrier, Encyclopedia of the eye, vol. 1. Oxford: Academic; 2010. p. 209–15.
Cunha-Vaz JG, Maurice DM. The active transport of fluorescein by the retinal vessels and the retina. J Physiol. 1967;191(3):467–86.
Dean M, Rzhetsky A, Allikmets R. The human ATP-binding cassette (ABC) transporter superfamily. Genome Res. 2001;11(7):1156–66.

Di Marco MP, Chen J, Wainer IW, Ducharme MP. A population pharmacokinetic-metabolism model for individualizing ciprofloxacin therapy in ophthalmology. Ther Drug Monit. 2004; 26(4):401–7.

Dorrell MI, Aguilar E, Friedlander M. Retinal vascular development is mediated by endothelial filopodia, a preexisting astrocytic template and specific R-cadherin adhesion. Invest Ophthalmol Vis Sci. 2002;43(11):3500–10.

Dorrell MI, Aguilar E, Jacobson R, Trauger SA, Friedlander J, Siuzdak G, Friedlander M. Maintaining retinal astrocytes normalizes revascularization and prevents vascular pathology associated with oxygen-induced retinopathy. Glia. 2010;58(1):43–54.

Duvvuri S, Majumdar S, Mitra AK. Role of metabolism in ocular drug delivery. Curr Drug Metab. 2004;5(6):507–15.

Eiferman RA, Stagner JI. Intraocular penetration of amikacin. Iris binding and bioavailability. Arch Ophthalmol. 1982;100(11):1817–9.

Eljarrat-Binstock E, Raiskup F, Stepensky D, Domb AJ, Frucht-Pery J. Delivery of gentamicin to the rabbit eye by drug-loaded hydrogel iontophoresis. Invest Ophthalmol Vis Sci. 2004; 45(8):2543–8.

Fernandes R, Suzuki K, Kumagai AK. Inner blood-retinal barrier GLUT1 in long-term diabetic rats: an immunogold electron microscopic study. Invest Ophthalmol Vis Sci. 2003;44(7):3150–4.

Fernandes R, Carvalho AL, Kumagai A, Seica R, Hosoya K, Terasaki T, Murta J, Pereira P, Faro C. Downregulation of retinal GLUT1 in diabetes by ubiquitinylation. Mol Vis. 2004;10:618–28.

Fernandes R, Gonçalves A, Cunha-Vaz J. Chapter 6: Blood-retinal barrier: the fundamentals. In: Deepak T, Gerald C, editors. Ocular drug delivery: barriers and application of nanoparticulate systems. Boca Raton: CRC Press/Taylor & Francis; 2012. p. 111–32.

Fojo AT, Ueda K, Slamon DJ, Poplack DG, Gottesman MM, Pastan I. Expression of a multidrug-resistance gene in human tumors and tissues. Proc Natl Acad Sci U S A. 1987;84(1):265–9.

Fruttiger M, Calver AR, Kruger WH, Mudhar HS, Michalovich D, Takakura N, Nishikawa S, Richardson WD. PDGF mediates a neuron-astrocyte interaction in the developing retina. Neuron. 1996;17(6):1117–31.

Gabelt BT, Kaufman PL. Section 4, Chapter 11: Production and flow of aqueous humor. In: Adler's physiology of the eye. 11th ed. Edinburgh: Elsevier Inc; 2011. p. 274–307.

Gao B, Wenzel A, Grimm C, Vavricka SR, Benke D, Meier PJ, Remè CE. Localization of organic anion transport protein 2 in the apical region of rat retinal pigment epithelium. Invest Ophthalmol Vis Sci. 2002;43(2):510–4.

Gardner TW, Antonetti DA, Barber AJ, LaNoue KF, Levison SW. Diabetic retinopathy: more than meets the eye. Surv Ophthalmol. 2002;47 Suppl 2:S253–62.

Gerhart DZ, Leino RL, Drewes LR. Distribution of monocarboxylate transporters MCT1 and MCT2 in rat retina. Neuroscience. 1999;92(1):367–75.

Ghiardi GJ, Gidday JM, Roth S. The purine nucleoside adenosine in retinal ischemia-reperfusion injury. Vision Res. 1999;39(15):2519–35.

Greenwood J. Characterization of a rat retinal endothelial cell culture and the expression of P-glycoprotein in brain and retinal endothelium in vitro. J Neuroimmunol. 1992;39(1–2):123–32.

Gupta SK(1), Velpandian T, Dhingra N, Jaiswal J. Intravitreal pharmacokinetics of plain and liposome-entrapped fluconazole in rabbit eyes. J Ocul Pharmacol Ther. 2000;16(6):511–8.

Gunda S, Hariharan S, Mitra AK. Corneal absorption and anterior chamber pharmacokinetics of dipeptide monoester prodrugs of ganciclovir (GCV): in vivo comparative evaluation of these prodrugs with Val-GCV and GCV in rabbits. J Ocul Pharmacol Ther. 2006;22(6):465–76.

Hagenbuch B, Meier PJ. The superfamily of organic anion transporting polypeptides. Biochim Biophys Acta. 2003;1609(1):1–18.

Hardberger RE, Hanna C, Goodart R. Effects of drug vehicles on ocular uptake of tetracycline. Am J Ophthalmol. 1975;80(1):133–8.

Hosoya K, Tomi M. Advances in the cell biology of transport via the inner blood-retinal barrier: establishment of cell lines and transport functions. Biol Pharm Bull. 2005;28(1):1–8.

Hosoya K, Kondo T, Tomi M, Takanaga H, Ohtsuki S, Terasaki T. MCT1-mediated transport of L-lactic acid at the inner blood-retinal barrier: a possible route for delivery of monocarboxylic acid drugs to the retina. Pharm Res. 2001;18(12):1669–76.

Hosoya K, Makihara A, Tsujikawa Y, Yoneyama D, Mori S, Terasaki T, Akanuma S, Tomi M, Tachikawa M. Roles of inner blood-retinal barrier organic anion transporter 3 in the vitreous/retina-to-blood efflux transport of p-aminohippuric acid, benzylpenicillin, and 6-mercaptopurine. J Pharmacol Exp Ther. 2009;329(1):87–93.

Jordán J, Ruíz-Moreno JM. Advances in the understanding of retinal drug disposition and the role of blood-ocular barrier transporters. Expert Opin Drug Metab Toxicol. 2013;9(9):1181–92.

Kaur C, Foulds WS, Ling EA. Blood-retinal barrier in hypoxic ischaemic conditions: basic concepts, clinical features and management. Prog Retin Eye Res. 2008;27(6):622–47.

Keren G, Alhalel A, Bartov E, Kitzes-Cohen R, Rubinstein E, Segev S, Treister G. The intravitreal penetration of orally administered ciprofloxacin in humans. Invest Ophthalmol Vis Sci. 1991;32(8):2388–92. PubMed PMID: 2071350.

Krishnamurthy P, Schuetz JD. Role of ABCG2/BCRP in biology and medicine. Annu Rev Pharmacol Toxicol. 2006;46:38–410.

Lee VHL, Robinson JR. Topical ocular drug delivery: recent developments and future challenges. J Ocul Pharmacol Ther. 1986;2(1):67–108.

Lee VH, Carson LW, Kashi SD, Stratford Jr RE. Metabolic and permeation barriers to the ocular absorption of topically applied enkephalins in albino rabbits. J Ocul Pharmacol. 1986; 2(4):345–52.

Lutty GA, McLeod DS. Retinal vascular development and oxygen-induced retinopathy: a role for adenosine. Prog Retin Eye Res. 2003;22(1):95–111.

Lynch MG, Brown RH, Goode SM, Schoenwald RD, Chien DS. Reduction of phenylephrine drop size in infants achieves equal dilation with decreased systemic absorption. Arch Ophthalmol. 1987;105(10):1364–5.

Mannermaa E, Vellonen KS, Urtti A. Drug transport in corneal epithelium and blood-retina barrier: emerging role of transporters in ocular pharmacokinetics. Adv Drug Deliv Rev. 2006; 58(11):1136–63.

Mayers M, Rush D, Madu A, Motyl M, Miller MH. Pharmacokinetics of amikacin and chloramphenicol in the aqueous humor of rabbits. Antimicrob Agents Chemother. 1991;35(9):1791–8.

McCarthy TJ. The effect of vehicle composition on the release of chloramphenicol from creams and eye ointments. S Afr Med J. 1975;49(31):1259–62.

Miller MH, Madu A, Samathanam G, Rush D, Madu CN, Mathisson K, Mayers M. Fleroxacin pharmacokinetics in aqueous and vitreous humors determined by using complete concentration-time data from individual rabbits. Antimicrob Agents Chemother. 1992;36(1):32–8.

Minamizono A, Tomi M, Hosoya K. Inhibition of dehydroascorbic acid transport across the rat blood-retinal and -brain barriers in experimental diabetes. Biol Pharm Bull. 2006;29(10): 2148–50.

Nagase K, Tomi M, Tachikawa M, Hosoya K. Functional and molecular characterization of adenosine transport at the rat inner blood-retinal barrier. Biochim Biophys Acta. 2006;1758(1): 13–9.

Nakamura K, Fujiki T, Tamura HO. Age, gender and region-specific differences in drug metabolising enzymes in rat ocular tissues. Exp Eye Res. 2005;81(6):710–5. Epub 2005 Jun 20.

Nakashima T, Tomi M, Katayama K, Tachikawa M, Watanabe M, Terasaki T, Hosoya K. Blood-to-retina transport of creatine via creatine transporter (CRT) at the rat inner blood-retinal barrier. J Neurochem. 2004;89(6):1454–61.

Nirmal J, Velpandian T, Biswas NR, Azad RV, Vasantha T, Bhatnagar A, Ghose S. Evaluation of the relevance of OCT blockade on the transcorneal kinetics of topically applied substrates using rabbits FIP 2010 World Congress in Association with AAPS, New Orleans USA. 2010. SA8208/T3427.

Nirmal J, Velpandian T, Singh SB, Biswas NR, Azad R, Thavaraj V, Mittal G, Bhatnagar A, Ghose S. Evaluation of the functional importance of organic cation transporters on the ocular disposition of its intravitreally injected substrate in rabbits. Curr Eye Res. 2012;37(12):1127–35. doi: 10.3109/02713683.2012.715715. Epub 2012 Aug 23.

Nirmal J, Singh SB, Biswas NR, Thavaraj V, Azad RV, Velpandian T. Potential pharmacokinetic role of organic cation transporters in modulating the transcorneal penetration of its substrates administered topically. Eye (Lond). 2013a;27(10):1196–203.

Nirmal J, Sirohiwal A, Singh SB, Biswas NR, Thavaraj V, Azad RV, Velpandian T. Role of organic cation transporters in the ocular disposition of its intravenously injected substrate in rabbits: implications for ocular drug therapy. Exp Eye Res. 2013b;116:27–35.

O'Day DM, Head WS, Robinson RD, Clanton JA. Bioavailability and penetration of topical amphotericin B in the anterior segment of the rabbit eye. J Ocul Pharmacol. 1986;2(4): 371–8.

Occhiutto ML, Freitas FR, Maranhao RC, Costa VP. Breakdown of the blood-ocular barrier as a strategy for the systemic use of nanosystems. Pharmaceutics. 2012;4(2):252–75.

Oh C, Saville BA, Cheng YL, Rootman DS. Compartmental model for the ocular pharmacokinetics of cyclosporine in rabbits. Pharm Res. 1995;12(3):433–7.

Pamulapati CR, Schoenwald RD. Ocular pharmacokinetics of a novel tetrahydroquinoline analog in rabbit: compartmental analysis and PK-PD evaluation. J Pharm Sci. 2012;101(1): 414–23.

Patton TF, Robinson JR. Influence of topical anesthesia on tear dynamics and ocular drug bioavailability in albino rabbits. J Pharm Sci. 1975;64(2):267–71.

Poitry-Yamate CL, Poitry S, Tsacopoulos M. Lactate released by Müller glial cells is metabolized by photoreceptors from mammalian retina. J Neurosci. 1995;15(7 Pt 2):5179–91.

Provis JM, Sandercoe T, Hendrickson AE. Astrocytes and blood vessels define the foveal rim during primate retinal development. Invest Ophthalmol Vis Sci. 2000;41(10):2827–36.

Runkle EA, Antonetti DA. The blood-retinal barrier: structure and functional significance. Methods Mol Biol. 2011;686:133–48.

Salminen L. Cloxacillin distribution in the rabbit eye after intravenous injection. Acta Ophthalmol. 1978;56(1):11–9.

Sasaki H, Yamamura K, Mukai T, Nishida K, Nakamura J, Nakashima M, Ichikawa M. Pharmacokinetic prediction of the ocular absorption of an instilled drug with ophthalmic viscous vehicle. Biol Pharm Bull. 2000;23(11):1352–6.

Schlosshauer B. Chapter 24: Blood–retina barriers. In: Handbook of neurochemistry and molecular neurobiology. New York: Springer US; 2007. p. 486–506.

Schmitt CJ, Lotti VJ, LeDouarec JC. Penetration of timolol into the rabbit eye. Measurements after ocular instillation and intravenous injection. Arch Ophthalmol. 1980;98(3):547–51.

Senthilkumari S, Velpandian T, Biswas NR, Saxena R, Ghose S. Evaluation of the modulation of P-glycoprotein (P-gp) on the intraocular disposition of its substrate in rabbits. Curr Eye Res. 2008a;33(4):333–43.

Senthilkumari S, Velpandian T, Biswas NR, Sonali N, Ghose S. Evaluation of the impact of P-glycoprotein (P-gp) drug efflux transporter blockade on the systemic and ocular disposition of P-gp substrate. J Ocul Pharmacol Ther. 2008b;24(3):290–300.

Senthilkumari S, Velpandian T, Biswas NR, Bhatnagar A, Mittal G, Ghose S. Evidencing the modulation of P-glycoprotein at blood-ocular barriers using gamma scintigraphy. Curr Eye Res. 2009;34(1):73–7.

Senthilkumari S, Lalitha P, Prajna NV, Haripriya A, Nirmal J, Gupta P, Velpandian T. Single and multidose ocular kinetics and stability analysis of extemporaneous formulation of topical voriconazole in humans. Curr Eye Res. 2010;35(11):953–60.

Sharma C, Velpandian T, Biswas NR, Nayak N, Vajpayee RB, Ghose S. Development of novel in silico model to predict corneal permeability for congeneric drugs: a QSPR approach. J Biomed Biotechnol. 2011;2011:483869. doi:10.1155/2011/483869. Epub 2011 Feb.

Shen J, Cross ST, Tang-Liu DD, Welty DF. Evaluation of an immortalized retinal endothelial cell line as an in vitro model for drug transport studies across the blood-retinal barrier. Pharm Res. 2003;20(9):1357–63.

Steinberg RH, Wood I. The relationship of the retinal pigment epithelium to photoreceptor outer segments in human retina. In: Marmor MF, editor. The retinal pigment epithelium. Cambridge/London: Harvard University Press; 1979. p. 32–44.

Takata K, Kasahara T, Kasahara M, Ezaki O, Hirano H. Ultracytochemical localization of the erythrocyte/HepG2-type glucose transporter (GLUT1) in cells of the blood-retinal barrier in the rat. Invest Ophthalmol Vis Sci. 1992;33(2):377–83.

Talluri RS, Samanta SK, Gaudana R, Mitra AK. Synthesis, metabolism and cellular permeability of enzymatically stable dipeptide prodrugs of acyclovir. Int J Pharm. 2008;361(1–2):118–24.

Tang-Liu DD, Liu S, Neff J, Sandri R. Disposition of levobunolol after an ophthalmic dose to rabbits. J Pharm Sci. 1987;76(10):780–3.

Ueno N, Refojo MF, Liu LH. Pharmacokinetics of the antineoplastic agent 1,3-bis(2-chloroethyl)-1-nitrosourea (BCNU) in the aqueous and vitreous of rabbit. Invest Ophthalmol Vis Sci. 1982;23(2):199–208.

Urtti A. Challenges and obstacles of ocular pharmacokinetics and drug delivery. Adv Drug Deliv Rev. 2006;58(11):1131–5.

Velpandian T. Intraocular penetration of antimicrobial agents in ophthalmic infections and drug delivery strategies. Expert Opin Drug Deliv. 2009;6(3):255–70.

van Rooyen MM, Coetzee JF, du Toit DF, van Jaarsveld PP. Intraocular concentration time relationships of subconjunctivally administered gentamicin. S Afr Med J. 1991;80(5):236–9.

Vinores SA. Assessment of blood-retinal barrier integrity. Histol Histopathol. 1995;10(1):141–54.

Xuguang S, Yanchuang L, Feng Z, Shiyun L, Xiaotang Y. Pharmacokinetics of chlorhexidine gluconate 0.02% in the rabbit cornea. J Ocul Pharmacol Ther. 2006;22(4):227–30.

Yao SY, Ng AM, Sundaram M, Cass CE, Baldwin SA, Young JD. Transport of antiviral 3′-deoxy-nucleoside drugs by recombinant human and rat equilibrative, nitrobenzylthioinosine (NBMPR)-insensitive (ENT2) nucleoside transporter proteins produced in Xenopus oocytes. Mol Membr Biol. 2001;18(2):161–7.

Zauberman H. Adhesive forces between the retinal pigment epithelium and sensory retina. In: Marmor MF, editor. The retinal pigment epithelium. Cambridge/London: Harvard University Press; 1979. p. 192–204.

Zhang Y, Yao Z, Kaila N, Kuebler P, Visich J, Maia M, Tuomi L, Ehrlich JS, Rubio RG, Campochiaro PA. Pharmacokinetics of ranibizumab after intravitreal administration in patients with retinal vein occlusion or diabetic macular edema. Ophthalmology. 2014;121(11):2237–46.

Chapter 4
Pharmacogenomics of Drugs in Ocular Therapeutics

Thirumurthy Velpandian and Govindasamy Kumaramanickavel

Abstract As genetic polymorphism is the key determinant for the expected therapeutic outcome, pharmacogenomics can be considered as one of the rationalized approaches in personalized medicine. Genetic variation in drug response can be attributed to the drug effector targets (Pharmacodynamics) or in the way of drug being handled by the body (Pharmacokinetics). Application of pharmacogenomics to ocular drug therapy cannot be isolated without considering the variation in the ocular kinetics of the drug in the therapeutic outcome. This chapter critically analyzes the growing importance and relevance of genetic polymorphism which can be attributed to the therapeutic efficacy due to altered pharmacological targets including the receptors of autonomic system, prostaglandins, carbonic anhydrase, vascular endothelial growth factor, complement Factor H and corticosteroids in the treatment of ocular disease.

4.1 Introduction

Genetic polymorphism deciding the fate of drugs for their expected therapeutic outcome is considered as one of the rationalized approaches gaining importance in personalized medicine. Understanding genetic diversity among species (both inter and intra) is the first step toward the adaptation of customized therapeutic options.

T. Velpandian, BPharm, MS(Pharmacol), PhD (✉)
Ocular Pharmacology and Pharmacy, Dr.Rajendra Prasad Centre for Ophthalmic Sciences, All India Institute of Medical Sciences, New Delhi, India
e-mail: tvelpandian@hotmail.com

G. Kumaramanickavel, MD
Department of Genetics and Molecular Biology, Narayana Nethralaya, Bangalore, India

Aditya Jyot Eye Hospital, Mumbai, India

T. Velpandian (ed.), *Pharmacology of Ocular Therapeutics*,
DOI 10.1007/978-3-319-25498-2_4

Factors affecting drug response during the treatment are very complicated to comprehend due to the intricacy of the individual causes. However, one among that cause is attributed to genetic factors. Drugs having high therapeutic index and not acting through specific molecular mechanisms are not suitable for the assessment using pharmacogenomics. Agents having lower therapeutic index, capable of causing intolerable toxicity, exaggerated pharmacological response-related adverse effects and acting through specific molecular pathways are the suitable candidates for pharmacogenomics.

4.2 Pharmacogenomics and Genetics

Pharmacogenomics is a branch of pharmacology concerned with the effect of genetic factors on reactions to drugs, whereas pharmacogenetics is the study of the role of inherited acquired variation in drug response (Weinshilboum and Wang 2006). However, at places in the literature, both pharmacogenetics and genomics are interchangeably used indicating the higher degree of overlapping boundaries of the two domains. The term pharmacogenetics has conventionally been used for years to explain the adverse effects arising by differential metabolism of drugs in selected population. The lack of either reduced or exaggerated action of drug or adverse effect can only be explained by the genetic polymorphism.

4.2.1 Fundamental Understanding of Pharmacogenomics

Therapeutic index for any drug is the ratio observed between the concentration of the drug required to produce 50 % of death (LD50) to the concentration of the drug causing 50 % of protective response (ED50) through a particular activity in a population of rats or mice. These animals are highly inbreed strains, closely related genetically. Despite being closely related, the differential drug responses for the death of 50 % of animals at a particular dose signify the fine levels of genetic variation among the animals responsible for making them as outliers against the specific activity. When it comes to population studies in large multicentric clinical trials, the degree of genetic variation in drug response is countered with placebo controls. However, when the drug is given to the patient suffering from a disease, the expected drug response for life-/function-saving attempts could be hampered due to the changes in genetic vulnerability. The differential responses in drug susceptibility due to genetic variation are further complicated when it comes to ophthalmic drugs. The presence of well-recognized barriers in the blood ocular interface causing lower levels of drugs in ocular tissues is one of the fundamental problems restricting the ocular availability of drugs for their pharmacological action (Velpandian 2009).

4.3 Genetic Variation in Drug Response: Positioning It for Ocular Therapy

Genetic polymorphism leading to discrepant drug responses for systemic diseases is explained by altered pharmacodynamics or pharmacokinetics. Pharmacodynamic changes are due to the genetic polymorphism causing altered targets for the binding site and altered expression of intracellular pathway involved in the working mechanism of the drug. Pharmacokinetic changes arise from the genetically altered pathways of drug absorption, efflux transport systems, distribution, metabolism, and excretion pathways. In case of ocular-specific drugs, systemic route is not a well-accepted strategy for achieving therapeutic concentration in ocular tissues due to the failures observed while rationalizing the attempts (Velpandian 2009). Intricacies involved in ocular structure, associated fluid dynamics, optical signal processing pathways, and genetic variations affecting the ultimate ocular functions in homeostasis as well as in pathology have been well established. Therefore, discussing pharmacogenomics for ocular diseases is highly limited by the type of diseases and therapeutic options available. The available distinct ocular drug administration pathways include topical administration of drugs as eye drops, intravitreal injections subconjunctival, sub-tenon, and retrobulbar injections. The therapeutic interventions available for the ocular diseases are quite restricted mostly to surgical approaches. Drug therapy for glaucoma and neovascular complications are the areas where the available major therapeutic options can be subjected for pharmacogenomic studies. Interestingly, the mechanism of action of drugs approved for the management of glaucoma shows variation which can be attributed to inter individual variability in drug response.

4.3.1 Ocular Pharmacokinetic Factors: Determinants of Dynamics

Pre-corneal factors are the major determinants of the outcome of drugs applied topically. After the topical administration, drugs classically take trans-corneal penetration to reach pharmacologically meaningful levels in the aqueous humor. Alternatively, trans-conjunctival pathway is also being taken by the drug molecules to reach ciliary epithelium. Presence of zona occludens in between the corneal epithelial cells makes paracellular transport of drugs through the cornea difficult. The major absorption pathway still relays on transcellular corneal route controlled by resistance from hydrophobic epithelium and hydrophilic stroma. Formulation factors such as viscosity, osmolarity, pH, and drop size are also the major extrinsic factors affecting aqueous bioavailability of drugs. Apart from this, corneal sensitivity for drugs, presence of preservatives, and levels of basal tear secretion further alter the ocular bioavailability of drugs (Lee and Robinson 1986).

Genetic polymorphism altering pharmacokinetic parameters such as absorption, metabolism, distribution, and elimination ultimately restricts the bioavailability of the drugs. However, the contribution of genetic polymorphism involved in the altered absorption of topically administered drugs has not been studied. Similarly, variations due to the retinal elimination of drugs are not assessed owing to the difficulties involved in their functional assessment. In addition there is lack of information on the tear concentration reached by drugs through lacrimal system after drug administration through systemic route.

4.4 Genetic Variation in the Drug Response for Antiglaucoma Agents

Glaucoma is classified as open-angle glaucoma and closed-angle glaucoma with respect to the status of the anterior chamber angle. It is further divided into primary and secondary subtypes. Primary open-angle glaucoma (POAG) is the most common subset, representing over 70 % of all the cases of glaucoma, and is characterized by an open anterior chamber angle, elevated IOP, and glaucomatous optic nerve changes. In this main type of glaucoma (POAG), more than 20 associated genetic loci have been reported. Yet only three causative genes have been identified in these loci, viz., myocilin (MYOC), optineurin (OPTN), and WD repeat domain 36 (WDR36). Concurrently mutations in these genes account for only a small percentage of the patients with POAG. It has been recognized that some of the glaucoma cases have a Mendelian inheritance pattern, and a considerable fraction of the cases result from a large number of variants in several genes each contributing toward cumulative effects (Fuse 2010). Genome-wide association studies (GWAS) have found about 27 genes related to POAG, but the pathological effects of these genes need to be investigated in more detail.

4.4.1 Drugs Acting Through Autonomic Functions

Pilocarpine, timolol, and brimonidine are the representative antiglaucoma agents known to act through sympathetic division of autonomic nervous system to reduce intraocular pressure. Sympathetic system-mediated transmission of neuronal impulses and its subsequent physiological actions are mediated chiefly through norepinephrine, epinephrine, and its associated receptors. Adrenoceptors are expressed by most cell types of the human body and are primary targets of the catecholamines, epinephrine, and norepinephrine (Ahles and Engelhardt 2014). As per the human genome studies, nine types of adrenoceptor genes are grouped into three broad families, namely, α1-, α2-, and β-adrenoceptors. Presence of α2- and β2-receptors in the ciliary process and epithelium of the eye and their role in the autoregulation of aqueous humor production have been well documented (Lapalus and Elena 1988).

Although at different body parts the gland secretion is under the control of cholinergic system, in ciliary process, it is under the influence of adrenergic system. In the perfusion model Kodama et al. (1985) reported that the beta blocker (timilol) at the minimal concentration of 0.05 microgram/ml was able to suppress aqueous humour production in enucleated rabbit eye up to 30 %, whereas cholinergic agent pilocarpine was ineffective.

Brimonidine is an α2-receptor agonist, while timolol is a β2-receptor antagonist. Predominately beta-blockers such as timolol, levobunolol, and carteolol are being used for the reduction of the formation of aqueous humor from the ciliary epithelium in glaucoma. Genetic polymorphism in the adrenergic receptors has been reported to change the affinity of ligand on its receptor (Green et al. 1993) and their metabolism (Arcavi and Benowitz 1993). Therefore, any genetic variation in the signal transduction pathway of the muscarinic and adrenergic receptors and drug transport across the cornea can have a profound impact on the activity of these agents in reducing intraocular pressure.

The beta-adrenergic receptors (ADRBs) are cell surface receptors that play central role in the sympathetic nervous system. Pharmacological targeting of two of these receptors, ADRB1 and ADRB2, represents a widely used therapeutic approach for common and important diseases including asthma, hypertension, and heart failure. Genetic variation in both ADRB1 and ADRB2 has been linked to both in-vitro and clinical disease phenotypes (Taylor 2007). As the ciliary and iris muscles are under the autonomic control, the intraocular pressure maintenance is extensively been modulated by autonomic control (Lanigan et al. 1989) in which the production of aqueous humor is under the control of adrenergic receptors ADRB1 and ADRB2 and its autoregulation is through alpha-2 adrenoceptors. The ADRB1, ADRB2, and ADRB3 adrenergic receptors are highly expressed in the eye, whereas ADRB1 and ADRB2 were specifically identified in the ciliary body, trabecular meshwork, and optic nerve head. Subjects with coding single nucleotide polymorphism rs1042714 in the ADRB2 gene (CC genotype) were significantly more likely to experience an IOP decrease of 20 % or more. This study also reported that the coding single nucleotide polymorphism in ADRB2 is associated with an increased likelihood of a clinically meaningful IOP response to topical beta-blockers (McCarty et al. 2008).

4.4.2 *Pilocarpine in Reducing IOP*

Pilocarpine apart from being used as antiglaucoma medications in ophthalmic preparations is also being used in oral preparations for the treatment of radiation-induced xerostomia and Sjögren syndrome. The major metabolic pathways of pilocarpine in human are hydrolysis and hydroxylation. The effect of PON1 polymorphism (Q192R) on pilocarpine hydrolase activity was analyzed using recombinant PON1 192Q and 192R and human plasma of volunteers. This result of this study showed that recombinant PON1 192R had higher catalytic efficiency than PON1 192Q. In human plasma, the activity of the R/R genotype was significantly higher than those of the Q/R and Q/Q genotypes. These result thus documented the polymorphism affecting pilocarpine hydrolase activity (Hioki et al. 2011).

Pilocarpine is also metabolized into pilocarpic acid by plasma esterase and to 3-hydroxypilocarpine by CYP2A6. Studies of genotyping analysis in Japanese patients (Endo et al. 2008) revealed that the poor metabolizers had two inactive CYP2A6 alleles, CYP2A6*4A, CYP2A6*7, CYP2A6*9, or CYP2A6*10. The apparent pilocarpine clearance was significantly lower in the poor metabolizers than in the comparatively nonpoor metabolizers.

4.4.3 Timolol in Reducing IOP and Causing Bradycardia

Several studies indicate altered beta-blocker metabolism-related pharmacokinetic profile to be responsible for its dynamic property. Thus, poor metabolizers of beta-blockers are expected to have a longer duration of activity when it is administered orally (Lennard et al. 1986). As topical timolol is the mainstay of glaucoma treatment, the impact of polymorphism affecting topically administered beta-blockers cannot be attributed to the liver metabolism. Fuchsjager-Mayrl et al. (2005) evaluated the functional importance of beta-2 adrenoceptor antagonist in reducing IOP among nonsmoking volunteers homozygous for the wild beta-2 adrenoceptor (Arg16/Gln27 ($n=24$)) and other two polymorphisms (Gly16/Gln27 ($n=47$) or Gly16/Glu27 ($n=18$). This study concluded that the ocular hypotensive effect of timolol ranged between 40–45% in all groups and was not significantly different between the three study groups ($p=0.979$). The results of this study concluded that polymorphism in beta-2 adrenoceptor metabolism does not influence the ocular hypotensive effects of topical beta adrenoceptor antagonists. However, the CYP2D6 poor metabolizers may be more prone to systemic adverse events than extensive metabolizers in case of topical timolol administration (Nieminen et al. 2005).

In POAG patients, CYP2D6 SNP Arg296Cys appeared to be correlative with the intersubject variability seen with timolol. Subjects with CC genotype tended to avoid timolol-induced bradycardia, and subjects with TT genotype tended to have poorer timolol-induced ocular hypotensive effects (Yang et al. 2009). Concurrently Yuan et al. (2010) reported that CYP2D6 SNP rs16947 may confer susceptibility to timolol-induced bradycardia. Patients with CC genotype were unlikely to suffer from timolol-induced bradycardia, whereas those with TT genotype were found to suffer from timolol-induced bradycardia.

4.4.4 Polymorphism in the Pressure Lower Effect of Prostaglandins

Currently, PGF2 alpha analogs are the groups of successful agents widely used in IOP control in glaucoma patients. Moreover, prostanoid FPA receptors exist in human trabecular meshwork, and any polymorphism in $F(2\alpha)$ is also expected to vary the pharmacodynamics of PG F(2α) analogs in glaucoma therapy. Sakurai et al. (2007) showed that rs3753380 and rs3766355, SNPs in the promoter, and intron 1 regions of the FP receptor gene correlate with response to short-term latanoprost treatment in normal volunteers. The genotype of these SNPs may be an important determinant of variability in response to latanoprost.

Organic anion transporter polypeptides (OATPs) which are responsible for topical penetration of prostaglandins into ocular tissues are also expected to play a role in establishing interindividual difference in drug concentrations and effects. Genetic polymorphism involved in the pharmacodynamics of prostaglandin analogs was evaluated in patients by analyzing the association between variants in the prostaglandin F(α) receptor (PTGFR), solute carrier organic anion transporter family 2A1 (SLCO2A1) genes, and intraocular pressure (IOP) in response to prostaglandin analogs. DNA samples were genotyped for the following SNPs: rs3753380 (promoter region) and rs3766355 (intronic region) of the prostaglandin F(2α) receptor gene and rs34550074 (Ala396Thr) of SLCO2A1 and correlated with mean change in IOP. This study interestingly revealed no indication for an association between SNPs in the prostaglandin F(2α) receptor gene or SLCO2A1 and IOP in response to prostaglandin analogs in a population of European descent (McCarty et al. 2012).

4.4.5 Polymorphism in Carbonic Anhydrase Causing Variation in Decreasing IOP

Change in taste of carbonated beverages is a common observation in the patients under the treatment with carbonic anhydrase inhibitors such as acetazolamide. Carbonic anhydrase (CA) activity plays an important role in controlling aqueous humor production in the eye and in regulating intraocular pressure. So far 14 isoforms of CA have been identified, of which CA II, CA IV, CA XII, and possibly CA XIV are expressed by the kidney (Schwartz 2002). Carbonic anhydrase enzymes (CAs, EC 4.2.1.1) are zinc-containing metalloproteins, which efficiently catalyze the reversible conversion of carbon dioxide to bicarbonate and release proton. These enzymes are essentially important for biological system and play several important physiological and pathophysiological functions (Imtaiyaz Hassan et al. 2013). CA inhibitors are widely used as a drug for the treatment of neurological disorders, antiglaucoma, anticancer and antiobesity agents. Interestingly, the interindividual variation in the response to acetazolamide has only been recently recognized in oral hygiene. Carbonic anhydrase VI (CA6) is a secreted enzyme that catalyzes the hydration of carbon hydroxide in saliva and other body fluids. CA6 has been implicated in taste, gastrointestinal dysfunctions, tooth erosion, and caries. Peres et al. (2010) analyzed the allele and genotype distribution of three polymorphisms in the coding sequences of (CA6) gene and checked for possible associations with salivary buffer and other related parameters in 245 children of 7–9 years. This study revealed that there was a positive association between buffer capacity and the rs2274327

(C/T) polymorphism. The allele T and genotype TT were significantly less frequent in individuals with the highest buffer capacity.

Oral acetazolamide is the standard care of treatment envisaged for the quick reduction in IOP in ocular emergencies. Apart from soluble isozymes CA II and CA I, histochemical studies confirmed the presence of a distinct membrane-associated carbonic anhydrase isoenzyme IV in the human eye (Hageman et al. 1991; Ridderstråle et al. 1994). Although CA-IV polymorphism has been documented well in the literature, studies about the change in IOP after systemic and topical administration of carbonic anhydrase inhibitors have not been conducted.

4.5 Role of Polymorphism in Response to Antiangiogenic Agents

Although the pathophysiology behind choroidal neovascularization observed in age-related macular degeneration has not been completely elucidated, the predominating factors responsible for the angiogenesis have been determined. The therapeutic modalities have also been developed based on the concept of neutralizing factors directly involved in angiogenesis or neovascularization. In this approach humanized monoclonal anti-VEGF antibodies (bevacizumab, ranibizumab), aptamers (pegaptanib), and soluble VEGF receptors (VEGF traps) are the popular approaches to control the neovascularization and macular edema. These agents also had a prominent role in pathological retinal neovascularization and macular edema arising due to diabetic complications. Intravitreal triamcinolone acetonide, a mineralocorticoid with antiangiogenic property, and photodynamic therapy are the other strategies followed for controlling neovascular complications.

4.5.1 Role of Various Factors Involved in AMD

Drusen is the pathological deposit found between the retinal pigmented epithelium (RPE) and Bruch's membrane. Drusen deposition has been recognized as a significant risk factor in the development of AMD. Altered clearance of drusen driven by changes in complement factor H has been reported to initiate the inflammatory response in AMD. These inflammatory reactions trigger upregulation of angiogenic factors and ultimately cause choroidal neovascularization. Treatment in AMD involves anti-VEGF agents mainly acting on the angiogenesis pathways. Polymorphism in CFH has been shown to predispose individual to AMD, while VEGF polymorphism has been shown to affect the outcome of pharmacological interventions. Hence, a knowledge on the genetics of these two key molecules would help in understanding and improvising AMD treatments.

4.5.2 *Vascular Endothelial Growth Factor and Its Polymorphism*

Vascular endothelial growth factor (VEGF) is the key regulator of physiological angiogenesis during embryogenesis, skeletal growth, and reproductive functions. VEGF has also been implicated in pathological angiogenesis associated with tumors and intraocular neovascular disorders. The VEGF gene is located on chromosome 6 at location 6p21.1. Its coding region spans approximately 14 Kb and consists of eight exons (Brogan et al. 1999; Tischer et al. 1991). VEGF belongs to a gene family that includes placental growth factor (PLGF), VEGFB, VEGFC, and VEGFD. Parapoxvirus genes have also been identified with homologs of VEGF and shown to have VEGF-like activities (Ferrara and Davis-Smyth 1997; Neufeld et al. 1999). Major role of VEGF-A is the formation of blood vessels during development or in pathological conditions, whereas VEGF-B plays a less pronounced role in the vascular system. VEGF-B seems to play a role only in the maintenance of newly formed blood vessels during pathological conditions (Zhang et al. 2009). VEGF-B also plays a protective role on neurons in the retina (Li et al. 2008). Importantly, VEGF-C and VEGF-D regulate lymphatic angiogenesis (Karkkainen et al. 2002; Stacker et al. 2002), emphasizing the unique role of this gene family in controlling growth and differentiation of multiple anatomic components of the vascular system.

Angiogenesis is an important host process that participates in choroidal neovascularization observed in age-related macular degeneration. Host variability in VEGF pathway can influence angiogenesis-dependent signaling, altering sensitivity to antiangiogenic drugs and prognosis. Numerous therapeutic agents targeting the VEGF pathway have been developed, viz., bevacizumab, ranibizumab, pegaptanib, and VEGF traps. Though these agents show promising efficacy, they are often very expensive, and apart from drug resistance, limited activity and severe toxicities also build complication in the therapeutic outcomes. There is a strong need for identification of markers enabling a prior selection of patients who are likely to benefit from these agents. These markers might also carry prognostic value and may help in decisions about the overall treatment approach to manage more or less aggressive tumors with varying degrees of angiogenic involvement. Numerous SNPs in the promoter, 5′, and 3′ untranslated regions (UTR) are present in VEGF. Single nucleotide polymorphism in VEGF molecule can result in different outcomes of anti-VEGF therapy in diseases like age-related macular degeneration (ARMD).

The importance of VEGF single nucleotide polymorphisms (SNP) in predicting the ARMD progression and anti-VEGF therapeutic response has been shown in numerous pharmacogenomics clinical studies. For example, some of the more frequent VEGF SNPs found to have association with the outcome of anti-VEGF therapy in ARMD are rs3025039 (936 C>T), rs699947 (−2578 C>A), rs833061 (−1498 C>T), rs1413711 (+674C>T), rs1413711 (+674C>T), rs1413711, rs943080, rs833069, rs3025000, rs699946, rs699946, rs1413711, rs3024997, and rs2010963 (−634 G >C) (Table 4.1).

Table 4.1 Studies comparing VEGF gene polymorphism and the clinical response to intravitreal anti-VEGF therapy in AMD

Gene	Population	Treatment	Duration of treatment	SNP (Allele)	Nucleotide variant	Response to anti-VEGF therapy	Reference
VEGF A	394/Korean	BVZ/RBZ	12–24 months	rs3025039	[C/T]	VA gain	Park et al. (2014)
	94/Spanish	RBZ	12 months	Rs699947	[A/C]	Improved VA	Cruz-Gonzalez et al. (2014)
				Rs833061	[C/T]	Improved VA	
	92/Brazilian	*RBZ*	*3 months*	Rs1413711	[A/G]	CRT improved	Veloso et al. (2014)
				Rs1413711	[A/G]	CRT improved	
				rs1413711 (CC)	[A/G]	No improvement in CRT	
	273/Korean	*RBZ*	*5 months*	Rs699947	[A/C]	Good response for visual improvement	Park et al. (2014)
	223/American	*RBZ*	*6 months*	rs943080 (TT)	[C/T]	No improvement in BCVA	Zhao et al. (2013)
	102/Korean	*RBZ*	*Monotherapy*	Rs833069	[A/G]	Significant decrease in CSMT, No change in BCVA	Chang et al. (2013)
	201/Australian	*BVZ/RBZ*	*12 months*	rs3025000 (TT or TC)	[C/T]	Better visual outcome at 6 months	Abedi et al. (2013)
	Italian	*BVZ*		rs699946 (G)	[C/T]	Respond better to BVZ than rs699946A	Agosta et al. (2012)
	104/Caucasian	*RBZ*	*6 months*	rs1413711	[A/G]	Influence short-term response to therapy	McKibbin et al. (2012)
	185/Austrian	*BVZ*	*42–1182 days*	rs3024997	[A/G]	Lower VA that other five snp taken	Boltz et al. (2012)
				rs2010963	[C/G]	Lower VA that other five snp taken	

4.5.3 Complement Factor H and Its Polymorphism

The recent revolution in age-related macular degeneration (AMD) genetics has demonstrated that genetic alterations affecting the alternative pathway of the complement cascade have a major influence on AMD risk. One of the two most important genetic loci is on chromosome 1 and contains genes encoding complement factor H (CFH). CFH is a blood-borne glycoprotein that is also produced locally by the RPE. This 155-kDa serum glycoprotein is composed of 20 complement control protein (CCP) domains, such that different regions of CFH recognize different ligands (Langford-Smith et al. 2014). CFH acts as a complement regulator and conveyor of host protection in two primary ways. CFH inhibits the formation of the alternative pathway C3 convertase by competing with factor B binding to C3b [or $C3(H_2O)$] via its CCP1–4 region; CFH also promotes the decay of existing C3 convertase by displacing factor Bb. In macular tissue, especially Bruch's membrane, relatively high levels of a truncated splice variant of CFH called factor H-like protein 1 (FHL-1) are present. There is an age-related loss of heparan sulfate from Bruch's membrane resulting in less available binding sites for FHL-1 (or CFH) to anchor to Bruch's membrane. This is compounded by the Y402H polymorphism in which CFH binds HS poorly. This ultimately results in complement activation and inflammation and thereby predisposes to AMD. Evidently supplementation with recombinant CFH has been proposed as a therapeutic strategy for AMD (Clark and Bishop 2014). The Y402H polymorphism in the complement regulatory protein factor H (CFH) can confer a >5-fold increased risk of developing AMD (Kelly et al. 2010). The importance of CFH single nucleotide polymorphisms (SNP) in predicting the ARMD progression and anti-VEGF therapeutic response has been shown in a number of pharmacogenomics clinical studies shown in Table 4.2.

4.5.4 Intravitreally Administered Glucocorticoids

Intravitreal route of administration minimizes the systemic side effects of glucocorticoids such as triamcinolone acetonide. Dexamethasone implants and fluocinolone acetonide are the alternatives available for intravitreal anti-VEGF therapy in ocular neovascular conditions. Corticosteroid treatments have emerged as an alternative therapy to conventional laser photocoagulation and other modalities for persistent diabetic macular edema.

Glucocorticoids are the most potent anti-inflammatory agents; however, a major factor limiting their clinical use is the wide variation in responsiveness to therapy. Five percent of the population are high steroid responders and develop an intraocular pressure (IOP) elevation of more than 15 mmHg above baseline (Razeghinejad and Katz 2012).

A meta-analysis reported that 32 % of individuals developed ocular hypertension (OHT) following 4-mg intravitreal triamcinolone, 66 and 79 % following 0.59 and 2.1 mg fluocinolone implant, respectively, and 11 and 15 % following

Table 4.2 Studies comparing the effect of CFH gene polymorphism with the clinical outcome after anti-VEGF therapy in different populations

Gene	Eyes and population	Treatment	Duration of treatment	SNP (Allele)	Nucleotide variant	Response to anti-VEGF therapy	Reference
CFH	128/Japanese	RBZ	24 months	162 V	[C/T]	Initial improvement but no visual progress	Hata et al. (2015)
	120/Japanese	RBZ	3 months	162 V	[C/T]	Retinal thickness decreased	Matsumiya et al. (2014)
				Y402H	[C/T]		
	193/Turkish	RZB	6 months	Y402H (CC)	[C/T]	Decrease in VA by 5 letter	Dikmetas et al. (2013)
				Y402H (TT)	[C/T]	Increase in VA by 5 letter	
				Y402H (TC)	[C/T]	–	
	365/American	BVZ/RBZ	24 months	rs1061170	[C/T]	No association with risk of AMD	Maguire et al. (2013)
	834/American	BVZ/RBZ		Y402H	[C/T]	No statistically significant differences in response by genotype	Piermarocchi and Miotto (2014)
	1510/Chinese	BVZ/RBZ		Y402H (TT)	[C/T]	Association treatment response with therapy	Chen et al. (2012)
	204/Swiss	RZB	24 months	rs1061170 (CT)	[C/T]	Significant favorable VA outcome	Menghini et al. (2012)
	420 eyes/Netherland	RZB	3 injections	6 high-risk alleles	[C/T]	Cumulative effect of high risk	Smailhodzic et al. (2012)
					[C/T]	Alleles in three of the genes are associated with poor response to therapy	
	Italian	BVZ/RBZ		rs1061170 CT	[C/T]	Improvement of visual acuity	Agosta et al. (2012)
	105/Japanese	RBZ	Monotherapy	Y402H	[C/T]	No clear association with therapy	Yamashiro et al. (2012)
	65/American	RBZ	12 months	Y402H	[C/T]	Associated with less improvement in VA	Francis (2011)

	104/Caucasian	RBZ		rs1061170	[C/T]	Influence short-term response to therapy	McKibbin et al. (2012)
	243/Swiss	RBZ	Avg 3.9 injection	p.Y402H (CC)	[C/T]	Decreased chance of positive treatment outcome	Kloeckener-Gruissem et al. (2011)
				p.Y402H (CT)	[C/T]	Increase chance of positive treatment outcome	
				p.Y402H (CT)	[C/T]	Increase chance of positive treatment outcome	
	156/American	RBZ	9 months	Y402H (rs1061170) (TT)	[C/T]	High risk of requiring additional RBZ	Lee et al. (2009)
	70/Tunician	BVZ	Until CNV was no longer active	Y402H	[C/T]	High association with AMD patients	Habibi et al. (2013)
					[C/T]	No significant association in response to BVZ	
	75/Korean	BVZ	Monotherapy	Y402H	[C/T]	No significant improvement in VA after 12 months	Kang et al. (2012)
	144/Chinese	BVZ		rs800292	[C/T]	Association in response to therapy	Tian et al. (2012)
	197/Australian	BVZ	Until CNV was no longer active	402HH	[C/T]	Worse outcome for distance and reading visual acuity	Nischler et al. (2011)
				402YH	[C/T]		
				402YY	[C/T]		
	86/American	BVZ	Until CNV was no longer active	Y402H (TT)	[C/T]	No improvement in VA after therapy than TT and TC genotype	Brantley et al. (2007)
				Y402H (TC)	[C/T]	No improvement in VA after therapy than TT and TC genotype	
				Y402H (CC)	[C/T]	Improvement in VA after therapy than TT and TC genotype	

0.35 and 0.7 mg dexamethasone implant, respectively. The common risk factors included preexisting glaucoma, higher baseline intraocular pressure (IOP), younger age, OHT following previous injection, uveitis, higher steroid dosage, and fluocinolone implant (Kiddee et al. 2013).

Glucocorticoid receptor polymorphisms (ER22/23EK, N363S, BclI, N766N, and single nucleotide polymorphisms (SNPs) within introns 3 and 4) were assessed in 52 patients (56 eyes) who underwent treatment with intravitreal triamcinolone acetonide (IVTA) for various retinal diseases. After removing the patients, those who are nonpolymorphic for ER22/23EK, N363S, and the intron 3 SNP, in the test population, the remaining were subjected for analysis for BclI, N766N, and intron 4 SNP. However, the small population did not record any statistically significant relationship between glucocorticoid receptor polymorphisms and IOP elevation following IVTA (Gerzenstein et al. 2008).

A retrospective case-controlled study in native Dutch patients (58 steroid responders and 44 nonresponders) genotyped three SNPs, viz., rs7759778 and rs1406945 in SFRS3 and rs2968909 in FKBP4 in patients who showed IOP more than 21 mmHg within 1 year of intravitreal triamcinolone of 4.0 mg. The patients were divided into an intraocular hypertension group (intraocular pressure >21 mmHg within a year after IVTA) and a non-intraocular hypertension group. Results of this study also did not confirm the role of genetic variants in the SFRS3 and FKBP4 genes in the pathogenesis of corticosteroid-induced ocular hypertension (Hogewind et al. 2012).

4.6 Future Directions for Pharmacogenomics

Polymorphism existing in muscarinic receptors (M1 and M2) and adrenergic receptors involved in other cardio, pulmonary, neuropsychiatric disorders and other disease conditions are well reported in the literature. However, its relevance to ocular pharmacogenomics is yet to be established. The practice of characterizing the genetic variation in the drug response must be incorporated during the clinical trials of the newer compounds to gain access to the knowledge of such effects in early stages of drug development. This can successfully avoid the expenses involved in reinstating clinical studies after the drug is brought into the market. But it should be noted that it is challenging to arrive at such an interpretation during the drug discovery stage itself due to the lack of conformity on the power of sample population used in the clinical studies. Hence, efforts should be made to identify and validate the type of genetic associations which can explain the type of variations that can be predicted during the drug evaluation stage. Although personalized medicine holds promise for the future about the possibilities of customizing medications based on individual genetic makeup, there are several concerns about their exploitation affecting fundamental rights of a human being. For the judicial application of pharmacogenomics in treatment options, appropriate regulatory framework for insurance policies and health care providers are of paramount importance.

References

Abedi F, Wickremasinghe S, Richardson AJ, Makalic E, Schmidt DF, Sandhu SS, Baird PN, Guymer RH. Variants in the VEGFA gene and treatment outcome after anti-VEGF treatment for neovascular age-related macular degeneration. Ophthalmology. 2013;120(1):115–21. doi:10.1016/j.ophtha.2012.10.006.

Agosta E, Lazzeri S, Orlandi P, Figus M, Fioravanti A, Di Desidero T, Sartini MS, Nardi M, Danesi R, Bocci G. Pharmacogenetics of antiangiogenic and antineovascular therapies of age-related macular degeneration. Pharmacogenomics. 2012;13(9):1037–53. http://doi.org/10.2217/pgs.12.77.

Ahles A, Engelhardt S. Polymorphic variants of adrenoceptors: pharmacology, physiology, and role in disease. Pharmacol Rev. 2014;66(3):598–637. http://doi.org/10.1124/pr.113.008219.

Arcavi L, Benowitz NL. Clinical significance of genetic influences on cardiovascular drug metabolism. Cardiovasc Drugs Ther: Int Soc Cardiovasc Pharmacother. 1993;7(3):311–24. Retrieved from http://www.ncbi.nlm.nih.gov/pubmed/8103355.

Boltz A, Ruiß M, Jonas JB, Tao Y, Rensch F, Weger M, Garhöfer G, Frantal S, El-Shabrawi Y, Schmetterer L. Role of vascular endothelial growth factor polymorphisms in the treatment success in patients with wet age-related macular degeneration. Ophthalmology. 2012;119(8):1615–20. doi:10.1016/j.ophtha.2012.02.001.

Brantley MA, Fang AM, King JM, Tewari A, Kymes SM, Shiels A. Association of complement factor H and LOC387715 genotypes with response of exudative age-related macular degeneration to intravitreal bevacizumab. Ophthalmology. 2007;114(12):2168–73. http://doi.org/10.1016/j.ophtha.2007.09.008.

Brogan IJ, Khan N, Isaac K, Hutchinson JA, Pravica V, Hutchinson IV. Novel polymorphisms in the promoter and 5' UTR regions of the human vascular endothelial growth factor gene. Hum Immunol. 1999;60(12):1245–9.

Chang W, Noh,DH, Sagong M and Kim T. Pharmacogenetic association with early response to intravitreal ranibizumab for age-related macular degeneration in a Korean population. Mol Vis. 2013;19:702–9.

Chen H, Yu K-D, Xu G-Z. Association between Variant Y402H in Age-Related Macular Degeneration (AMD) Susceptibility Gene CFH and Treatment Response of AMD: A Meta-Analysis. PLoS One. 2012;7(8):e42464. http://doi.org/10.1371/journal.pone.0042464.

Clark S, Bishop P. Role of factor H and related proteins in regulating complement activation in the macula, and relevance to age-related macular degeneration. J Clin Med. 2014;4(1):18–31. http://doi.org/10.3390/jcm4010018.

Cruz-Gonzalez F, Cabrillo-Estévez L, López-Valverde G, Cieza-Borrella C, Hernández-Galilea E, González-Sarmiento R. Predictive value of VEGF A and VEGFR2 polymorphisms in the response to intravitreal ranibizumab treatment for wet AMD. Graefes Arch Clin Exp Ophthalmol. 2014;252(3):469–75. doi:10.1007/s00417-014-2585-7.

Dikmetas O, Kadayıfcılar S, Eldem B. The effect of CFH polymorphisms on the response to the treatment of age-related macular degeneration (AMD) with intravitreal ranibizumab. Mol Vis. 2013;19:2571–8. Retrieved from http://www.pubmedcentral.nih.gov/articlerender.fcgi?artid=3869644&tool=pmcentrez&rendertype=abstract.

Endo T, Nakajima M, Fukami T, Hara Y, Hasunuma T, Yokoi T, Momose Y. Genetic polymorphisms of CYP2A6 affect the in-vivo pharmacokinetics of pilocarpine. Pharmacogenet Genomics. 2008;18(9):761–72. http://doi.org/10.1097/FPC.0b013e328303c034.

Ferrara N, Davis-Smyth T. The biology of vascular endothelial growth factor. Endocr Rev. 1997;18(1):4–25. http://doi.org/10.1210/edrv.18.1.0287.

Francis PJ. The influence of genetics on response to treatment with ranibizumab (Lucentis) for age-related macular degeneration: the Lucentis Genotype Study (an American Ophthalmological Society thesis). Trans Am Ophthalmol Soc. 2011;109:115–56. Retrieved from http://www.pubmedcentral.nih.gov/articlerender.fcgi?artid=3259677&tool=pmcentrez&rendertype=abstract.

Fuchsjager-Mayrl G, Markovic O, Losert D, Lucas T, Wachek V, Muller M, Schmetterer L. Polymorphism of the beta-2 adrenoceptor and IOP lowering potency of topical timolol in healthy subjects. Mol Vis. 2005;11:811–5. Retrieved from http://www.ncbi.nlm.nih.gov/pubmed/16205624.

Fuse N. Genetic bases for glaucoma. Tohoku J Exp Med. 2010;221(1):1–10.

Gerzenstein SM, Pletcher MT, Cervino ACL, Tsinoremas NF, Young B, Puliafito CA, Fini ME, Schwartz SG. Glucocorticoid receptor polymorphisms and intraocular pressure response to intravitreal triamcinolone acetonide. Ophthalmic Genet. 2008;29(4):166–70. http://doi.org/10.1080/13816810802320217.

Green SA, Cole G, Jacinto M, Innis M, Liggett SB. A polymorphism of the human beta 2-adrenergic receptor within the fourth transmembrane domain alters ligand binding and functional properties of the receptor. J Biol Chem. 1993;268(31):23116–21. Retrieved from http://www.ncbi.nlm.nih.gov/pubmed/7901205.

Habibi I, Sfar I, Kort F, Aounallah-Skhiri H, Chebil A, Chouchene I, Bouraoui R, Limaiem R, Largheche L, Jendoubi-Ayed S, Makhlouf M, Ben Abdallah T, Ayed K, El Matri L, Gorgi Y. Y402H polymorphism in complement factor H and age-related macular degeneration in the Tunisian population. Ophthalmic Res. 2013;49(4):177–84. http://doi.org/10.1159/000345068.

Hageman GS, Zhu XL, Waheed A, Sly WS. Localization of carbonic anhydrase IV in a specific capillary bed of the human eye. Proc Natl Acad Sci U S A. 1991;88(7):2716–20. Retrieved from http://www.pubmedcentral.nih.gov/articlerender.fcgi?artid=51309&tool=pmcentrez&rendertype=abstract.

Hata M, Tsujikawa A, Miyake M, Yamashiro K, Ooto S, Oishi A, Nakanishi H, Takahashi A, Yoshimura N. Two-year visual outcome of ranibizumab in typical neovascular age-related macular degeneration and polypoidal choroidal vasculopathy. Graefes Arch Clin Exp Ophthalmol. 2015;253(2):221–7. http://doi.org/10.1007/s00417-014-2688-1.

Hioki T, Fukami T, Nakajima M, Yokoi T. Human paraoxonase 1 is the enzyme responsible for pilocarpine hydrolysis. Drug Metab Dispos. 2011;39(8):1345–52. http://doi.org/10.1124/dmd.111.038141.

Hogewind BF, Micheal S, Bakker B, Hoyng CB, den Hollander AI. Analysis of single nucleotide polymorphisms in the SFRS3 and FKBP4 genes in corticosteroid-induced ocular hypertension. Ophthalmic Genet. 2012;33(4):221–4. http://doi.org/10.3109/13816810.2012.716488.

Imtaiyaz Hassan M, Shajee B, Waheed A, Ahmad F, Sly WS. Structure, function and applications of carbonic anhydrase isozymes. Bioorg Med Chem. 2013;21(6):1570–82. http://doi.org/10.1016/j.bmc.2012.04.044.

Kang HK, Yoon MH, Lee DH, Chin HS. Pharmacogenetic influence of LOC387715/HTRA1 on the efficacy of bevacizumab treatment for age-related macular degeneration in a Korean population. Korean J Ophthalmol: KJO. 2012;26(6):414–22. http://doi.org/10.3341/kjo.2012.26.6.414.

Karkkainen MJ, Mäkinen T, Alitalo K. Lymphatic endothelium: a new frontier of metastasis research. Nat Cell Biol. 2002;4(1):E2–5. http://doi.org/10.1038/ncb0102-e2.

Kelly U, Yu L, Kumar P, Ding J-D, Jiang H, Hageman GS, Arshavsky VY, Frank MM, Hauser MA, Rickman CB. Heparan sulfate, including that in Bruch's membrane, inhibits the complement alternative pathway: implications for age-related macular degeneration. J Immunol. 2010;185(9):5486–94. http://doi.org/10.4049/jimmunol.0903596.

Kiddee W, Trope GE, Sheng L, Beltran-Agullo L, Smith M, Strungaru MH, Baath J, Buys YM. Intraocular pressure monitoring post intravitreal steroids: a systematic review. Surv Ophthalmol. 2013;58(4):291–310. doi:10.1016/j.survophthal.2012.08.003.

Kloeckener-Gruissem B, Barthelmes D, Labs S, Schindler C, Kurz-Levin M, Michels S, Fleischhauer J, Berger W, Sutter F, Menghini M. Genetic association with response to intravitreal ranibizumab in patients with neovascular AMD. Invest Ophthalmol Vis Sci. 2011;52(7):4694–702. http://doi.org/10.1167/iovs.10-6080.

Kodama T, Reddy VN, Macri FJ. Pharmacological study on the effects of some ocular hypotensive drugs on aqueous humor formation in the arterially perfused enucleated rabbit eye. Ophthalmic Res. 1985;17(2):120–4. Retrieved from http://www.ncbi.nlm.nih.gov/pubmed/3982786.

Langford-Smith A, Keenan TD, Clark SJ, Bishop PN, Day AJ. The role of complement in age-related macular degeneration: heparan sulphate, a ZIP code for complement factor H? J Innate Immun. 2014;6(4):407–16. doi:10.1159/000356513.

Lanigan LP, Clark CV, Hill DW. Intraocular pressure responses to systemic autonomic stimulation. Eye. 1989;3(Pt 4):477–83. http://doi.org/10.1038/eye.1989.72.

Lapalus P, Elena PP. Neurotransmitters and intraocular pressure. Fundam Clin Pharmacol. 1988;2(4):305–25. Retrieved from http://www.ncbi.nlm.nih.gov/pubmed/2906034.

Lee VHL, Robinson JR. Topical ocular drug delivery: recent developments and future challenges. J Ocul Pharmacol Ther. 1986;2(1):67–108.

Lee AY, Raya AK, Kymes SM, Shiels A, Brantley MA. Pharmacogenetics of complement factor H (Y402H) and treatment of exudative age-related macular degeneration with ranibizumab. Br J Ophthalmol. 2009;93(5):610–3. http://doi.org/10.1136/bjo.2008.150995.

Lennard MS, Tucker GT, Silas JH, Woods HF. Debrisoquine polymorphism and the metabolism and action of metoprolol, timolol, propranolol and atenolol. Xenobiotica. 1986;16(5):435–47. Retrieved from http://www.ncbi.nlm.nih.gov/pubmed/2874665.

Li Y, Zhang F, Nagai N, Tang Z, Zhang S, Scotney P, Lennartsson J, Zhu C, Qu Y, Fang C, Hua J, Matsuo O, Fong GH, Ding H, Cao Y, Becker KG, Nash A, Heldin CH, Li X. VEGF-B inhibits apoptosis via VEGFR-1-mediated suppression of the expression of BH3-only protein genes in mice and rats. J Clin Invest. 2008;118(3):913–23. http://doi.org/10.1172/JCI33673.

Maguire MG, Daniel E, Shah AR, Grunwald JE, Hagstrom SA, Avery RL, Huang J, Martin RW, Roth DB, Castellarin AA, Bakri SJ, Fine SL, Martin DF. Incidence of choroidal neovascularization in the fellow eye in the comparison of age-related macular degeneration treatments trials. Ophthalmology. 2013;120(10):2035–41. http://doi.org/10.1016/j.ophtha.2013.03.017.

Matsumiya W, Honda S, Yanagisawa S, Miki A, Nagai T, Tsukahara Y. Evaluation of clinical and genetic indicators for the early response to intravitreal ranibizumab in exudative age-related macular degeneration. Pharmacogenomics. 2014;15(6):833–43. http://doi.org/10.2217/pgs.14.51.

McCarty CA, Burmester JK, Mukesh BN, Patchett RB, Wilke RA. Intraocular pressure response to topical beta-blockers associated with an ADRB2 single-nucleotide polymorphism. Archiv Ophthalmol. 2008;126(7):959–63. http://doi.org/10.1001/archopht.126.7.959.

McCarty CA, Berg R, Patchett R, Wilke RA, Burmester JK. Lack of association between polymorphisms in the prostaglandin F2α receptor and solute carrier organic anion transporter family 2A1 genes and intraocular pressure response to prostaglandin analogs. Ophthalmic Genet. 2012;33(2):74–6. http://doi.org/10.3109/13816810.2011.628357.

McKibbin M, Ali M, Bansal S, Baxter PD, West K, Williams G, Cassidy F, Inglehearn CF. CFH, VEGF and HTRA1 promoter genotype may influence the response to intravitreal ranibizumab therapy for neovascular age-related macular degeneration. Br J Ophthalmol. 2012;96(2):208–12. http://doi.org/10.1136/bjo.2010.193680.

Menghini M, Kloeckener-Gruissem B, Fleischhauer J, Kurz-Levin MM, Sutter FKP, Berger W, Barthelmes D. Impact of loading phase, initial response and CFH genotype on the long-term outcome of treatment for neovascular age-related macular degeneration. PLoS One. 2012;7(7):e42014. http://doi.org/10.1371/journal.pone.0042014.

Neufeld G, Cohen T, Gengrinovitch S, Poltorak Z. Vascular endothelial growth factor (VEGF) and its receptors. FASEB J: Off Publ Fed Am Soc Exp Biol. 1999;13(1):9–22. Retrieved from http://www.ncbi.nlm.nih.gov/pubmed/9872925.

Nieminen T, Uusitalo H, Mäenpää J, Turjanmaa V, Rane A, Lundgren S, Ropo A, Rontu R, Lehtimäki T, Kähönen M. Polymorphisms of genes CYP2D6, ADRB1 and GNAS1 in pharmacokinetics and systemic effects of ophthalmic timolol. A pilot study. Eur J Clin Pharmacol. 2005;61(11):811–9. http://doi.org/10.1007/s00228-005-0052-4.

Nischler C, Oberkofler H, Ortner C, Paikl D, Riha W, Lang N, Patsch W, Egger SF. Complement factor H Y402H gene polymorphism and response to intravitreal bevacizumab in exudative age-related macular degeneration. Acta Ophthalmol. 2011;89(4):e344–9. http://doi.org/10.1111/j.1755-3768.2010.02080.x.

Park UC, Shin JY, Kim SJ, Shin ES, Lee JE, McCarthy LC, Newcombe PJ, Xu CF, Chung H, Yu HG. Genetic factors associated with response to intravitreal ranibizumab in Korean patients with neovascular age-related macular degeneration. Retina. 2014;34(2):288–97. doi:10.1097/IAE.0b013e3182979e1e.

Peres RC, Camargo G, Mofatto LS, Cortellazzi KL, Santos MC, Nobre-dos-Santos M, Bergamaschi CC, Line SR. Association of polymorphisms in the carbonic anhydrase 6 gene with salivary buffer capacity, dental plaque pH, and caries index in children aged 7–9 years. Pharmacogenomics J. 2010;10(2):114–9. http://doi.org/10.1038/tpj.2009.37.

Piermarocchi S, Miotto S. Re: Hagstrom et al.: Pharmacogenetics for genes associated with age-related macular degeneration in the comparison of AMD treatments trials (CATT) (Ophthalmology 2013;120:593–9). Ophthalmology. 2014;121(8):e43–4. http://doi.org/10.1016/j.ophtha.2013.12.044.

Razeghinejad MR, Katz LJ. Steroid-induced iatrogenic glaucoma. Ophthal Res. 2012;47(2): 66–80. http://doi.org/10.1159/000328630.

Ridderstråle Y, Wistrand PJ, Brechue WF. Membrane-associated CA activity in the eye of the CA II-deficient mouse. Invest Ophthalmol Vis Sci. 1994;35(5):2577–84. Retrieved from http://www.ncbi.nlm.nih.gov/pubmed/8163345.

Sakurai M, Higashide T, Takahashi M, Sugiyama K. Association between genetic polymorphisms of the prostaglandin F2alpha receptor gene and response to latanoprost. Ophthalmology. 2007;114(6):1039–45. http://doi.org/10.1016/j.ophtha.2007.03.025.

Schwartz GJ. Physiology and molecular biology of renal carbonic anhydrase. J Nephrol. 2002;15 Suppl 5:S61–74.

Smailhodzic D, Muether PS, Chen J, Kwestro A, Zhang AY, Omar A, Van de Ven JP, Kirchhof B, Hoyng CB, Klevering BJ, Koenekoop RK, Fauser S, den Hollander AI. Cumulative effect of risk alleles in CFH, ARMS2, and VEGFA on the response to ranibizumab treatment in age-related macular degeneration. Ophthalmology. 2012;119(11):2304–11. http://doi.org/10.1016/j.ophtha.2012.05.040.

Stacker SA, Achen MG, Jussila L, Baldwin ME, Alitalo K. Lymphangiogenesis and cancer metastasis. Nat Rev Cancer. 2002;2(8):573–83. http://doi.org/10.1038/nrc863.

Taylor MR. Pharmacogenetics of the human beta-adrenergic receptors. Pharmacogenomics J. 2007;7(1):29–37. Epub 2006 Apr 25.

Tian J, Qin X, Fang K, Chen Q, Hou J, Li J, Yu W, Chen D, Hu Y, Li X. Association of genetic polymorphisms with response to bevacizumab for neovascular age-related macular degeneration in the Chinese population. Pharmacogenomics. 2012;13(7):779–87. http://doi.org/10.2217/pgs.12.53.

Tischer E, Mitchell R, Hartman T, Silva M, Gospodarowicz D, Fiddes JC, Abraham JA. The human gene for vascular endothelial growth factor. Multiple protein forms are encoded through alternative exon splicing. J Biol Chem. 1991;266(18):11947–54.

Veloso CE, de Almeida LN, Recchia FM, Pelayes D, Nehemy MB. VEGF gene polymorphism and response to intravitreal ranibizumab in neovascular age-related macular degeneration. Ophthalmic Res. 2014;51(1):1–8.

Velpandian T. Intraocular penetration of antimicrobial agents in ophthalmic infections and drug. Expert Opin Drug Deliv. 2009;6(3):255–70. doi:10.1517/17425240902798119.

Weinshilboum RM, Wang L. Pharmacogenetics and pharmacogenomics: development, science, and translation. Ann Rev Genom Hum Genet. 2006;7:223–45. http://doi.org/10.1146/annurev.genom.6.080604.162315.

Yang Y, Wu K, Yuan H, Yu M. Cytochrome oxidase 2D6 gene polymorphism in primary open-angle glaucoma with various effects to ophthalmic timolol. J Ocul Pharmacol Ther. 2009;25(2): 163–71. doi:10.1089/jop.2008.0028.

Yamashiro K, Tomita K, Tsujikawa A, Nakata I, Akagi-Kurashige Y, Miyake M, Ooto S, Tamura H, Yoshimura N. Factors associated with the response of age-related macular degeneration to intravitreal ranibizumab treatment. Am J Ophthalmol. 2012;154(1):125–36. http://doi.org/10.1016/j.ajo.2012.01.010.

Yuan H, Yu M, Yang Y, Wu K, Lin X, Li J. Association of CYP2D6 single-nucleotide polymorphism with response to ophthalmic timolol in primary open-angle Glaucoma – a pilot study. J Ocul Pharmacol Ther. 2010;26(5):497–501. doi:10.1089/jop.2010.0013.

Zhang F, Tang Z, Hou X, Lennartsson J, Li Y, Koch AW, Scotney P, Lee C, Arjunan P, Dong L, Kumar A, Rissanen TT, Wang B, Nagai N, Fons P, Fariss R, Zhang Y, Wawrousek E, Tansey G, Raber J, Fong GH, Ding H, Greenberg DA, Becker KG, Herbert JM, Nash A, Yla-Herttuala S, Cao Y, Watts RJ, Li X. VEGF-B is dispensable for blood vessel growth but critical for their survival, and VEGF-B targeting inhibits pathological angiogenesis. Proc Natl Acad Sci U S A. 2009;106(15):6152–7. http://doi.org/10.1073/pnas.0813061106.

Zhao L, Grob S, Avery R, Kimura A, Pieramici D, Lee J, Rabena M, Ortiz S, Quach J, Cao G, Luo H, Zhang M, Pei M, Song Y, Tornambe P, Goldbaum M, Ferreyra H, Kozak I, Zhang K. Common variant in VEGFA and response to anti-VEGF therapy for neovascular age-related macular degeneration. Curr Mol Med. 2013;13(6):929–34.

Chapter 5
The Biochemistry of the Eye

Narayanasamy Angayarkanni, Karunakaran Coral, Subramaniam Rajesh Bharathi Devi, and Aluru Venkata Saijyothi

Abstract Biochemical pathways involved in maintaining the functions of various ocular structures are very unique in nature. Therefore, understanding ocular biochemistry is of immense importance while exploring the changes during pathological conditions. These changes play a significant role on the scope of converting the biochemical manifestations into therapeutic opportunities. Current knowledge regarding the ocular biochemistry of these structures is ever expanding to be limited within a single chapter. Prudent efforts of this chapter is to review the molecular construct of the tissues of the eye and their characteristic metabolism, discussed under the subtitles as: cornea; lens, iris, ciliary body and aqueous humor; sclera; uvea; vitreous, retina and the retinal pigment epithelium.

5.1 Biochemistry of the Cornea

The cornea is a transparent convex tissue, sensitive due to rich unmyelinated nerve endings and accounts for two-thirds of the refractive nature of the eye with a refractive index of 1.376. It is around 0.5 mm in thickness and 11.5 mm in diameter. It is limited at its periphery by the corneal limbus, where the transparent cornea ends and the opaque sclera begins. The tissue is immune privileged as it is avascular and is

N. Angayarkanni (✉) • K. Coral • S.R. Bharathi Devi • A.V. Saijyothi
RS Mehta Jain Department of Biochemistry and Cell Biology, Vision Research Foundation, Sankara Nethralaya, Chennai, India
e-mail: angayar07@gmail.com

T. Velpandian (ed.), *Pharmacology of Ocular Therapeutics*,
DOI 10.1007/978-3-319-25498-2_5

nourished by the tear and aqueous humor. The structural arrangement of the tissue layers enables the refraction of the light.

The human cornea consists primarily of three layers: outer epithelium, middle stroma, and inner endothelium. There are two other acellular layers, the Bowman's layer that separates the epithelium from stroma and the Descemet's membrane that separates endothelium from stroma. Recently a novel, well-defined, acellular layer in the pre-Descemet's cornea (Dua's layer) that separates along the last row of keratocytes is reported as the 6th layer (Dua et al. 2014).

The ectoderm after the lens formation, forms the epithelium of the cornea. The neural crest cells migrate to form the endothelium, while a few migrate to become the keratoblasts. These keratoblasts proliferate and synthesize hyaluran to form the stromal matrix in the embryonic state. They further differentiates into keratocytes, which then synthesizes collagen and proteoglycan, replacing the hyaluran-water environment of the extra cellular matrix (ECM), finally forming the stroma of the adult cornea (Hassell and Birk 2010).

5.1.1 The Corneal Epithelium: The Regenerative Layer

It is the outermost layer consisting of four to five layers of stratified nonkeratinized squamous epithelial cells and a single basal layer (~50 μm). The basal columnar cells regenerate as they are mitotically active and are anchored to the basement membrane through an adhesion complex. Maintenance of the adult corneal epithelium is a dynamic process, incorporating constant cell production, movement, and loss. Turnover of epithelial cells occurs every 5–7 days by displacement of the top layer which that slough off into the tear, while the basal cells move toward the surface that form two to three layers of wing-shaped polyhedral cells. These cells undergo terminal differentiation and desquamation and subsequently form the top layer. The outermost layer of the epithelium is in intimate contact with the tear film via the glycocalyx that keeps the surface moist. This is important in light transmission, preventing damage due to drying and in acting as effective barrier against pathogen entry. The epithelium which is continuous between the cornea and the conjunctiva, has differential characteristics in these tissues. Unlike epidermis, the corneal epithelium do not lose their nucleus and extensively keratinize (Beebe and Masters 1996). Tight junctions between the epithelial cells ensure a polarized epithelium with limited trans cellular permeability.

According to the conventional hypothesis, slowly dividing limbal epithelial stem cells (LESCs), located in the basal limbal epithelium, maintain the corneal epithelium. However, recently, an alternative view proposes that corneal epithelial stem cells scattered throughout the basal layer of the corneal epithelium are responsible for homeostasis of the tissue and that LESCs are active only during wound healing (Yoon et al. 2014).

5.1.2 The Stromal Matrix

The middle stromal layer of the cornea is made of packed collagen fibrils arranged as orthogonal layers of collagen or lamellae with sparsely distributed keratocytes. Stroma constitutes 90 % of the corneal thickness. Fibrils of 25–30 nm diameter are regularly packed within lamellae, and there are 200 such lamellae, each 1.5–2.5 μm thick. This lattice-like structure ensures minimal light scattering and is responsible for the corneal transparency. The stromal keratocyte cells are sparsely distributed among the collagen lamella, and they extend projections toward other keratocytes. These cells secrete collagen and other extracellular matrix components (ECM) to maintain the stroma (Hassell and Birk 2010).

The excessive proliferation of the stromal keratocytes in the central cornea than in the periphery gives the refractive shape to the cornea (Rada et al. 1996). Insulin like growth factors namely, IGF I and II play an important role in the postnatal stromal development of the cornea (Kane et al. 2009). The keratocytes respond to growth factors for the ECM turnover especially during wound healing. Fibroblast growth factor, FGF2 and the Transforming growth factor, TGF-beta act on keratocytes and induce myofibroblast formation. TGF-beta induces the expression of smooth muscle actin, collagen, and proteoglycan. Posttranslational modifications play a role in the structure and function of the various ECM proteins. The hydration of the stroma which is ~3.5 mg H_2O/mg dry tissue makes the stroma relatively transparent. The stromal ECM consist primarily of collagen I and V, where collagen V is involved in collagen assembly (Birk et al. 1986). Collagen is synthesized in the rough endoplasmic reticulum of the cell as procollagen and is secreted into the ECM. The proteases at the cell surface remove the N- and C-terminal non-helical, globular ends. The resulting collagen molecules then arrange laterally in a staggered array to form collagen fibrils of various lengths and diameters. Specific lysine and hydroxylysine residues in the N- and C-telopeptides are oxidatively deaminated by lysyl oxidase enzyme (LOX) to produce reactive aldehydes that undergo a series of non-enzymatic condensation reactions to form covalent intra- and inter-molecular cross-links. The major reducible cross-links are dehydro-hydroxylysinonorleucine (deH-HLNL) and dehydrohistidinohydroxymerodesmosine (deH-HHMD). A non-reducible cross-link, histidinohydroxylysinonorleucine (HHL), UV-resistant stable tri-functional cross-link are seen in mature cornea (Fig. 5.1).

Decorin (Li et al. 1992), lumican (Blochberger et al. 1992; Kao et al. 2006), keratocan (Chakravarti 2006; Corpuz et al. 1996), and mimecan (Funderburgh et al. 1997) are the four major proteoglycans that regulate the stromal collagen fibril formation and its stabilization. These corneal proteoglycans belong to the small leucine-rich type proteoglycan gene family. The polypeptide chain of the core protein is coiled into a tight spiral with a leucine-rich region located at every 360°, thereby aligning all the leucine-rich regions on one surface of the coil. These aligned leucine-rich regions interact with the collagen molecules to regulate fibril formation (Hassell and Birk 2010).

The core protein of the corneal stromal proteoglycans, namely, decorin, has a single 55–60 kDa chondroitin/dermatan sulfate chain, while lumican, keratocan, and osteoglycin/mimecan have 2–3 keratan sulfate chains of 10–15 kDa each, that

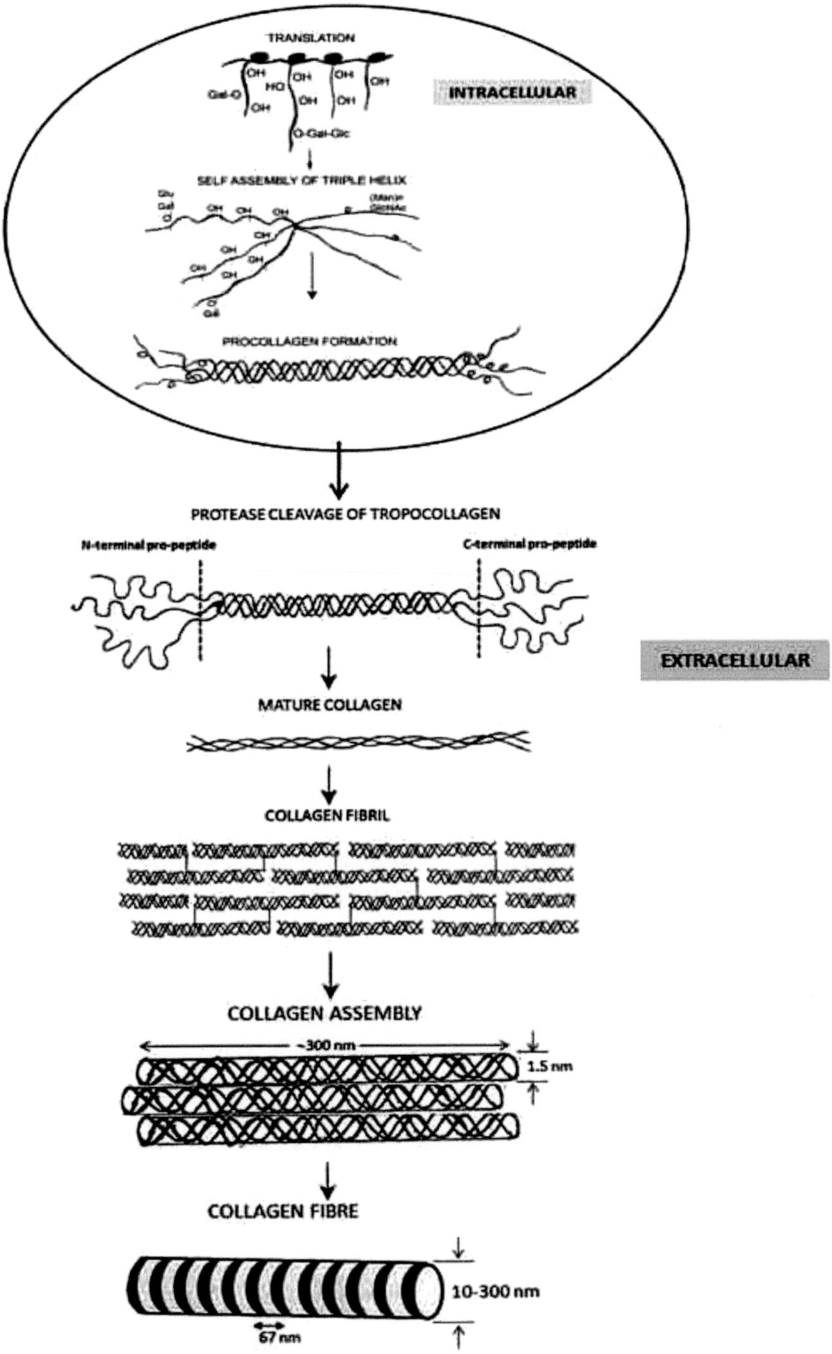

Fig. 5.1 Collagen Biosynthesis: It involves synthesis of pro-α and β chains, self-assembly of pro-collagens, secretion, cleavage of pro-peptides and self-assembly into fibril

regulate the spacing between the fibrils. Keratan sulfate (KS) is an important constituent of several collagen-rich tissues and is the major glycosaminoglycan (GAG) in the cornea, where it is N-linked to asparagine residues on the core protein by the corneal Glc-NAc 6-*O*-sulfotransferase enzyme (Akama et al. 2001). The sulfate groups of the keratan sulfate are essential to maintain the hydration level in cornea and for the solubility of the proteoglycan. Mutations resulting in defective proteoglycans lead to corneal dystrophies (Yasutaka Hayashida, *PNAS* 2006).

5.1.3 Endothelium: The Pump and the Barrier Function

The inner most layer of the cornea is the endothelium that forms a uniform monolayer of hexagonal cells (5 μ thick) with a cell density of around 2500 cells/mm^2. The endothelium functions as both a barrier to fluid movement into the cornea and an active pump to move the fluid out of the cornea, ensuring corneal transparency. The barrier function was first demonstrated in the nineteenth century by Leber (Stocker and Reichle 1974). The function, as metabolic pump, discovered almost a century later in 1972, when Maurice DM (Freeman 1972) demonstrated that the endothelium possessed active, energy-dependent fluid pump that moved water from the corneal stroma into the anterior chamber. This ensures corneal transparency. The number of endothelial cells is therefore critical (at least around 400–500/mm^2) for the optimal pump activity. Steady-state hydration occurs when the endothelial pump rate equals the GAG-driven leak (Maurice et al. 1981). A "pump-leak" mechanism where the active transport properties of the endothelium represent the "pump" and the stromal swelling pressure represents the "leak" was established (Riley 1969a, b). For the pump to function, Na^+/K^+-ATPase activity and the presence of HCO_3^-, Cl^-, and carbonic anhydrase activities are required. The pump requires Na^+/K^+-ATPase activity that actively transports Na^+ from the stroma to the anterior chamber and forms a diffusing gradient for water, thereby maintaining a constant stromal hydration. Several basolateral (stromal side) anion transporters, apical (facing the aqueous humor) ion channels, and water channels have been identified. Numerous anion transport mechanisms have been identified in the endothelium, namely, basolateral Na(+)/2HCO(3)(−) cotransport, Na(+)/K(+)/2Cl(−) cotransport, Cl(−)/HCO(3)(−) exchange, and apical anion channels permeable to both Cl(−) and HCO(3)(−), apart from the carbonic anhydrase-mediated CO_2-diffusive mode of apical HCO_3^- flux and apical Ca^{2+}-sensitive chloride channel (Bonanno 2003, 2012). The barrier function of the endothelium is in a dynamic regulation where the tight junctions and the adherent junctions play an integral role in addition to the Pumps and the channels (Srinivas, 2010).

Cellular glucose uptake is promoted by the glucose transporters present on both the apical and basolateral endothelial cell membranes (Kumagai et al. 1994). Eighty-five percent of glucose consumed in the cornea is converted to lactic acid (Riley 1969a). Epithelium is impermeable to lactate, and therefore in the cornea, it is about twice the concentration (~13 mM) to that in the aqueous humor (~7 mM), resulting in a large gradi-

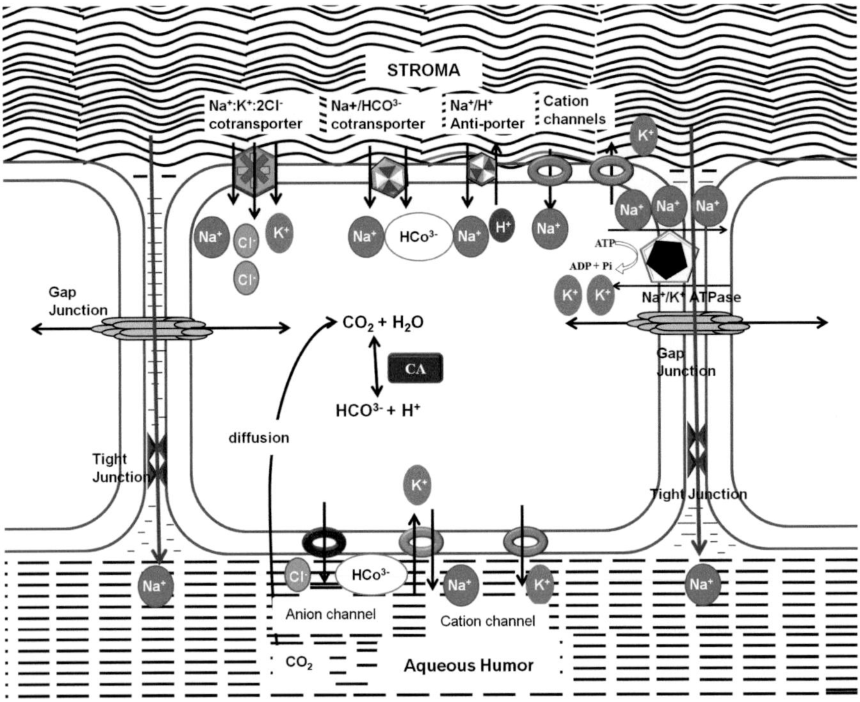

Fig. 5.2 Pump Leak Mechanism of stromal hydration: Stromal hydration is maintained by the pumps in the endothelium, ATP-driven Na^+/K^+ ATPase; $Na^+:K^+:2Cl^-$ co-transporter; Na^+/HCO^{3-} co-transporter; Na^+/H^+ anti-porter; selective and nonselective cationic and anionic channels

ent for lactate flux from cornea to anterior chamber across the endothelium. Lactate: H(+) cotransport was demonstrated in the endothelium (Giasson and Bonanno 1994) (Fig. 5.2).

Corneal endothelium has a high density of aquaporin (AQP1) located on both apical and basolateral membranes (Kuang et al. 2004). AQP1 is present for the passive movement of the water for faster stromal hydration as in physiological situations such as eye closure (which swells the cornea by ~4 %) or exposure to hypo-osmotic conditions as in swimming (Bonanno 2012).

There is no mitotic activity of the corneal endothelial cells as these are inhibited in the G1 phase. There is 0.3–0.6 % loss of endothelial cells per year which is compensated by the migration of the neighboring cells or spreading to a pleomorphic shape. Cell loss is critical for the pump activity and can result in corneal edema, bullous keratopathy, and the loss of visual acuity. Cell loss occurs in trauma, refractive surgeries, penetrating keratoplasty, corneal dystrophies, diabetes, and glaucoma. Corneal endothelial dystrophy is a chronic progressive endogenous degeneration of the corneal endothelium, partly due to genetic predisposition (Joyce 2012). Therefore, current researches explore the proliferative capacity of these corneal endothelial cells.

The corneal endothelial dystrophies are congenital hereditary endothelial dystrophy 1 (CHED1), congenital hereditary endothelial dystrophy 2 (CHED2), posterior polymorphous corneal dystrophy (PPCD), and Fuchs endothelial corneal dystrophy (FECD) (Weiss et al. 2008). However, the molecular pathologies remain largely unknown. Genetic factors, chronic oxidative stress, mitochondrial damage, extracellular matix changes, endoplasmic reticulum (ER) stress changes, and apoptosis contribute to the pathology of FECD. Early- and late-onset FECD are distinct corneal conditions with the similar clinical and phenotypic characteristics but different genetic risk factors (Schmedt et al. 2012). Two types of congenital hereditary endothelial dystrophy (CHED) have been described: CHED1, which is autosomal dominant, and CHED2, which is autosomal recessive. The major differences between CHED1 and CHED2 lie on the onset, mode of inheritance, genetic mutations, and associated conditions. Mutations of 25 types in different locations of the *SLC4A11* gene that codes for BTR1 (bicarbonate transport-related protein) or NaBC1 are known (Schmedt et al. 2012). Genetic defects in *SLC4A11* disrupt the fluid flux across corneal endothelium necessary for maintenance of healthy corneal hydration. However, the mechanism by which the mutation leads specifically to atrophy of corneal endothelium is still not clear (Hemadevi et al. 2008; Vithana et al. 2006). Posterior polymorphous corneal dystrophy (PPCD) is a rare non-progressive disorder that affects corneal endothelium and the DM (Henriquez et al. 1984). Mutations in the genes, VSX1 (visual system homebox 1), TCF8, and CO8A2 seem to have genetic heterogeneity (Schmedt et al. 2012).

5.1.4 The Limbus

Between the cornea and the sclera is the limbus, a zone of approximately 1 mm that surrounds the cornea and is the site for surgical incisions for cataract and glaucoma. In the limbus, the stem cells for the epithelium as well as vascular elements reside in providing nutrients to the avascular cornea. The vasculature of the limbus derives in primates primarily from the anterior ciliary arteries (Van Buskirk 1989). The limbus has two important functions in maintaining a healthy corneal epithelium. It is the source of stem cells for the corneal epithelium; it also acts as a barrier separating the clear avascular corneal epithelium from the surrounding vascular conjunctival tissue. This microenvironment can be altered due to disease leading to limbal stem cell deficiency, when the corneal surface becomes replaced by hazy conjunctival tissue. The causes of limbal stem cell deficiency include, chemical injuries to the eye, inflammatory diseases, and hereditary diseases (Ahmad 2012).

5.1.5 Basement Membrane

Basement membranes are specialized acellular matrix that not only plays a role in separating the cellular layers but also connect them through the molecular matrix. Corneal epithelial basement membrane modulates the epithelial-to-stroma and stroma-to-epithelial interactions by regulating cytokines and growth factor movement from one cell layer to the other. In cornea, the basement membrane is present between epithelial cells and stroma. After 8 weeks of gestation, the epithelium is separated out from stroma by basement membrane which is avascular. The lamina lucida and lamina densa are the adjacent layers. The basement membrane is chiefly composed of the laminin, apart from collagen, heparan sulfate proteoglycans (HSPG), and nidogens. The composition varies from the limbal region to the central cornea. Laminins are heterotrimeric glycoproteins that are most abundant with different isoforms playing distinct roles. The gene defect has been associated with corneal diseases such as keratoconus, Fuchs dystrophy, and bullous keratopathy. Fibronectin, thrombospondin, matrilin, tenascin C, and nidogens 1 and 2 are the other major basement membrane matrix proteins that act as link proteins to laminin. The anchored proteoglycans such as perlecan, a complex multi-domain HSPG, can bind to various but discrete molecules. It regulates the availability of fibroblast growth factors (FGF), bone morphogenic proteins (BMP), platelet-derived growth factor (PDGF), vascular endothelial growth factors (VEGF), transforming growth factor β-1 (TGF-β1), and insulin-like growth factors (IGF) to bind to their receptors thereby mediates the cell signaling for migration, proliferation, and differentiation of a variety of cells. Perlecan is crucial for corneal epithelium formation and differentiation. Perlecan-deficient mice show epithelial defects. Mutations are reported in integrin, keratins, collagen subtypes, laminin, and many of the basement membrane proteins (Alarcon et al. 2009; Torricelli et al. 2013).

The hemidesmosome (HD) link is a complex of extracellular transmembrane and cytoplasmic molecules that form structural link between the intracellular keratin intermediate filament of cytoskeleton of the basal epithelial cell and the underlying basement membrane. The basement membrane zone has the hemidesmosome and the lamina lucida and lamina densa, which is the uppermost region of the stroma (Borradori and Sonnenberg 1999). Basement membrane normally functions as a barrier to the penetration of epithelial TGF-β1 and PDGF into the stroma. Loss of basement membrane leads to penetration of these factors that promote myofibroblasts development. Thus, basement membrane functions as the regulating barrier, limiting the fibrotic responses in injury, by regulating molecular interaction between the epithelium and the stroma. It plays a role in maintaining homeostasis of the matrix by downregulating wound healing signaling, modulation of epithelial cell growth proliferation and differentiation (Singh et al. 2011). Basement membrane also acts as a barrier to the bacterial penetration (Alarcon et al. 2009).

5.1.6 Descemet's Membrane

Descemet's membrane is a thick basement membrane (5–10 μm). Descemet's membrane like other basement membranes consists of two distinct layers, a posterior layer adjacent to the endothelium and an anterior layer formed by collagen lamellae and proteoglycans (Kabosova et al. 2007).

5.1.7 *Innervations in Cornea*

An important characteristic of the cornea is its heavy innervations, with around 300 times the number of nerve endings per square mm of the skin. These are sensory nerves derived from the ciliary nerves of the trigeminal ganglion ophthalmic branch. The nerves penetrate the cornea through the peripheral stroma in a radial pattern and shed their myelin sheet, surrounded only by Schwann cell sheaths. They subdivide several times into smaller side branch and then advance to the epithelium to form the basal epithelial nerve plexes. The absence of a myelin sheath on central corneal axons is necessary to maintain corneal transparency. Corneal nerves exert a trophic effect on the epithelium and maintain the health of corneal epithelium. Dysfunction of the nerve causes degenerative neurotrophic keratitis resulting in decreased mitotic activity of the basal epithelial cells, decreased epithelial thickness, increased epithelial permeability, loss of cellular glycogen stores, decreased oxygen uptake rates, and altered hypoxic swelling responses. Table 5.1 shows the various trophic factors released by the corneal nerve endings and their response (Muller et al. 2003).

Table 5.1 Neuropeptides and nerve growth factors in the cornea

S. No.	Name of the factor	Effect/acts on	Reference
1	Substance P	Stimulation of corneal epithelial cell proliferation	Garcia-Hirschfeld et al. (1994)
		Migration	Nishida et al. (1996)
		Adhesion	Nakamura et al. (1998a, b), Chikama et al. (1999), Araki-Sasaki et al. (2000)
2	Calcitonin gene-related peptide	Colocalizes with SP in ocular nerve fibers; epithelial renewal and wound repair	Jones and Marfurt (1991, 1998), Muller and Klooster (2001) Mertaniemi et al. (1995)
3	Norepinephrine	Stimulates corneal epithelial cell proliferation and migration	Voaden (1971), Murphy et al. (1998)
		Some other studies suggest that adrenergic nerves exert inhibitory influences on epithelial cell proliferation and migration	Friedenwald and Buschke (1944), Reidy et al. (1994)
	Catecholamines	Stimulate epithelial chloride ion transport from stroma to tears in rabbit cornea	Klyce and Crosson (1985)

(continued)

Table 5.1 (continued)

S. No.	Name of the factor	Effect/acts on	Reference
4	Acetylcholine	Stimulates epithelial cell DNA synthesis	Cavanagh and Colley (1982), Colley et al. (1985)
		Increases cyclic GMP production	Cavanagh and Colley (1982) Walkenbach and Ye (1991)
		Activates the phosphoinositide cycle	Proia et al. (1986)
		Cholinergic stimulation of keratinocytes, promotes cell-to-cell cell-to-substrate adhesion and cell motility	Grando et al. (1995), Zia et al. (1997)
5	Vasoactive intestinal polypeptide	Stimulates corneal epithelial cell production of nerve growth factor	Campbell et al. (2001)
6	Neurotensin	Increases keratocyte proliferation and viability and decreases keratocyte apoptosis in cultured human corneal keratocytes	Bourcier et al. (2002)
7	Met-enkephalin	An inhibitor of wound healing	Zagon et al. (1998)
8	Neurotrophin 3 (NT-3) Neurotrophin 4/5 (NT-4) Brain-derived neurotrophic factor (BDNF)	Binds with TrkB and initiates signal transduction cascade leading to gene transcription	Patapoutian et al. (1999), Dechant and Barde (2002)
9	Nerve growth factor	Homeostasis and regeneration of epithelium and stroma in human cornea	Lambiase et al. (1998, 2000)
		Anti-inflammatory and healing promoting in murine immune corneal ulcers with stromal melting	Bonini et al. (2000)
		Enhances migration of corneal epithelial cells for wound healing	Murphy et al. (2001)
		Regulate corneal epithelial stem cells	Schermer et al. (1986), Touhami et al. (2002)
10	Ciliary neurotrophic factor	Released in response to oxidative stress by corneal Endothelial cells via VIP synthesis in sympathetic ganglia	Koh (2002), Koh and Waschek (2000), Pitts et al. (2001)
		Neurite outgrowth of peripheral sensory nerves	White et al. (2000)
11	Glial cell-derived neurotrophic factor	Synthesized by keratocytes in stroma to modulate the function of corneal epithelial cells	You et al. (2001), Ebner et al. (2001)
		Migration of corneal epithelial cells in Boyden chambers and in an in vitro wound healing assay and induced MAP-kinase signaling	

5.1.8 Innate Immunity of the Cornea

Though the cornea is avascular, during injury there is an inflammatory response characterized by stromal cell infiltration of polymorphonuclear neutrophils (PMNs) that come from the limbal vessels followed by a cascade of events involving anti-inflammatory mediators. If inflammation is not resolved, then corneal fibrosis, pigmentation, and neovascularization take place, resulting in corneal scarring and disruption of the blood ocular barrier, resulting in chronic immune-mediated uveitis (Grahn and Cullen 2000).

Ocular immune system protects the eye from infection and regulates healing processes following injuries. The eye is an immune-privileged site and is endowed with remarkable properties that permit the long-term survival of foreign tumor and tissue grafts due to multiple anatomical, physiological, and immunoregulatory processes. Innate immune responses provide an inherent barrier against corneal infection while also serving as a primary mode of defense that is present from birth. The most evident is the tear film that coats the cornea and conjunctiva and serves several important functions such as lubrication, supply of oxygen, and protection against a range of potential pathogens. Ocular tissues and fluids express a wide variety of anti-inflammatory and immunosuppressive molecules, including lysozyme, lactoferrin, lipocalin, calcitonin gene-related peptide, somatostatin, and complement regulatory proteins. Table 5.2 lists the various antimicrobial proteins and peptides in the tear.

Toll-like receptors present at the ocular surface render additional immune barrier by triggering the earliest immune response to the invading pathogens. The TLRs act by modulating the adaptive immune response which is mediated by MyD88 (myeloid differentiation factor 88). Additionally, certain TLRs can also induce TRIF {TIR [Toll/IL (interleukin)-1 receptor] domain-containing adaptor protein which induces IFN (interferon) β}-dependent signaling (Kenny and O'Neill 2008). The activation of these intracellular signaling pathways induces the expression of cytokines, chemokines, and adhesion molecules.

Around, 10 TLRs (TLR1–TLR10) have been shown to be present in humans (Akira et al. 2001; Yu and Hazlett 2006). Different TLRs play a key role in the regulation of the response to infectious agents in the cornea: TLR4 and TLR5 are involved in Gram-negative; TLR2 in Gram-positive bacterial infections, TLR2 and TLR4 are activated in fungal keratitis; TLR3, TLR7, and TLR8 are involved in viral infections. Both the bacterial and viral genomes are able to activate a TLR9 response. Lambiase et al. have reviewed the scope of toll-like receptors at ocular surface (Lambiase et al. 2011).

Reports suggest that TLRs may become therapeutic targets in inflammatory ocular diseases, associated with the possibility to use extracellular TLR agonists. Pharmacological modulation of TLR intracellular signaling pathways may allow novel therapeutic strategies for avoiding the detrimental effects of prolonged inflammation at the ocular surface. The evaluation of TLR-modulating molecules in human diseases has already started with several ongoing clinical trials (Hennessy et al. 2010). There is a rapidly growing literature on TLRs in the cornea and conjunctiva, opening the possibility of targeting these molecules in the management of ocular surface diseases.

Table 5.2 Antimicrobial proteins and peptides in tear

Protein/peptide	Composition	Effective against	Mode of action	References
Lysozyme	20–30 %	Gram-positive bacteria	Hydrolysis of 1,4-beta-linkages between *N*-acetylmuramic acid and *N*-acetyl-D-glucosamine in the peptidoglycan	Sack et al. (2001) Aho et al. (1996) Albert (2008)
		Fungi	Cleaves chitodextrins in fungal cell wall	Lee-Huang et al. (1999)
Lactoferrin	20–30 %	Bacteria, fungi, and viruses	Binds divalent cations including iron depriving the bacteria of essential growth nutrient Acts as cationic detergent and disrupts the cell membrane of some bacteria, fungi, and virus	Janssen and van Bijsterveld (1983) Sack et al. (2001) Farnaud and Evans (2003)
Lipocalin	25 % reflex tear	Bacteria and fungi	Binds to microbial siderophores Protects ocular surface from microbial cysteine proteases	van't Hof et al. (1997), Fluckinger et al. (2004) Dartt (2011)
Secretory Immunoglobulin A	Major Ig in tear		Neutralize pathogen preventing their host attachment Binds to lectin-like adhesion molecule of pathogens Chemotactic to phagocytic neutrophils	Lan et al. (1998, 1999), Campos-Rodriguez et al. (2004), Mantis et al. (2011)
Complement fragments	Low levels in basal tear. Not present in reflex tear		Alternate complement pathway activation leading to formation of membrane attack complex	Willcox et al. (1997)
Cytokeratin 6A		Bacteria	Induce cell wall/membrane permeabilization, inhibit bacterial motility	Tam et al. (2012)

Table 5.2 (continued)

Protein/peptide	Composition	Effective against	Mode of action	References
Secretory phospholipase A (sPLA2)	Major tear protein	Gram-positive bacteria	Binds to the anionic bacterial surface, kills via its lipolytic enzymatic activity. hydrolyzes the sn-2-fatty acyl moiety from phospholipids	Buckland et al. (2000) Nevalainen et al. (2008)
Secretory leukocyte protease inhibitor (SLPI)	Reflex tears, higher amount in closed eye tears	Active against both Gram-positive and negative bacteria, fungi, and HIV	High cationic charge, binds anionic bacterial surface, inhibits neutrophil elastase	Franken et al. (1989) Sallenave (2010), Sathe et al. (1998)
Elafin	Low concentration	Bacteria	Directly antimicrobial	Sallenave (2010)
Bactericidal/ permeability-increasing protein (BPI)	Low concentration	Gram-negative bacteria	Bind LPS and kill	Peuravuori et al. (2006) Holweg et al. (2011)
β-lysin		Gram-positive bacteria	Targets the bacterial cell membrane. Inhibits bacterial catalase and peroxidase	Ford et al. (1976)
Surfactant protein (SP) A and D [members of C-type collectins)		Gram-negative bacteria	Bind pathogens and regulate host defense, block microbial traversal in the cornea	Wu et al. (2003) Ni et al. (2005), Awasthi (2010), Alarcon et al. (2011)
Antimicrobial peptides (AMPs) (<50 amino acids)		Bacteria	Disruption of microbial cell membranes leading to cell death	Choi et al. (2012)
α-Defensins, β- defensins	Basal and reflex tears		Direct antimicrobial activity	Haynes et al. (1999), Garreis et al. (2010)
Glycoproteins				
MUC1, MUC4, MUC16 Gel-forming MUC5Ac			Trap pathogens helping to move them to the lacrimal drainage pathway, facilitating their removal from the surface	Paulsen and Berry (2006), Spurr-Michaud et al. (2007), Mantelli and Argueso (2008)

5.1.9 Growth Factors in Corneal Wound Healing

5.1.9.1 Epithelial Growth Factor (EGF)

It is a family of 13 growth factors that includes EGF, TGF-α, and heparin binding EGF (HB-EGF). The receptor, namely, EGFR, acts as a cell surface receptor. Four related receptor tyrosine kinases include EGFR/erbB1/HER1, erbB2/HER2, erbB3/HER3, and erbB4/HER4 (Schultz et al. 1991), all of which have been detected in the corneal epithelium. EGF is secreted by platelets, macrophages, and fibroblasts and act on epithelial cells (Hynes et al. 2001). Heterodimerization of EGF receptor tyrosine kinases results in the activation of the signaling cascade resulting in corneal epithelial migration, thereby promoting epithelial wound healing (Fig. 5.3).

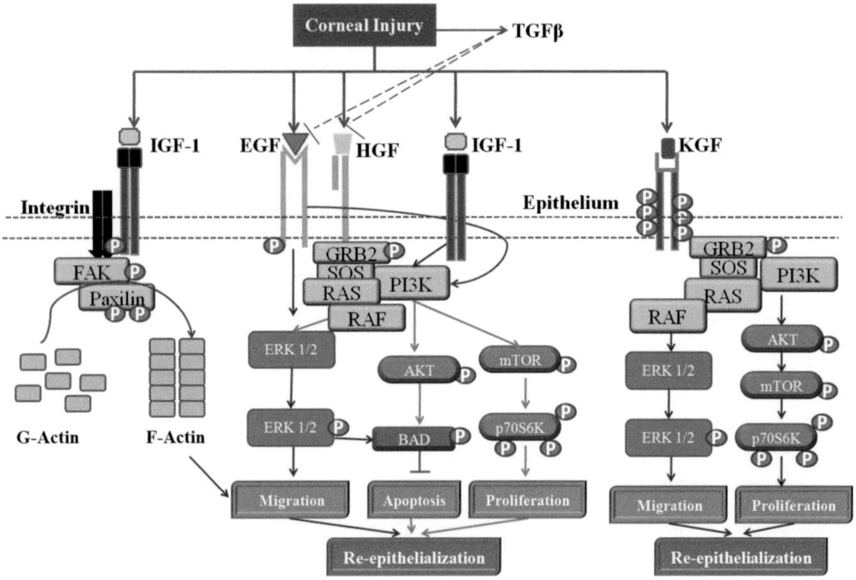

Fig. 5.3 Interplay of Growth factors in Corneal Wound healing: The growth factors, EGF, HGF, KGF and IGF-1 promotes cell proliferation through the activation of the Pi3K-AKT pathway. EGF enhances migration through the ERK1/2 pathway. IGF-1 and Substance-P (S-P) synergistically activate integrin-5 mediated actin polymerization via Fak-Paxilin t promote migration of the epithelial cells. KGF in limbal epithelium promotes migration and proliferation through the ERK1/2 and PI3K pathway. TGFβ secreted by epithelium can prevent re-epithelization by inhibiting EGF and HGF signaling

5.1.9.2 Keratinocyte Growth Factor (KGF)

Keratinocyte growth factor (28 kDa), a fibroblast growth factor known as FGF-7, is a potent mitogen for the corneal epithelial cells. It is produced by the conjunctival and the stromal fibroblasts (Wilson et al. 1999). However, KGF exerts paracrine effect on the corneal and the limbal epithelial cells, increases cell proliferation, thereby promoting wound healing effect. KGF activates Ras-MAPK and PI3K/p70 S6 pathways in the corneal epithelial cells and the p38 pathway in the limbal epithelial cells (Chandrasekher et al. 2001; Cheng et al. 2009).

5.1.9.3 Hepatocyte Growth Factor (HGF)

Hepatocyte growth factor (69 kDa of α-chain and a 34 kDa of β-chain) produced by mesenchymal cells stimulates the tyrosine activity of high-affinity receptor, c-Met, a proto-oncogene product expressed in epithelial cells (Bottaro et al. 1991). HGF is produced mainly by fibroblasts and has a paracrine action on the epithelium. While KGF is produced in the limbal cornea, HGF is produced more centrally. HGF-facilitates corneal epithelial cell migration and proliferation and inhibits apoptosis (Yu et al. 2010). HGF activates Ras-MAPK pathways via the receptor-Grb2/Sos complex (Liang et al. 1998). HGF is also reported to transactivate EGFR (Spix et al. 2007).

5.1.9.4 Insulin-like Growth Factor-1 (IGF-1)

Insulin-like growth factor-1 and its receptors are expressed by both epithelial cells and fibroblasts of the cornea (Li and Tseng 1995). IGF has been shown to induce all migration through activation of PI3K/AKT pathway, while in corneal epithelial cell it enhances proliferation and inhibits apoptosis (Lee et al. 2006). IGF-1 increases chemotaxis in the corneal fibroblasts (Yanai et al. 2006). IGF seems to have a synergistic effect with substance P in corneal wound healing (Nakamura et al. 1997) and upregulates FAK, paxilllin, and integrin alpha 5 (Nakamura et al. 1998a, b). IGF also a plays a role in cell communication via gap junctions through connexin 43 expression in fibroblasts (Ko et al. 2009). Insulin is present in human tear film, and its receptors are seen in the corneal epithelial, keratocytes, and conjunctival cells. Systemic and topical application of insulin promotes re-epithelialization in the cornea.

5.1.9.5 Transforming Growth Factor-β (TGF-β)

TGF-β family has three members, TGF-β1, TGF-β2, and TGF-β3. They regulate cell proliferation, extracellular matrix synthesis, angiogenesis, immune response, apoptosis, and differentiation (Andresen and Ehlers 1998; Roberts 2002). Latent

TGF-β binding proteins (LTBPs) regulate TGF-β bioavailability, activity, and secretion. TGF-β 1 and TGF-β 2 are seen in the corneal epithelium and stroma and tear fluid with higher levels of TGF-β2. The TGF-β receptors RI and RII are located in the epithelial, stromal, and endothelial layers of the cornea (Andresen et al. 1997; Nishida et al. 1994). While TGF-β1 and TGF-β 2 inhibit corneal, endothelial cell proliferation, they stimulate stromal fibroblast proliferation (Yanai et al. 2006; Kay et al. 1998). TGF-β1 delays re-epithelialization, increases keratocyte proliferation, and promotes myofibroblast differentiation. It increases the connective tissue growth factor (CTGF) levels and ends up in increased collagen synthesis and scar formation as seen in the corneal fibroblasts (Folger et al. 2001). Corneal fibrosis and haze in Photorefractive Keratectomy (PRK) is inhibited by TGF- β inhibition as shown in rabbits (Jester et al. 1997).

Corneal epithelial cell proliferation promoted by KGF and HGF is inhibited by TGF-beta, while in keratocytes it promotes the growth-promoting effect of EGF, thus functioning based on other growth factors in the environment. EGFR is transactivated by GPCR (G protein-coupled receptor), a central mediator that converges multiple extracellular signals in corneal epithelial wound healing. The two major signaling pathways are ERK and PI3K/AKT. Non-EGF family growth factors, namely, insulin, IGF, and HGF, also activate ERK and PI3K pathways in endothelial cells (Hongo et al. 1992; Honma et al. 1997).

Chemical signals in the injury process are the cellular proteins now termed as "alarmins," that include high mobility group box 1 and heat shock proteins, antimicrobial peptides at the site of injury as a defense to inhibit further damage by release of lipid autocoids, lysophosphatidic acid, adenosine, and other nucleotides which can further act as alarmins (Yu et al. 2010). Many purinoreceptors are expressed by the corneal epithelial cells. Release of high levels of ATP by the injured cells can activate the P2Y receptors that results in EGFR transactivation via GPCR activation and calcium wave signaling that in turn promotes wound healing (Yin et al. 2007).

5.1.10 Lipids in Cornea

The neutral lipids form the major composition in human cornea, which is 34 %. This includes cholesterol, cholesterol esters, and triglycerides followed by the sphingolipids (24 %) and the gangliosides (10 %) (Feldman 1967). The phospholipids in cornea include phosphatidyl choline, phosphatidyl ethanolamine, and sphingomyelins (Rodrigues et al. 1983). The fatty acids predominantly seen are oleic acid, palmitic acid, and stearic acid (Tschetter 1966).

The tear film lipid layer consists of a mixture of nonpolar lipids (wax esters, cholesterol, and cholesterol esters), which is 60–70 % of the layer; the rest is composed of phospholipids, glycolipids, and a small amount of free fatty acids, including omega fatty acids and mono- and diglycerides (Andrews 1970; Tiffany

1987). Tear lipids arrive from meibomian glands and the accessory sebaceous gland of Zeis. The phospholipids secreted by the meibomian gland act as amphiphilic molecules to form an interphase between the outer nonpolar lipid layer and the inner aqueous layer (Pucker and Haworth 2015). Dietary intake of omega fatty acids and its topical application is shown to be effective against dry eye (Roncone et al. 2010).

Corneal arcus results from lipid infiltration into the peripheral cornea in humans. These lipids are cholesterol-rich lipid particles deficient in apolipoprotein (apo)-B (Cogan and Kuwabara 1959). Lipid keratopathy is another condition common in women, often associated with hypercholesterolemia with cholesterol esters as droplets deposited in the stroma by lipid-overloaded fibroblasts (Gaynor et al. 1996). Corneal neovascularization can pave way for lipid access to the cornea; herpetic keratitis and chemical injuries produce severe lipid keratopathy (Forsius 1961). Another disease, granular corneal dystrophy, an autosomal dominant heritable condition, is characterized by granular deposits in the cornea and shows an increase in phospholipids with no changes in cholesterol (Rodrigues et al. 1983). Lipids are known to be involved in the pathology of dry eye with the loss of the lipid layer thickness being associated with the severity of the dry eye (Foulks 2007).

Injury to the cornea stimulates the release of platelet activation factor (PAF), a bioactive lipid that activates phospholipoase A2 (PLA2). This results in the release of arachidonic acid (AA) as well as its conversion to prostaglandins (PGD), thromboxanes (TX), and lipoxygenase (LOX) derivatives (Bazan 1987; Bazan et al. 1985a, b) in all the three layers of the cornea. Cycloxygenase-1 (COX-1) is expressed throughout the cornea, whereas COX-2 is predominantly expressed close to the wound (Amico et al. 2004). Laser in situ keratomileusis (LASIK), which damages the stroma, induces expression of COX-2 in the central epithelium and in the keratocytes adjacent to the wound (Miyamoto et al. 2004). COX-2 metabolites contribute to tissue damage and neovascularization. LOX derivatives from arachidonic acid, 12- and 15-hydroxy/hydroperoxy eicosatetraenoic acids, and lipoxin A4 resolvins (RvE1) from eicosapentaenoic acid (EPA) and neuroprotectin D1 (NPD1) from docosahexaenoic acid (DHA) potentiate repair and regeneration. Stimulation of the cornea with pigment epithelial-derived factor in the presence of DHA gives rise to the synthesis of NPD1, a derivative of LOX activity, and increases regeneration of corneal nerves (Kenchegowda and Bazan 2010).

15-hydroxy/hydroperoxyeicosatetraenoic acid [15(S)-HETE] formed from arachidonic acid (AA) by LOX action has a protecting effect from the dry eye (Gamache et al. 2002) and promotes mucin secretion (Jackson et al. 2001). While LOX derivatives are protective agents in the cornea, PAF plays a central role in mediating corneal inflammation, cell death, and neovascularization.

Corneal injury causes altered levels of growth factors that activate 12/15-LOX. Prostaglandins show a variety of effects in cornea through the eicosanoids (Table 5.3). A balance of pro- and anti-inflammatory levels of bioactive lipids decides the fate of corneal injury.

Table 5.3 Lipid mediators in corneal injury

Lipid	Source/site of action	Mode of action	References
Eicosanoids: PGD2	Conjunctival epithelium	Causes epithelial defects though chemotaxis of eosinophils in the conjunctiva.	Fujishima et al. (2005)
PGE2	Corneal endothelium Myofibroblasts	Inhibit endothelial cell proliferation. Causes corneal nerve stimulation.	Kawamura et al. (2008), Chen et al. (2003), Belmonte et al. (2004)
Prostaglandins (PG): Cytosolic PLA2 (cPLA2) α and γ; secretory PLA2s (sPLA): GIII, GX, and GXIIIA	Seen in the corneal epithelium and tears PLA2 activation occurs in the epithelium after stimulation by platelet-activated factor (PAF)	Provides antibacterial protection after corneal injury. cPLA2α releases. In corneal injury that increases COX and LOX metabolites. PAF, a bioactive lipid that activates PLA2 increases after corneal injury. Activators of MMPs in the cornea and conjunctiva.	Landreville et al. (2004) Hurst and Bazan (1995) Bazan et al. (1991) Ottino and Bazan (2001)
Oxidized lipids HETEs: 15(S)-HETE: a product of 15-lipoxygenase (LOX) Other oxidized lipids: leukotrienes, lipoxins, and hepoxilins Lipoxin A4 (LxA4), another product of 12/15-LOX	Corneal epithelium Human and monkey corneas express 15-LOX-1 in the cytoplasm and 15-LOX-2 in the cytoplasm and nucleus of mouse/rabbit corneas ALX in human corneal endothelial cells	HETE brings about PKC alpha translocation to plasma membrane via MAPK/ERK and cPlA2 when stimulated by EGF. HGF. 12(S)- and 15(S)-HETEs act as lipid mediators in the cornea for the proliferation. EGF released after corneal injury increases epithelial proliferation through induction of 12/15-LOX. Stimulate epithelial wound healing LxA4 synthesis is stimulated by EGF. LxA4 and epi-LxA4 act through a G protein-coupled receptor (ALX/FPR2).	Sharma et al. (2005) Liminga et al. (1994), Ottino et al. (2003) Wilson et al. (1994, 1999) Gronert et al. (2005) Kenchegowda et al. (2009), He et al. (2008)
Cytochrome P450 monooxygenase: two main compounds are formed: 12-R-hydroxyeicosatetraenoic acid [12(R)-HETE], and its degraded product, 12-R-hydroxyeicosatrienoic acid [12(R)-HETrE]	Cornea and tear	12(R)- HETrE is a potent inflammatory and angiogenic mediator in hypoxia (contact lens wear/chemical injuries) in the cornea. Increases in human tears during inflammation. These compounds diffuse across the stroma and inhibit the endothelial Na^+/K^+ -ATPase.	Schwartzman et al. (1985), Conners et al. (1995, 1997) Mieyal et al. (2001), Williams et al. (1996)

Platelet activation factor (PAF)	All corneal cells except fibroblasts. It is increased by growth factors that are upregulated in injury: KGF, TGF-beta, and HGF	Inflammatory mediator through PAF-R receptor coupled to G proteins. Inhibits epithelial wound healing PAF activates MMP-1, MMP-9, and uPA PAF attracts PMNs and other leukocytes to the site of injury PAF activates MAPK-ERK1/2 PAF also triggers the Ca^{2+} influx in corneal epithelial cells that could also be involved in cPLA2 activation PAF induces stromal keratocyte apoptosis by activation of NF-κB	Sugimoto et al. (1992), Ma and Bazan (2000) Bazan et al. (1993), Bazan and Ottino (2002), Tao et al. (1995, 1996) He et al. (2006) Bazan and Varner (1997), Bazan et al. (1997), Wilson and Kim (1998) Ma (2001)
ω-3 Fatty acids and their derivatives α-Linolenic acid and to the elongation and desaturation products: eicosapentaenoic acid (20:5, EPA) and docosahexaenoic acid (22:6, DHA) Derivatives of EPA: 5,12,18-R-trihydroxy-eicosapentaenoic acid called resolvin E1 (RvE1) DHA derivative: neuroprotectin D1 (NPD1: 10R, 17S-dihydroxy-docosa-4Z,7Z,11E,13E,15Z,19Z- hexaenoic acid)	Animal models: corneal inflammation Dry eye In the cornea, DHA is a minor component of membrane phospholipids In the cornea, neurotrophins as well as the corresponding Trk-receptors are expressed in epithelial cells and keratocytes	Blocks PMN infiltration and reduces leukocyte-mediated tissue injury Increases tear production as well as epithelial cell density Reduces corneal neovascularization by reducing infiltrated neutrophils/macrophages and the gene expression of inflammatory cytokines A role in regenerating corneal innervation and has a synergistic effect with PEDF Promotes epithelial cell proliferation	Serhan et al. (2008) Li et al. (2008), ARVO Serhan et al. (2008), Esquenazi et al. (2005) Cortina et al. (2010) Lambiase et al. (2000), Cortina et al. (2010), Bazan and Bazan (1984)

5.1.11 The Lacrimal Functional Unit and the Tear Film Dynamics

The tear film is considered a vital structure whose main role is to protect the ocular surface from external environment, infectious agents, and desiccation. The multiple functions of tear fluids include: lubrication of the eyelids, formation of a smooth and even layer over the cornea and conjunctiva, providing antibacterial systems for the ocular surface and nutrients for the epithelium, act as a vehicle for the entry of polymorphonuclear leukocytes in case of injury, and washing away the toxic irritants (Lemp and Blackman 1981; Braun et al. 2015).

Tear film is a trilaminar structure consisting of: (1) a thin anterior lipid layer (0.1 μ) originating from the meibomian glands which contains both polar and nonpolar lipids; (2) an intermediate aqueous layer (7 μ) originating from the lacrimal glands, which contains water soluble substances, including electrolytes, proteins, retinol, immunoglobulins, and enzymes- and (3) innermost mucous layer (0.02–0.04 μ) – secreted by conjunctival goblet cells and lacrimal gland acinar cells and containing components loosely bound to glycocalyx of the corneal and conjunctival epithelial cells.

Tear is composed of 98 % water and 2 % solids, like proteins, lipids, carbohydrates, and salts. The total tear volume produced is around 6.2 μl, ranging from 3.4 to 10.7 μl. The thickness of tear film is 6–7 μm; the pH slightly basic, i.e., 7.5; and the osmolarity is 300–334 milli osmolar (Jordan and Baum 1980). Sodium, potassium, chloride, bicarbonate, magnesium, and calcium salts are found in the tear. The chloride concentration is more in tears compared to the serum (Van Haeringen 1981). Tear has metabolites such as glucose, urea, lactate, pyruvate, ascorbate, retinol, free amino acids, uric acid and bilirubin.

The tear film is thus a complex mixture of proteins, lipids, mucus, salts, enzymes, and other metabolites produced from multiple sources such as the lacrimal gland, meibomian gland, goblet cells, and accessory lacrimal glands of the ocular surface. Glands of Krause located in the lamina propria of the conjunctival fornices (superior and inferior), Moll glands at the base of the lashes anterior to the meibomian glands and Wolfring located above the superior border of the upper lid tarsus contributes to the secretion of components into the lacrimal fluid (Lamberts et al. 1994). The lacrimal gland is a paired, almond-shaped gland, one for each eye that secretes the aqueous layer of the tear film. They are situated in the upper, outer portion of each orbit, in the lacrimal fossa of the orbit formed by the frontal bone (Walcott 1998). The lacrimal glands secrete lacrimal fluid as a result of neuronal stimuli, which flows through the main excretory ducts into the space between the eyeball and lids and during blinking of eyes. The lacrimal fluid is spread across the surface of the eye accumulating in the lacrimal lake and is drawn into the puncta by capillary action, flowing through the lacrimal canaliculi to the inner corner of the eyelids entering the lacrimal sac, then to the nasolacrimal duct, and then finally into the nasal cavity. Lacrimal functional unit (LFU) is an integrated system including lacrimal gland, ocular surface, lids, and sensory and motor nerves, to carry out its function. The lacrimal glands consist of a tubular secretory epithelium organized into lobes that drain into ducts. It is a multilobular tissue composed of acinar, ductal, and myoepithelial cells. The acinar cells account for 80 % of the cells present in the lacrimal gland and are the sites for synthesis, storage, and secretion of proteins. Several tear proteins like lysozyme, lactoferrin, growth factors such as epidermal growth factor and transforming growth factor are crucial to the homeostasis of the ocular surface.

Ductal cells: These cells modify the primary fluid secreted by the acinar cells to secrete water and electrolytes. Myoepithelial cells contain multiple processes, which surround the basal area of the acinar and ductal cells. They contain a smooth muscle actin that helps to contract and force the fluid out of the ducts and onto the ocular surface similar to salivary and mammary glands. Other cell types present in the lacrimal gland includes plasma cells, B and T cells, dendritic cells, macrophages, bone marrow-derived monocytes, and mast cells. Immunoglobulin A (IgA)-positive plasma cells are the majority of the mononuclear cells in the lacrimal gland (Dua et al. 1994; Wieczorek et al. 1988). These cells synthesize and secrete IgA, which is then transported into acinar and ductal cells and are secreted by these epithelial cells as secretory IgA.

5.1.11.1 Neural Control of Tear Secretion

The lacrimal gland is innervated by the parasympathetic and sympathetic nervous system (Botelho et al. 1966; Sibony et al. 1988). Nerves are located in close proximity to acinar, ductal, and myoepithelial cells as well as blood vessels, and they control a wide variety of lacrimal gland functions (Botelho et al. 1966; Sibony et al. 1988). Stimulation of lacrimal gland secretion occurs through a neural reflex arc originating from the ocular surface (Botelho 1964). Stimuli to the ocular surface activate afferent sensory nerves in the cornea and conjunctiva which in turn activates efferent parasympathetic and sympathetic nerves in the lacrimal gland to stimulate secretion.

Neurotransmitters and neuropeptides released by the lacrimal gland nerves include acetylcholine, vasoactive intestinal peptide (VIP), norepinephrine, neuropeptide Y (NPY), substance P (SP), and calcitonin gene-related peptide (CGRP). These neuromediators interact with specific receptors present on the surface of lacrimal gland cells to initiate a specific response (Hodges and Dartt 2003). Acetylcholine and norepinephrine are the most potent stimuli of for the secretion of lacrimal gland proteins, water, and electrolytes (Dartt 2004; Hodges and Dartt 2003). Acetylcholine binds to cholinergic M3 muscarinic receptors, and norepinephrine binds to α- and β-adrenergic receptors (Hodges and Dartt 2003; Mauduit et al. 1993) leading to respective stimulation.

5.1.11.2 Hormonal Control of Tear Secretion

Hormones from the hypothalamic-pituitary-gonadal axis has a profound impact on lacrimal gland structure and function. Adrenocorticotropic hormone (ACTH), alpha-melanocyte-stimulating hormone (a-MSH), prolactin, androgens, estrogens, and progestins influence lacrimal gland functions (Leiba et al. 1990; Mircheff et al. 1992;

Sullivan et al. 1996). In addition, glucocorticoids, retinoic acid, insulin, and glucagon affect various aspects of the lacrimal gland (Petersen 1976; Rocha et al. 2000; Ubels et al. 1994). Arginine vasopressin, a peptide produced in the posterior pituitary, has physiologic role in fluid homeostasis, is present in the lacrimal gland acinar and ductal cells (Djeridane 1994). Androgens are potent hormones that stimulate the secretion of secretory IgA, an important component of the mucosal immune system of the eye (Sullivan et al. 1996). Androgens accounts for many of the gender-related differences seen in the lacrimal gland (Azzarolo et al. 1997; Sullivan et al. 1999).

Protein and water secretion by lacrimal gland (Walcott 1998): A number of proteins is synthesized and secreted by the lacrimal gland acinar cells. The secretion of these proteins is stimulated by the neurotransmitters and neuropeptides found in the neurons that innervate the gland (Dartt 2004). The acinar cells have receptors for acetylcholine (muscarinic M3), VIP, and norepinephrine and receptors for peptides of the proenkephalin family as well as other peptides such as neuropeptide Y, adrenocorticotropic hormone, and alpha-melanocyte-stimulating hormone. The acinar cells are extensively coupled by gap junctions. Second messengers produced by activation of these receptors, such as Ca^{2+} and inositol trisphosphate (IP3), diffuse from stimulated cells to adjacent non-stimulated ones, causing them to become activated, which further leads to protein secretion.

Water is the one of the major secretory products of the lacrimal gland. This water moves through the interstitial spaces of the gland into the lumen of the gland where it is mixed with the other secretory products. This water movement is accomplished by osmosis, which depends on the movement of ions from the acinar cells into the lumen (Dartt 2009). The acinar cell surface membrane is differentiated into basolateral and apical domain, which are separated by the junctional complex. The apical domain contains water channels (aquaporin 5), which facilitates the movement of water across the epithelium. In addition, Cl^- and K^+ channels are present to allow the movement of solute across the epithelium. The basolateral membranes contain large number of Na^+ pumps (Mircheff 1989), Na^+/K^+-ATPase, which actively move K^+ into the cell and Na^+ out of the cell, maintains the gradients. It is this gradient (more Na^+ outside and K^+ inside) that provides the motive force for the movement of ions and water across the epithelium. In addition, there are several coupled transport systems (porters) driven by the concentration gradients created by the Na^+ pump and by the activity of carbonic anhydrase. The basolateral membranes also have ion channels, specifically for K^+, Cl^-, and Ca^{2+} as well as more general cation and anion channels. This link between ion channels and their permeability and the movement of water may form the underlying mechanism of dry eyes.

5.1.11.3 Tear Proteins

Normal tears contain a total protein concentration of 6–10 mg/ml of tear and at least 80 tear proteins (Gachon et al. 1982) as reported. Major tear proteins include lysozyme, lactoferrin, secretory immunoglobulin A (sIg A), serum albumin (Li et al. 2005), lipocalin (Glasgow et al. 1995; Redl et al. 1992; Schoenwald et al. 1998), lipophilin (Lehrer et al. 1998) and tear-specific prealbumin (TSP), lacrimal proline-rich proteins (LPRR4) (Aluru et al. 2012), defensins, zinc-alpha-glycoprotein, mammaglogulins, and heat shock proteins originating from the lacrimal gland. Measured levels of proteins such as β2 microglobulin, cystatins, substance P, epidermal growth factor (EGF), transforming growth factor β1 and β2 (TGFβ1 and β2), plasmin, tryptase, and α1 antitrypsin change depending on the conditions. Other proteins include, mucins, antiproteinases, and bactericidal protein β-lysine (Ford et al. 1976). Growth factors, EGF, TGF-β1 and β2 are present in normal tear fluids and have been associated with corneal wound healing (Grus et al. 2001).

The glycoproteins in the tear includes orosomucoid, α1-glycoprotein, transferrin, ceruloplasmin, Zn-α2-glycoprotein, and mucous glycoproteins which contribute to the high viscous nature of the ocular mucus. The viscosity of human tears reduces during blinking, but between each blink it raises and thus stabilizes the tear film.

5.1.11.4 Tear Enzymes

A large number of enzymes including glucose-metabolizing enzymes, antiproteases, collagenases, matrixmetalloproteases, and other proteolytic enzymes are present in tears. During infections of the eye or in corneal ulcerations, the levels of some of these enzymes like α1-antitrypsin and α2-microglobulin are increased (Ford et al. 1976).

5.1.11.5 Tear Lipids

It includes free fatty acids, free sterols, triglycerides, diesters, polar lipids, and hydrocarbons. Meibomian secretion with its hydrophobic nature, functions as a barrier that prevents spill over of tears. The lipid layer reduces the rate of evaporation from an open eye, provides lubrication for the eyelid/ocular interface, and contributes to the optical properties of the tear film (McCulley and Shine 2001; McCulley and Shine 2003; Nicolaides et al. 1989).

5.1.12 Mucins in Tear

Glycoproteins are abundantly expressed, especially in the conjunctival cells and are abundantly found in tears. 424 glycogenes have been identified by the gene chip array of the conjunctival epithelium. Mucins are high-molecular-weight glycoproteins, and the carbohydrate-binding proteins form the major component of the tear glycoproteins (Mantelli and Argueso 2008). They have a characteristic property of tandem repeats of amino acids rich in serine and threonine to which O-glycan is attached (Gendler and Spicer 1995). Apical cell layers of the corneal epithelium produce mucin. MUC5AC is the major secreted mucin of the conjunctival goblet cells. The transmembrane mucins, MUC1, MUC4, and MUC16, are produced by the epithelium (Guzman-Aranguez et al. 2010).

Mucins along with galectin-3 promote barrier integrity and prevent bacterial adhesion. Galectin-3 is the most abundantly expressed carbohydrate-binding protein in human conjunctival epithelium, while galectin-8 and galectin-9 are found in much lower concentrations (Mantelli and Argueso 2008). Oligomerization of galectin-3 results in lattices that resist lateral movement of membrane components on the glycocalyx (Pablo Argüeso et al. 2013). Human tear mucins consist primarily of α2-6 sialyl core 1 (Galβ1-3GalNAcα1-Ser/Thr) (Guzman-Aranguez et al. 2009). However, in the conjunctiva, α2-3 sialyl core 1 is seen. The glycosylated mucins are hydrophilic and are responsible for the water-binding capacity that prevents ocular surface drying. In addition to mucins, glycosyltransferases, proteoglycans, glycan degradation proteins, and Notch signaling molecules are expressed on the ocular surface. They act as receptors for the pathogens, thereby trapping and removing pathogens from the epithelial surfaces. They prevent barrier function by preventing endocytosis (Guzman-Aranguez et al. 2012). Thus, lubrication and clearance of pathogens and debris are the major functions of the mucins and other glycoproteins in the tear.

5.2 Biochemistry of Lens

The lens of the vertebrate eye is a unique organ in that it is nonvascularized and noninnervated (Bloemendal 1981). The entire organ is composed of cells of surface ectodermal origin at various stages of differentiation surrounded by a basal lamina, the lens capsule (Duncan 1981; Bloemendal 1981). The epithelial cells ranging from 9 to 17 mm in diameter (Brown and Bron 1987) remain quiescent in the central epithelium (nondividing phase), surrounded by a germinative dividing zone of cells which divide toward the equatorial area (dividing phase) and terminally differentiate (differentiating phase) into long, transparent fiber cells in the equatorial region (Papaconstantinou 1967; Piatigorsky 1981). The transition of lens cortex into fiber cells during the developmental stages is characterized by biochemical changes which includes the synthesis of fiber-specific proteins, α- and β-crystallins, and arid morphologic changes such as cell elongation, loss of cellular organelles, and disintegration of the nucleus (Worgul et al. 1989). The single monolayer of anterior epithelial cells in the mature lens represents a very static population and is essential for maintaining the metabolic homeostasis and transparency of the entire lens (Spector et al. 1995). Anteriorly, they form an epithelial monolayer, while internally they are represented by shells of concentrically arranged fully differentiated fiber cells, which form the bulk of the lens (Winkler and Riley 1991). Thus, the lens continually grows throughout life and maintains its distinct polarity with the monolayer of epithelial cells covering only the anterior half of the fibers (McAvoy and Chamberlain 1989).

5.2.1 *Glucose Metabolism in the Lens*

The deeper fibers which make up most of the adult lens are organelle-free, while most of superficial fibers are metabolically active and are nucleated. Since the lens must be a transparent and colorless medium, the energy required for its growth and transparency is derived chiefly from glucose. To maintain transparency, the lens cannot be endowed with pigmented oxidative enzymes of the cytochrome system or the riboflavin-containing group. Thus, in the lens, glucose is catabolized primarily to lactic acid, and is not appreciably combusted to CO_2 (Kinoshita et al. 1961). Anaerobic glycolysis yields about 70 % of the ATP (Winkler and Riley 1991). Aerobic incubation done in the absence of glucose indicates that the aerobic phase of metabolism is capable of providing energy to a certain degree. To support the energy-utilizing mechanisms, the Krebs cycle and the oxygen-utilizing mechanisms are sufficiently active to consume enough endogenous substrates (Piere and van Heyningen 1956). The ability of the lens to synthesize sorbitol is an unusual feature of lens glucose metabolism. The lens is rendered a favorite site for sorbitol production due to reasons like high pentose shunt activities, relatively high aldose reductase, and low hexokinase (Van Hayningen 1962).

5.2.2 *Sorbitol Metabolism and Aldose Reductase*

During normoglycemia, glucose entering the cell is rapidly phosphorylated by the enzyme hexokinase and enters the Embden-Meyerhof pathway, providing the major aerobic energy source for the cell (Kador et al. 1985). This pathway is fully saturated at normal glucose levels, and hence if hyperglycemia occurs, the excessive glucose cannot be metabolized by this pathway. The enzyme aldose reductase (AR) has a much lower affinity for glucose than hexokinase, and significant amounts of glucose enter the sorbitol (or polyol) pathway only when its levels are raised. AR converts glucose to the alcohol sorbitol, which is then further oxidized to fructose by the enzyme sorbitol dehydrogenase (Kador et al. 1985)

5.2.3 *Transport of Fluid by Lens Epithelium*

The lens is an avascular tissue which is thought to be nourished by diffusion. Yet, the metabolic consumption of nutrients by the lens cannot be attributed to simple diffusion of nutrients into the lens (Harris et al. 1955). Studies have shown lens fibre cells membranes to be rich in ion channels (K^+, Na^+, Ca^{2+}), water channels (aquaporins), pumps (Na^+/K^+-ATPase) (Mathias and Rae 2004), and specific transporters for small molecules such as glucose and amino acids (Lim et al. 2006, 2007). Four mechanisms that govern the solute transfer from the aqueous and vitreous humors to the lens fibers in order of relevance are as follows:

(i) Na^+ -leak conductance drives the paracellular transport of water, small molecules, and ions along the intercellular spaces between epithelial and FCs.
(ii) Specific carriers and transporters to bring about membrane transport of such solutes from the intercellular spaces to the fiber cytoplasm.
(iii) Gap-junctional coupling mediating solute flux between superficial and deeper fibers, efflux of waste products in the equator, and electrical coupling of fibers driven by Na^+/K^+ -ATPase.
(iv) Caveoli and coated vesicles for the transcellular transfer (Paterson and Delamere 2004).

5.2.4 Lens Crystallins

The structural proteins abundantly seen in the lens that are evolutionarily related to stress proteins are the two crystallin gene families which comprise of the α-crystallins and the βγ-crystallins. α-Crystallins which possess chaperone-like activity in vitro are molecular chaperones that prevent aberrant protein interactions. Their activity includes remodeling and protecting the cytoskeleton, inhibition of apoptosis, and enhancement of the resistance of cells to stress. Binding to proapoptotic proteins such as p53 may be the possible mechanism of action for inhibition of apoptosis in lens (Jolly and Morimoto 2000); α -Crystallins are known to prevent undesired interactions and aggregation of cytoskeletal proteins (Horwitz 2003). Proteins of the βγ-crystallin family proteins are suggested to affect lens development, and its expression is seen in tissues outside the lens. Of the transcription factors regulating expression of different crystallin genes in lenses of different species, the most commonly studied are Pax-6, retinoic acid receptors, maf, Sox, CREB, and AP-1 (Cui et al. 2004; Cvekl and Piatigorsky 1996; Cvekl et al. 1994). Recent work demonstrates that targeted disruption of a DNA repair molecule, Nbs, affects transcription of crystallins (Yang et al. 2006).

5.2.5 Connexins in Lens

Connexins [Cx] are a family of membrane proteins that have two extracellular loops, one intracellular loop, four transmembrane domains and intracellular C as well as terminus N-terminus. In mammals, almost all cell types express one or more Cx isoforms. Cx43 is the most ubiquitous (Beyer et al. 1987; Dupont et al. 1988). Cx46 is present in lens (Paul et al. 1991) and lung (Abraham et al. 1999). Mammalian lens express three connexin isoforms. Cx43 and Cx50 is expressed by cortical epithelial cells (Dahm et al. 1999), whereas nuclear fiber cells express Cx46 and Cx50 (Tenbroek et al. 1992) and Cx50 (Kistler et al. 1985; White et al. 1992). Cx46 and Cx50 expressed by mature fiber cells are needed for the coupling of both peripheral and interior fiber cells (Baldo et al. 2001; Gong et al. 1998; Martinez-Wittinghan et al. 2004) and for maintaining lens transparency (Benedek 1971; Mathias et al. 1997; Hejtmancik 2008).

5.2.6 *Aquaporins in Lens*

The predominant membrane protein present in mature fibers is aquaporin 0 [AQP0], also called the major intrinsic protein [MIP]. AQP0 functions as a water channel at a pH of 6.5 and forms thin junctions of 11–13 nm thickness between the lens fibers at low calcium concentrations (Nemeth-Cahalan and Hall 2000); it also acts as an adhesion molecule interacting with Cx50 for the differentiation of lens fibers and to enhance gap junction formation (Engel et al. 2008; Kumari and Varadaraj 2009; Yu and Jiang 2004; Liu et al. 2011). Studies show that MIP (AQP0) expression in the adult bovine lens is seen in thin, asymmetric membrane interactions set apart from the thicker, symmetric junctions containing connexins (Gruijters et al. 1987).

5.2.7 *Apoptosis in Lens Epithelial Cells*

Programmed cell death or apoptosis is one of the features of the early steps in eye development associated with morphogenesis. Suppression of programmed cell death in the later stages is essential for tissue differentiation, and in the adult, factors inducing inflammatory cell apoptosis maintain the immune-privileged status of the eye (Lang 1997). Fibroblast growth factor is one of the components that acts during morphogenesis to bring about suppression of apoptosis in cells of the lens lineage (Bozanic et al. 2003). Human cataract patients have a significant percentage of apoptotic epithelial cells, while normal human lenses of similar age do not (Li et al. 1995a), and lens epithelial cell apoptosis can be activated by oxidative stress (Spector et al. 1995) and calcimycin (Li et al. 1995b) that cause cataract.

5.2.8 *Epithelial to Mesenchymal Transition (EMT)*

The transition process by which epithelial cells undergo phenotypic changes, acquire mesenchymal properties and increase their ability to migrate and/or synthesize interstitial matrices is called as EMT. In the lens, this happens commonly after injury as seen in cataract extraction, leading to fibrosis of the lens capsule. Wnt pathway has been shown to be involved in EMT and fibrosis of epithelial cells (He et al. 2009; Konigshoff et al. 2008). Wnt3a, a member of the Wnt family, is found to induce the accumulation of β-catenin and thereby the activation of the canonical Wnt signaling pathway (Nalesso et al. 2011). Transforming growth factor β (TGFβ) has been reported to induce the EMT of lens epithelial cells and promotes Wnt expression during cataract development (Chong et al. 2009).

5.2.9 Advanced Glycation End Products (AGE) in Aging Lens

Proteins when exposed to reducing sugars for a long time leads to accumulation of advanced glycation end products (AGEs) due to nonenzymatic glycation. Proteins like collagens and crystallins, which are long-lived are found to be subjected to this modification. This has been reported as the etiology in diseases like cataracts, diabetic complications, and arteriosclerosis. AGEs may alter cellular functions resulting in fibrosis in lens epithelial cells (Hong et al. 2000).

5.2.10 Antioxidants

Superoxide is converted to hydrogen peroxide by superoxide dismutases, in most tissues of the body, including the lens. Since hydrogen peroxide produces hydroxyl radical OH, it can become highly toxic. Catalase and glutathione peroxidase prevent this toxicity by a system of antioxidant molecules, wherein glutathione plays a vital role (Lou 2003). Ascorbate plays an important part in lens biology, both as an antioxidant and as a UV filter when present in aqueous medium (Varma et al. 1979; Hegde and Varma 2004; Devamanoharan et al. 1991).

5.3 Biochemistry of the Uvea

The uvea is otherwise called as uveal coat/tract or vascular tunic and is comprised of the iris, ciliary body, and choroid, of which the iris and ciliary body lie in the anterior segment, while the choroid spans the entire eye ball between the retina and sclera. The uveal vasculature functions for the nutrition and gas exchange by direct perfusion into the iris and ciliary body and indirectly to the lens, sclera, and retina. Moreover, the uvea helps in reducing the light reflection within the eye, by light absorption, and hence improves the image quality. The most important function of the uvea includes the secretion of aqueous humor by the ciliary process.

The inner surface of the ciliary body which has two layers of epithelium forms the aqueous humor. This epithelium has an inner nonpigmented layer and outer pigmented layer. The ciliary capillaries are highly fenestrated, and the ultrafiltrate of the blood fills the stroma which is formed by the active transport of ions. From the stroma, selective transport of solutes occurs producing osmotic flux producing the AH.

Uveitis is a group of intraocular disorders involving inflammation of the uvea and, in few cases, other related ocular structures that cause about 10 % of blindness (Agrawal et al. 2010), of which about 50 % have bilateral vision impairment (Durrani et al. 2004). Uveitis can be classified as anterior, intermediary, and posterior uveitis; iridocyclitis is the inflammation at the anterior uvea (iris and ciliary body). In case of inflammation of the iris alone, it is referred to as iritis. Inflammation at ciliary body is cyclitis, which is intermediate uveitis. Acute anterior uveitis starts with an intense inflammation around the cornea. The case of posterior uveitis may be bilateral, associated with painless loss of vision. When an inflammation in the vitreous is involved, floaters may be present that are aggregates of inflammatory cells suspended in the vitreous. Loss of vision may be generally due to cataract, opacity in the vitreous, chorioretinal scarring, cystoid macular edema, secondary glaucoma, retinal vascular occlusions, inflammatory optic neuropathy, and retinal detachment (Guly and Forrester 2010; Lowder and Char 1984). Posterior uveitis refers to inflammation in the choroid called as choroiditis, and when the adjacent layer to the uvea is also involved, the condition is termed as retinochoroiditis/uveoretinitis. When the retina is involved, in case of retinal blood vessels, it is called retinal vasculitis, vitritis (vitreous), and when the optic nerve is involved, it is papillitis (Char and Schlaegel 1982).

Various causes have been attributed to the onset of uveitis as drug induced, traumatic, infection induced, and autoimmunity. Uveitis in some cases is found to be generally coupled with many systemic diseases, namely, Behcet's syndrome, juvenile idiopathic arthritis, sarcoidosis, masquerade syndrome, and infectious diseases like tuberculosis. In about half the cases, it is considered to be idiopathic, and no systemic association is found. In such cases uveitis is presumed to be autoimmune (Rothova et al. 1992). The management of uveitis is determined by the presence or absence of infection or is noninfective and by the likelihood of a threat to sight (Guly and Forrester 2010). The immune response elicited to the infection is considered in part to be responsible for the inflammation and thus the consequent ocular damage and visual loss. Hence topical and systemic steroids are often used in addition to suppress inflammation in patients with infection-related uveitis.

5.3.1 Iris

The human iris is a thin, visible circular structure of eye responsible for controlling the diameter and size of the pupil, thus the amount of light reaching the retina. Iris bounds by the dark pupil and white sclera. It suspends in the aqueous humor behind the cornea but present in front of the lens (Davis-Silberman and Ashery-Padan 2008).

The iris divides the space between the lens and the cornea into the anterior chamber (between the cornea and the iris) and posterior chambers (between the iris and the lens). The periphery of the iris attaches to its root at the iridocorneal angle of the anterior chamber that merges with the tissue of the ciliary body and trabecular meshwork. The human iris formation begins at third month of gestation and completes by the 8 months of gestation, but the pigmentation continues till the first year after birth. The size of the iris varies from person to person with an average size of 12 mm in diameter ranges from 10.2 to 13.0 mm in diameter (Eagle 1988).

The iris consists of four layers:

1. The anterior layer
2. Stroma
3. Sphincter muscle fibers and dilator muscle fibers
4. The posterior pigment epithelium

The anterior layer is a visible part of the iris which is lightly pigmented. Heavily pigmented melanocytes are present in this layer. The stroma consists of loose connective tissue containing fibroblasts, melanocytes, and collagen fibers. The eye color depends on the melanin pigment content within the stroma and the anterior layer. The involuntary smooth muscle sphincter pupillae or circular muscle lies within the stroma, close to the pupil margin and is about 0.75–1 mm in diameter and 0.1–1.7 mm in thickness.

The dilator pupillae muscles (radial muscles) form a flat sheet beneath the stroma and extends from the iris to the sphincter. These two smooth muscles control the size of the pupil that regulates the amount of light entering the eye.

The posterior epithelium includes two layers of cells that are heavily pigmented. Both anterior and posterior surfaces of the iris provide highly complex and unique iris patterns to individuals. The iris is a well-protected organ, and the iris patterns are stable over many years. Therefore the iris pattern is suitable for individual identification (Eagle 1988).

The important reaction in iris epithelium is formation of melanin pigment. Synthesis of iris melanosome pigment melanin is initiated by converting tyrosine to dihydroxyphenylalanine by the enzyme tyrosinase. Mutation in tyrosinase gene results in ocular albinism.

Recent studies with iris organ culture shows, apart from the differential modulation of tyrosinase transcription, several other factors can contribute to the variability of iris darkening due to certain topical prostaglandin analog therapies. Other enzymes that are involved in the biosynthesis of melanin include 5, 6-dihydroxyindole carboxylic acid oxidase and dopachrome tautomerase. Differential expression of each of these enzymes also alters the formation of melanin. Therefore, variations in each of these serve as potential targets for modulating iridial melanocyte responsiveness to latanoprost (Lindsey et al. 2001).

Iris is the major site to produce prostaglandins that regulates various functions such as smooth muscle contraction, intraocular pressure, and blood-aqueous barrier penetration (Dröge et al. 2003).

Aniridia is a rare, congenital ocular disorder with the characteristics of incomplete formation of the iris caused by the mutations of the paired box gene-6 (PAX6) (Liu et al. 2015).

Fernández-López E et al. reported in their case study first time a sutureless artificial iris implant fixed in the ciliary sulcus after cataract surgery, and they suggest artificial iris will be a promising device for treating photophobia in congenital aniridia (Fernández-López et al. 2015).

5.3.2 Ciliary Body

Human ocular ciliary body (CB) is located between ora serreta and iris which is multifunctional. Ciliary body consists of ciliary muscle and epithelial layer. The epithelial layer is again in two forms, namely, pigmented epithelial layer (PE) and nonpigmented epithelial layer (NPE). The anterior portion of CB continues with iris epithelium; posteriorly NPE continues with neural retina and PE with retinal pigment epithelium. The important function of ciliary epithelium is to produce aqueous humor. Aqueous humor is required to build up the intraocular pressure (IOP) that maintains the eye shape and also nourishes avascular eye tissues, like the lens and cornea. Ciliary muscle helps for proper accommodation of lens (Janssen et al. 2012).

CB synthesizes and expresses multiple neuroendocrine proteins such as neurotensin, natriuretic peptides, and somatostatin, steroid-converting enzymes, transferrin, transthyretin, angiotensin, and growth factors(Coca-Prados and Escribano 2007); these endocrine molecules play role in regulating IOP, the composition of the aqueous humor. The ocular microenvironment of blood-aqueous barrier is anti-inflammatory, minimizes ocular tissue damage, and restores vision clarity (Taylor 2009). The aqueous humor is rich in soluble immunomodulatory factors produced by pigmented epithelium that includes CD86, TGF-beta, and TSP1 (Sugita 2009). NPE and PE also involved in a variety of metabolic process, including lipid and vitamin metabolism showed by gene functional studies. Janssen et al showed the gene expression profiles and functional annotations of the NPE and PE which were highly similar. They found that most important functionalities of the NPE and PE were related to developmental processes, neural nature of the tissue, endocrine and metabolic signaling, and immunological functions. A total of 1576 genes differed statistically significantly between NPE and PE. From these genes, at least 3 were cell specific for the NPE and 143 for the PE. They also observed high expression in the (N)PE of 35 genes that were previously implicated in molecular mechanisms related to glaucoma (Janssen et al. 2012). The CB is also involved in several pathologies. The most important are glaucoma, anterior uveitis/iridocyclitis, (pseudo) exfoliation syndrome, and uveal melanoma (Janssen et al. 2012).

Aqueous humor production depends on the interaction of complex mechanisms within the ciliary body that involves blood flow, transcapillary exchange, and transport processes in the ciliary epithelium.

The enzyme ATPase, present predominantly in nonpigmented epithelium (Cole 1964), is responsible for sodium transport to the posterior chamber and for aqueous formation. It is not a simple dialysate or ultrafiltrate of the blood plasma (Kinsey 1951). An active mechanism demanding high metabolic energy is required for the continuous aqueous production by the ciliary processes.

An ultrafiltration from the capillaries of ciliary processes together with secretory mechanism in the ciliary epithelium produces aqueous humor. The secretory mechanism involves active transport of electrolytes, coupled with fluid transport and carbonic anhydrase action. The produced aqueous humor consists of two chambers of unequal volume, the anterior and posterior and the communication between these two occurs through the pupil. Aqueous humor secreted by ciliary processes flows into the posterior chamber from which it flows into the anterior chamber and drains into extraocular venous systems (McCaa 1982).

5.3.2.1 Trabecular Meshwork

The aqueous outflow determining structure in the anterior chamber includes ciliary muscle and trabecular meshwork (TM). The TM and Schlemm's canal (SC) are located in the iridocorneal angle. SC is a circumferential channel which accounts for 70–90 % of AH outflow. The endothelial cell lining the SC is the major determinant of the intra ocular pressure (IOP) since it is the primary site of resistance to the AH outflow. It is recently speculated to have features of lymphatic and blood vascular nature (Ramos et al. 2007; Truong et al 2014). The TM is a porous connective tissue (300×50–150 μm) with a lamellar arrangement, and the SC is arranged circumferentially (25 mm long) (Hogan et al. 1971). The filtering portion of TM has three regions, namely, uveal meshwork, corneoscleral meshwork, and juxtacanalicular region (JCT). There is also a non-filtering anterior part that protrudes under the cornea (Tamm 2009). The uveal meshwork form irregular intratrabecular fenestrations (Lutjen-Drecoll and Rohen 2001). The trabecular meshwork contains three-dimensional elastic fiber that connects the inner wall of Schlemm's canal anteriorly, the ciliary body internally, and the choroid and ciliary muscle posteriorly (Overby et al. 2014). The outer layer of cells in TM act primarily as pre-filters and are aggressively phagocytic, removing cellular debris from AH before the fluid moves deeper into the less porous JCT and SC. The endothelial cells play a metabolic role in regulating the AH outflow dynamics. Both adrenergic and sympathetic fibers are present in the TM which increase the outflow facility after adrenoreceptor stimulation (Wax and Molinoff 1987). The contractile property of AH aids in aqueous outflow regulation.

5.3.2.2 Aqueous Humor Formation

Aqueous humor is a transparent watery fluid present in the anterior chamber secreted by ciliary processes of the ciliary body, a musculoepithelial structure, which is located behind the iris. It maintains the intraocular pressure, i.e., the product of the rate of aqueous production and the rate of aqueous drainage. The rate of aqueous humor formation is 2–3 μl/min. The fluid enters into the posterior chamber and flows back through the space between the lens and the iris and enters the non-vascularized tissues of the anterior chamber through the pupil (Rasmussen and Kaufman 2014).

AH forms through passive diffusion, ultrafiltration, and active secretion (Sit 2014). The plasma ultrafiltrate gets accumulated in the stroma which contributes to the AH in the posterior chamber (Civan and Macknight 2004). About 90 % of the aqueous humor formation is through active secretion from the nonpigmented ciliary epithelial cells (Mark 2010). The transport of fluid across osmotic pressure is through the water channel aquaporins (AQPs), namely, AQP1 and AQP4 (Yamaguchi et al. 2006). The ATP required for this transport is supplied by the Na^+ /K^+ -ATPase, an enzyme located in both the nonpigmented and pigmented ciliary epithelia (To et al. 2001). This can be inhibited by glycosides, vanadate, and acetozolamide and thus gains pharmacological interest (Goel et al. 2010). Another enzyme of pharmacological attention is carbonic anhydrase which is in the nonpigmented and pigmented ciliary epithelia transports bicarbonates. This aids in pH regulation by affecting Na^+ ions and helps for active ion transport (Maren 1976).

Apart from electrolytes, carbohydrates, glutathione, urea, proteins, and amino acids are the major constituents in AH. The protein levels are 200 times less in AH compared to plasma, and this is mainly made up of glycoproteins and immunoglobulins like Ig G, Ig M, and Ig A (Allansmith et al. 1973). Free amino acids are present in AH attributing to the active transport (Dickinson et al. 1968). The levels of urea and glucose reflect 80 % of plasma concentration (Reiss et al. 1986). Matrix enzymes like collagenase are also found in AH which helps in the ECM maintenance and contribute to TM resistance pathway (Vadillo-Ortega et al. 1989). Glutathione and ascorbate are the two important antioxidants present in AH, which protect the tissues from light-induced oxidative damage. Ascorbate levels are 50 times more compared to plasma (Leite et al. 2009).

The ciliary, iris epithelium, and the tight junctions of the iris endothelial cells contribute to the blood-aqueous barrier.

5.3.2.3 Aqueous Humor Outflow Pathway

Aqueous humor leaves the anterior chamber through the well-structured tissue, trabecular meshwork, and it reaches the Schlemm's canal, which drains into the aqueous veins through the conventional pathway (Goel et al. 2010). On the other hand, aqueous humor leaves the eye by diffusion through intercellular spaces among the ciliary muscle fibers through the uveoscleral or non-conventional pathway by diffusion through intercellular spaces among ciliary muscle fibers (Bill 1975). The trabecular meshwork plays an important role in providing most of the flow resistance to aqueous humor outflow. Modification of the trabecular meshwork resistance is responsible for the regulation of intraocular pressure.

Through the trabecular meshwork pathway AH reaches the Schlemm's canal and drains via the aqueous veins. This flow of AH through TM is dependent on the outflow resistance which is measured as μl/minute/mL of Hg (Stamer and Acott 2012). Through the TM, maximum amount of AH drains. The layers present in the TM are uveal meshwork formed by the iris and ciliary body stroma with large intercellular spaces, followed by corneoscleral meshwork which has lamellar endothelial-like cells which have collagen and elastic fibers. Their intercellular spaces are narrow and offer resistance to aqueous outflow. The next layer is called juxtacanalicular or cribriform meshwork which is rich in extracellular matrix and very narrow intercellular space. The AH has to then cross the endothelial cell lined by the Schlemm's canal (Epstein and Rohen 1991). This is done by either the paracellular route or transcellular route. There are autonomic and sensory innervations to form neurotransmitters which influence the permeability of TM (Ruskell 1976).

Glaucoma is a condition in which the aqueous humor builds up in the eye leading to increase in the intraocular pressure that consequently damages the optic nerve and nerve fibers from the retina. Normal intraocular pressure ranges from 12 to 22 mmHg. Ocular hypertension is a condition in which the person has high IOP (intraocular pressure) and does not show symptoms of glaucoma. The signs and symptoms of glaucoma include progressive visual field loss, optic nerve changes, and loss of vision which occurs gradually over a long period of time (Tektas and Lutjen-Drecoll 2009). Primary open-angle glaucoma is the most common type of glaucoma (Tektas and Lutjen-Drecoll 2009). People with normal-tension glaucoma have open, normal-appearing angles. In normal-tension glaucoma, optic nerve fibers get damaged even though there is a normal intraocular pressure. It may be considered one of the autoimmune diseases. Primary angle-closure glaucoma is the physical obstruction of trabecular meshwork by the iris (Tektas and Lutjen-Drecoll 2009). Plateau iris glaucoma is a condition where in the anterior chamber, angle closes due to pupillary dilation without iris block. Mixed glaucoma is the combination of primary open-angle glaucoma and primary angle-closure glaucoma. Secondary open-angle glaucoma is characterized by the aqueous outflow resistance between the trabecular meshwork and anterior chamber in pre-trabecular and trabecular form. Glaucomas are treated by applying drops which enhance aqueous draining or reduce aqueous secretion such as beta-blockers to reduce AH secretion (Cheng et al. 2012), alpha-adrenergic agonists (Chew et al. 2014), carbonic anhydrase inhibitors (Scozzafava and Supuran 2014), prostaglandin F2α analogs (Alm 2014), and cholinergic agents or miotic to increase the TM outflow pathway, e.g., pilocarpine and Carbachol (Lee and Higginbotham 2005).

Laser trabeculoplasty is done to treat open-angle glaucoma. A high-energy laser beam is used to open clogged drainage canals and help fluid drain more easily from the eye. Laser surgery for glaucoma initially lowers pressure in the eye. Overtime, however the intraocular pressure may begin to rise (Leahy and White 2015). In trabeculectomy and drainage implants, the fluid is directed to a bleb on the outer layer of the eyeball where it can be absorbed (SooHoo et al. 2014). Laser peripheral iridotomy surgery is used in the treatment of angle-closure glaucoma. In iridotomy, a small hole is created in the iris using a laser so that the fluid can flow through it and leaves the eye. After surgery in the affected eye, the other eye is also recommended for iridotomy because of the high risk that its drainage will also close in the future (Ng et al. 2012).

5.3.2.4 Aqueous Humor Proteomics in Glaucoma

Proteomic analysis of aqueous humor has been done in primary open-angle glaucoma and is suggested as a tool for diagnosis (Izzotti et al. 2010). The proteome can reflect the metabolic changes in the surrounding tissue and therefore can give clues on the pathogenic mechanisms in glaucoma.

TGF-β is known to be elevated in the aqueous humor in all types of glaucoma. This can be secreted from one or more tissues surrounding the anterior segment, including the ciliary epithelium, iris, lens epithelium, corneal endothelium, and trabecular meshwork and it is also possible that the elevated levels of TGF-β in glaucomatous TM tissues could be derived in part from the aqueous humor (Tovar-Vidales et al. 2011).

The differentially expressed aqueous humor proteins in buphthalmic rabbits, a model for "developmental glaucoma," revealed significant differential expression of several AH proteins in these rabbits based on LC-MS/MS platform (Edward and Bouhenni 2011).

A proteomic analysis of the aqueous humor compositions of "POAG patients" revealed that the protein composition in aqueous humor was significantly different in POAG patients versus non-POAG patients. 2D followed by LC/MS/MS analysis revealed increase in prostaglandins, caspase 14, transthyretin, albumin, cystatin C, albumin, and transferrin (Duan et al. 2010).

Proteomic analysis of the pseudoexfoliation material similarly suggests that extracellular matrix and stress response proteins are associated with "pseudoexfoliation glaucoma" (Lee 2008). Apart from aqueous humor and trabecular meshwork cells, protein profiling at the level of tear has been done that revealed an inflammatory tear protein profile present in "chronically medicated glaucomatous eyes" and are different from that found in primary dry eye. This study describes the drug effect on the treatment profile (Wong et al. 2011).

Gene expression patterns of trabecular meshwork and Schlemm's canal were shown to be similar to those of circulating leukocytes. The same study reported on the extensive alterations in characteristic protein expression patterns of circulating leukocytes for "normal-tension and primary open-angle glaucoma" (Golubnitschaja et al. 2007; Zhao et al. 2004).

5.3.2.5 Aqueous Humor Metabolites in Glaucoma

Reactive oxygen species (ROS) play a fundamental role in the pathophysiology of many diseases, including glaucoma. The iron-catalyzed formation of ROS is a major player in these processes. Erdumus et al have reported decreased serum antioxidants and increased serum superoxide dismutase (SOD) levels in patients with POAG indicating that antioxidant system dysfunction may be involved in the etiopathogenesis (Erdurmus et al. 2011). Studies have found that hepcidin, a prohormone produced in the liver, is expressed in other eye tissues, such as in Muller cells, photoreceptor cells, and retinal pigmented epithelium (RPE). It is increased in aqueous humor of POAG patients, with an expression pattern similar to that of ferroportin (Sorkhabi et al. 2010). It is also widely accepted that mitochondria might play a pivotal role in the pathophysiology of glaucoma (Kong et al. 2009). Low citrate has been reported in the plasma of glaucoma patients (Fraenkl et al. 2011). Citrate is an important molecule in the energy production cycle in mitochondria, and reduced mitochondrial activity might also lead to a decreased citrate production resulting in lower blood citrate levels. Oxidative DNA damage may induce human trabecular meshwork degeneration, leading to increase IOP. Increased levels of 8-hydroxy deoxyguanosine, (8-OHdG), an indicator of DNA damage, was seen in human trabecular meshwork specimens collected from patients with primary open-angle glaucoma (POAG) (Sacca et al. 2005). Patients with PACG also had high 8-OHdG concentrations (Chang et al. 2011). Apart from oxidative stress and DNA damage, aqueous amino acids levels are also reportedly altered. Individual amino acids, namely, threonine, serine, asparagine, glutamine, methionine, tyrosine, phenylalanine, histidine, tryptophan, and arginine, were reported to be higher in aqueous of glaucomas than in the cataract patients (Hannappel et al. 1985). Plasma levels of homocysteine were also increased in pseudoexfoliative glaucoma (PXG) patients and POAG patients (Turgut et al. 2010). Higher levels of hydroxyproline reported in aqueous indicative of increased collagen turnover is reported in pseudoexfoliation syndrome (PXF) in syndrome (Yagci et al. 2007).

5.4 Biochemistry of Sclera

The sclera is the white, fibrous, opaque protective external tunic of the eye rich in elastin and collagen fibers. It extends from the anterior to posterior chambers, i.e., limbus (corneoscleral junction) to the cribriform plate (optic nerve head). The type I collagen irregularity contributes to the opaqueness of the sclera (Keeley et al. 1984). The layers of sclera are episclera, stroma, lamina fusca, and endothelium. The sclera is continuous with the dura mater and cornea. It contributes to the maximal connective tissue layer of the eye, providing resistance against the internal and external stresses and acts as a support harboring extraocular muscular insertions. A healthy sclera appears normal and white, while one with inflammation has the scleral blood vessels engorged. While the episclera is vasculairsed, the scleral stroma is avascular receiving the nutrients from the episcleral and he underlying choroidal vasculatures. The sclera is richly supplied with nerves. The posterior ciliary nerves enters the sclera near the optic nerve.

The metabolic requirement of the sclera is low and has low turnover of the collagen. Scleral matrix is made up of scaffold of protein fibrils, collagen and elastin, and interfibrillar proteoglycans and glycoproteins, which surround a diffuse population of cells. The human sclera contains predominantly collagen which is about 50–75 % depending upon the different techniques done for estimating (Keeley et al. 1984).

The Tenon's capsule fibroblasts synthesize the collagen (Gross 1999). These include the different types of collagen such as I, II ,V, and VI with type I followed by type III as the predominant ones, and are restricted to the outermost sclera (Heathcote 1994). The collagen fibrils of the sclera range from 25 to 300 nm as observed by electron microscopy (Komai and Ushiki 1991). There are thinner fibrils in the lamina cribrosa, trabecular meshwork, and corneoscleral angle (Albon et al. 1995). This is attributed to adaptation and the required elasticity (Parry and Craig 1984). Type XII is associated with type I fibrils in human sclera as a different isoform (Anderson et al. 2000). The elastin component of the sclera aids as additional supporting system for the collagen network. Elastin contains amino acids like alanine, valine, isoleucine, and leucine. It contains little hydroxyproline and hydroxylysine unlike collagen. It contains cross-links, namely, desmosine and isodesmosine. The elastin fibers are abundant in the inner stromal region near the extraocular muscles. There are four times more elastin in the lamina cribrosa and peripapillary sclera compared to the equatorial region (Quigley et al. 1991). The sclera matrix consists of proteoglycans. The main proteoglycans mostly belong to small leucine-rich repeat family members, namely, Decorin and Biglycan (Friedman et al. 2000). Decorin has been found to play an important role in development and wound healing, and reduced synthesis is found and seen in the development of myopia (Rada et al. 2000). Lumican found in the sclera by immunohistochemical studies is involved in regulating collagen fibrillogenesis and has been linked with high myopia in humans. Lumican deficiency causes scleral anomalies (Austin et al. 2002). Recent studies have revealed the presence of perlecan, agrin, prolargin, versican, aggregan, mimecan, and fibromodulin in scleral layers as revealed by immunofluoresence staining (Keenan, et al. 2012). These studies reveal that electron dense filaments of the decorin distribute along the collagen fibrils with a periodic pattern (Kimura et al. 1995). The C-terminal region of collagen type I binds to decorin and is also associated with type VI collagen (Keene et al. 1987).

Sclera exhibits low cellularity compared to most vascularized tissues, and the only cell is the scleral fibrocyte. Sclerocytes can undergo rapid transformation into active fibroblasts following insult like trauma, surgery, postoperative scarring and topical application of drugs, and neoplasia to the sclera. Histiocytes, blast cells, granulocytes, lymphocytes, and plasma cells can also be seen in the sclera occasionally. In inflammatory stimulus, these cells enter from blood vessels of the choroid and episclera and arrive to the site of insult. Scleral cells respond to growth factors like platelet-derived growth factor (PDGF), transforming growth factor, fibroblast growth factor, thymocyte-derived growth factors, IL-1 and interferon gamma.

Scleritis is a chronic ocular inflammatory condition of the sclera. Scleritis is marked with redness in the sclera that is diffuse or localized in a pie-shaped area. The etiology of this condition varies from idiopathic, confined to the eye to systemic autoimmune diseases and in rare cases due to infection or drug reaction as well as due to a tumor or surgical complications. Infectious scleritis can be primary or secondary to keratitis or endophthalmitis. Surgery, trauma, and the use of corticosteroids are considered as major predisposing factors (Ramenaden and Raiji 2013;

Smith et al. 2007). With non-necrotizing scleritis, there is no much threat to vision unless there is presence of uveitis or keratitis. In case of necrotizing scleritis, much visible necrosis of sclera can be viewed along with the exposure of the underlying uvea, which is more often coupled with rheumatoid arthritis or systemic vasculitis (Smith et al. 2007; Sainz de la Maza and Foster 1994). Watson and Hayray (Watson and Hayreh 1976) defined five distinct classifications of scleritis, namely:

(a) Anterior scleritis which involves inflammation in the anterior sclera that can be diffused or nodular or can be non-inflammatory necrotizing scleritis
(b) Scleromalacia perforans: Inflammatory necrosis of anterior sclera
(c) Posterior scleritis: Inflammation of posterior sclera
(d) Sclerokeratitis: Inflammation of sclera that occurs in association with cornea
(e) Episcleritis: Inflammation of sclera and conjunctiva

5.4.1 Molecular Derangement in Uveitis

Uveitis phenotypes can differ significantly, and most types of uveitis are believed to be polygenic with complex inheritance patterns. In uveitis there is a strong association of HLA-B27 with acute anterior uveitis and HLA-A29 with birdshot chorioretinopathy (Martin et al. 2003). The genomic analysis of serum, aqueous, and vitreous of Fuchs uveitis-affected patients showed the presence of rubella virus-specific antibody and its gene, speculating the probable involvement of the virus in chronic inflammation of this disease (Cimino et al. 2013). Studies suggest that uveitis shares some of its pathogenic mechanisms associated with other autoimmune diseases and conclude the "common gene, common pathway" hypothesis for autoimmune disorders (Mattapallil et al. 2008). The study involving rat model of experimental autoimmune uveitis (EAU) recognized three quantitative trait loci (QTL) linked with EAU on rat chromosomes 4, 12, and 10 (Eau1, Eau2, and EAU2) (Pennesi and Caspi 2002). Using microsatellite markers of resistant and susceptible MHC class II-matched rat strains, new possible QTLs on rat chromosomes 2, 3, 7, 10, and 19 (Eau4-Eau9) were identified that direct susceptibility to uveitis. Also a protective allele was identified in the uveitis-susceptible rat strain in the Eau5 locus at D7Wox18, and epistatic interactions between QTLs influenced the severity. These identified regions were found to colocalize with the genetic determinants of other autoimmune disease models and to the syntenic regions recognized on human chromosomes 4q21-31, 5q31-33, 16q22-24, 17p11-q12, 20q11-13, and 22q12-13, from patients suffering from autoimmune disorders.

Autoimmune uveitis encompassing inflammatory triggers occurs with relapse. The mechanism of the reaction and the molecular agents eliciting relapse has remained unexplored. To understand this, studies have used the only spontaneously occurring uveitis model equine recurrent uveitis (ERU), for proteomics and molecular analysis, since it very closely resembles the human autoimmune uveitis. In autoimmune uveitis, autoreactive T cells cross the blood-retinal barrier and damage the inner eye tissues. Studies have identified CRALBP (cellular retinaldehyde-binding protein) as a novel antigen (Deeg et al. 2006). Anti-CRALBP antibody was significantly elevated in the sera of affected individuals (Deeg et al. 2007c). Malate dehydrogenase, IRBP (iron-responsive element binding protein), the highly antigenic S-antigen (aka S-arrestin) and recoverin are the other identified proteins (Deeg et al. 2007b, 2008). Increase in VEGF and lowered PEDF (pigment epithelium-derived factor) with blood-retinal barrier breakdown aid autoreactive T cell infiltration (Deeg et al. 2007a). Increased incidences of IgG4 hc, IgM, alpha-2HS-glycoprotein, serotransferrin, and complement factor B, with decreased levels of IgG5 hc, apolipoprotein A-IV, apolipoprotein H, and high-molecular-weight kininogen, are reported (Zipplies et al. 2010). Based on immunohistochemistry analysis, increase in the complement activation products B/Ba, B/Bb, Bb neoantigen, iC3b, and C3d with no difference in C5b-9 levels is reported. Macrophage involvement in the inflammatory process of autoimmune uveitis is reported (Zipplies et al. 2010). Additionally differential expression of several cellular proteins such as MMPs and TIMP-2 (matrix metalloproteinase and their inhibitors) and potassium ion channels and decreased osteopontin and fibronectin have been reported (Deeg et al. 2011; Eberhardt et al. 2012; Hofmaier et al. 2011; Zayas-Santiago et al. 2014).

5.5 Biochemistry of the Vitreous, Retina and Retinal Pigment Epithelium

5.5.1 The Vitreous

The vitreous humor occupies a large portion of the eye posteriorly: behind the lens and in front of the retina. It is a clear jelly-like substance that fills the eye and gives a shape. The vitreous is divided into three compartments, namely, vitreous base, central vitreous, and cortical vitreous. Concentration and arrangement of collagens differ in all the three layers. The concentration of collagen is about 300 μg/ml and it is highly insoluble. It contains predominantly type II collagen with lower amounts of type IX, type V/XI collagen (de Smet et al. 2013). Collagen is arranged from anterior to posterior direction with denser arrangement of collagen fibers in the vitreous base and cortical vitreous, while the central part has very thin collagen fibrils. The vitreous base covers the dorsal side of the lens, and ends at the region of ora serrata, where the neurosensory retina begins. The cortical vitreous begins at the retina and maintains the strong attachment through inner limiting lamina (ILL). Collagen fibers run parallel to the ILL and acts like strong glue over the retina, to spread over the RPE. The less dense central vitreous makes the bulk of vitreous zone with the collagen fibers running from anterior to posterior direction from anterior to posterior part (Bishop 2000; Le Goff and Bishop 2008). Hence, this arrangement of collagen fibers making a contact over the inner surface acts like a substratum for lens ciliary body and retina. It also acts as a shock absorber.

The vitreous is composed of 98–99 % water with collagen gel fibril and in between with a network of very long molecules of hyaluron (HA) which render the viscoelastic property to the vitreous (Swann 1987). The viscoelastic property of the vitreous is required for protecting the retina from shock. The hyaluronic acid and collagen interaction gives transparency and hydration and the spacing arrangements decrease light scattering in the vitreous (Bishop 2000).

The vitreous contains heterotypic collagen fibril formed by the co-assembly of type II, IX, V, and XI collagen. Among the total collagen content of the vitreous, type II constitutes (60–75 %), type IX (25 %), type V, VI, and XI collagen constituting minor quantities. These *collagenase* core is bound with HA attracts the counter ions and water and swells the vitreous. It also space the collagen fibers apart from clumping and makes the vitreous a transparent medium for the passage of light. *Chondroitin* sulfate is also found in the vitreous, decorating type XI collagen. There are also few noncollagenous proteins present in the vitreous, namely, albumin, transferrin, lactoferrin which can be seen in gel electrophoresis (Nguyen and Fife 1986).

The glycosaminoglycan present in the vitreous is hyaluronic acid with a molecular weight of 3000 kDa. The HA-collagen interaction comes from the electron microscopic observation of vitreous. These interactions are found to occur through chondroitin sulfate chains and collagen fibrils (Theocharis et al. 2008). Concentration of HA in the human vitreous is between 65 and 400 μg/ml (Balzas 1984).

There are a few cells in the vitreous called as hyalocytes which are more towards the peripheral part of the vitreous. They are star-shaped stellate cells with oval nuclei measuring 10–15 μm (Sommer et al. 2009) and are considered as specialized form of macrophages. They are known to synthesize extracellular matrix and regulate vitreous immunology in inflammation. The hyalocytes play a major role as antigen-presenting cells (Sakamoto and Ishibashi 2011). In vitro the hyalocytes can be cultured, and they response to inflammatory molecules by secreting urokinase-type plasminogen activator and vascular endothelial growth factor (Hata et al. 2008). Hyalocytes are present in epiretinal membrane and contribute to the inflammatory mechanism (Joshi et al. 2013).

Formation of Vitreous Humor

Separation of neural and surface ectoderm at 3rd to 4th week of gestation forms the vitreous cavity and it is filled with collagenous-like material. Mesodermal cells enter into this vitreous cavity, forms hyaloid vessels, and it is branched throughout the vitreous cavity. Fibroblast and phagocyte cells from the outer most layer of this vessel latter differentiate into hyalocytes. A cellular-material-like collagen formed after 6th week of gestation. Hyaloid vessels regress as the fetus develops and are not seen in adults (Jack 1972; Linsenmayer et al. 1982).

Vitreal Proteomics

The vitreous is a stagnant structure unlike aqueous which is continuously produced and drained. The vitreous is having close interaction with the various cells of the eyes such as the retinal layers and RPE and therefore is a repository of molecules from the tissues around. Skeie et al. showed that the protein prolife of vitreous differs in the substructures and also showed the presence of various intracellular proteins like Glial fibrilary acidic protein (GFAP, from glial cells), Rhodopsin (from Rods), RPE-specific protein RPE-65. This group also reported the presence of complement proteins and damage-associated molecular patterns (DAMPs) in the healthy human cadaver vitreous, and these molecules amplify inflammation in response to the changes in the vitreal milieu during disease conditions (Skeie et al. 2015). Hence, knowing the vitreous proteome helps in understating the disease process, such as in diabetic retinopathy (DR), age-related macular degeneration (ARMD), and other vitreo-retinal pathologies.

Vitreal proteomics have revealed the presence of proteins involved in WNT, MAPK signaling pathway, m*etalloproteases* metabolism, and transporters. Since most of these proteins have appeared full length (Skeie et al. 2015; Murthy et al. 2014), it is suggested that the vitreous might be stagnant without synthesis and drainage. Vitreous profile of patients with diabetic macular edema (DME) showed that plasma k*allikrein*-kinin system is a contributing factor for disease pathogenesis (Kita et al. 2015). It showed upregulated hemopexin and downregulated clusterin, transerythrin, and crystalline-S in DME compared to diabetic retinopathy (DR) (Hernández et al. 2013). Vitreous proteome also reflected the difference in the expression of proteins in DR that includes angiopoietin-related protein 6, apolipoprotein A-I, estrogen receptor alpha, angiotensinogen, complement C3, complement factor I, prothrombin, alpha-1-antitrypsin, and antithrombin III. Decreased levels of proteins like calsyntenin-1, interphotoreceptor retinoid-binding protein, and neuroserpin were also revealed (Kim et al. 2007; Gao et al. 2008; Merchant and Klein 2009; Wang et al. 2013).

Vitreous Metabolome

Metabolomic analysis revels that vitreal cortex is rich in lactate, glutamine, and creatine. The metabolome profile shows characteristics of anaerobic glycolysis in the retina, conversion of glutamate to glutamine to prevent excitotoxicty, ROS scavenging, and ATP restoration. The vitreous base is rich especially in ascorbate, *betaine*, and alanine. Ascorbate helps to maintain oxygen gradient and maintains low oxygenation at ciliary body and lens. Betaine helps in osmoregulation. Core area of the vitreous is rich in acetate and glucose. Glucose concentration of the vitreous is similar to the serum concentration, and hence, it goes up during hyperglycemic episode. Glucose is utilized to produce energy, and it diffuses to the cortex where it can be metabolized more rapidly (Locci et al. 2014).

Vitreous metabolite profile also differs during pathological conditions. Barba et al. reported on the elevated level of acetate in the cases of DR due to type 1 diabetes (Barba et al. 2010). Vitreous concentration of oxaloacetate, glucose, and urea are more in the lens-induced *uveitis* than chronic uveitis, thus showing that metabolite profile helps to identify subtype of diseases (Young et al. 2009). It is also helpful in forensic science to identify the time and cause of death such as in intoxication, dehydration, and hyperglycemia (Palmiere and Mangin 2012; Madea 2013; Costa et al. 2014).

As aging occurs, the vitreous liquefies and aggregates. Liquefaction of vitreous or synchisis begins at middle age and slowly progresses towards late age. Aggregation of vitreous is called syneresis which is due to the conformation change of HA-collagen interaction (Johnson 2010, 2013). Liquefaction occurs in the central vitreous due to over production of free radicals which affects the glycosaminoglycans and chondroitin sulfate concentration (Kamei and Totani 1982).

5.5.2 The Retina

The retina is a highly complex structure where several types of cells communicate through countless molecules for visual information. The most central part of the macula is fovea, a central 0.35 mm wide depression, and represents the retinal region of greatest visual acuity. The central 500 mm of the fovea contains no retinal capillaries (foveal avascular zone), making the fovea dependent on blood supply from the choriocapillaris. The extreme retinal periphery is thin enough to be supplied by diffusion from the choroidal circulation, while the rest has retinal circulation.

The blood-retinal barrier (BRB) is composed of both inner and outer barrier. The outer blood-retinal barrier consists of the choriocapillary basement membrane, Bruch's membrane, and the intercellular junctions of the retinal pigment epithelium (RPE), to regulate the movement of solutes and nutrients from the choroid to the subretinal space. In contrast, the inner BRB, similar to the blood-brain barrier (BBB) is located in the inner retinal microvasculature and comprises the microvascular endothelium which lines these vessels. The tight junctions located between these cells mediate highly selective diffusion of molecules from the blood to the retina, and the barrier is essential in maintaining retinal homeostasis (Campbell and Humphries 2012). The retina comprises six neuronal cell types and one glial cell type that are derived from a common progenitor cell. Each type of cell plays a unique role in the retina. These include photoreceptor cells (rods and cones), horizontal cells, bipolar cells, amacrine cells, interplexiform cells, and ganglion cells.

Photoreceptors cells are specialized cells classified into rods and cones based on their structure. They are composed of photosensitive membrane at distal end, a large synaptic terminal end, and cell organelles in the central region. The rods are slender, cylindrical structures that fill the subretinal spaces between their larger cone neighbors and stretch into the pigment epithelium cells of the retina. The differentiation of cells into rods is mediated by retinoic acid, sonic hedgehog, and activin (Levine et al. 1997; Ebrey and Koutalos 2001). The rod's outer segments contain the light-sensitive pigment rhodopsin, a vitamin A derivative (11-cis-retinal) coupled to a protein (opsin), which resides within the membrane of disks that are stacked on top of one another within the rod's outer segment. The outer and inner segments of photoreceptors are surrounded by processes of the RPE cells which provide a number of supportive functions, including the regeneration of bleached photo pigment and the uptake and degradation of disks which are periodically shed by rods and cones into the subretinal space. The proximal ends of the photoreceptors contain the synaptic machinery which releases glutamate, an excitatory chemical neurotransmitter which interacts with glutamate receptors found in the second-order neurons, the bipolar cells, and the horizontal cells. The photoreceptors and bipolar cells in the retina exhibit "ribbon synapse," wherein there is continuous release of the neurotransmitter, glutamate (tonic release) modulated only by the graded changes in the membrane potential, unlike the action-potential-driven bursts of release, as seen in conventional synapse. The photoreceptor cells and the bipolar cells exhibit syntaxin 3 expression that regulates synaptic vesicle fusion reaction, calcium sensitivity, and transmitter release (Morgans 2000). Rods are most sensitive and function for vision under scotopic conditions (in low light), and cones are responsible for vision under photopic conditions (in bright light) and underlie the visual acuity and color vision. This signal from photoreceptor is then transferred to retinal neurons residing within the inner nuclear layer (INL). Bipolar cells transmit this signal radially from the outer retina to the ganglion cell layer (GCL). The Müller glial cells extend across the entire thickness of the retina. Visual information then converges upon the dendrites of the ganglion cell types, which is transmitted to the nerve fiber layer (NFL) collected at the optic nerve head. This in turn is transmitted through the optic nerve to the brain (Poche and Reese 2009).

The horizontal cells are the interneurons and together with amacrine cells lie within the inner nuclear layer (Poche and Reese 2009). There are 13 types of bipolar cells that add details to the information delivered to the brain originated from the photoreceptors. Fine details like contrast and composition of colors are encoded by these cells (Euler et al. 2014). They are classified into two types: metabotropic (ON) or ionotropic (OFF) receptor, based on their response to glutamate released by the photoreceptors. With light, the photoreceptor hyperpolarizes and releases less glutamate that leads to the depolarization of the ON bipolar cells, while OFF bipolar cells respond by hyperpolarizing (Ayoub and Copenhagen 1991).

Amacrine cells are interneurons in the inner nuclear layer and are the second synaptic retinal layer that influences retinal signal processing (Santiago Ramón y Cajal 1892). There are about 40 different types of amacrine cells, classified based on their receptive field, their localization in the inner plexiform layer (IPL), and by neurotransmitter type. Most are inhibitory using either gamma-aminobutyric acid (GABA) or glycine as neurotransmitters. Functionally they are involved in the complex process of retinal image, specifically adjusting image brightness and in detecting motion (Balasubramanian and Gan 2014). Many functions of amacrine cells are not well understood. But the feed-forward inhibition onto the ganglion cells forms the prominent action of amacrine cells (Trenholm and Awatramani 2015).

Ganglion cells are neurons located near the inner surface of the retina and are the final output neurons of the vertebrate retina. They vary in size and respond to visual stimulation. Ganglion cells collect visual information from bipolar cells and amacrine cells and transmit it to the brain. Based on their projections and functions, there are at five main classes, namely, Parasol (Magnocellular, or M pathway); Midget (Parvocellular, or P pathway); Bistratified (Koniocellular, or K pathway); photosensitive ganglion cells (melanopsin ganglion cells); and superior colliculus for eye movements (saccades) (Sanes and Masland 2015).

The retina has the glial cells, namely, the Muller cells, microglia, and astroglial cells. The Muller cells are the major glial cells, located in the inner nuclear layer and extend from the internal limiting membrane to the bases of the rods and cones, where they form junctional complexes called the outer limiting membrane. They are involved in the metabolic regulation of the retina apart from giving structural support and are involved in the transcellular movement of ions, water, and bicarbonate. Muller cells de-differentiate to neuronal (astrocytes) progenitor cells during injury that helps in the regeneration of photoreceptors (Reichenbach and Bringmann 2013). Microglia are phagocytic cells in the retina required for neuronal homeostasis and innate immune defense. The immunological potential of microglia is comparable with blood monocytes and macrophages (Pena-Altamira et al. 2015).

The final common pathway for expressing retinal processing is the ganglion cell, whose axon goes to the brain. A variety of ganglion cell types are present in each retina and vary according to the size of the dendritic tree and soma, the sublamination pattern within the inner plexiform layer (IPL), and the complexity of dendritic branching. The dendrites of ganglion cells receive synaptic inputs from bipolar and amacrine cells. Their synaptic currents converge onto the cell body. The impulse-generating site for each ganglion cell is probably located within the initial segment region of the axon (Moore and O'Brien 2015).

The Biochemistry of Retinal Functions in Vision

The outer segments of the rods and cones contain a region filled with membrane-bound disks, which contain proteins bound to the chromophore 11-*cis*-retinal. In rod cells, the protein which binds the chromophore retinal is *opsin*, and the bound complex of 11-*cis*-retinal plus opsin is known as *rhodopsin*, or visual purple. 11-*cis*-retinal has a maximum absorbance in the ultraviolet part of the spectrum, but the maximum absorbance for rhodopsin is 500 nm. The chromophore undergoes *isomerization* to all-*trans*-retinal. As the protein changes its conformation, it initiates a cascade of biochemical reactions that result in the closing of Na^+ channels in the cell membrane. When the Na^+ channels are closed, a large potential difference builds up across the plasma membrane. This potential difference is passed on to adjoining nerve cell as an electrical impulse at the synaptic terminal. The nerve cell carries this impulse to the brain, where the visual information is interpreted. Light absorption by rhodopsin leads to closure of the channels and hyperpolarization (Ryan 2006).

Synapse is the point of connection between the end foot of one neuron and the membrane of another. Synapses are classified into two types, namely, chemical and electrical synapses. Chemical synapses are seen in mammals, whereas electrical synapses are found in the brains of invertebrates. In chemical synapse, the nerve impulse at the end foot of an axon triggers the release of a chemical agent called neuromodulator substance. Neurotransmitters are defined as a neuroactive compound released from the nerve. These compounds produce rapid changes in the cell which results in hyper- or depolarization of postsynaptic membranes (Hoon et al. 2014). Glycine is an important neurotransmitter in the processing of auditive information through cochlear nuclei, the superior oliva complex, and the inferior colliculus (Zafra et al. 1997), and in the processing of visual information in retinal ganglion cells. Glycinergic synaptic transmission is detected in Golgi cells of the cerebellum (Dieudonne 1995). The glycine-mediated neurotransmission plays an important role in storage of the transmitter in synaptic vesicles and neuron depolarization. Functional glycinergic transmission appears early in brain development, and activation of glycine and gamma-aminobutyric acid (GABA) receptors depolarizes neurons during the last prenatal period and early postnatal days (Cherubini et al. 1991; Flint et al. 1998; Aragon and Lopez-Corcuera 2003).

Glutamic acid is one of the proteinogenic amino acids. It is a nonessential amino acid and has a side chain carboxylic acid functional group. The carboxylate anions and salts of glutamic acid are known as glutamates. Glutamate is the most abundant excitatory neurotransmitter in the nervous system and it plays a key role in long-term potentiation. The continuous "tonic" release of glutamate is sustained by the active calcium channels. The cone photoreceptor shows that there is segregation of the calcium influx (voltage-gated calcium channels) and efflux (plasma membrane calcium ATPase) sites. While there is continuous influx of calcium into photoreceptor terminals in darkness, calcium extrusion is balanced by the influx through the channels (Morgans 2000).

The neuromodulator dopamine is found in one or more types of amacrine cell in the mammalian retina. It is characteristic of large cell body and a dense plexus of dendrites in stratum S1 of the inner plexiform layer. Holes or "rings" in the plexus of criss-crossing stained dendrites are sites of amacrine cell bodies or large amacrine dendrites. Different types of dopamine have been reported. Type 1 dopamine cell (A18) is known to synapse upon the AII rod amacrine cell and upon A8 and A17 cells. It also provides ascending processes to the outer plexiform layer which are known to synapse on the GABAergic interplexiform cell (Kolb et al. 1991). Glutamate and dopamine colocalize to the A18 cell type (type 1 CA cell), and serotonin has also been found to coexist in the same amacrine cells in cat retina (Wassle and Chun 1988). The dopamine type 1 cell exhibits glutamate, GABA, and histamine H1 receptors (Frazao et al. 2011).

A second type of dopamine amacrine cell has also been described in primate (Mariani and Hokoc 1988) (Crooks and Kolb 1992), in rabbit and mouse retinas. The type 2 CA cell has dendrites stratifying in stratum 3 of the IPL. It can be revealed in transgenetic mouse retina labeled with green fluorescent protein (GFP) (Contini et al. 2010). Both D1 and D2 receptor types have been found on neurons of the inner and outer retina in many vertebrates. It is thought that both D1 and D2 receptors are coupled by gap junctions, because of dopamine's known action in cyclic AMP regulation of gap junction channels. Thus, D1 receptors have been demonstrated in association with horizontal cells of the OPL and amacrine and ganglion cells of the inner retina. D2 receptors are also found in the inner retina but mostly are associated with photoreceptors in the outer nuclear layer, outer limiting membrane, and retinal pigment epithelium. D1 and D2 receptors are robust on ganglion cell bodies, despite the fact that the dopamine amacrine cell is not known to make direct synapses upon ganglion cells. However, several ganglion cell types are connected to amacrine cells via gap junctions and the dopamine effect is probably via diffusion of dopamine from DA cells to the site partners of electrical coupling acting through both D1 and D2 receptors. The best known effect of dopamine on gap junctions is that upon AII to AII amacrine cell gap junctions and AII to cone bipolar gap junctions. Dopamine particularly affects the former homologous gap junctions, while the gas transmitter, nitric oxide, affects the heterologous gap junction involving the ON cone bipolar gap junction (Massey and Miller 1988).

Acetylcholine (ACh) is found in a mirror symmetric pair of amacrine cells in the vertebrate retina. It is reported that ACh starburst amacrine cells colocalize GABA (Vaney and Young 1988). Starburst amacrine cells are excitatory with ACh release early in development of the retina, and this release is necessary for the development of retinal waves.

Serotonin is one of the neurotransmitters and is reported to exist in two types in the rabbit retina. One of these is A17 cell or the reciprocal amacrine cell of the rod system in the rabbit. Serotonin coexists with GABA in the A17 cell and the latter is thought to be the releasable transmitter (Schutte and Weiler 1987). A few cold-blooded vertebrates have a bistratified amacrine cell and a bipolar cell type that participates in the off mechanism of retinal processing through seratonin (Hurd and Eldred 1993). Adenosine purine nucleotide is a neuromodulator in the mammalian retina. Immunocytochemistry studies reported that the presence of adenosine in the amacrine and ganglion cell layers (Blazynski and Perez 1991). It colocalizes with GABA, acetylcholine, and serotonin.

Substance P (SP) is a neuropeptide belonging to the tachykinin family that includes neurokinin A, neuropeptide K, and neurokinin B. It is reported as a neurotransmitter in the vertebrate retina (Kolb et al. 1995). In the human retina, they appear as large-field cells with large cell bodies lying in normal or displaced positions on either side of the IPL.

Lipids in Retina

Unesterified (free) cholesterol is predominantly found in brain (14 mg/g wet weight), while other organs contains 2–3 mg/g, including retina, which is the part of central nervous system (Dietschy and Turley 2004; Bjorkhem 2006; Bretillon et al. 2007). Fliesler and Schroepfer reported that cholesterol accounts for at least 98 % of the total sterols of whole retina and >99 % of the total sterols of rod outer segment (ROS) membranes (Fliesler and Schroepfer 1982). Staining for HMG-CoA reductase showed that Müller cells, rod inner segments, and RPE cells can synthesis cholesterol de novo (Rodwell et al. 1976). However, compared to the major cholesterogenic tissues (i.e., liver and intestine), the rate of cholesterol synthesis in the mature brain and retina is relatively slow (Fliesler et al. 1993; Keller et al. 2004). Cholesterol appears to be broadly distributed in all layers of the neural retina (Bretillon et al. 2008), although the inner plexiform layer is found to be relatively enriched in cholesterol compared with the outer segment layer (Francis 1955; Curcio et al. 2005). A high-cholesterol environment, such as that present in the basal disks, has been found to reduce the efficiency of the phototransduction cascade by hindering activation of rhodopsin and impairing the cyclic nucleotide phosphodiesterase activity that hydrolyzes cGMP (Albert and Boesze-Battaglia 2005). The retina can take up circulating LDL-borne cholesterol, in contrast to the exclusion by the brain. Using labeled LDL particles, it was shown that LDL can cross Bruch's membrane and reach the RPE (Gordiyenko et al. 2004). LDL-R (LDL receptor) has been localized to the endothelial cells of the choriocapillaris, photoreceptor inner segments, retinal ganglion cells, and Müller cells (Tserentsoodol et al. 2006b). Low-density lipoprotein receptor (LRP-1) has been identified in retinal ganglion cells (Shi et al. 2008) that helps in the uptake of cholesterol.

5.5.2.1 The Retinal Pigment Epithelium

The retinal pigment epithelium (RPE) is a monolayer of highly specialized pigmented cells lying as a single sheet of hexagonally arranged cuboidal cells on Bruch's membrane sandwiched between the neural retina and the choriocapillaris. It is derived embryologically from the same neural tube tissue that forms the sensory retina. The RPE cells are highly polarized where the apical membrane interdigitates the outer segment of photoreceptors in the subretinal space and the basolateral membrane appends on the multilayered Bruch's membrane (Fig. 5.4). RPE has no photoreceptive functions or neural functions, but it is necessary for the support and viability of the photoreceptors. Moreover, RPE is indispensable for the development of the retina and secretes growth factors necessary for the survival and differentiation of the photoreceptor (Stiemke et al. 1994; Adamis et al. 1993). In addition, RPE executes assortment of functions such as the absorption of scattered light, phagocytosis of photoreceptor outer segments, transportation of nutrients, retinoid recycling, protection against reactive oxygen species, and more importantly the blood-retinal barrier to preserve the photosensitive retinal cells. Consequently, there are many inherited retinal degeneration conditions linked to RPE-specific gene dysfunction and similarly some mutations in the photoreceptors which could affect the RPE survival. Human adult eye has approximately 3.5 million RPE cells (Bok 1993). Anterior to the ora serrata, the RPE continues as the ciliary pigment epithelium. The apical surface of the RPE interfaces with the outer segments of the photoreceptors, while the basal domain is attached firmly to the underlying Bruch's membrane (BM). The brown color of the RPE is imparted by its melanin granules. The highest concentration of pigment is found in the peripheral retina and the lowest in the macula area (Weiter et al. 1986). The retina and the RPE are separated by a potential space called the subretinal space. The retina is not firmly attached to the pigment epithelium except at the optic disk and ora serrata; attachments in other places are weak and can be easily disrupted. The apical side has numerous long microvilli (3–7 μm in length), which interdigitate with the rods and cones of the retina and partially envelope them. These interdigitations along with the extracellular matrix

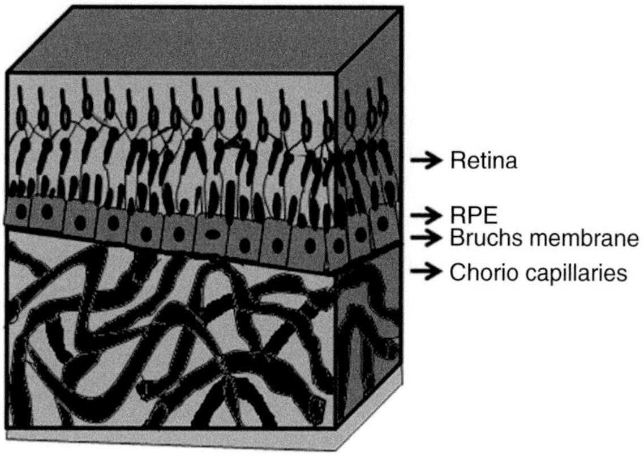

Fig. 5.4 Pictorial representation of RPE-Bruch's membrane-choriocapillaris

and neural cell adhesion molecule (N-CAM) expressed by the RPE on the apical side allow some degree of adhesion between retina and RPE (Fig. 5.4).

Apical Basal Arrangement of RPE

The RPE cells are joined near the apical side by tight junctions (zonula occludens), which form a part of the blood-retinal barrier. The apical cytoplasm contains microfilaments and microtubules and also the greatest concentration of melanin granules. The basal infoldings are 1 μm, and they help in the attachment of RPE to BM of choroid by expression of integrins. The small convoluted infoldings also increase the surface area for absorption and secretion. Laterally the RPE has specialized junctions called the tight junctions – zona occludens (ZO-1) – and adherent junctions cadherins, connexin, and desmosomes.

The apical surfaces of RPE cells face the photoreceptors and contain both long and short microvilli. The apical surface of the RPE and the rod and cone outer segments are coated with an extracellular matrix called interphotoreceptor matrix (IPM) (Marmor 1988). The IPM also serves as a medium for the exchange of metabolites between the outer segments of the photoreceptors and the RPE (Clark and Hall 1986). Due to the lack of tight attachment beneath the neural retina and the RPE, the neural retina becomes detached from the RPE under certain conditions. Detachment simultaneously disrupts the photoreceptors and RPE and can eventually lead to the loss of vision (Zayit-Soudry et al. 2007). The apical membrane of the RPE is rich in Na^+/K^+-ATPase which, together with other ionic transport mechanisms, moves water out of the subretinal space. The apical location of the Na^+/K^+-ATPase along with the epithelium of the choroid plexus is a unique feature among epithelia, as this pump is normally located basally. The removal of subretinal fluid by the RPE is thought to provide the major motive force for adhesion of the neural retina to the RPE (Clark and Hall 1986; Marshall 1987). As part of the photoreceptor renewal process, the apical processes of the RPE continually phagocytize the distal portions of the outer segments of rods and cones (Clark and Hall 1986; Marshall 1987). The basal plasma membrane of the RPE cell has numerous infoldings and lies on a basement membrane which is secreted by the RPE (Clark and Hall 1986) itself. These infoldings are very useful for facilitating ion movement in transporting epithelia such as the RPE, as they increase the surface area of the cell. The basal surface of the RPE express integrins $\alpha3\beta1$, $\alpha6\beta1$, and $\alpha5\beta3$ and mediate attachment to the basement membrane (BM), a fibroelastic layer which separates the photoreceptor- RPE unit from its blood supply derived from the choriocapillaris (Clark and Hall 1986). BM is permeable to small molecules and some macromolecules and is thought to contribute to the blood-retinal barrier (Pino and Essner 1981).

The basal and lateral membranes are usually referred as a single functional unit, called as basolateral. The lateral domain of the adjacent RPE cells is connected by apical zonula occludens, i.e., tight junctions, and zonula adherens, i.e., adherens junction (Fine 1961). These junctions seal off the subretinal space where the exchange of macromolecules with the choriocapillaris takes place. The zonula occludens between adjacent RPE cells form a "tight" intercellular junction due to interaction between the extracellular domains of adjacent occluding molecules leading to high transepithelial resistance and an intact blood-retinal barrier. Tight junctions are also responsible for the sequestration of molecules into the apical and basal plasma membrane domains. The cytoplasmic domain of occludin interacts with other proteins including ZO-1 and ZO-2 to form complex and interacts with the actin cytoskeleton for various signal transduction pathways.

The adherens junctions play a role in maintenance of the polygonal shape of the RPE and the organization of the cytoskeleton actin (Sandig and Kalnins 1988). Gap junctions are also present in the basolateral membrane called connexins which are important for the exchange of ions and metabolites between cells. Basal membrane also expresses integrins and show focal adhesion points with the extracellular matrix (Docherty et al. 1984).

5.5.2.2 Functions of RPE

The Antioxidant Activity of the Melanin Pigment

The RPE has numerous and varied functions. RPE is the first tissue to become pigmented (melanin) (Dorey et al. 1990), and hence it is named as pigmented epithelial cells. The ellipsoidal melanin granules called melanosomes are one of the most conspicuous cytoplasmic components in RPE (Feeney-Burns et al. 1984). Within the adult RPE cell, the melanin granules are located in the apical portion of the cell, adjacent to the rod outer segment. Melanin granules function to reduce light scattering. By absorbing radiant energy (visible and ultraviolet spectrum) and dissipates it as heat. In addition melanin can bind redox-active metal ions and sequester them in an inactive state, thus preventing oxidative damage to the retina by these potential photosensitizing agents (Sarna 1992). The absorption of light by melanin acts as an effective antioxidant to protect the RPE cells and regulate their metabolic activity; in fact, RPE cells high in melanin content exhibit significantly less formation of lipofuscin than cells low or devoid of in melanin (Nilsson et al. 2003). In case of an intense oxidative insult, structural or functional changes in RPE melanin may lead to loss of antioxidant capacity (Sarna 1992). Tyrosinase, a copper-containing enzyme, catalyzes the oxidation of tyrosine to melanin. The RPE is capable of synthesizing tyrosinase and producing melanosomes. In contrast to the epidermal melanosomes, the melanosomes of the RPE remain within the cell and are not transferred to other cells. Within the eye, the melanin concentration of RPE cells decreases between the periphery and posterior pole and increases in the macular region (Weiter et al. 1986). With age, melanin content decreases in the RPE cells, and melanin granules become more uniformly distributed within the cytoplasm.

The human RPE is normally well protected against oxidative damage. Pigment granules, however, are known to undergo an age-related change. Granules become increasingly complex with ageing, due to fusion of melanin with lipofuscin, forming, melanolipofuscin. In the aging RPE, oxidative changes in melanin generate reactive oxygen species upon excitation with blue light.

Phagocytosis of the Shed Rod Outer Segment

One of the critical functions of the RPE is to phagocytose and degrade the rod outer segment (ROS) which is shed diurnally from the distal end of the photoreceptors. Two specific mechanisms for RPE phagocytosis are proposed, a slow, nonspecific process and a rapid receptor-mediated uptake of shed ROS. The receptor-mediated uptake is a multistep process which involves recognition-attachment, internalization, and degradation (Stossel 1974). Receptor ligand binding interaction between shed ROS and RPE microvilli is the first step of the phagocytic process (Bok 1993). Several studies have reported that α5β5 integrin is a functional ROS receptor (Finnemann and Rodriguez-Boulan 1999). Others studies suggest that it is mediated by the receptor tyrosine kinase, c-met, and its ligand GAS-6 (Hall et al. 2001). Binding of the ROS is followed by invagination of plasma membrane around the outer segment fragment, leading to its ingestion into a phagosome. An actin network forms at the site of attachment that extend into pseudopods which surround and engulf the fragments to form the phagosome which are transported basally (Rakoczy et al. 1994). After this, the phagosomes fuse with the lysosomes and are degraded. The lysosomal enzymes hydrolyze the sequestered outer segments into small molecules that diffuse out of the RPE and are reused within the cell. Cathepsin D is the most important enzyme that degrades rhodopsin, the major glycosylated protein present in the outer segment; another enzyme is cysteine protease cathepsin S (Rakoczy et al. 1994).

With age and pathological changes in human eye, deficient degradation of the outer segment material within the phagolysosomes may lead to the formation of lipofuscin granules (Feeney-Burns et al. 1984; Tate et al. 1995).

Blood-Retinal Barrier, Transport, and Ionic Pumps

The blood-retinal barrier (BRB) is formed by the endothelial cells of retinal blood vessels (inner blood-retinal barrier) and the retinal pigment epithelial cells (outer blood-retinal barrier). The multilayered neural retina is separated by the subretinal space from the retinal pigment epithelium (RPE) monolayer, which separates the outer surface of the neural retina from the choroid. Under physiologic conditions, the retina is firmly attached to the RPE. Because of their specialized functions, the RPE cells have unique morphologic and functional polarity properties. Only selected nutrients are exchanged between the choroid and retina; the transcellular and paracellular passage of other molecules across the RPE is restricted. One feature of RPE cells is the predominant apical localization of Na^+/K^+-ATPase, which regulates intracellular Na^+ and K^+ homeostasis (Quinn and Miller 1992).

Anatomically the outer blood-retinal barrier is formed by the RPE, which controls the exchange of fluid and molecules between the fenestrated choriocapillaris and the outer retina. Two major components of RPE barrier function are the tight junctions between the RPE cells and the polarized distribution of RPE membrane proteins (Anderson and Van Itallie 1995). Since tight junction inhibits intercellular diffusion, molecular exchanges predominantly occur across the RPE cells themselves. Nevertheless, tight junctions are dynamic structures, and their permeability can be modified by specific physiological conditions as well as by certain pharmacological agents (Balda et al. 1991). Furthermore diffusible factors secreted from the neural retina, or RPE-derived growth factors (such as hepatocyte growth factor), may be involved in the regulation of the structure and function of RPE tight junctions (Balda et al. 1991; Cereijido et al. 1993). The regulation of transepithelial transport is dependent on the asymmetric distribution of cellular proteins (Drubin and Nelson 1996). This polarity of the epithelial cells changes upon interaction with the environment. In RPE the Na^+/K^+-ATPase is localized at the apical cell membrane, and cytoskeletal proteins like ankyrin and fodrin known to be associated with the ATPase are localized apically, whereas in most other epithelial cells they are localized basolaterally (Gundersen et al. 1991). RPE cells have receptors in their basal and lateral membranes for nutrient that arrive through the choriocapillaries that must be transported toward the outer retina, such as retinol and its binding protein. Human RPE expresses the protons coupled monocarboxylate transporters (MCT1 and MCT3). MCT1 is seen in the apical membrane, while MCT3 in the basolateral membrane. The coordinated activities of these two transporters facilitate the flux of lactate and from the retina to the choroid (Robey et al. 1992).

P-glycoprotein is another protein that contributes to the normal transport function of RPE cells. The protein is expressed in cultured and native human RPE cells on the apical and basolateral membrane surface (Kennedy and Mangini 2002). The basolateral expression of P-glycoprotein serves to clear the unwanted metabolites from the subretinal space, thus serving a protective function to the neural retina. There is evidence that apical P-glycoprotein can mediate ATP efflux, function as a lipid translocase, modulate volume-sensitive chloride ion efflux and steroid secretion, transport retinoids (Kennedy and Mangini 2002).

The movement of water and catabolites from the retina toward the choriocapillaries is important for the nutrition of the retina, for maintenance of ocular pressure, and possibly for maintenance of retinal attachment to the RPE (Miller et al. 1982). In conjunction with passive forces, active transport of solutes across the RPE contributes to the movement of water out of the eye. The apical surface of the RPE cells also shows specialized molecular mechanisms for these functions. Aquaporin 1 is a hexahelical integral membrane protein that functions as a constitutive channel for water transport expressed in human fetal and adult RPE where it facilitates water movement across the RPE monolayer (Stamer et al. 2003).

Fluid movement from the retina to the choroids is not blocked by ouabain (Miller et al. 1982), a Na^+/K^+-ATPase inhibitor, suggesting that this enzyme is not involved in the removal of water from the subretinal space. The regulation of pH across the pigment epithelium is thought to involve three apical and two basolateral transporters that provide pathways for the transport of Na^+ and HCO_3^-. Breakdown of the blood-retinal barrier has serious consequences for the health of the eye and is present in many types of retinopathies (Gariano et al. 1996).

The Visual Cycle

The visual cycle regenerates the chromophore of the rod and cone opsins through a series of metabolic reactions for light absorption in the photoreceptors (Wald 1935). 11-cis Retinal undergoes conformational changes upon absorption of a photon and modified to all-trans retinal which is then deposited into the lumen of the rod outer segment disk. The ATP-binding cassette family protein, ABCA4 (a flippase), preferentially binds the N-retinyldiene-phosphatidylethanolamine form of all-trans retinal and transports it to the cytoplasmic side of the disks (Sun and Nathans 1997; Sun et al. 1999; Ahn et al. 2000; Molday et al. 2000; Beharry et al. 2004). The retinol dehydrogenases present in the cytoplasm of the rod outer segment reduce the all-trans retinal to all-trans retinol (Rattner et al. 2000) and trafficked to the microvilli of RPE by interphotoreceptor retinol-binding protein (IRBP) (Bridges et al. 1984). Further, the cellular retinol-binding protein (CRBP) carries the all-trans retinol to the endoplasmic reticulum where the retinoid cycle enzymes are present. The lecithin-retinol acyltransferase (LRAT) esterifies the all-trans retinol to all-trans retinyl esters (Kawaguchi et al. 2007), which is further hydrolyzed and isomerized by retinal pigment epithelial-specific protein 65 kDa (RPE65) to form 11-cis retinol (Redmond et al. 2005; Jin et al. 2005a, b). Finally, the cellular retinaldehyde-binding protein (CRALBP) aids the specific retinaldehyde dehydrogenase 5 (RDH5) in the oxidation of 11-cis retinol to form 11-cis retinal, the end product of the retinoid cycle (Saari and Bredberg 1982). Eventually, IRBP binds the 11-cis retinal and transports it to the photoreceptors for the regeneration of photoactive rhodopsin. In case of dark to light adaptation, a sudden surge of 11-cis retinal is required to meet the higher turnover rate. There are distinct pools of 11-cis retinal present, for instance, in the rod outer segment or in the subretinal space apart from the visual cycle which can compensate the demand (Strauss 2005). Thus, RPE plays an indispensable role in the visual cycle of rods. In contrast to the rod visual cycle, cone opsins recycle through Muller glial cells and probably partly using the RPE as well (Wang et al. 2008). However, the mechanism of cone visual cycle is largely unknown.

The function of chaperone RPE65 is very crucial for the visual cycle. Many clinical and experimental data strongly suggested the role of RPE65 in the retinol isomerization cycle (Iseli et al. 2002; Katz and Redmond 2001; Gu et al. 1997). Apart from that, the most critical function of RPE65 is acclimatizing the visual cycle for dark and light adaptation (Xue et al. 2004). There are two forms of RPE65, the membrane-bound RPE65 (mRPE65) which is a chaperone for all-trans-retinyl esters and the soluble form (sRPE65) which is a chaperone for vitamin A. The sRPE65 is not palmitoylated, whereas mRPE is triply palmitoylated. When the visual cycle is not very active, mRPE65 is converted into sRPE65 by LRAT which inhibits further synthesis of chromophore. Thus, the palmitoylation switch of RPE65, regulates the visual cycle (Xue et al. 2004).

Secretion of Growth Factors and Cytokines

RPE are known to secrete a wide variety of growth factors and cytokines under physiological and pathological conditions. While many studies have been performed delineating the regulation and effect of these factors on cultured cells in disease states, little is known about their role in the resting RPE monolayer. Secreted cytokines and growth factors in the monolayer may act in an autocrine or paracrine fashion on the cell of origin or adjacent RPE, or they may have paracrine effects on adjacent photoreceptors or choroidal cells. Chemokines and inflammatory cytokines are secreted in significant amounts only after RPE activation. RPE monolayer reveals expression of TGF-β2, bFGF, aFGF, FGF-5, HGF, and PDGF-A as well as their corresponding receptors. Local production of TGF-β by the RPE monolayer could have multiple effects including maintenance of an anti-inflammatory state, inhibition of cellular proliferation, and stimulation of phagocytosis. FGFs typically enhance RPE cell proliferation and migration, but in the monolayer, bFGF may be acting as a survival-promoting factor for RPE cells (Jin et al. 2005a, b). Vascular endothelial growth factor (VEGF) and its receptors are expressed by RPE; however, expression of VEGF in the resting monolayer appears to be low, while it is increased during altered conditions of vitreoretinal pathologies (Blaaugeers et al. 1999; Coral et al. 2013).

5.5.2.3 Retinal Pigment Epithelium in Pathology

Once differentiated, the RPE does not renew itself by cell division; it continues to carry out its versatile functions throughout the lifetime of the individual unless such processes are lost due to disease. Because of the diverse functions of the RPE and its importance in retinal integrity, any alterations in the normal functioning of the RPE may result in either visual impairment or blindness. Alterations in RPE function may occur either as a result of diseases which specifically affect the RPE, such as age-related macular degeneration and central serous retinopathy (CSR) (Wang et al. 2008), or due to secondary changes resulting from retinal diseases such as retinitis pigmentosa (RP) (Sahel et al. 2010) and proliferative vitreoretinopathy (Tosi et al. 2014) and proliferative diabetic retinopathy (PDR) (Heng et al. 2013; Kaviarasan et al. 2015).

References

Abraham V, Chou ML, DeBolt KM, Koval M. Phenotypic control of gap junctional communication by cultured alveolar epithelial cells. Am J Physiol. 1999;276:L825–34.

Adamis AP, Shima DT, Yeo KT, Yeo TK, Brown LF, Berse B, D'Amore PA, Folkman J. Synthesis and secretion of vascular permeability factor/vascular endothelial growth factor by human retinal pigment epithelial cells. Biochem Biophys Res Commun. 1993;193:631–8.

Agrawal RV, Murthy S, Sangwan V, Biswas J. Current approach in diagnosis and management of anterior uveitis. Indian J Ophthalmol. 2010;58(1):11–9. doi:10.4103/0301-4738.58468.

Ahmad S. Concise review: limbal stem cell deficiency, dysfunction, and distress. Stem Cells Transl Med. 2012;1:110–5.
Ahn J, Wong JT, Molday RS. The effect of lipid environment and retinoids on the ATPase activity of ABCR, the photoreceptor ABC transporter responsible for Stargardt macular dystrophy. J Biol Chem. 2000;275:20399–405.
Aho HJ, Saari KM, Kallajoki M, Nevalainen TJ. Synthesis of group II phospholipase A2 and lysozyme in lacrimal glands. Invest Ophthalmol Vis Sci. 1996;37(9):1826–32.
Akama TO, Nakayama J, Nishida K, Hiraoka N, Suzuki M, McAuliffe J, Hindsgaul O, Fukuda M, Fukuda MN. Human corneal GlcNac 6-O-sulfotransferase and mouse intestinal GlcNac 6-O-sulfotransferase both produce keratan sulfate. J Biol Chem. 2001;276:16271–8.
Akira S, Takeda K, Kaisho T. Toll-like receptors: critical proteins linking innate and acquired immunity. Nat Immunol. 2001;2(8):675–80. 90609 [pii]. doi:10.1038/90609.
Alarcon I, Kwan L, Yu C, Evans DJ, Fleiszig SM. Role of the corneal epithelial basement membrane in ocular defense against Pseudomonas aeruginosa. Infect Immun. 2009;77:3264–71.
Alarcon I, Tam C, Mun JJ, LeDue J, Evans DJ, Fleiszig SM. Factors impacting corneal epithelial barrier function against pseudomonas aeruginosa traversal. Invest Ophthalmol Vis Sci. 2011;52(3):1368–77. iovs.10-6125 [pii]. doi:10.1167/iovs.10-6125.
Albert AD, Boesze-Battaglia K. The role of cholesterol in rod outer segment membranes. Prog Lipid Res. 2005;44(2–3):99–124.
Albon J, Karwatowski WJ, Avery N, Easty DL, Duance VC. Changes in the collagenous matrix of the aging human lamina cribrosa. Br J Ophthalmol. 1995;79:368–75.
Allansmith MR, Whitney CR, McClellan BH, Newman LP. Immunoglobulins in the human eye. Location, type, and amount. Arch Ophthalmol. 1973;89:36–45.
Alm A. Latanoprost in the treatment of glaucoma. Clin Ophthalmol. 2014;8:1967–85.
Aluru SV, Agarwal S, Srinivasan B, Iyer GK, Rajappa SM, Tatu U, et al. Lacrimal Proline Rich 4 (LPRR4) Protein in the Tear Fluid Is a Potential Biomarker of Dry Eye Syndrome. PLoS ONE 2012;7(12):e51979.
Amico C, Yakimov M, Catania MV, Giuffrida R, Pistone M, Enea V. Differential expression of cyclooxygenase-1 and cyclooxygenase-2 in the cornea during wound healing. Tissue Cell. 2004;36(1):1–12. doi:S0040816603000831 [pii].
Andresen JL, Ehlers N. Chemotaxis of human keratocytes is increased by platelet-derived growth factor-BB, epidermal growth factor, transforming growth factor-alpha, acidic fibroblast growth factor, insulin-like growth factor-I, and transforming growth factor-beta. Curr Eye Res. 1998;17(1):79–87.
Andresen JL, Ledet T, Ehlers N. Keratocyte migration and peptide growth factors: the effect of PDGF, bFGF, EGF, IGF-I, aFGF and TGF-beta on human keratocyte migration in a collagen gel. Curr Eye Res. 1997;16(6):605–13.
Anderson JM, Van Itallie CM. Tight junctions and the molecular basis for regulation of paracellular permeability. Am J Physiol. 1995;269:G467–75.
Anderson S, SandarRaj S, Fite D, Wessel H, SundarRaj N. Developmentally regulated appearance of spliced variants of type XII collagen in the cornea. Invest Ophthalmol Vis Sci. 2000;41:55–63.
Andrews JS. Human tear film lipids. I. Composition of the principal non-polar component. Exp Eye Res. 1970;10:223–27.
Aragon C, Lopez-Corcuera B. Structure, function and regulation of glycine neurotransporters. Eur J Pharmacol. 2003;479(1–3):249–62.
Austin BA, Coulon C, Liu CY, Kao WW, Rada JA. Altered collagen fibril formation in the sclera of lumican-deficient mice. Invest Ophthalmol Vis Sci. 2002;43:1695–701.
Awasthi S. Surfactant protein (SP)-A and SP-D as antimicrobial and immunotherapeutic agents. Recent Pat Antiinfect Drug Discov. 2010;5(2):115–23. doi:BSP/PRI/EPUB/00003 [pii].
Ayoub GS, Copenhagen DR. Application of a fluorometric method to measure glutamate release from single retinal photoreceptors. J Neurosci Methods. 1991;37(1):7–14.
Azzarolo AM, Mircheff AK, Kaswan RL, Stanczyk FZ, Gentschein E, Becker L, Nassir B, Warren DW. Androgen support of lacrimal gland function. Endocrine. 1997;6:39–45.

Balasubramanian R, Gan L. Development of retinal amacrine cells and their dendritic stratification. Curr Ophthalmol Rep. 2014;2(3):100–6.

Balda MS, Gonzalez-Mariscal L, Contreras RG, Macias-Silva M, Torres-Marquez ME, Garcia-Sainz JA, Cereijido M. Assembly and sealing of tight junctions: possible participation of G-proteins, phospholipase C, protein kinase C and calmodulin. J Membr Biol. 1991;122:193–202.

Baldo GJ, Gong X, Martinez-Wittinghan FJ, Kumar NM, Gilula NB, et al. Gap junctional coupling in lenses from alpha[8] connexin knockout mice. J Gen Physiol. 2001;118(5):447–56.

Balzas EA. Functional anatomy of the vitreous. In: Duane TD, Jaeger EA (eds). Biomedical Foundations of Ophthalmology, vol 1, Ch 17 Harper and Row: Philadelphia, 1984, pp 1–16.

Barba I, Garcia-Ramírez M, Hernández C, Alonso MA, Masmiquel L, et al. Metabolic fingerprints of proliferative diabetic retinopathy: an 1H-NMRbased metabonomic approach using vitreous humor. Invest Ophthalmol Vis Sci. 2010; 51: 4416–21.

Bazan HE. Corneal injury alters eicosanoid formation in the rabbit anterior segment in vivo. Invest Ophthalmol Vis Sci. 1987;28(2):314–9.

Bazan HE, Bazan NG. Composition of phospholipids and free fatty acids and incorporation of labeled arachidonic acid in rabbit cornea. Comparison of epithelium, stroma and endothelium. Curr Eye Res. 1984;3(11):1313–9.

Bazan H, Ottino P. The role of platelet-activating factor in the corneal response to injury. Prog Retin Eye Res. 2002;21(5):449–64. doi:S1350946202000113 [pii].

Bazan HE, Varner L. A mitogen-activated protein kinase (MAP-kinase) cascade is stimulated by platelet activating factor (PAF) in corneal epithelium. Curr Eye Res. 1997;16(4):372–9.

Bazan HE, Birkle DL, Beuerman R, Bazan NG. Cryogenic lesion alters the metabolism of arachidonic acid in rabbit cornea layers. Invest Ophthalmol Vis Sci. 1985a;26(4):474–80.

Bazan HE, Birkle DL, Beuerman RW, Bazan NG. Inflammation-induced stimulation of the synthesis of prostaglandins and lipoxygenase-reaction products in rabbit cornea. Curr Eye Res. 1985b;4(3):175–9.

Bazan HE, Reddy ST, Lin N. Platelet-activating factor (PAF) accumulation correlates with injury in the cornea. Exp Eye Res. 1991;52(4):481–91.

Bazan HE, Tao Y, Bazan NG. Platelet-activating factor induces collagenase expression in corneal epithelial cells. Proc Natl Acad Sci U S A. 1993;90(18):8678–82.

Bazan HE, Tao Y, DeCoster MA, Bazan NG. Platelet-activating factor induces cyclooxygenase-2 gene expression in corneal epithelium. Requirement of calcium in the signal transduction pathway. Invest Ophthalmol Vis Sci. 1997;38(12):2492–501.

Beebe DC, Masters BR. Cell lineage and the differentiation of corneal epithelial cells. Invest Ophthalmol Vis Sci. 1996;37:1815–25.

Beharry S, Zhong M, Molday RS. N-retinylidene-phosphatidylethanolamine is the preferred retinoid substrate for the photoreceptor-specific ABC transporter ABCA4 (ABCR). J Biol Chem. 2004;279:53972–9.

Belmonte C, Acosta MC, Gallar J. Neural basis of sensation in intact and injured corneas. Exp Eye Res. 2004;78(3):513–25.

Benedek GB. Theory of transparency of the eye. Appl Opt. 1971;10(3):459–73. doi:16827 [pii].

Beyer EC, Paul DL, Goodenough DA. Connexin43: a protein from rat heart homologous to a gap junction protein from liver. J Cell Biol. 1987;105(6 Pt 1):2621–9.

Bill A. Blood circulation and fluid dynamics in the eye. Physiol Rev. 1975;55:383–417.

Birk DE, Fitch JM, Linsenmayer TF. Organization of collagen types I and V in the embryonic chicken cornea. Invest Ophthalmol Vis Sci. 1986;27:1470–7.

Bishop PN. Structural macromolecules and supramolecular organisation of the vitreous gel. Progress in retinal and eye research. 2000; 19(3): 323–44.

Bjorkhem I. Crossing the barrier: oxysterols as cholesterol transporters and metabolic modulators in the brain. J Intern Med. 2006;260(6):493–508.

Blazynski C, Perez MT. Adenosine in vertebrate retina: localization, receptor characterization, and function. Cell Mol Neurobiol. 1991;11(5):463–84.

Blochberger TC, Vergnes JP, Hempel J, Hassell JR. cDNA to chick lumican (corneal keratan sulfate proteoglycan) reveals homology to the small interstitial proteoglycan gene family and expression in muscle and intestine. J Biol Chem. 1992;267:347–52.

Bloemendal H, editor. Molecular and cellular biology of the eye lens. New York: John Wiley; 1981.
Bok D. The retinal pigment epithelium: a versatile partner in vision. J Cell Sci Suppl. 1993; 17:189–95.
Bonanno JA. Identity and regulation of ion transport mechanisms in the corneal endothelium. Prog Retin Eye Res. 2003;22:69–94.
Bonanno JA. Molecular mechanisms underlying the corneal endothelial pump. Exp Eye Res. 2012;95:2–7.
Bonini S, Lambiase A, Rama P, Caprioglio G, Aloe L. Topical treatment with nerve growth factor for neurotrophic keratitis. Ophthalmology. 2000;107(7):1342–7.
Borradori L, Sonnenberg A. Structure and function of hemidesmosomes: more than simple adhesion complexes. J Invest Dermatol. 1999;112:411–8.
Botelho SY. Tears and the lacrimal gland. Sci Am. 1964;211:78–86.
Botelho SY, Hisada M, Fuenmayor N. Functional innervation of the lacrimal gland in the cat. Origin of secretomotor fibers in the lacrimal nerve. Arch Ophthalmol. 1966;76:581–8.
Bottaro DP, Rubin JS, Faletto DL, Chan AM, Kmiecik TE, Vande Woude GF, Aaronson SA. Identification of the hepatocyte growth factor receptor as the c-met proto-oncogene product. Science. 1991;251(4995):802–4.
Bourcier T, Rondeau N, Paquet S, Forgez P, Lombet A, Pouzaud F, Rostene W, Borderie V, Laroche L. Expression of neurotensin receptors in human corneal keratocytes. Invest Ophthalmol Vis Sci. 2002;43(6):1765–71.
Bozanic D, Tafra R, Saraga-Babic M. Role of apoptosis and mitosis during human eye development. Eur J Cell Biol. 2003;82(8):421–29. S0171-9335(04)70313-1 [pii]. doi:10.1078/0171-9335-00328.
Braun RJ, King-Smith PE, Begley CG, Li L, Gewecke NR. Dynamics and function of the tear film in relation to the blink cycle. Prog Retin Eye Res. 2015;45:132–64.
Bretillon L, Diczfalusy U, et al. Cholesterol-24S-hydroxylase (CYP46A1) is specifically expressed in neurons of the neural retina. Curr Eye Res. 2007;32(4):361–6.
Bretillon L, Acar N, et al. ApoB100,LDLR-/- mice exhibit reduced electroretinographic response and cholesteryl esters deposits in the retina. Invest Ophthalmol Vis Sci. 2008;49(4):1307–14.
Bridges CD, Alvarez RA, Fong SL, Gonzalez-Fernandez F, Lam DM, Liou GI. Visual cycle in the mammalian eye. Retinoid-binding proteins and the distribution of 11-cis retinoids. Vision Res. 1984;24:1581–94.
Brown NA, Bron AJ. An estimate of the human lens epithelial cell size in vivo. Exp Eye Res. 1987;44:899–906.
Buckland AG, Heeley EL, Wilton DC. Bacterial cell membrane hydrolysis by secreted phospholipases A(2): a major physiological role of human group IIa sPLA(2) involving both bacterial cell wall penetration and interfacial catalysis. Biochim Biophys Acta. 2000;1484(2–3): 195–206. doi:S1388-1981(00)00018-4 [pii].
Campbell M, Humphries P. The blood-retina barrier: tight junctions and barrier modulation. Adv Exp Med Biol. 2012;763:70–84.
Campos-Rodriguez R, Oliver-Aguillon G, Vega-Perez LM, Jarillo-Luna A, Hernandez-Martinez D, Rojas-Hernandez S, Rodriguez-Monroy MA, Rivera-Aguilar V, Gonzalez-Robles A. Human IgA inhibits adherence of acanthamoeba polyphaga to epithelial cells and contact lenses. Can J Microbiol. 2004;50(9):711–18. w04-057 [pii]. doi:10.1139/w04-057.
Cavanagh HD, Colley AM. Cholinergic, adrenergic, and PGE1 effects on cyclic nucleotides and growth in cultured corneal epithelium. Metab Pediatr Syst Ophthalmol. 1982;6(2):63–74.
Cereijido M, Gonzalez-Mariscal L, Contreras RG, Gallardo JM, Garcia-Villegas R, Valdes J. The making of a tight junction. J Cell Sci Suppl. 1993;17:127–32.
Chakravarti S. Focus on molecules: keratocan (KERA). Exp Eye Res. 2006;82:183–4.
Chandrasekher G, Kakazu AH, Bazan HE. HGF- and KGF-induced activation of PI-3K/p70 s6 kinase pathway in corneal epithelial cells: its relevance in wound healing. Exp Eye Res. 2001;73(2):191–202. S0014-4835(01)91026-7 [pii]. doi:10.1006/exer.2001.1026.

Chang D, Sha Q, Zhang X, Liu P, Rong S, Han T, Liu P, Pan H. The evaluation of the oxidative stress parameters in patients with primary angle-closure glaucoma. PLoS One. 2011;6: e27218.

Char DH, Schlaegel Jr TF. Chapter 39: General factors in uveitis. In: Duane TD, editor. Clinical ophthalmology. 4th ed. Philadelphia: Harper & Row; 1982. p. 1–7.

Cherubini E, Gaiarsa JL, et al. GABA: an excitatory transmitter in early postnatal life. Trends Neurosci. 1991;14(12):515–9.

Chen KH, Hsu WM, Chiang CC, Li YS. Transforming growth factor-beta2 inhibition of corneal endothelial proliferation mediated by prostaglandin. Curr Eye Res. 2003;26(6):363–70.

Cheng JW, Cheng SW, Gao LD, Lu GC, Wei RL. Intraocular pressure-lowering effects of commonly used fixed-combination drugs with timolol: a systematic review and meta-analysis. PLoS One. 2012;7:e45079.

Chew SK, Skalicky SE, Goldberg I. Brinzolamide plus brimonidine for the treatment of glaucoma: an update. Expert Opin Pharmacother. 2014;15:2461–71.

Choi KY, Chow LN, Mookherjee N. Cationic host defence peptides: multifaceted role in immune modulation and inflammation. J Innate Immun. 2012;4(4):361–70. 000336630 [pii]. doi:10.1159/000336630.

Chong CC, Stump RJ, Lovicu FJ, McAvoy JW. TGFbeta promotes Wnt expression during cataract development. Exp Eye Res. 2009;88(2):307–13. S0014-4835(08)00254-6 [pii] doi:10.1016/j.exer.2008.07.018.

Cimino L, Aldigeri R, Parmeggiani M, Belloni L, Zotti CA, Fontana L, et al. Searching for viral antibodies and genome in intraocular fluids of patients with Fuchs uveitis and non-infectious uveitis. Graefes Arch Clin Exp Ophthalmol. 2013;251(6):1607–12.

Civan MM, Macknight AD. The ins and outs of aqueous humour secretion. Exp Eye Res. 2004;78:625–31.

Clark VM, Hall MO. RPE cell surface proteins in normal and dystrophic rats. Invest Ophthalmol Vis Sci. 1986;27:136–44.

Coca-Prados M, Escribano J. New perspectives in aqueous humor secretion and in glaucoma: the ciliary body as a multifunctional neuroendocrine gland. Prog Retin Eye Res. 2007;26(3): 239–62. doi:10.1016/j.preteyeres.2007.01.002.

Cogan DG, Kuwabara T. Arcus senilis; its pathology and histochemistry. AMA Arch Ophthalmol. 1959;61(4):553–60.

Cole DF. Location of ouabain-sensitive adenosine triphosphatase in ciliary epithelium. Exp Eye Res. 1964;3:72–5.

Conners MS, Stoltz RA, Webb SC, Rosenberg J, Dunn MW, Abraham NG, Laniado-Schwartzman M. A closed eye contact lens model of corneal inflammation. Part 1: increased synthesis of cytochrome P450 arachidonic acid metabolites. Invest Ophthalmol Vis Sci. 1995;36(5): 828–40.

Conners MS, Urbano F, Vafeas C, Stoltz RA, Dunn MW, Schwartzman ML. Alkali burn-induced synthesis of inflammatory eicosanoids in rabbit corneal epithelium. Invest Ophthalmol Vis Sci. 1997;38(10):1963–71.

Contini M, Lin B, et al. Synaptic input of ON-bipolar cells onto the dopaminergic neurons of the mouse retina. J Comp Neurol. 2010;518(11):2035–50.

Coral K, Madhavan J, Pukhraj R, Angayarkanni N. High glucose induced differential expression of lysyl oxidase and its isoform in ARPE-19 cells. Curr Eye Res. 2013;38(1):194–203.

Corpuz LM, Funderburgh JL, Funderburgh ML, Bottomley GS, Prakash S, Conrad GW. Molecular cloning and tissue distribution of keratocan. Bovine corneal keratan sulfate proteoglycan 37A. J Biol Chem. 1996;271:9759–63.

Cortina MS, He J, Li N, Bazan NG, Bazan HE. Neuroprotectin D1 synthesis and corneal nerve regeneration after experimental surgery and treatment with PEDF plus DHA. Invest Ophthalmol Vis Sci. 2010;51(2):804–10. iovs.09-3641 [pii]. doi:10.1167/iovs.09-3641.

Costa JL, Morrone AR, Resende RR, Chasin AAM, Tavares MFM. Development of a method for the analysis of drugs of abuse in vitreous humor by capillary electrophoresis with diode array detection (CE-DAD). J Chromatogr B Biomed Sci Appl. 2014;945–946:84–91

Cui W, Tomarev SI, Piatigorsky J, Chepelinsky AB, Duncan MK. Mafs, Prox1, and Pax6 can regulate chicken betaB1-crystallin gene expression. J Biol Chem. 2004;279(12):11088–95. M312414200 [pii]. doi:10.1074/jbc.M312414200.

Curcio CA, Presley JB, et al. Esterified and unesterified cholesterol in drusen and basal deposits of eyes with age-related maculopathy. Exp Eye Res. 2005;81(6):731–41.

Cvekl A, Piatigorsky J. Lens development and crystallin gene expression: many roles for Pax-6. Bioessays. 1996;18(8):621–30. doi:10.1002/bies.950180805.

Cvekl A, Sax CM, Bresnick EH, Piatigorsky J. A complex array of positive and negative elements regulates the chicken alpha A-crystallin gene: involvement of Pax-6, USF, CREB and/or CREM, and AP-1 proteins. Mol Cell Biol. 1994;14(11):7363–76.

Dahm R, Van Marle J, Prescott AR, Quinlan RA. Gap junctions containing alpha8-connexin [MP70] in the adult mammalian lens epithelium suggests a reevaluation of its role in the lens. Exp Eye Res. 1999;69(1):45–56.

Dartt DA. Interaction of EGF family growth factors and neurotransmitters in regulating lacrimal gland secretion. Exp Eye Res. 2004;78:337–45.

Dartt DA. Neural regulation of lacrimal gland secretory processes: relevance in dry eye diseases. Prog Retin Eye Res. 2009;28:155–77.

Davis-Silberman N, Ashery-Padan R. Iris development in vertebrates; genetic and molecular considerations. Brain Res. 2008;1192(March):17–28. doi:10.1016/j.brainres.2007.03.043.

Deeg CA, Amann B, Raith AJ, Kaspers B. Inter- and intramolecular epitope spreading in equine recurrent uveitis. Invest Ophthalmol Vis Sci. 2006;47(2):652–6.

Deeg CA, Altmann F, Hauck SM, Schoeffmann S, Amann B, Stangassinger M, Ueffing M. Down-regulation of pigment epithelium-derived factor in uveitic lesion associates with focal vascular endothelial growth factor expression and breakdown of the blood-retinal barrier. Proteomics. 2007a;7(9):1540–8.

Deeg CA, Hauck SM, Amann B, Kremmer E, Stangassinger M, Ueffing M. Major retinal autoantigens remain stably expressed during all stages of spontaneous uveitis. Mol Immunol. 2007b;44(13):3291–6. doi:10.1016/j.molimm.2007.02.027.

Deeg CA, Raith AJ, Amann B, Crabb JW, Thurau SR, Hauck SM, et al. CRALBP is a highly prevalent autoantigen for human autoimmune uveitis. Clin Dev Immunol. 2007c;2007:39245.

Deeg CA, Hauck SM, Amann B, Pompetzki D, Altmann F, Raith A, et al. Equine recurrent uveitis – a spontaneous horse model of uveitis. Ophthalmic Res. 2008;40(3–4):151–3.

Deeg CA, Eberhardt C, Hofmaier F, Amann B, Hauck SM. Osteopontin and fibronectin levels are decreased in vitreous of autoimmune uveitis and retinal expression of both proteins indicates ECM re-modeling. PLoS One. 2011;6(12):e27674.

De Smet MD, Gad Elkareem AM, Zwinderman AH. The vitreous, the retinal interface in ocular health and disease. Ophthalmologica Journal international d'ophtalmologie International journal of ophthalmology Zeitschrift fur Augenheilkunde. 2013; 230(4): 165–78.

Devamanoharan PS, Henein M, Morris S, et al. Prevention of selenite cataract by vitamin C. Exp Eye Res. 1991;52(5):563–8.

Dickinson JC, Durham DG, Hamilton PB. Ion exchange chromatography of free amino acids in aqueous fluid and lens of the human eye. Invest Ophthalmol. 1968;7:551–63.

Dietschy JM, Turley SD. Thematic review series: brain Lipids. Cholesterol metabolism in the central nervous system during early development and in the mature animal. J Lipid Res. 2004;45(8):1375–97.

Dieudonne S. Glycinergic synaptic currents in Golgi cells of the rat cerebellum. Proc Natl Acad Sci U S A. 1995;92(5):1441–5.

Djeridane Y. Immunohistochemical evidence for the presence of vasopressin in the rat harderian gland, retina and lacrimal gland. Exp Eye Res. 1994;59:117–20.

Docherty RJ, Edwards JG, Garrod DR, Mattey DL. Chick embryonic pigmented retina is one of the group of epithelioid tissues that lack cytokeratins and desmosomes and have intermediate filaments composed of vimentin. J Cell Sci. 1984;71:61–74.

Dorey CK, Torres X, Swart T. Evidence of melanogenesis in porcine retinal pigment epithelial cells in vitro. Exp Eye Res. 1990;50:1–10.

Dröge MJ, van Sorge AA, van Haeringen NJ, Quax WJ, Zaagsma J. Alternative splicing of cyclooxygenase-1 mRNA in the human iris. Ophthalmic Res. 2003;35(3):160–3.
Drubin DG, Nelson WJ. Origins of cell polarity. Cell. 1996;84:335–44.
Dua HS, Gomes JA, Jindal VK, Appa SN, Schwarting R, Eagle Jr RC, Donoso LA, Laibson PR. Mucosa specific lymphocytes in the human conjunctiva, corneoscleral limbus and lacrimal gland. Curr Eye Res. 1994;13:87–93.
Dua HS, Faraj LA, Said DG, Gray T, Lowe J. Re: Jester et al.: Lessons in corneal structure and mechanics to guide the corneal surgeon (Ophthalmology 2013;120:1715–1717). Ophthalmology. 2014;121:e18.
Duan X, Xue P, Wang N, Dong Z, Lu Q, Yang F. Proteomic analysis of aqueous humor from patients with primary open angle glaucoma. Mol Vis. 2010;16:2839–46.
Duncan G, editor. Mechanisms of cataract formation in the human lens. London: Academic; 1981.
Dupont E, el Aoumari A, Roustiau-Sévère S, Briand JP, Gros D. Immunological characterization of rat cardiac gap junctions: presence of common antigenic determinants in heart of other vertebrate species and in various organs. J Membr Biol. 1988;104(2):119–28.
Durrani OM, Tehrani NN, Marr JE, Moradi P, Stavrou P, Murray PI. Degree, duration and causes of visual loss in uveitis. Br J Ophthalmol. 2004;88:1159–62.
Eagle RC. Iris pigmentation and pigmented lesions: an ultrastructural study. Trans Am Ophthalmol Soc. 1988;86:581–687.
Eberhardt C, Amann B, Stangassinger M, Hauck SM, Deeg CA. Isolation, characterization and establishment of an equine retinal glial cell line: a prerequisite to investigate the physiological function of Müller cells in the retina. J Anim Physiol Anim Nutr. 2012;96(2):260–9.
Ebrey T, Koutalos Y. Vertebrate photoreceptors. Prog Retin Eye Res. 2001;20(1):49–94.
Edward DP, Bouhenni R. Anterior segment alterations and comparative aqueous humor proteomics in the buphthalmic rabbit (an American Ophthalmological Society thesis). Trans Am Ophthalmol Soc. 2011;109:66–114.
Engel A, Fujiyoshi Y, Gonen T, Walz T. Junction-forming aquaporins. Curr Opin Struct Biol. 2008;18(2):229–35. S0959-440X(07)00196-0 [pii]. doi:10.1016/j.sbi.2007.11.003.
Epstein DL, Rohen JW. Morphology of the trabecular meshwork and inner-wall endothelium after cationized ferritin perfusion in the monkey eye. Invest Ophthalmol Vis Sci. 1991;32:160–71.
Erdurmus M, Yagci R, Atis O, Karadag R, Akbas A, Hepsen IF. Antioxidant status and oxidative stress in primary open angle glaucoma and pseudoexfoliative glaucoma. Curr Eye Res. 2011;36:713–8.
Esquenazi S, Bazan HE, Bui V, He J, Kim DB, Bazan NG. Topical combination of NGF and DHA increases rabbit corneal nerve regeneration after photorefractive keratectomy. Invest Ophthalmol Vis Sci. 2005;46(9):3121–27. 46/9/3121 [pii]. doi:10.1167/iovs.05-0241.
Euler T, Haverkamp S, et al. Retinal bipolar cells: elementary building blocks of vision. Nat Rev Neurosci. 2014;15(8):507–19.
Farnaud S, Evans RW. Lactoferrin – a multifunctional protein with antimicrobial properties. Mol Immunol. 2003;40(7):395–405. doi:S0161589003001524 [pii].
Feeney-Burns L, Hilderbrand ES, Eldridge S. Aging human RPE: morphometric analysis of macular, equatorial, and peripheral cells. Invest Ophthalmol Vis Sci. 1984;25:195–200.
Feldman GL. Human ocular lipids: their analysis and distribution. Surv Ophthalmol. 1967;12(3):207–43.
Fernández-López E, Pascual FP, Pérez-López M, Quevedo AM, Martínez CP. Sutureless artificial iris after phacoemulsification in congenital aniridia. Optom Vis Sci. 2015;92(4 Suppl 1): S36–9. doi:10.1097/OPX.0000000000000527.
Fine BS. Limiting membranes of the sensory retina and pigment epithelium. An electron microscopic study. Arch Ophthalmol. 1961;66:847–60.
Finnemann SC, Rodriguez-Boulan E. Macrophage and retinal pigment epithelium phagocytosis: apoptotic cells and photoreceptors compete for alphavbeta3 and alphavbeta5 integrins, and protein kinase C regulates alphavbeta5 binding and cytoskeletal linkage. J Exp Med. 1999;190:861–74.
Fliesler SJ, Schroepfer Jr GJ. Sterol composition of bovine retinal rod outer segment membranes and whole retinas. Biochim Biophys Acta. 1982;711(1):138–48.

Fliesler SJ, Florman R, et al. In vivo biosynthesis of cholesterol in the rat retina. FEBS Lett. 1993;335(2):234–8.
Flint AC, Liu X, et al. Nonsynaptic glycine receptor activation during early neocortical development. Neuron. 1998;20(1):43–53.
Fluckinger M, Haas H, Merschak P, Glasgow BJ, Redl B. Human tear lipocalin exhibits antimicrobial activity by scavenging microbial siderophores. Antimicrob Agents Chemother. 2004;48(9):3367–72. 48/9/3367 [pii]. doi:10.1128/AAC.48.9.3367-3372.2004.
Folger PA, Zekaria D, Grotendorst G, Masur SK. Transforming growth factor-beta-stimulated connective tissue growth factor expression during corneal myofibroblast differentiation. Invest Ophthalmol Vis Sci. 2001;42(11):2534–41.
Ford LC, DeLange RJ, Petty RW. Identification of a nonlysozymal bactericidal factor (beta lysin) in human tears and aqueous humor. Am J Ophthalmol. 1976;81(1):30–3.
Forsius H. Lipid keratopathy. A clinical and serum lipid chemical study of sixteen cases. Acta Ophthalmol (Copenh). 1961;39:273–83.
Foulks GN. The correlation between the tear film lipid layer and dry eye disease. Surv Ophthalmol. 2007;52(4):369–74. S0039-6257(07)00057-4 [pii]. doi:10.1016/j.survophthal.2007.04.009.
Fraenkl SA, Muser J, Groell R, Reinhard G, Orgul S, Flammer J, Goldblum D. Plasma citrate levels as a potential biomarker for glaucoma. J Ocul Pharmacol Ther. 2011;27:577–80.
Francis CM. Lipids in the retina. J Comp Neurol. 1955;103(2):355–83.
Franken C, Meijer CJ, Dijkman JH. Tissue distribution of antileukoprotease and lysozyme in humans. J Histochem Cytochem. 1989;37(4):493–8.
Frazao R, McMahon DG, et al. Histamine elevates free intracellular calcium in mouse retinal dopaminergic cells via H1-receptors. Invest Ophthalmol Vis Sci. 2011;52(6):3083–8.
Freeman RD. Oxygen consumption by the component layers of the cornea. J Physiol. 1972;225:15–32.
Friedman JS, Ducharme R, Raymond V, Walter MA. Isolation of a novel iris-specific and leucine-repeat protein (oculoglycan) using differential selection. Invest Opthalmol Vis Sci. 2000;41: 2059–66.
Fujishima H, Fukagawa K, Okada N, Takano Y, Tsubota K, Hirai H, Nagata K, Matsumoto K, Saito H. Prostaglandin D2 induces chemotaxis in eosinophils via its receptor CRTH2 and eosinophils may cause severe ocular inflammation in patients with allergic conjunctivitis. Cornea. 2005;24(8 Suppl):S66–70.
Funderburgh JL, Corpuz LM, Roth MR, Funderburgh ML, Tasheva ES, Conrad GW. Mimecan, the 25-kDa corneal keratan sulfate proteoglycan, is a product of the gene producing osteoglycin. J Biol Chem. 1997;272:28089–95.
Gachon AM, Richard J, Dastugue B. Human tears: normal protein pattern and individual protein determinations in adults. Curr Eye Res. 1982;2:301–8.
Gamache DA, Wei ZY, Weimer LK, Miller ST, Spellman JM, Yanni JM. Corneal protection by the ocular mucin secretagogue 15(S)-HETE in a rabbit model of desiccation-induced corneal defect. J Ocul Pharmacol Ther. 2002;18(4):349–61. doi:10.1089/10807680260218515.
Gao BB, Chen X, Timothy N, Aiello LP, Feener EP. Characterization of the vitreous proteome in diabetes without diabetic retinopathy and diabetes with proliferative diabetic retinopathy. J Proteome Res. 2008;7(6):2516–25.
Garcia-Hirschfeld J, Lopez-Briones LG, Belmonte C. Neurotrophic influences on corneal epithelial cells. Exp Eye Res. 1994;59(5):597–605.
Gariano RF, Kalina RE, Hendrickson AE. Normal and pathological mechanisms in retinal vascular development. Surv Ophthalmol. 1996;40:481–90.
Garreis F, Schlorf T, Worlitzsch D, Steven P, Brauer L, Jager K, Paulsen FP. Roles of human beta-defensins in innate immune defense at the ocular surface: arming and alarming corneal and conjunctival epithelial cells. Histochem Cell Biol. 2010;134(1):59–73. doi:10.1007/s00418-010-0713-y.
Gaynor PM, Zhang WY, Salehizadeh B, Pettiford B, Kruth HS. Cholesterol accumulation in human cornea: evidence that extracellular cholesteryl ester-rich lipid particles deposit independently of foam cells. J Lipid Res. 1996;37(9):1849–61.

Gendler SJ, Spicer AP. Epithelial mucin genes. Annu Rev Physiol. 1995;57:607–34.
Giasson C, Bonanno JA. Facilitated transport of lactate by rabbit corneal endothelium. Exp Eye Res. 1994;59:73–81.
Glasgow BJ, Abduragimov AR, Farahbakhsh ZT, Faull KF, Hubbell WL. Tear lipocalins bind a broad array of lipid ligands. Curr Eye Res. 1995;14:363–72.
Goel M, Picciani RG, Lee RK, Bhattacharya SK. Aqueous humor dynamics: a review. Open Ophthalmol J. 2010;4:52–9.
Golubnitschaja O, Yeghiazaryan K, Wunderlich K, Schild HH, Flammer J. Disease proteomics reveals altered basic gene expression regulation in leukocytes of Normal-Tension and Primary Open-Angle glaucoma patients. Proteomics. 2007;1:1316–23.
Gong X, Baldo GJ, Kumar NM, Gilula NB, Mathias RT. Gap junctional coupling in lenses lacking alpha3 connexin. Proc Natl Acad Sci U S A. 1998;95(26):15303–8.
Gordiyenko N, Campos M, et al. RPE cells internalize low-density lipoprotein (LDL) and oxidized LDL (oxLDL) in large quantities in vitro and in vivo. Invest Ophthalmol Vis Sci. 2004;45(8):2822–9.
Grahn BH, Cullen CL. Equine phacoclastic uveitis: the clinical manifestations, light microscopic findings, and therapy of 7 cases. Can Vet J. 2000;41(5):376–82.
Gronert K, Maheshwari N, Khan N, Hassan IR, Dunn M, Laniado Schwartzman M. A role for the mouse 12/15-lipoxygenase pathway in promoting epithelial wound healing and host defense. J Biol Chem. 2005;280(15):15267–78. M410638200 [pii]. doi:10.1074/jbc.M410638200.
Gross RL. Collagen type I and III synthesis by Tenon's capsule fibroblasts in culture: individual patient characteristics and response to mitomycin C, 5-fluorouracil and ascorbic acid. Trans Am Ophthalmol Soc. 1999;97:513–43.
Gruijters WT, Kistler J, Bullivant S, Goodenough DA. Immunolocalization of MP70 in lens fiber 16–17 nm intercellular junctions. J Cell Biol. 1987;104(3):565–72.
Grus FH, Sabuncuo P, Augustin AJ. Analysis of tear protein patterns of dry-eye patients using fluorescent staining dyes and two-dimensional quantification algorithms. Electrophoresis. 2001;22:1845–50.
Gu SM, Thompson DA, Srikumari CR, Lorenz B, Finckh U, Nicoletti A, Murthy KR, Rathmann M, Kumaramanickavel G, Denton MJ, Gal A. Mutations in RPE65 cause autosomal recessive childhood-onset severe retinal dystrophy. Nat Genet. 1997;17:194–7.
Guly CM, Forrester JV. Investigation and management of uveitis. BMJ (Clin Res ed). 2010;341:c4976.
Gundersen D, Orlowski J, Rodriguez-Boulan E. Apical polarity of Na, K-ATPase in retinal pigment epithelium is linked to a reversal of the ankyrin-fodrin submembrane cytoskeleton. J Cell Biol. 1991;112:863–72.
Guzman-Aranguez A, Mantelli F, Argüeso P. Mucin-type O-glycans in Tears of Normal Subjects and Patients with Non-Sjögren's Dry Eye. Investigative Ophthalmology & Visual Science. 2009;50(10):4581–7.
Guzman-Aranguez A, Argüeso P. Structure and biological roles of mucin-type O-glycans at the ocular surface., Ocul Surf. 2010;8(1):8–17. http://www.ncbi.nlm.nih.gov/pubmed/20105403.
Hall MO, Prieto AL, Obin MS, Abrams TA, Burgess BL, Heeb MJ, Agnew BJ. Outer segment phagocytosis by cultured retinal pigment epithelial cells requires Gas6. Exp Eye Res. 2001;73:509–20.
Hannappel E, Pankow G, Grassl F, Brand K, Naumann GO. Amino acid pattern in human aqueous humor of patients with senile cataract and primary open-angle glaucoma. Ophthalmic Res. 1985;17:341–3.
Harris JE, Hauschildt JD, Nordquist LT. Transport of glucose across the lens surfaces. Am J Ophthalmol. 1955;39(2 Pt 2):161–9.
Hassell JR, Birk DE. The molecular basis of corneal transparency. Exp Eye Res. 2010;91: 326–35.

Hata Y, Sassa Y, Kita T, Miura M, Kano K, Kawahara S, et al. Vascular endothelial growth factor expression by hyalocytes and its regulation by glucocorticoid. The British journal of ophthalmology. 2008;92(11):1540–4.
Haynes RJ, Tighe PJ, Dua HS. Antimicrobial defensin peptides of the human ocular surface. Br J Ophthalmol. 1999;83(6):737–41.
He J, Bazan NG, Bazan HE. Alkali-induced corneal stromal melting prevention by a novel platelet-activating factor receptor antagonist. Arch Ophthalmol. 2006;124(1):70–78. 124/1/70 [pii]. doi:10.1001/archopht.124.1.70.
He W, Dai C, Li Y, Zeng G, Monga SP, Liu Y. Wnt/beta-catenin signaling promotes renal interstitial fibrosis. J Am Soc Nephrol. 2009;20(4):765–76. ASN.2008060566 [pii]. doi:10.1681/ASN.2008060566.
Heathcote JG. Collagen and its disorders. In: Garner A, Klintworth GK, editors. Pathobiology of ocular disease. A dynamic approach. 2nd ed. New York: Marcel Dekker; 1994. p. 1033–84.
Hegde KR, Varma SD. Protective effect of ascorbate against oxidative stress in the mouse lens. Biochim Biophys Acta. 2004;1670:12–8. doi:S0304416503002253 [pii].
Hejtmancik JF. Congenital cataracts and their molecular genetics. Semin Cell Dev Biol. 2008;19(2):134–49. S1084-9521(07)00161-9 [pii]. doi:10.1016/j.semcdb.2007.10.003.
Hemadevi B, Veitia RA, Srinivasan M, Arunkumar J, Prajna NV, Lesaffre C, Sundaresan P. Identification of mutations in the SLC4A11 gene in patients with recessive congenital hereditary endothelial dystrophy. Arch Ophthalmol. 2008;126:700–8.
Heng LZ, Comyn O, Peto T, Tadros C, Ng E, Sivaprasad S, Hykin PG. Diabetic retinopathy: pathogenesis, clinical grading, management and future developments. Diabet Med. 2013;30: 640–50.
Hennessy EJ, Parker AE, O'Neill LA. Targeting toll-like receptors: emerging therapeutics? Nat Rev Drug Discov. 2010;9(4):293–307.
Henriquez AS, Kenyon KR, Dohlman CH, Boruchoff SA, Forstot SL, Meyer RF, Hanninen LA. Morphologic characteristics of posterior polymorphous dystrophy. A study of nine corneas and review of the literature. Surv Ophthalmol. 1984;29:139–47.
Hernández C, García-Ramírez M, Colomé N, Corraliza L, García-Pascual L, Casado J et al. Identification of new pathogenic candidates for diabetic macular edema using fluorescence-based difference gel electrophoresis analysis. Diabetes Metab Res Rev. 2013;29(6):499–506.
Hodges RR, Dartt DA. Regulatory pathways in lacrimal gland epithelium. Int Rev Cytol. 2003;231:129–96.
Hofmaier F, Hauck SM, Amann B, Degroote RL, Deeg CA. Changes in matrix metalloproteinase network in a spontaneous autoimmune uveitis model. Invest Ophthalmol Vis Sci. 2011;52(5): 2314–20.
Hogan MJ, Alvarado JA, Weddell JE. Histology of the human eye: an atlas and textbook. Philadelphia: W. B. Saunders Company; 1971.
Holweg A, Schnare M, Gessner A. The bactericidal/permeability-increasing protein (BPI) in the innate defence of the lower airways. Biochem Soc Trans. 2011;39(4):1045–50. BST0391045 [pii]. doi:10.1042/BST0391045.
Hong SB, Lee KW, Handa JT, Joo CK. Effect of advanced glycation end products on lens epithelial cells in vitro. Biochem Biophys Res Commun. 2000;275(1):53–9. S0006-291X(00)93245-5 [pii]. doi:10.1006/bbrc.2000.3245.
Hongo M, Itoi M, Yamaguchi N, Imanishi J. Distribution of epidermal growth factor (EGF) receptors in rabbit corneal epithelial cells, keratocytes and endothelial cells, and the changes induced by transforming growth factor-beta 1. Exp Eye Res. 1992;54(1):9–16.
Honma Y, Nishida K, Sotozono C, Kinoshita S. Effect of transforming growth factor-beta1 and -beta2 on in vitro rabbit corneal epithelial cell proliferation promoted by epidermal growth factor, keratinocyte growth factor, or hepatocyte growth factor. Exp Eye Res. 1997;65(3):391–96. S0014-4835(97)90338-9 [pii]. doi:10.1006/exer.1997.0338.
Hoon M, Okawa H, et al. Functional architecture of the retina: development and disease. Prog Retin Eye Res. 2014;42:44–84.
Horwitz J. Alpha-crystallin. Exp Eye Res. 2003;76:145–53. doi:S0014483502002786 [pii].

Hurd 2nd LB, Eldred WD. Synaptic microcircuitry of bipolar and amacrine cells with serotonin-like immunoreactivity in the retina of the turtle, Pseudemys scripta elegans. Vis Neurosci. 1993;10(3):455–71.
Hurst JS, Bazan HE. Platelet-activating factor preferentially stimulates the phospholipase A2/cyclooxygenase cascade in the rabbit cornea. Curr Eye Res. 1995;14(9):769–75.
Hynes NE, Horsch K, Olayioye MA, Badache A. The ErbB receptor tyrosine family as signal integrators. Endocr Relat Cancer. 2001;8(3):151–9.
Iseli HP, Wenzel A, Hafezi F, REme CE, Grimm C. Light damage susceptibility and RPE65 in rats. Exp Eye Res. 2002;75:407–13.
Izzotti A, Longobardi M, Cartiglia C, Sacca SC. Proteome alterations in primary open angle glaucoma aqueous humor. J Proteome Res. 2010;9:4831–8.
Jackson 2nd RS, Van Dyken SJ, McCartney MD, Ubels JL. The eicosanoid, 15-(S)-HETE, stimulates secretion of mucin-like glycoprotein by the corneal epithelium. Cornea. 2001; 20(5):516–21.
Jack RL. Ultrastructure of the hayaloid vasucalr system. Arch Opthalmol. 1972;87(5):555–67
Janssen PT, van Bijsterveld OP. Origin and biosynthesis of human tear fluid proteins. Invest Ophthalmol Vis Sci. 1983;24(5):623–30.
Janssen SF, Gorgels TG, Bossers K, Ten Brink JB, Essing AH, Nagtegaal M, van der Spek PJ, Jansonius NM, Bergen AA. Gene expression and functional annotation of the human ciliary body epithelia. PloS One. 2012;7(9):e44973. doi:10.1371/journal.pone.0044973.
Jester JV, Barry-Lane PA, Petroll WM, Olsen DR, Cavanagh HD. Inhibition of corneal fibrosis by topical application of blocking antibodies to TGF beta in the rabbit. Cornea. 1997; 16(2):177–87.
Jin M, Li S, Moghrabi WN, Sun H, Travis GH. Rpe65 is the retinoid isomerase in bovine retinal pigment epithelium. Cell. 2005a;122:449–59.
Jin M, Yaung J, Kannan R, He S, Ryan SJ, Hinton DR. Hepatocyte growth factor protects RPE cells from apoptosis induced by glutathione depletion. Invest Ophthalmol Vis Sci. 2005b;46:4311–9.
Johnson MW. Posterior vitreous detachment: evolution and complications of its early stages. American journal of ophthalmology. 2010; 149(3): 371–82 e1.
Johnson MW. How should we release vitreomacular traction: surgically, pharmacologically, or pneumatically? American journal of ophthalmology. 2013;155(2):203–5 e1.
Jolly C, Morimoto RI. Role of the heat shock response and molecular chaperones in oncogenesis and cell death. J Natl Cancer Inst. 2000;92:1564–72.
Joshi M, Agrawal S, Christoforidis JB. Inflammatory mechanisms of idiopathic epiretinal membrane formation. Mediators of inflammation. 2013;2013:192582.
Jordan A, Baum J. Basic tear flow. Does it exist? Ophthalmology. 1980;87:920–30.
Joyce NC. Proliferative capacity of corneal endothelial cells. Exp Eye Res. 2012;95:16–23.
Kabosova A, Azar DT, Bannikov GA, Campbell KP, Durbeej M, Ghohestani RF, Jones JC, Kenney MC, Koch M, Ninomiya Y, Patton BL, Paulsson M, Sado Y, Sage EH, Sasaki T, Sorokin LM, Steiner-Champliaud MF, Sun TT, Sundarraj N, Timpl R, Virtanen I, Ljubimov AV. Compositional differences between infant and adult human corneal basement membranes. Invest Ophthalmol Vis Sci. 2007;48:4989–99.
Kador PF, Kinoshita JH, Sharpless NE. Aldose reductase inhibitors: a potential new class of agents for the pharmacological control of certain diabetic complications. J Med Chem. 1985;28(7): 841–9.
Kamei A, Totani A. Isolation and characterization of minor glycosaminoglycans in the rabbit vitreous body. Biochemical and biophysical research communications. 1982;109(3):881–7.
Kane BP, Jester JV, Huang J, Wahlert A, Hassell JR. IGF-II and collagen expression by keratocytes during postnatal development. Experimental Eye Research. 2009;89(2):218–23.
Kao WW, Funderburgh JL, Xia Y, Liu CY, Conrad GW. Focus on molecules: lumican. Exp Eye Res. 2006;82:3–4.
Katz ML, Redmond TM. Effect of Rpe65 knockout on accumulation of lipofuscin fluorophores in the retinal pigment epithelium. Invest Ophthalmol Vis Sci. 2001;42:3023–30.

Kaviarasan K, Jithu M, Arif Mulla M, Sharma T, Sivasankar S, Das UN, Angayarkanni N. Low blood and vitreal BDNF, LXA and altered Th1/Th2 cytokine balance are potential risk factors for diabetic retinopathy. Metabolism. 2015;64(9):958–66.

Kawaguchi R, Yu J, Honda J, Hu J, Whitelegge J, Ping P, Wiita P, Bok D, Sun H. A membrane receptor for retinol binding protein mediates cellular uptake of vitamin A. Science. 2007;315:820–5.

Kawamura A, Tatsuguchi A, Ishizaki M, Takahashi H, Fukuda Y. Expression of microsomal prostaglandin E synthase-1 in fibroblasts of rabbit alkali-burned corneas. Cornea. 2008;27(10):1156–63. 00003226-200812000-00012 [pii]. doi:10.1097/ICO.0b013e318180e53e.

Kay EP, Lee MS, Seong GJ, Lee YG. TGF-beta S stimulate cell proliferation via an autocrine production of FGF-2 in corneal stromal fibroblasts. Curr Eye Res. 1998;17(3):286–93.

Keeley FW, Morin JD, Vesely S. Characterisation of collagen from normal human sclera. Exp Eye Res. 1984;39:533–42.

Keenan TD, Clark SJ, Unwin RD, Ridge LA, Day AJ, Bishop PN. Mapping the differential distribution of proteoglycan core proteins in the adult human retina, choroid, and sclera. Invest Ophthalmol Vis Sci. 2012;53:7528–38.

Keene DR, Sakai LY, Bächinger HP, Burgeson RE. Type III collagen can be present on banded collagen fibrils regardless of fibril diameter. J Cell Biol. 1987;105:2393–402.

Keller RK, Small M, et al. Enzyme blockade: a nonradioactive method to determine the absolute rate of cholesterol synthesis in the brain. J Lipid Res. 2004;45(10):1952–7.

Kenchegowda S, Bazan HE. Significance of lipid mediators in corneal injury and repair. J Lipid Res. 2010;51(5):879–91.

Kennedy BG, Mangini NJ. P-glycoprotein expression in human retinal pigment epithelium. Mol Vis. 2002;8:422–30.

Kenny EF, O'Neill LA. Signalling adaptors used by toll-like receptors: an update. Cytokine. 2008;43(3):342–9.

Kim T, Kim SJ, Kim K, Kang UB, Lee C, Park KS. Profiling of vitreous proteomes from proliferative diabetic retinopathy and nondiabetic patients. Proteomics. 2007;7(22):4203–15.

Kimura S, Kobayashi M, Nakamura M, Hirano K, Awaya S, Hoshino T. Immunoelectron microscopic localization of decorin in aged human corneal and scleral stroma. J Electron Microsc. 1995;44:445–9.

Kinoshita JH, Kern HL, Merola LO. Factors affecting the cation transport of calf lens. Biochim Biophys Acta. 1961;47:458–66.

Kinsey VE. The chemical composition and the osmotic pressure of the aqueous humor and plasma of the rabbit. J Gen Physiol. 1951;34(3):389–402.

Kistler J, Kirkland B, Bullivant S. Identification of a 70,000-D protein in lens membrane junctional domains. J Cell Biol. 1985;101(1):28–35.

Kita T, Clermont AC, Murugesan N, Zhou Q, Fujisawa K, Ishibashi T, et al. Plasma kallikrein-kinin system as a VEGF-independent mediator of diabetic macular edema. Diabetes. 2015;64(10):3588–99.

Klyce SD, Crosson CE. Transport processes across the rabbit corneal epithelium: a review. Curr Eye Res. 1985;4(4):323–31. doi:10.3109/02713688509025145.

Ko JA, Yanai R, Morishige N, Takezawa T, Nishida T. Upregulation of connexin43 expression in corneal fibroblasts by corneal epithelial cells. Invest Ophthalmol Vis Sci. 2009;50(5):2054–60. iovs.08-2418 [pii]. doi:10.1167/iovs.08-2418.

Koh SW. Ciliary neurotrophic factor released by corneal endothelium surviving oxidative stress ex vivo. Invest Ophthalmol Vis Sci. 2002;43(9):2887–96.

Koh SW, Waschek JA. Corneal endothelial cell survival in organ cultures under acute oxidative stress: effect of VIP. Invest Ophthalmol Vis Sci. 2000;41(13):4085–92.

Kolb H, Cuenca N, et al. Postembedding immunocytochemistry for GABA and glycine reveals the synaptic relationships of the dopaminergic amacrine cell of the cat retina. J Comp Neurol. 1991;310(2):267–84.

Kolb H, Fernandez E, et al. Substance P: a neurotransmitter of amacrine and ganglion cells in the vertebrate retina. Histol Histopathol. 1995;10(4):947–68.

Komai Y, Ushiki T. The three-dimensional organisation of collagen fibrils in the human cornea and sclera. Invest Ophthalmol Vis Sci. 1991;32:2244–58.

Kong GY, Van Bergen NJ, Trounce IA, Crowston JG. Mitochondrial dysfunction and glaucoma. J Glaucoma. 2009;18:93–100.
Konigshoff M, Balsara N, Pfaff EM, Kramer M, Chrobak I, Seeger W, Eickelberg O. Functional Wnt signaling is increased in idiopathic pulmonary fibrosis. PLoS One. 2008;3(5):e2142. doi:10.1371/journal.pone.0002142.
Kuang K, Yiming M, Wen Q, Li Y, Ma L, Iserovich P, Verkman AS, Fischbarg J. Fluid transport across cultured layers of corneal endothelium from aquaporin-1 null mice. Exp Eye Res. 2004;78:791–8.
Kumagai AK, Glasgow BJ, Pardridge WM. GLUT1 glucose transporter expression in the diabetic and nondiabetic human eye. Invest Ophthalmol Vis Sci. 1994;35:2887–94.
Kumari SS, Varadaraj K. Intact AQP0 performs cell-to-cell adhesion. Biochem Biophys Res Commun. 2009;390(3):1034–39. S0006-291X(09)02094-4 [pii]. doi:10.1016/j.bbrc.2009.10.103.
Lamberts DW, Smolin G, Thoft RA. Physiology of the tear film. New York: The Cornea Little Brown & Co; 1994. p. 439–55.
Lambiase A, Bonini S, Micera A, Rama P, Aloe L. Expression of nerve growth factor receptors on the ocular surface in healthy subjects and during manifestation of inflammatory diseases. Invest Ophthalmol Vis Sci. 1998;39(7):1272–5.
Lambiase A, Manni L, Bonini S, Rama P, Micera A, Aloe L. Nerve growth factor promotes corneal healing: structural, biochemical, and molecular analyses of rat and human corneas. Invest Ophthalmol Vis Sci. 2000;41(5):1063–9.
Lambiase A, Micera A, Sacchetti M, Mantelli F, Bonini S. Toll-like receptors in ocular surface diseases: overview and new findings. Clin Sci (Lond). 2011;120(10):441–50. CS20100425 [pii]. doi:10.1042/CS20100425.
Lan JX, Willcox MD, Jackson GD, Thakur A. Effect of tear secretory IgA on chemotaxis of polymorphonuclear leucocytes. Aust N Z J Ophthalmol. 1998;26 Suppl 1:S36–9.
Lan J, Willcox MD, Jackson GD. Effect of tear-specific immunoglobulin a on the adhesion of pseudomonas aeruginosa I to contact lenses. Aust N Z J Ophthalmol. 1999;27(3–4):218–20.
Landreville S, Coulombe S, Carrier P, Gelb MH, Guerin SL, Salesse C. Expression of phospholipases A2 and C in human corneal epithelial cells. Invest Ophthalmol Vis Sci. 2004;45(11):3997–4003. 45/11/3997 [pii]. doi:10.1167/iovs.04-0084.
Lang RA. Apoptosis in mammalian eye development: lens morphogenesis, vascular regression and immune privilege. Cell Death Differ. 1997;4(1):12–20. 4400211 [pii]. doi:10.1038/sj.cdd.4400211.
Le Goff MM, Bishop PN. Adult vitreous structure and post natal changes. Eye (Lond). 2008;22(10):1214–22.
Leahy KE, White AJ. Selective laser trabeculoplasty: current perspectives. Clin Ophthalmol. 2015;9:833–41.
Lee RK. The molecular pathophysiology of pseudoexfoliation glaucoma. Curr Opin Ophthalmol. 2008;19:95–101.
Lee DA, Higginbotham EJ. Glaucoma and its treatment: a review. Am J Health Syst Pharm. 2005;62:691–9.
Lee HK, Lee JH, Kim M, Kariya Y, Miyazaki K, Kim EK. Insulin-like growth factor-1 induces migration and expression of laminin-5 in cultured human corneal epithelial cells. Invest Ophthalmol Vis Sci. 2006;47(3):873–82. 47/3/873 [pii]. doi:10.1167/iovs.05-0826.
Lee-Huang S, Huang PL, Sun Y, Kung HF, Blithe DL, Chen HC. Lysozyme and RNases as anti-HIV components in beta-core preparations of human chorionic gonadotropin. Proc Natl Acad Sci U S A. 1999;96(6):2678–81.
Lehrer RI, Xu G, Abduragimov A, Dinh NN, Qu XD, Martin D, Glasgow BJ. Lipophilin, a novel heterodimeric protein of human tears. FEBS Lett. 1998;432:163–7.
Leiba H, Garty NB, Schmidt-Sole J, Piterman O, Azrad A, Salomon Y. The melanocortin receptor in the rat lacrimal gland: a model system for the study of MSH (melanocyte stimulating hormone) as a potential neurotransmitter. Eur J Pharmacol. 1990;181:71–82.
Leite MT, Prata TS, Kera CZ, Miranda DV, de Moraes Barros SB, Melo Jr LA. Ascorbic acid concentration is reduced in the secondary aqueous humour of glaucomatous patients. Clin Experiment Ophthalmol. 2009;37:402–6.

Lemp MA, Blackman HJ. Ocular surface defense mechanisms. Ann Ophthalmol. 1981;13: 61–3.
Lemp MA, Blackman HJ. Ocular surface defense mechanisms. Ann Ophthalmol. 1981;13:61–3.
Levine EM, Roelink H, et al. Sonic hedgehog promotes rod photoreceptor differentiation in mammalian retinal cells in vitro. J Neurosci. 1997;17(16):6277–88.
Li DQ, Tseng SC. Three patterns of cytokine expression potentially involved in epithelial-fibroblast interactions of human ocular surface. J Cell Physiol. 1995;163(1):61–79.
Li W, Vergnes JP, Comeut PK, Hassell JR. cDNA clone to chick corneal chondroitin/dermatan sulfate proteoglycan reveals identity to decorin. Arch Biochem Biophys. 1992;296:192–7.
Li W-C, Kuszak JR, Dunn K, Wang R-R, Ma W-C, Wang G-M, Spector A, Leib M, Cotliar AM, Weiss M, Espy J, Howard G, Farris RL, Auran J, Donn A, Hofelt A, Mackay C, Merriam J, Mittle R, Smith TR. Lens epithelial cell apoptosis appears to be a common cellular basis for non-congenital cataract development in humans and animals. J Cell Biol. 1995a;130(1): 169–81.
Li W-C, Kuszak JR, Wang G-M, Wu Z-Q, Spector A. Calcimycin-induced lens epithelial cell apoptosis contributes to cataract formation. Exp Eye Res. 1995b;61(1):91–8. Jolly, C., Morimoto, R.I., 2000.
Li N, Wang N, Zheng J, Liu XM, Lever OW, Erickson PM, Li L. Characterization of human tear proteome using multiple proteomic analysis techniques. J Proteome Res. 2005;4:2052–61.
Liang Q, Mohan RR, Chen L, Wilson SE. Signaling by HGF and KGF in corneal epithelial cells: Ras/MAP kinase and Jak-STAT pathways. Invest Ophthalmol Vis Sci. 1998;39(8):1329–38.
Lim J, Lorentzen KA, Kistler J, Donaldson PJ. Molecular identification and characterisation of the glycine transporter (GLYT1) and the glutamine/glutamate transporter (ASCT2) in the rat lens. Exp Eye Res. 2006;83(2):447–55. S0014-4835(06)00162-X [pii]. doi:10.1016/j.exer.2006.01.028.
Lim J, Li L, Jacobs MD, Kistler J, Donaldson PJ. Mapping of glutathione and its precursor amino acids reveals a role for GLYT2 in glycine uptake in the lens core. Invest Ophthalmol Vis Sci. 2007;48(11):5142–51. 48/11/5142 [pii]. doi:10.1167/iovs.07-0649.
Liminga M, Hornsten L, Sprecher HW, Oliw EH. Arachidonate 15-lipoxygenase in human corneal epithelium and 12- and 15-lipoxygenases in bovine corneal epithelium: comparison with other bovine 12-lipoxygenases. Biochim Biophys Acta. 1994;1210(3):288–96.
Lindsey JD, Jones HL, Hewitt EG, Angert M, Weinreb RN. Induction of tyrosinase gene transcription in human iris organ cultures exposed to latanoprost. Arch Ophthalmol. 2001;119(6): 853–60.
Linsenmayer TF, Gibney E, Little CD. Type II collagen in the early embryonic chick cornea and vitreous: immunoradiochemical evidence. Exp Eye Res. 1982;34(3):371–9.
Liu J, Xu J, Gu S, Nicholson BJ, Jiang JX. Aquaporin 0 enhances gap junction coupling via its cell adhesion function and interaction with connexin 50. J Cell Sci. 2011;124(Pt 2):198–206. jcs.072652 [pii]. doi:10.1242/jcs.072652.
Liu Q, Wan W, Liu Y, Liu Y, Hu Z, Guo H, Xia K, Jin X. A novel PAX6 deletion in a Chinese family with congenital aniridia. Gene. 2015;563(1):41–4. doi:10.1016/j.gene.2015.03.001.
Locci E, Scano P, Rosa MF, Nioi M, Noto A, et al. A metabolomic approach to animal vitreous humor topographical composition: a pilot study. PLoS One. 2014;9(5):e97773.
Lou MF. Redox regulation in the lens. Prog Retin Eye Res. 2003;22(5):657–82. doi:S1350946203000508 [pii].
Lowder CY, Char DH. Uveitis-a review. West J Med. 1984;140:421–32.
Lutjen-Drecoll E, Rohen JW. Functional morphology of the trabecular meshwork. In: Tasman W, Jaeger EA, editors. Duane's foundations of clinical ophthalmology. Philadelphia: J.B. Lippincott Company; 2001. p. 1–30.
Ma X, Bazan HE. Increased platelet-activating factor receptor gene expression by corneal epithelial wound healing. Invest Ophthalmol Vis Sci. 2000;41(7):1696–702.
Madea B. Estimation of time since death. Encyclopedia of forensic sciences. 2nd ed. Elsevier: Academic press, CA, USA; 2013. p. 229–38.
Mantelli F, Argueso P. Functions of ocular surface mucins in health and disease. Curr Opin Allergy Clin Immunol. 2008;8(5):477–83.

Mantis NJ, Rol N, Corthesy B. Secretory IgA's complex roles in immunity and mucosal homeostasis in the gut. Mucosal Immunol. 2011;4(6):603–11. mi201141 [pii]. doi:10.1038/mi.2011.41.

Maren TH. The rates of movement of Na+, Cl-, and HCO-3 from plasma to posterior chamber: effect of acetazolamide and relation to the treatment of glaucoma. Invest Ophthalmol. 1976;15:356–64.

Mark HH. Aqueous humor dynamics in historical perspective. Surv Ophthalmol. 2010;55:89–100.

Marmor MF. New hypotheses on the pathogenesis and treatment of serous retinal detachment. Graefes Arch Clin Exp Ophthalmol. 1988;226:548–52.

Marshall J. The ageing retina: physiology or pathology. Eye. 1987;1(Pt 2):282–95.

Martin TM, Kurz DE, Rosenbaum JT. Genetics of uveitis. Ophthalmol Clin North Am. 2003;16(4):555–65.

Martinez-Wittinghan FJ, Sellitto C, White TW, Mathias RT, Paul D, Goodenough DA. Lens gap junctional coupling is modulated by connexin identity and the locus of gene expression. Invest Ophthalmol Vis Sci. 2004;45(10):3629–37. 45/10/3629 [pii]. doi:10.1167/iovs.04-0445.

Mathias RT, Rae JL. The lens: local transport and global transparency. Exp Eye Res. 2004;78(3):689–98.

Mathias RT, Rae JL, Baldo GJ. Physiological properties of the normal lens. Physiol Rev. 1997;77(1):21–50.

Mattapallil MJ, Sahin A, Silver PB, Sun SH, Chan CC. Common genetic determinants of uveitis shared with other autoimmune disorders. J Immunol. 2008;180(10):6751–9.

Mauduit P, Jammes H, Rossignol B. M3 muscarinic acetylcholine receptor coupling to PLC in rat exorbital lacrimal acinar cells. Am J Physiol. 1993;264:C1550–60.

Maurice DM, McCulley JP, Schwartz BD. The use of cultured endothelium in keratoplasty. Vision Res. 1981;21:173–4.

Mcavoy JW, Chamberlain CG. Fibroblast growth factor (FGF) induces different responses in lens epithelial cells depending on its concentration. Development. 1989;107(2):221–8.

McCaa CS. The eye and visual nervous system: anatomy, physiology and toxicology. Environ Health Perspect. 1982;44(April):1–8.

McCulley JP, Shine WE. The lipid layer: the outer surface of the ocular surface tear film. Biosci Rep. 2001;21:407–18.

McCulley JP, Shine WE. Meibomian gland function and the tear lipid layer. Ocul Surf. 2003;1:97–106.

Merchant ML, Klein JB. Proteomics and diabetic retinopathy. Clin Lab Med. 2009;29(1):139–49.

Mieyal PA, Dunn MW, Schwartzman ML. Detection of endogenous 12-hydroxyeicosatrienoic acid in human tear film. Invest Ophthalmol Vis Sci. 2001;42(2):328–32.

Miller SS, Hughes BA, Machen TE. Fluid transport across retinal pigment epithelium is inhibited by cyclic AMP. Proc Natl Acad Sci U S A. 1982;79:2111–5.

Mircheff AK. Lacrimal fluid and electrolyte secretion: a review. Curr Eye Res. 1989;8:607–17.

Mircheff AK, Warren DW, Wood RL, Tortoriello PJ, Kaswan RL. Prolactin localization, binding, and effects on peroxidase release in rat exorbital lacrimal gland. Invest Ophthalmol Vis Sci. 1992;33:641–50.

Miyamoto T, Saika S, Okada Y, Kawashima Y, Sumioka T, Fujita N, Suzuki Y, Yamanaka A, Ohnishi Y. Expression of cyclooxygenase-2 in corneal cells after photorefractive keratectomy and laser in situ keratomileusis in rabbits. J Cataract Refract Surg. 2004;30(12):2612–7.

Molday LL, Rabin AR, Molday RS. ABCR expression in foveal cone photoreceptors and its role in Stargardt macular dystrophy. Nat Genet. 2000;25:257–8.

Moore KB, O'Brien J. Connexins in neurons and glia: targets for intervention in disease and injury. Neural Regen Res. 2015;10(7):1013–7.

Muller LJ, Marfurt CF, Kruse F, Tervo TM. Corneal nerves: structure, contents and function. Exp Eye Res. 2003;76:521–42.

Murthy KR, Goel R, Subbannayya Y, Jacob HK, Murthy PR, Manda SS, et al. Proteomic analysis of human vitreous humor. Clin Proteomics. 2014;11(1):29.

Nakamura M, Ofuji K, Chikama T, Nishida T. Combined effects of substance P and insulin-like growth factor-1 on corneal epithelial wound closure of rabbit in vivo. Curr Eye Res. 1997;16(3):275–8.

Nakamura M, Chikama T, Nishida T. Up-regulation of integrin alpha 5 expression by combination of substance P and insulin-like growth factor-1 in rabbit corneal epithelial cells. Biochem Biophys Res Commun. 1998a;246(3):777–82. doi:S0006291X98987046 [pii].

Nakamura M, Nagano T, Chikama T, Nishida T. Up-regulation of phosphorylation of focal adhesion kinase and paxillin by combination of substance P and IGF-1 in SV-40 transformed human corneal epithelial cells. Biochem Biophys Res Commun. 1998b;242(1):16–20. doi:S0006291X97978992 [pii].

Nalesso G, Sherwood J, Bertrand J, Pap T, Ramachandran M, De Bari C, Pitzalis C, Dell'accio F. WNT-3A modulates articular chondrocyte phenotype by activating both canonical and noncanonical pathways. J Cell Biol. 2011;193(3):551–64. jcb.201011051 [pii]. doi:10.1083/jcb.201011051.

Nemeth-Cahalan KL, Hall JE. pH and calcium regulate the water permeability of aquaporin 0. J Biol Chem. 2000;275(10):6777–82.

Nevalainen TJ, Graham GG, Scott KF. Antibacterial actions of secreted phospholipases A2. Review. Biochim Biophys Acta. 2008;1781(1–2):1–9. S1388-1981(07)00232-6 [pii]. doi:10.1016/j.bbalip.2007.12.001.

Ng WS, Ang GS, Azuara-Blanco A. Laser peripheral iridoplasty for angle-closure. Cochrane Database Syst Rev. 2012;(2):CD006746.

Nguyen BQ, Fife RS. Vitreous contains a cartilage-related protein. Exp Eye Res. 1986;43(3):375–82.

Ni M, Evans DJ, Hawgood S, Anders EM, Sack RA, Fleiszig SM. Surfactant protein D is present in human tear fluid and the cornea and inhibits epithelial cell invasion by pseudomonas aeruginosa. Infect Immun. 2005;73(4):2147–56.

Nicolaides N, Santos EC, Smith RE, Jester JV. Meibomian gland dysfunction. III. Meibomian gland lipids. Invest Ophthalmol Vis Sci. 1989;30:946–51.

Nilsson SE, Sundelin SP, Wihlmark U, Brunk UT. Aging of cultured retinal pigment epithelial cells: oxidative reactions, lipofuscin formation and blue light damage. Doc Ophthalmol. 2003;106:13–6.

Nishida K, Kinoshita S, Yokoi N, Kaneda M, Hashimoto K, Yamamoto S. Immunohistochemical localization of transforming growth factor-beta 1, -beta 2, and -beta 3 latency-associated peptide in human cornea. Invest Ophthalmol Vis Sci. 1994;35(8):3289–94.

Ottino P, Bazan HE. Corneal stimulation of MMP-1, -9 and uPA by platelet-activating factor is mediated by cyclooxygenase-2 metabolites. Curr Eye Res. 2001;23(2):77–85.

Ottino P, Taheri F, Bazan HE. Growth factor-induced proliferation in corneal epithelial cells is mediated by 12(S)-HETE. Exp Eye Res. 2003;76(5):613–22. doi:S0014483503000034 [pii].

Overby DR, Bertrand J, Schicht M, Paulsen F, Stamer WD, Lutjen-Drecoll E. The structure of the trabecular meshwork, its connections to the ciliary muscle, and the effect of pilocarpine on outflow facility in mice. Invest Ophthalmol Vis Sci. 2014;55:3727–36.

Palmiere C, Mangin P. Postmortem chemistry update part I. Int J Legal Med. 2012;126:187–98.

Papaconstantinou J. Molecular aspects of lens cell differentiation. Science. 1967; 156(3773):338–46.

Parry DAD, Craig AS. Growth and development of collagen fibrils in connective tissue. In: Ruggeri A, Motta P, editors. Ultrastructure of the connective tissue matrix. Boston: Martinus Nijhoff; 1984. p. 34–64.

Patapoutian A, Backus C, Kispert A, Reichardt LF. Regulation of neurotrophin-3 expression by epithelial-mesenchymal interactions: the role of Wnt factors. Science. 1999; 283(5405):1180–3.

Paterson CA, Delamere NA. ATPases and lens ion balance. Exp Eye Res. 2004;78:699–703.

Paul DL, Ebihara L, Takemoto LJ, Swenson KI, Goodenough DA. Connexin46, a novel lens gap junction protein, induces voltage-gated currents in nonjunctional plasma membrane of Xenopus oocytes. J Cell Biol. 1991;115(4):1077–89.

Paulsen FP, Berry MS. Mucins and TFF peptides of the tear film and lacrimal apparatus. Prog Histochem Cytochem. 2006;41(1):1–53.
Pena-Altamira E, Prati F, et al. Changing paradigm to target microglia in neurodegenerative diseases: from anti-inflammatory strategy to active immunomodulation. Expert Opin Ther Targets. 2015;15:1–14.
Pennesi G, Caspi RR. Genetic control of susceptibility in clinical and experimental uveitis. Int Rev Immunol. 2002;21(2–3):67–88.
Petersen OH. Electrophysiology of mammalian gland cells. Physiol Rev. 1976;56:535–77.
Peuravuori H, Aho VV, Aho HJ, Collan Y, Saari KM. Bactericidal/permeability-increasing protein in lacrimal gland and in tears of healthy subjects. Graefes Arch Clin Exp Ophthalmol. 2006;244(2):143–8.
Piatigorsky J. Lens differentiation in vertebrates. A review of cellular and molecular features. Differentiation. 1981;19(3):134–53.
Piere A, van Heyningen R. Metabolism of the lens. In: Biochemistry of the eye. Oxford: Blackwell Scientific Publications; 1956.
Pino RM, Essner E. Permeability of rat choriocapillaris to hemeproteins. Restriction of tracers by a fenestrated endothelium. J Histochem Cytochem. 1981;29:281–90.
Pitts RL, Wang S, Jones EA, Symes AJ. Transforming growth factor-beta and ciliary neurotrophic factor synergistically induce vasoactive intestinal peptide gene expression through the cooperation of Smad, STAT, and AP-1 sites. J Biol Chem. 2001;276(23):19966–73.
Poche RA, Reese BE. Retinal horizontal cells: challenging paradigms of neural development and cancer biology. Development. 2009;136(13):2141–51.
Pucker AD, Haworth KM. The presence and significance of polar meibum and tear lipids. Ocul Surf. 2015;13(1):26–42.
Quigley HA, Dorman-Pease ME, Brown AE. Quantitative study of collagen and elastin of the optic nerve head and sclera in human and experimental monkey glaucoma. Curr Eye Res. 1991;10:877–88.
Quinn RH, Miller SS. Ion transport mechanisms in native human retinal pigment epithelium. Invest Ophthalmol Vis Sci. 1992;33:3513–27.
Rada JA, Fini ME, Hassell JR. Regionalized growth patterns of young chicken corneas. Invest Ophthalmol Vis Sci. 1996;37:2060–7.
Rada JA, Nickla DL, Troilo D. Decreased proteoglycan synthesis associated with form deprivation myopia in mature primate eyes. Investigative Ophthalmology & Visual Science. 2000:41; 2050–58.
Rakoczy PE, Mann K, Cavaney DM, Robertson T, Papadimitreou J, Constable IJ. Detection and possible functions of a cysteine protease involved in digestion of rod outer segments by retinal pigment epithelial cells. Invest Ophthalmol Vis Sci. 1994;35:4100–8.
Ramenaden ER, Raiji VR. Clinical characteristics and visual outcomes in infectious scleritis: a review. Clin Ophthalmol (Auckland, NZ). 2013;7:2113–22.
Ramos RF, Hoying JB, Witte MH, Daniel Stamer W. Schlemm's canal endothelia, lymphatic, or blood vasculature? J Glaucoma. 2007;16:391–405.
Rasmussen CA, Kaufman PL. Exciting directions in glaucoma. Can J Ophthalmol. 2014; 49:534–43.
Rattner A, Smallwood PM, Nathans J. Identification and characterization of all-trans-retinol dehydrogenase from photoreceptor outer segments, the visual cycle enzyme that reduces all-transretinal to all-trans-retinol. J Biol Chem. 2000;275:11034–43.
Redl B, Holzfeind P, Lottspeich F. cDNA cloning and sequencing reveals human tear prealbumin to be a member of the lipophilic-ligand carrier protein superfamily. J Biol Chem. 1992;267:20282–7.
Redmond TM, Poliakov E, Yu S, Tsai JY, Lu Z, Gentleman S. Mutation of key residues of RPE65 abolishes its enzymatic role as isomerohydrolase in the visual cycle. Proc Natl Acad Sci U S A. 2005;102:13658–63.
Reichenbach A, Bringmann A. New functions of Muller cells. Glia. 2013;61(5):651–78.

Reiss GR, Werness PG, Zollman PE, Brubaker RF. Ascorbic acid levels in the aqueous humor of nocturnal and diurnal mammals. Arch Ophthalmol. 1986;104:753–5.
Riley MV. Aerobic glycolysis in the ox cornea. Exp Eye Res. 1969a;8:201–4.
Riley MV. Glucose and oxygen utilization by the rabbit cornea. Exp Eye Res. 1969b;8:193–200.
Roberts AB. The ever-increasing complexity of TGF-beta signaling. Cytokine Growth Factor Rev. 2002;13(1):3–5.
Robey HL, Hiscott PS, Grierson I. Cytokeratins and retinal epithelial cell behaviour. J Cell Sci. 1992;102(Pt 2):329–40.
Rocha EM, de M Lima MH, Carvalho CR, Saad MJ, Velloso LA. Characterization of the insulin-signaling pathway in lacrimal and salivary glands of rats. Curr Eye Res. 2000;21:833–42.
Rodrigues MM, Streeten BW, Krachmer JH, Laibson PR, Salem Jr N, Passonneau J, Chock S. Microfibrillar protein and phospholipid in granular corneal dystrophy. Arch Ophthalmol. 1983;101(5):802–10.
Rodwell VW, Nordstrom JL, et al. Regulation of HMG-CoA reductase. Adv Lipid Res. 1976;14:1–74.
Roncone M, Bartlett H, Eperjesi F. Essential fatty acids for dry eye: a review. Cont Lens Anterior Eye. 2010;33(2):49–54; quiz 100. S1367-0484(09)00153-2 [pii]. doi:10.1016/j.clae.2009.11.002.
Rothova A, Buitenhuis HJ, Meenken C, Brinkman CJ, Linssen A, Alberts C, et al. Uveitis and systemic disease. Br J Ophthalmol. 1992;76:137–41.
Ruskell GL. The source of nerve fibres of the trabeculae and adjacent structures in monkey eyes. Exp Eye Res. 1976;23:449–59.
Ryan SJ. Retina. Philadelphia: [Great Britain], Elsevier/Mosby; 2006.
Saari JC, Bredberg L. Enzymatic reduction of 11-cis-retinal bound to cellular retinal-binding protein. Biochim Biophys Acta. 1982;716:266–72.
Sacca SC, Pascotto A, Camicione P, Capris P, Izzotti A. Oxidative DNA damage in the human trabecular meshwork: clinical correlation in patients with primary open-angle glaucoma. Arch Ophthalmol. 2005;123:458–63.
Sack RA, Nunes I, Beaton A, Morris C. Host-defense mechanism of the ocular surfaces. Biosci Rep. 2001;21(4):463–80.
Sahel J, Bonnel S, Mrejen S, Paques M. Retinitis pigmentosa and other dystrophies. Dev Ophthalmol. 2010;47:160–7.
Sainz de la Maza M, Foster CS. Ocular prognosis of scleritis and systemic vasculitic diseases. Excerpta Medica, International Congress Series. 1994;1068:373–76.
Sakamoto T, Ishibashi T. Hyalocytes: essential cells of the vitreous cavity in vitreoretinal pathophysiology? Retina. 2011;31(2):222–8.
Sallenave JM. Secretory leukocyte protease inhibitor and elafin/trappin-2: versatile mucosal antimicrobials and regulators of immunity. Am J Respir Cell Mol Biol. 2010;42(6):635–43. 2010-0095RT [pii]. doi:10.1165/rcmb.2010-0095RT.
Sandig M, Kalnins VI. Subunits in zonulae adhaerentes and striations in the associated circumferential microfilament bundles in chicken retinal pigment epithelial cells in situ. Exp Cell Res. 1988;175:1–14.
Sanes JR, Masland RH. The types of retinal ganglion cells: current status and implications for neuronal classification. Annu Rev Neurosci. 2015;38:221–46.
Sarna T. Properties and function of the ocular melanin – a photobiophysical view. J Photochem Photobiol B. 1992;12:215–58.
Schmedt T, Silva MM, Ziaei A, Jurkunas U. Molecular bases of corneal endothelial dystrophies. Exp Eye Res. 2012;95:24–34.
Schoenwald RD, Vidvauns S, Wurster DE, Barfknecht CF. The role of tear proteins in tear film stability in the dry eye patient and in the rabbit. Adv Exp Med Biol. 1998;438:391–400.
Schultz G, Rotatori DS, Clark W. EGF and TGF-alpha in wound healing and repair. J Cell Biochem. 1991;45(4):346–52. doi:10.1002/jcb.240450407.

Schutte M, Weiler R. Morphometric analysis of serotoninergic bipolar cells in the retina and its implications for retinal image processing. J Comp Neurol. 1987;260(4):619–26.
Schwartzman ML, Abraham NG, Masferrer J, Dunn MW, McGiff JC. Cytochrome P450 dependent metabolism of arachidonic acid in bovine corneal epithelium. Biochem Biophys Res Commun. 1985;132(1):343–51. doi:0006-291X(85)91028-9 [pii].
Scozzafava A, Supuran CT. Glaucoma and the applications of carbonic anhydrase inhibitors. Subcell Biochem. 2014;75:349–59.
Serhan CN, Yacoubian S, Yang R. Anti-inflammatory and proresolving lipid mediators. Annu Rev Pathol. 2008;3:279–312.
Sharma GD, Ottino P, Bazan NG, Bazan HE. Epidermal and hepatocyte growth factors, but not keratinocyte growth factor, modulate protein kinase calpha translocation to the plasma membrane through 15(S)-hydroxyeicosatetraenoic acid synthesis. J Biol Chem. 2005; 280(9):7917–24.
Shi Z, Rudzinski M, et al. Alpha2-macroglobulin is a mediator of retinal ganglion cell death in glaucoma. J Biol Chem. 2008;283(43):29156–65.
Sibony PA, Walcott B, McKeon C, Jakobiec FA. Vasoactive intestinal polypeptide and the innervation of the human lacrimal gland. Arch Ophthalmol. 1988;106:1085–8.
Singh V, Santhiago MR, Barbosa FL, Agrawal V, Singh N, Ambati BK, Wilson SE. Effect of TGFbeta and PDGF-B blockade on corneal myofibroblast development in mice. Exp Eye Res. 2011;93:810–7.
Sit AJ. Intraocular pressure variations: causes and clinical significance. Can J Ophthalmol. 2014;49:484–8.
Skeie MJ, Roybal NC, Mahajan BV. Proteomic insight into the molecular function of the vitreous. PLoS One. 2015;10(5):e0127567.
Smith JR, Mackensen F, Rosenbaum JT. Therapy insight: scleritis and its relationship to systemic autoimmune disease. In nature clinical practice. Rheumatology. 2007;3(4):219–26.
Sommer F, Brandl F, Weiser B, Tesmar J, Blunk T, Gopferich A. FACS as useful tool to study distinct hyalocyte populations. Exp Eye Res. 2009;88(5):995–9.
SooHoo JR, Seibold LK, Radcliffe NM, Kahook MY. Minimally invasive glaucoma surgery: current implants and future innovations. Can J Ophthalmol (Journal canadiend'ophtalmologie). 2014;49:528–33.
Sorkhabi R, Ghorbanihaghjo A, Javadzadeh A, Motlagh BF, Ahari SS. Aqueous humor hepcidin prohormone levels in patients with primary open angle glaucoma. Mol Vis. 2010;16: 1832–6.
Spector A, Wang GM, Wang RR, Li WC, Kleiman NJ. A brief photochemically induced oxidative insult causes irreversible lens damage and cataract. II. Mechanism of action. Exp Eye Res. 1995;60(5):483–93.
Spix JK, Chay EY, Block ER, Klarlund JK. Hepatocyte growth factor induces epithelial cell motility through transactivation of the epidermal growth factor receptor. Exp Cell Res. 2007;313(15):3319–25.
Spurr-Michaud S, Argueso P, Gipson I. Assay of mucins in human tear fluid. Exp Eye Res. 2007;84(5):939–50.
Srinivas SP. Dynamic Regulation of Barrier Integrity of the Corneal Endothelium. Optometry and vision science: official publication of the American Academy of Optometry. 2010;87(4): E239–54.
Stamer WD, Acott TS. Current understanding of conventional outflow dysfunction in glaucoma. Curr Opin Ophthalmol. 2012;23:135–43.
Stamer WD, Bok D, Hu J, Jaffe GJ, McKay BS. Aquaporin-1 channels in human retinal pigment epithelium: role in transepithelial water movement. Invest Ophthalmol Vis Sci. 2003;44:2803–8.
Stiemke MM, Landers RA, al-Ubaidi MR, Rayborn ME, Hollyfield JG. Photoreceptor outer segment development in Xenopus laevis: influence of the pigment epithelium. Dev Biol. 1994;162:169–80.

Stocker FW, Reichle K. Theodor Leber and the endothelium of the cornea. Am J Ophthalmol. 1974;78:893–6.
Stossel TP. Phagocytosis (third of three parts). N Engl J Med. 1974;290:833–9.
Strauss O. The retinal pigment epithelium in visual function. Physiol Rev. 2005;85:845–81.
Sugimoto T, Tsuchimochi H, McGregor CG, Mutoh H, Shimizu T, Kurachi Y. Molecular cloning and characterization of the platelet-activating factor receptor gene expressed in the human heart. Biochem Biophys Res Commun. 1992;189(2):617–24.
Sugita S. Role of ocular pigment epithelial cells in immune privilege. Arch Immunol Ther Exp. 2009;57(4):263–8. doi:10.1007/s00005-009-0030-0.
Sullivan DA, Block L, Pena JD. Influence of androgens and pituitary hormones on the structural profile and secretory activity of the lacrimal gland. Acta Ophthalmol Scand. 1996;74:421–35.
Sullivan DA, Wickham LA, Rocha EM, Krenzer KL, Sullivan BD, Steagall R, Cermak JM, Dana MR, Ullman MD, Sato EH, Gao J, Rocha FJ, Ono M, Silveira LA, Lambert RW, Kelleher RS, Tolls DB, Toda I. Androgens and dry eye in Sjogren's syndrome. Ann N Y Acad Sci. 1999;876:312–24.
Sun H, Nathans J. Stargardt's ABCR is localized to the disc membrane of retinal rod outer segments. Nat Genet. 1997;17:15–6.
Sun H, Molday RS, Nathans J. Retinal stimulates ATP hydrolysis by purified and reconstituted ABCR, the photoreceptor-specific ATP-binding cassette transporter responsible for Stargardt disease. J Biol Chem. 1999;274:8269–81.
Swann DA. Biochemistry of the vitreous. Bull Soc Belge Ophtalmol. 1987;223(Pt 1):59–72.
Tam C, Mun JJ, Evans DJ, Fleiszig SM. Cytokeratins mediate epithelial innate defense through their antimicrobial properties. J Clin Invest. 2012;122(10):3665–77.
Tamm ER. The trabecular meshwork outflow pathways: structural and functional aspects. Exp Eye Res. 2009;88:648–55.
Tao Y, Bazan HE, Bazan NG. Platelet-activating factor enhances urokinase-type plasminogen activator gene expression in corneal epithelium. Invest Ophthalmol Vis Sci. 1996;37(10):2037–46.
Tate Jr DJ, Miceli MV, Newsome DA. Phagocytosis and H2O2 induce catalase and metallothionein gene expression in human retinal pigment epithelial cells. Invest Ophthalmol Vis Sci. 1995;36:1271–9.
Taylor AW. Ocular immune privilege. Eye. 2009;23(10):1885–9. doi:10.1038/eye.2008.382.
Tektas OY, Lutjen-Drecoll E. Structural changes of the trabecular meshwork in different kinds of glaucoma. Exp Eye Res. 2009;88:769–75.
Tenbroek E, Arneson M, Jarvis L, Louis C. The distribution of the fiber cell intrinsic membrane proteins MP20 and connexin46 in the bovine lens. J Cell Sci. 1992;103(Pt 1):245–57.
Theocharis DA, Skandalis SS, Noulas AV, Papageorgakopoulou N, Theocharis AD, Karamanos NK. Hyaluronan and chondroitin sulfate proteoglycans in the supramolecular organization of the mammalian vitreous body. Connect Tissue Res. 2008;49(3):124–8.
Tiffany JM. The lipid secretion of the meibomian glands. Adv Lipid Res. 1987;22:1–62.
To CH, Do CW, Zamudio AC, Candia OA. Model of ionic transport for bovine ciliary epithelium: effects of acetazolamide and HCO. Am J Physiol Cell Physiol. 2001;280:C1521–30.
Torricelli AA, Singh V, Santhiago MR, Wilson SE. The corneal epithelial basement membrane: structure, function, and disease. Invest Ophthalmol Vis Sci. 2013;54:6390–400.
Tosi GM, Marigliani D, Romeo N, Toti P. Disease pathways in proliferative vitreoretinopathy: an ongoing challenge. J Cell Physiol. 2014;229(11):1577–83.
Tovar-Vidales T, Clark AF, Wordinger RJ. Transforming growth factor-beta2 utilizes the canonical Smad-signaling pathway to regulate tissue transglutaminase expression in human trabecular meshwork cells. Exp Eye Res. 2011;93:442–51.
Trenholm S, Awatramani GB. Origins of spontaneous activity in the degenerating retina. Front Cell Neurosci. 2015;9:277.
Truong TN, Li H, Hong YK, Chen L. Novel characterization and live imaging of Schlemm's canal expressing Prox-1. PLoS One. 2014;9:e98245.

Tschetter RT. Lipid analysis of the human cornea with and without arcus senilis. Arch Ophthalmol. 1966;76(3):403–5.

Tserentsoodol N, Sztein J, et al. Uptake of cholesterol by the retina occurs primarily via a low density lipoprotein receptor-mediated process. Mol Vis. 2006;12:1306–18.

Turgut B, Kaya M, Arslan S, Demir T, Guler M, Kaya MK. Levels of circulating homocysteine, vitamin B6, vitamin B12, and folate in different types of open-angle glaucoma. Clin Interv Aging. 2010;5:133–9.

Ubels JL, Dennis M, Lantz W. The influence of retinoic acid on growth and morphology of rat exorbital lacrimal gland acinar cells in culture. Curr Eye Res. 1994;13:441–9.

Vadillo-Ortega F, Gonzalez-Avila G, Chevez P, Abraham CR, Montano M, Selman-Lama M. A latent collagenase in human aqueous humor. Invest Ophthalmol Vis Sci. 1989;30:332–5.

Van Buskirk EM. The anatomy of the limbus. Eye (Lond). 1989;3(Pt 2):101–8.

Van Haeringen NJ. Clinical biochemistry of tears. Surv Ophthalmol. 1981;26:84–96.

Van Hayningen R. The sorbital pathway in the lens. Exp Eye Res. 1962;1:396–404.

van't Hof W, Blankenvoorde MF, Veerman EC, Amerongen AV. The salivary lipocalin von Ebner's gland protein is a cysteine proteinase inhibitor. J Biol Chem. 1997;272(3):1837–41.

Varma SD, Kumar S, Richards RD. Light-induced damage to ocular lens cation pump: prevention by vitamin C. Proc Natl Acad Sci U S A. 1979;76(7):3504–6.

Vithana EN, Morgan P, Sundaresan P, Ebenezer ND, Tan DT, Mohamed MD, Anand S, Khine KO, Venkataraman D, Yong VH, Salto-Tellez M, Venkatraman A, Guo K, Hemadevi B, Srinivasan M, Prajna V, Khine M, Casey JR, Inglehearn CF, Aung T. Mutations in sodium-borate cotransporter SLC4A11 cause recessive congenital hereditary endothelial dystrophy (CHED2). Nat Genet. 2006;38:755–7.

Walcott B. The lacrimal gland and its veil of tears. News Physiol Sci. 1998;13:97–103.

Wald G. Carotenoids and the visual cycle. J Gen Physiol. 1935;19:351–71.

Wang M, Munch IC, Hasler PW, Prunte C, Larsen M. Central serous chorioretinopathy. Acta Ophthalmol. 2008;86:126–45.

Wang H, Feng L, Hu J, Xie C, Wang F. Differentiating vitreous proteomes in proliferative diabetic retinopathy using high-performance liquid chromatography coupled to tandem mass spectrometry. Exp Eye Res. 2013;108:110–9.

Wassle H, Chun MH. Dopaminergic and indoleamine-accumulating amacrine cells express GABA-like immunoreactivity in the cat retina. J Neurosci. 1988;8(9):3383–94.

Watson PG, Hayreh SS. Scleritis and episcleritis. Br J Ophthalmol. 1976;60:163–91.

Wax MB, Molinoff PB. Distribution and properties of beta-adrenergic receptors inhuman iris-ciliary body. Invest Ophthalmol Vis Sci. 1987;28(3):420–30.

Weiss JS, Kruth HS, Kuivaniemi H, Tromp G, Karkera J, Mahurkar S, Lisch W, Dupps WJ, PS Jr W, Winters RS, Kim C, Rapuano CJ, Sutphin J, Reidy J, Hu FR, da Lu W, Ebenezer N, Nickerson ML. Genetic analysis of 14 families with Schnyder crystalline corneal dystrophy reveals clues to UBIAD1 protein function. Am J Med Genet A. 2008;146A:271–83.

Weiter JJ, Delori FC, Wing GL, Fitch KA. Retinal pigment epithelial lipofuscin and melanin and choroidal melanin in human eyes. Invest Ophthalmol Vis Sci. 1986;27:145–52.

White TW, Bruzzone R, Goodenough DA, Paul DL. Mouse Cx50, a functional member of the connexin family of gap junction proteins, is the lens fiber protein MP70. Mol Biol Cell. 1992;3(7):711–20.

Wieczorek R, Jakobiec FA, Sacks EH, Knowles DM. The immunoarchitecture of the normal human lacrimal gland. Relevancy for understanding pathologic conditions. Ophthalmology. 1988;95:100–9.

Willcox MD, Morris CA, Thakur A, Sack RA, Wickson J, Boey W. Complement and complement regulatory proteins in human tears. Invest Ophthalmol Vis Sci. 1997;38(1):1–8.

Williams KK, Woods WD, Edelhauser HF. Corneal diffusion and metabolism of 12(R)-hydroxyeicosatetraenoic acid (12(R)HETE). Curr Eye Res. 1996;15(8):852–9.

Wilson SE, Kim WJ. Keratocyte apoptosis: implications on corneal wound healing, tissue organization, and disease. Invest Ophthalmol Vis Sci. 1998;39(2):220–6.

Wilson SE, He YG, Weng J, Zieske JD, Jester JV, Schultz GS. Effect of epidermal growth factor, hepatocyte growth factor, and keratinocyte growth factor, on proliferation, motility and differentiation of human corneal epithelial cells. Exp Eye Res. 1994;59(6):665–78. S0014-4835(84)71152-3 [pii]. doi:10.1006/exer.1994.1152.

Wilson SE, Chen L, Mohan RR, Liang Q, Liu J. Expression of HGF, KGF, EGF and receptor messenger RNAs following corneal epithelial wounding. Exp Eye Res. 1999;68(4):377–97. S0014-4835(98)90603-0 [pii]. doi:10.1006/exer.1998.0603.

Winkler BS, Riley MV. Relative contributions of epithelial cells and fibers to rabbit lens ATP content and glycolysis. Invest Ophthalmol Vis Sci. 1991;32(9):2593–8.

Wong TT, Zhou L, Li J, Tong L, Zhao SZ, Li XR, Yu SJ, Koh SK, Beuerman RW. Proteomic profiling of inflammatory signaling molecules in the tears of patients on chronic glaucoma medication. Invest Ophthalmol Vis Sci. 2011;52:7385–91.

Worgul BV, Merriam GR, Medvedovsky C. Cortical cataract development: an expression of primary damage to the lens epithelium. Lens Eye Toxic Res. 1989;6(4):559–71.

Wu H, Kuzmenko A, Wan S, Schaffer L, Weiss A, Fisher JH, Kim KS, McCormack FX. Surfactant proteins A and D inhibit the growth of gram-negative bacteria by increasing membrane permeability. J Clin Invest. 2003;111(10):1589–602. doi:10.1172/JCI16889.

Xue L, Gollapalli DR, Maiti P, Jahng WJ, Rando RR. A palmitoylation switch mechanism in the regulation of the visual cycle. Cell. 2004;117:761–71.

Yagci R, Ersoz I, Aydin B, Beyaz E, Gurel A, Durmus M, Duman S. Aqueous humor and serum concentration of hydroxyproline in pseudoexfoliation syndrome. J Glaucoma. 2007; 16:225–9.

Yamaguchi Y, Watanabe T, Hirakata A, Hida T. Localization and ontogeny of aquaporin-1 and -4 expression in iris and ciliary epithelial cells in rats. Cell Tissue Res. 2006;325:101–9.

Yanai R, Yamada N, Inui M, Nishida T. Correlation of proliferative and anti-apoptotic effects of HGF, insulin, IGF-1, IGF-2, and EGF in SV40-transformed human corneal epithelial cells. Exp Eye Res. 2006;83(1):76–83. S0014-4835(06)00065-0 [pii]. doi:10.1016/j.exer.2005.10.033.

Yang YG, Frappart PO, Frappart L, Wang ZQ, Tong WM. A novel function of DNA repair molecule Nbs1 in terminal differentiation of the lens fibre cells and cataractogenesis. DNA Repair (Amst). 2006;5(8):885–93. S1568-7864(06)00122-4 [pii]. doi:10.1016/j.dnarep.2006.05.004.

Yasutaka H, Tomoya OA, Nicola B, Philip L, Robert DY, Keith MM, Briedgeen K, Clare EH, Bruce C, Akira T, Jun N, Michiko NF, Yasuo T, Kohji N, and Andrew JQ. Matrix morphogenesis in cornea is mediated by the modification of keratan sulfate by GlcNAc 6-O-sulfotransferase. PNAS. 2006;103(36):13333–38.

Yin J, Xu K, Zhang J, Kumar A, Yu FS. Wound-induced ATP release and EGF receptor activation in epithelial cells. J Cell Sci. 2007;120(Pt 5):815–25. jcs.03389 [pii]. doi:10.1242/jcs.03389.

Yoon JJ, Ismail S, Sherwin T. Limbal stem cells: central concepts of corneal epithelial homeostasis. World J Stem Cells. 2014;6:391–403.

You L, Ebner S, Kruse FE. Glial cell-derived neurotrophic factor (GDNF)-induced migration and signal transduction in corneal epithelial cells. Invest Ophthalmol Vis Sci. 2001;42(11): 2496–504.

Young SP, Nessim M, Falciani F, Trevino V, Banerjee SP, Scott RA, et al. Metabolomic analysis of human vitreous humor differentiates ocular inflammatory disease. Mol Vis. 2009;15:1210–7.

Yu FS, Hazlett LD. Toll-like receptors and the eye. Invest Ophthalmol Vis Sci. 2006;47(4): 1255–63. 47/4/1255 [pii]. doi:10.1167/iovs.05-0956.

Yu XS, Jiang JX. Interaction of major intrinsic protein (aquaporin-0) with fiber connexins in lens development. J Cell Sci. 2004;117(Pt 6):871–80. jcs.00945 [pii]. doi:10.1242/jcs.00945.

Yu FS, Yin J, Xu K, Huang J. Growth factors and corneal epithelial wound healing. Brain Res Bull. 2010;81(2–3):229–35. S0361-9230(09)00270-6 [pii]. doi:10.1016/j.brainresbull.2009.08.024.

Zafra F, Aragon C, et al. Molecular biology of glycinergic neurotransmission. Mol Neurobiol. 1997;14(3):117–42.

Zagon IS, Sassani JW, Wu Y, McLaughlin PJ. The autocrine derivation of the opioid growth factor, [Met5]-enkephalin, in ocular surface epithelium. Brain Res. 1998;792(1):72–8. doi:S0006-8993(98)00123-1 [pii].

Zayas-Santiago A, Agte S, Rivera Y, Benedikt J, Ulbricht E, Karl A, et al. Unidirectional photoreceptor-to-Müller glia coupling and unique K+ channel expression in Caiman retina. PLoS One. 2014;9(5):e97155. doi:10.1371/journal.pone.0097155.

Zayit-Soudry S, Moroz I, Loewenstein A. Retinal pigment epithelial detachment. Surv Ophthalmol. 2007;52:227–43.

Zhao X, Ramsey KE, Stephan DA, Russell P. Gene and protein expression changes in human trabecular meshwork cells treated with transforming growth factor-beta. Invest Ophthalmol Vis Sci. 2004;45:4023–34.

Zipplies JK, Hauck SM, Schoeffmann S, Amann B, van der Meijden CH, Stangassinger M, et al. Kininogen in autoimmune uveitis: decrease in peripheral blood stream versus increase in target tissue. Invest Ophthalmol Vis Sci. 2010;51(1):375–82.

Chapter 6
Drugs Acting Through Autonomic System for Ocular Use

Nabanita Halder, Rohit Saxena, Swati Phuljhele, and Thirumurthy Velpandian

Abstract Autonomic nervous system plays a pivotal role in controlling ocular functions starting from aperture and focus control to the production of aqueous humour. It also controls the intrinsic functions and blood supply to various ocular tissues through cholinergic and adrenergic receptors. Cholinergic and adrenergic agonists and antagonists are major class of drugs used in diagnostic and therapeutic purposes in ophthalmology. This chapter is an attempt to review the autonomic nervous system innervations to the ocular structures, their role in carrying out physiological functions of eye and drugs acting through this system as diagnostic, palliative and curative strategies in various ophthalmic conditions.

6.1 Introduction

The structure of autonomic nervous system was morphologically explained by Galen in AD 130–200. He described the presence of a "sixth cranial nerve" which is currently known as ninth (glossopharyngeal) along with tenth (vagus) and eleventh (accessory nerves) and the sympathetic chain as well. He also exhibited the presence of superior and inferior cervical ganglion, the semilunar ganglion, and the rami communicantes which can be found in Traite des nerfs of Tissot in 1778

N. Halder, PhD (✉) • T. Velpandian, BPharm, MS(Pharmacol), PhD
Ocular Pharmacology and Pharmacy, Dr. Rajendra Prasad Center for Ophthalmic Sciences, All India Institute of Medical Sciences, New Delhi 110 029, India
e-mail: nabanitah.aiims@gmail.com

R. Saxena, MD • S. Phuljhele
Ophthalmology, Dr. Rajendra Prasad Center for Ophthalmic Sciences, All India Institute of Medical Sciences, New Delhi, India

T. Velpandian (ed.), *Pharmacology of Ocular Therapeutics*,
DOI 10.1007/978-3-319-25498-2_6

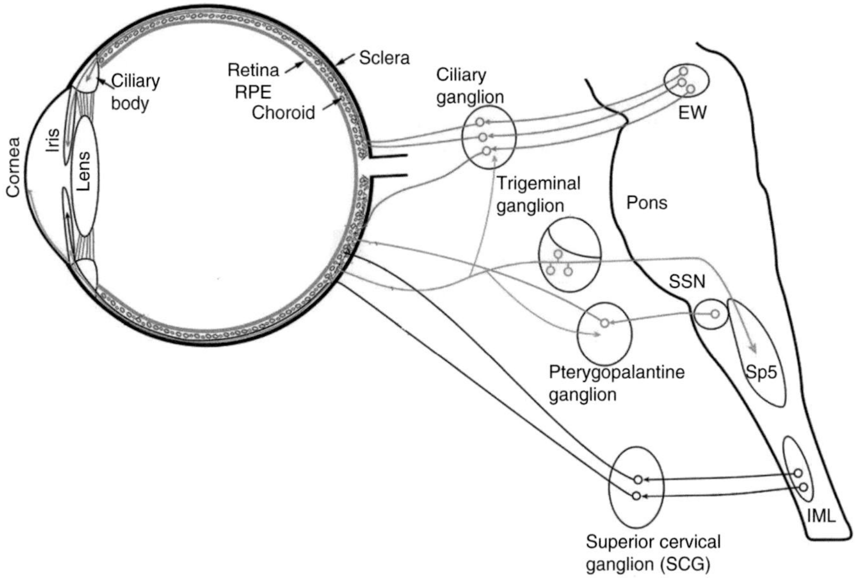

Fig. 6.1 Autonomic and trigeminal ocular projections in the eye (Adapted with permission from McDougal and Gamlin (2015))

(Ackerknecht 1974). However, the therapeutic and diagnostic application of drugs through autonomic nervous system came to ophthalmology in the early nineteenth century (refer to the Chap. 1).

Ocular functions are highly influenced by the autonomic nervous system. Functionally, they control the muscle responsible for pupillary diameter of the iris (aperture control), muscles responsible for lens curvature (focus control), and production of aqueous humor. Apart from this it also controls the blood supply to the iris, ciliary body, retina, choroid, and optic nerve. Trigeminal and autonomic projections controlling ocular functions are shown in Fig. 6.1. The eye receives its parasympathetic innervations through postganglionic ciliary ganglion and sympathetic innervations through superior cervical ganglion. Apart from this local, intrinsic control has been achieved by trigeminal sensory fibers at many regions of the eye and neurons within ciliary and pterygopalatine ganglia at many regions of the eye. The cornea is innervated by the sensory fibers of the trigeminal nerve which is capable of stimulating lacrimation by the interconnections with the lacrimal gland through pterygopalatine ganglia. Presence of endothelial alpha- and beta-receptors in the cornea has been shown to modulate the corneal thickness by their respective agonists (Nielsen and Nielsen 1985). Extensive information regarding autonomic control of the eye can be read by the excellent review of McDougal and Gamlin (2015) and Kardon (2005). Presence of cholinergic and adrenergic receptors in various parts of the eye and their functional significance are shown in Table 6.1.

Table 6.1 Presence and function of autonomic receptors in the structures of the eye

Structure	Sympathetic receptors	Response	Para-sympathetic receptors	Response
Iris-radial muscle	α1	Mydriasis	–	–
Iris-spincter muscle	–	–	M3 & M2	Miosis
Ciliary muscle	β	Relaxation (far vision)	M3 & M2	Contraction (near vision)
Ciliary epithelium	α2	Decrease production of aqueous humor	M1 & M2	Unknown
	B2	Production of aqueous humor		
Lacrimal glands	α1	Secretion (+)	M3 & M2	Secretion (3+)
Corneal epithelium	B2	Epithelial wound healing	M2, M4 & M5	Unknown
	α1	Cl-transport		
Corneal endothelium	β2	Corneal hydration	M2, M4 & M5	Unknown
Trabecular meshwork	β2	Decreased resistance	M3	Increased resistance
Retina and choroid (blood vessels)	β	Vascular control	M1–M5	
Conjunctiva			M3	Goblet cell secretion
Retinal pigmented epithelium	A1 & β2	H_2O transport	–	

6.2 Autonomic Control on the Pupil

Iris circular and radial muscles are innervated by postganglionic parasympathetic and sympathetic nerves respectively. Upon the activation of sympathetic nerves, norepinephrine is released from the postganglionic nerve ending, causing radial muscles of the iris to get contracted, causing mydriasis, whereas parasympathetic activation releases acetylcholine (ACh) from postganglionic nerve terminals causing miosis. The mechanism of them causing mydriasis and miosis are shown in Fig. 6.2. The dynamic equilibrium between both of the nervous systems determines pupillary diameter based upon the amount of light reaching the retina. The normal human eye can dilate the pupil from 1.5 to 8 mm in diameter and this change is expected to modulate the depth of focus, optical aberration, retinal illumination, and diffraction. Coordinated performance of the iris aperture along with focal length adjustment rendered by ciliary muscles by autonomic control is required for the optimum performance of visual system at different conditions. When the dynamic equilibrium exists between the sympathetic and parasympathetic system, pharmacological agents are used to achieve mydriasis or miosis by stimulating the appropriate autonomic

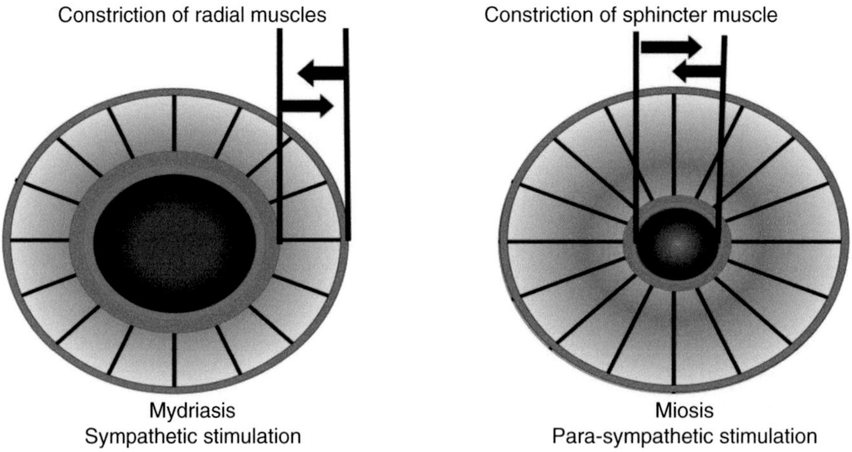

Fig. 6.2 Showing the effect of adrenergic (sympathetic) and cholinergic (parasympathetic) stimulation on pupillary diameter causing mydriasis and miosis respectively

receptors. Phenylephrine is an alpha-1 agonist capable of stimulating the contraction of iris radial muscle and cause mydriasis but atropine which is a muscarinic blocker is capable of removing the influence of cholinergic stimuli-induced contraction on iris circular muscle (sphincter muscle), thereby causing the domination of existing tone of sympathetic system leading to mydriasis. Dapiprazole is a selective α(1)-adrenoreceptor antagonist approved to reverse the mydriasis induced by atropine.

Similarly, miosis can be induced by the stimulation circular muscles of the iris (sphincter muscle) using cholinomimetic-like pilocarpine or cholinesterase inhibitors and α(1)-adrenoreceptor blocker dapiprazole. Dapiprazole causes miosis by removing the action of sympathetic tone on radial muscles of the iris, leading to the shift of equilibrium to cholinergic tone (Bartlett and Classe 1992).

Apart from the presence of acetylcholine (neurotransmitter of cholinergic nerves) and norepinephrine (neurotransmitter of sympathetic nerves), other neurotransmitters and neuropeptides such as VIP, neuropeptide Y, nitric oxide synthase (for nitric oxide), and ATP were identified in the postganglionic neurons; they are not exploited so far by any pharmacological means for diagnostic or therapeutic potential. However, they are reported to be involved in the intrinsic pathways in controlling blood supply, aqueous humor dynamics, and other functions (Neuhuber and Schrodl 2011). The list of adrenergic and cholinergic receptors identified in various ocular structures and their functional importance are shown in Table 6.1. Apart from the classical autonomic pathway, morphine is known to stimulate parasympathetic pathway through the Edinger-Westphal nucleus, causing miosis in the iris.

Anisocoria is a condition commonly manifested by the unequal sizes of pupils. This could vary from simple to life-threatening conditions. Pupillary inequality is usually identified by their reaction in both dim and bright illuminations before initiating further clinical proceedings. Once the dysfunctioning of pupils is confirmed, differential diagnostic procedure is opted in neuro-ophthalmology in defining the underlying condition. It is aided by a handful of drugs like pilocarpine, hydroxylamphetamine, cocaine, phenylephrine, and morphine.

6.3 Autonomic Control Over Accommodation

Accommodation in the eye is primarily due to the strong influence of the parasympathetic system. The lens in the anterior segment is enclosed in a lens capsule and suspended by the specialized fibers called zonules from the ciliary body. Ciliary muscles are clarified into outer longitudinal, middle radial, and inner circular layers. In normal conditions influence of the parasympathetic system makes the ciliary circular muscles to contract, causing zonules to relax and thereby causing the lens to become convex and move a little toward the anterior segment. This action fixes the lens toward for near vision, called accommodation. When the radial muscle is pulled by sympathetic stimulation, stretched zonules cause reduction in curvature, leading to the lens adjustment for far vision. Antimuscarinic drugs like atropine abolish the effect of accommodation, causing the lens to fix for far vision. One of the mechanisms put forward for sympathomimetic agents is that their action on ciliary radial muscle puts traction on scleral spur, causing a decreased resistance in trabecular meshwork in reducing intraocular pressure.

6.4 Autonomic Control Over Lacrimal Secretion

Contribution of lacrimal gland secretion plays an important role in the formation of precorneal tear fluid. Parasympathetic innervation through M3 receptors plays a major role in the lacrimation and it is modulated by the sympathetic system. The lacrimal gland is reported to have transcellular Cl^- secretion in the acinus which involves Cl^--selective channels in the apical plasma membrane (Mircheff 1989). Muscarnic agonist carbachol increases transepithelial Cl^- fluxes that attribute to lacrimal fluid production (Selvam et al. 2013). Interestingly, some degree of cross-talk between purinergicP2 receptors and M3 and α1D-adrenergic receptors are reported to influence tear secretion (Murakami et al. 2000). Purinergic receptor subtypes are known to play divergent physiological functions in various structures like in corneal wound repair, modulating trabecular remodeling, visual processing in the retina, etc. (Sanderson et al. 2014). Pilocarpine is known to stimulate lacrimation through muscarinic receptors of the lacrimal gland and atropine is known to block lacrimal secretion and causes dry eye. Antihistaminics are known to have antimuscarinic side effects which are mediated through M3 receptor responsible for glandular secretion. Therefore, the lacrimal, P2Y(2), receptor subtype gains pharmacological importance due to its involvement in sharing the tear secretion pathway like carbachol. Topical instillation of P2Y(2) receptor agonist (diquafosol) has been reported to increase in net Cl^-, fluid transport, and glycoprotein release onto the ocular surface (Fujihara et al. 2001; Mundasad et al. 2001).

6.5 Autonomic Control Over Aqueous Humor Production and IOP Control

In the anterior segment of the eye, aqueous humor produced by the ciliary processes is secreted into the posterior chamber and it reaches into anterior chamber through the pupil. From the anterior chamber, majority of the aqueous humor (80–95 %) drains into the canal of Schlemm to the episcleral venular plexus and finally it drains into systemic circulation. Apart from this route, it also routes through unconventional uveoscleral pathway. The rate of production of aqueous humor and its disappearance through drainage pathways together determines intraocular pressure and finally development of glaucoma. Production of aqueous humor comes under the influence of the sympathetic system through beta-receptors which is regulated by presynaptic α2 receptors (autoreceptors) in the sympathetic nerve endings. The classical regulation of intraocular pressure is achieved by blocking β2 adrenergic receptors or by stimulating presynaptic α2 receptors. Apart from this mechanism, directly or indirectly acting sympathomimetics widen the trabecular meshwork by creating a traction in the scleral spur through ciliary muscles. Epinephrine has also been reported to increase uveoscleral flow, which is likely through stimulating beta-2-adrenergic receptors (Almand Nilsson 2009).

The sympathetic system supplies to tissues of eyes through its various receptors and thus may produce diverse effects depending on the receptor activated. It supplies the pupil dilator muscle and brings about mydriasis through α1 receptor. It also produces the contraction of Muller's muscle through the same receptors. The sympathetic system has dual effect on aqueous production wherein it enhances the aqueous humor formation through ß2 receptors while inhibiting formation through α2 receptors. It also relaxes the ciliary body muscle through its ß2 receptors. The parasympathetic ocular effects are produced through muscarinic receptors. This includes supply to the sphincter papillae muscle, causing miosis and contraction of the ciliary body muscle, leading to accommodation and enhanced drainage of aqueous humor.

6.6 Autonomic Control Over Blood Circulation and Neuroprotection

Alpha-2 adrenergic agonists, in addition to their pressure-lowering effects in the eye, may act directly upon retinal neurons, including retinal ganglion cells. Alpha-2A expression was identified in the human retina, on ganglion cells, and cells in the inner and outer nuclear layers (Kalapesi et al. 2005), whereas only a few clinical studies so far showed any benefit of neuroprotection in glaucoma (Evans et al. 2003; Sena and Lindsley 2013). Presence and involvement of β-adrenergic system in angiogenic processes has been implicated in infantile hemangiomas, retinopathy of prematurity, and cancer (Filippi et al. 2015). As the neurotransmitters of the autonomic nervous system such as acetylcholine and norepinephrine are vasoactive substances, therefore, presence of adrenergic and cholinergic receptors at the cornea, iris, ciliary body, retina, and choroid is expected to play a significant role on their vascular tone and cellular homeostasis (Mori et al. 2010; Toda et al. 1996; Casini et al. 2014). However, the current knowledge available is not enough to speculate the pharmacological utilization of these receptors in various ophthalmic conditions.

6.7 Drugs Acting Through Sympathetic Nervous System

Adrenergic agonists and antagonists are the major class of drugs which have been extensively used in ophthalmology. Norepinephrine, epinephrine, and dopamine are the three major adrenergic neurotransmitters of the sympathetic division of the autonomic nervous system. These amines work by activating adrenergic receptors, namely, alpha- and beta-receptors, present in various tissues of the eye which are primarily innervated by postganglionic sympathetic nerves. The distribution of these receptors is mentioned in Table 6.1.

Adrenergic agonists can be classified into directly acting, indirectly acting, and mixed-acting agents. Drugs such as epinephrine which can directly stimulate the receptors by binding to one or more receptors are known as directly acting. Drugs which can increase the release of responsible neurotransmitter from presynaptic vesicles to augment the effect of the sympathetic innervations are known as indirectly acting such as cocaine. Drugs which can perform both the actions of direct and indirect activation are known as mixed acting (Fig. 6.1).

The eye has both alpha- and beta-adrenergic receptors. Adrenergic receptors are present in corneal epithelium, endothelium, iris radial and sphincter muscles, trabecular meshwork, ciliary epithelium, ciliary muscles, lacrimal gland, and retinal pigment epithelium (Table 6.1). The adrenergic system plays a vital role in maintaining the tonicity of this part for the physiological processes of the eye through constriction and dilation. Thus, this system has been a subject for manipulation for various diagnostic, palliative, and curative strategies in ophthalmic conditions.

6.7.1 Directly Acting Sympathomimetics

6.7.1.1 Epinephrine (Alpha 1 Agonist)

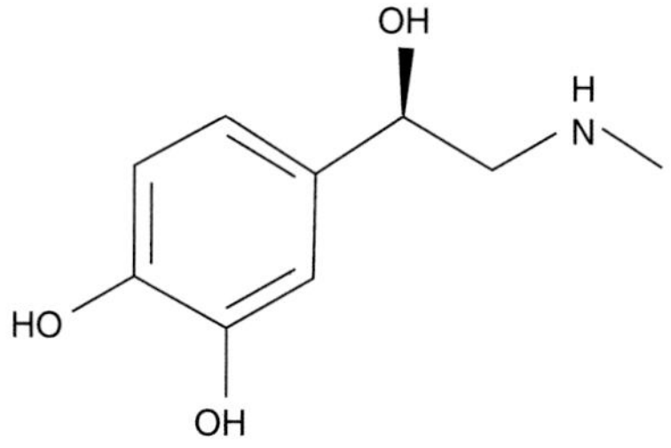

The first hormone ever isolated was epinephrine, which was an iron complex and marketed in 1900 by Farbwerke Hoechst as Suprarenin (Sneader 2001). Epinephrine was also known as adrenaline which is a nonselective but potent stimulant of both alpha- and beta-receptors (α1, α2, α3, β1, and β2). Epinephrine is chiefly secreted through the medulla of the adrenal gland and in the synapses of nerve cells, where it acts as a neurotransmitter (Fig. 6.5a).

Mechanism of Action and Therapeutic Use
Epinephrine binds to alpha- and beta-receptors present in ciliary bodies and the iris. It causes vasoconstriction of the ciliary vessels, resulting in decreased production of aqueous humor through ciliary bodies. It also reduces the aqueous production by ciliary epithelium and facilitates the outflow through trabecular meshwork. This finally reduces the intraocular pressure in the eye. It also causes constriction of the radial muscle of the iris, resulting in miosis. Due to this property and site of action, epinephrine is extensively used in glaucoma and in iritis patients. It is also used before ophthalmic surgery to avoid synechiae.

Dosage
Epinephrine comes in 0.1, 0.5, 1 and 2 % ophthalmic solution for the topical instillation in glaucoma patients. It is recommended to use as a single drop (0.5 or 1 %) 1–2 times daily.

Side Effects
Burning, allergy, reactive hyperemia, headache, and deposition of black oxidation products in the conjunctiva and cornea are the common side effects of topically instilled epinephrine. Angle-closure glaucoma can be induced in the persons who anatomically has narrow iridocorneal angle. A study by Ballin et al. in 1966 reported that the topical ocular use of epinephrine has been shown to be correlated with an increased frequency of cardiac extrasystoles; thus it has to be used cautiously in patients with history of heart disease, hyperthyroidism, or abnormal sensitivity to the systemic effects of epinephrine.

6.7.1.2 Dipivefrin

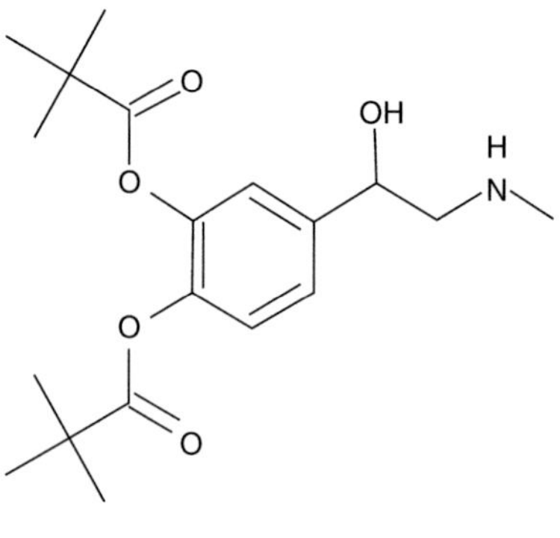

Dipivefrin is an ester analogue and is a prodrug of epinephrine which is formed by the diesterification of pivalic acid and epinephrine. The addition of pivaloyl groups to the epinephrine molecule makes it more lipophilic and hence increases the permeability of this molecule into the anterior chamber of the eye once instilled topically. This drug is widely used to treat open angle glaucoma.

Mechanism of Action and Therapeutic Use
Due to its high lipophilicity, it penetrates into the cornea and there it is hydrolyzed by the esterases to convert into its active constituent of epinephrine. The mechanism of action of dipivefrin is as similar as the parent drug epinephrine. It acts by stimulating α- and/or β2-adrenergic receptors, leading to a decrease in aqueous production and an increase of outflow facility. In comparison to its native molecule epinephrine, dipivefrin is having better penetration, ocular tolerance, and longer-lasting effect. Due to this property, dipivefrin is usually preferred over epinephrine.

Dosage
Dipivefrin is commercially available as 0.1 % ophthalmic solution recommended for once a day use in glaucoma patients, as it is a longer-acting adrenergic receptor agonist.

Side Effects
Side effects include photosensitivity, conjunctival hyperemia, burning, allergy, and hypersensitivity. Caution has to be taken with patients showing hypersensitivity to epinephrine.

6.7.1.3 Phenylephrine

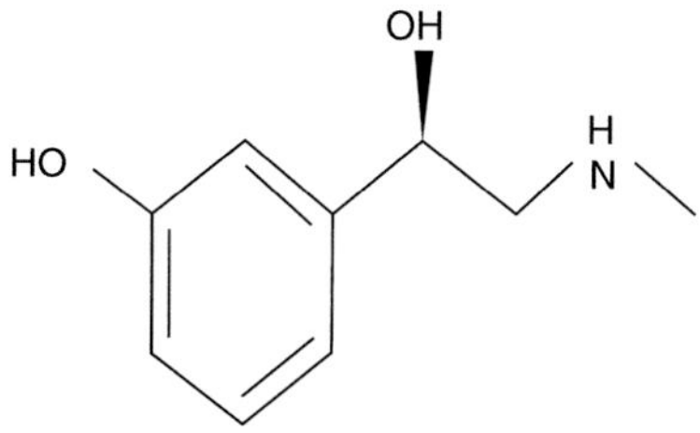

Phenylephrine is a sympathomimetic amine that selectively acts predominantly on alpha-one adrenergic receptors. It is a noncatecholamine and it differs from epinephrine chemically only in lacking hydroxyl group at position 4 on the benzene ring. It activates beta-receptors as well but only at high concentration. So its vasoconstrictor effect is mediated generally through activation of alpha-receptors.

Mechanism of Action and Therapeutic Use
Phenylephrine binds and activates alpha-1 receptors present at the radial muscles of the iris. Activation of alpha-1 receptors at the radial muscles causes radial muscle contraction, resulting in dilation of the pupil (mydriasis). Phenylephrine is a commonly used mydriatic instilled before the examination of the retina.

Dosage

Phenylephrine is used as topical mydriatic ophthalmic solution in the concentration of 0.12, 2.5, and 10 %. This is usually used in conjunction with the tropicamide for the fastest mydriatic effect.

Side Effects

Side effects include hyperemia, burning, allergy, photosensitivity, and hypersensitivity. As it is a potent vasoconstrictor, systemic absorption can cause rise in blood pressure; hence care should be taken with hypertensive patients.

6.7.2 Mixed-Acting Sympathomimetics

6.7.2.1 Ephedrine

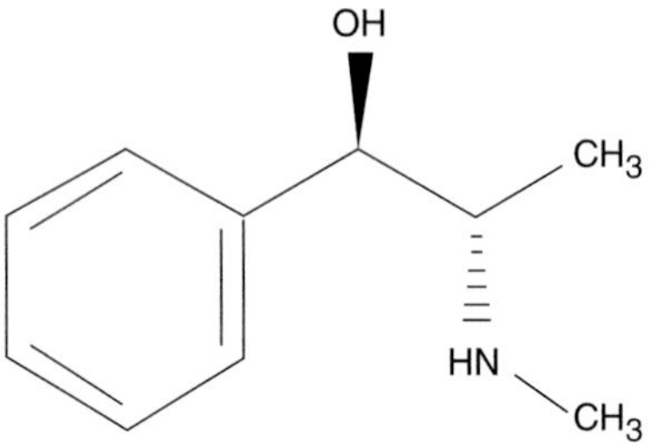

Ephedrine is a mixed-acting sympathomimetic drug which has affinity toward both alpha- and beta-adrenergic receptors. Structurally it is similar to epinephrine, but chemically, ephedrine is an alkaloid which is found in various plants in the genus *Ephedra*. It mainly enhances the activity of norepinephrine at presynaptic synapses and on adrenergic receptors.

Mechanism of Action and Therapeutic Use

Ephedrine acts on adrenergic receptor alpha and beta postsynaptically by increasing the presynaptic activity of norepinephrine at the presynapses. It causes mydriasis by increasing vasoconstriction effect of norepinephrine on the alpha-receptor present at the iris radial muscle. Study reported that ephedrine is less effective in causing mydriasis in colored individuals than the whites (Obianwu and Rand 1965). It has been speculated by Angenent and Koetle (1953) that the poor mydriatic action of the compound in deeply pigmented human iris may lack enough norepinephrine as the precursor of this neurotransmitter, i.e., dopamine may be diverted to form melanin in the dark iris.

Ephedrine is primarily used as mydriatic for ophthalmic use. Since better options are available, this is not commonly used now.

Side Effects
Tachyphylaxis is the common phenomenon for the ephedrine use.

6.7.3 Indirectly Acting Sympathomimetics

6.7.3.1 Hydroxyamphetamine

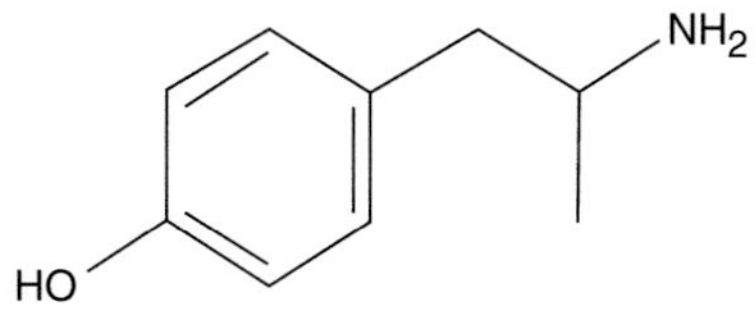

Hydroxyamphetamine is an indirectly acting sympathomimetic drug which is a major metabolite of amphetamine. It is produced after hydroxylation of amphetamine through the CYP2D6 member of cytochrome P450 superfamily.

Mechanism of Action and Therapeutic Use
It acts by decreasing the serotonin and monoamine oxidase metabolism. Inhibition of monoamine oxidases prevents the metabolism of catecholamine in the presynaptic terminal, thus indirectly increasing the amount of norepinephrine at the synaptic cleft. This further antagonizes the action of adrenergic receptors. Adrenergic receptors are present widely in iridial and ciliary bodies. Application of hydroxyamphetamine topically causes mydriasis by increasing the catecholamine at the presynaptic cleft. As this drug does not stimulate the effector cells directly, it has some very important application at diagnosing Horner's syndrome (oculosympathetic palsy or OSP) in ophthalmic condition. By 1971, hydroxyamphetamine was commercially available in the market for distinguishing between postganglionic and preganglionic or central causes of OSP. Location of lesion in Horner's disease is diagnosed by instilling the drug topically to induce mydriasis. If the lesion is present preganglionically, then the mydriasis would happen, as postganglionically neurons are intact to release the norepinephrine, whereas postganglionic neuron lesion results in less or no norepinephrine being released, and mydriasis will be incomplete or absent in response to topical hydroxyamphetamine (Smit 2010).

Dosage
Hydroxyamphetamine is commercially available as 1 % ophthalmic solution alone and with conjunction with 0.25 % tropicamide. This ophthalmic preparation is extensively used by the ophthalmologist for the diagnosis and localization of Horner's syndrome.

Side Effects
The common side effects after instillation include change in color vision, dry mouth, headache, increased sensitivity to light, and burning and stinging sensation in the eye.

6.7.3.2 Cocaine

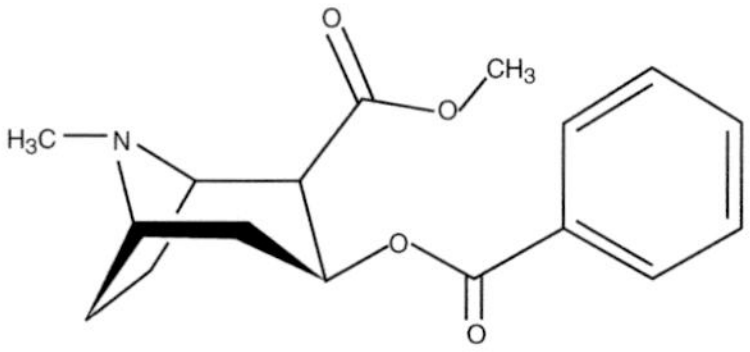

Cocaine is produced from the leaves of the coca plant (*Erythroxylum coca*). It is an ester of benzoic acid and methylecgonine. It is one of the directly acting sympathomimetics used often for mydriasis and local anesthetic effect.

Mechanism of Action and Therapeutic Use

Cocaine inhibits the reuptake of the neurotransmitter, namely, norepinephrine, dopamine, and serotonin, at postganglionic sympathetic nerve endings. Accumulation of neurotransmitter at the synaptic cleft stimulates the adrenergic receptors. When given topically in the eye, radial muscle of the pupil contracts and causes mydriasis. Cocaine is used from a long time for the diagnosis of anisocoria produced by Horner's syndrome. Sympathetic innervation disturbance anywhere will result in less or no neurotransmitter release at the synaptic cleft, and cocaine in that case would not be able to produce mydriasis, which is a confirmation tool for the anisocoria that resulted from Horner's syndrome (Smit 2010). Besides this action, cocaine also inhibits the nerve impulses; thus it is also used as local anesthetic.

Dosage

Cocaine is available in 1–4 % ophthalmic solution for the diagnosis of anisocoria and for local anesthesia prior to ophthalmic surgeries such as lid surgery. Cocaine 2–10 % has been the gold standard in the diagnosis of unilateral Horner's syndrome for more than 30 years (Smit 2010).

Side Effects

Although no evident side effects have been seen for topically applied cocaine ophthalmic solution, systemic absorption can cause nervousness, excitement, euphoria, confusion, agitation, and restlessness.

6.7.4 Topical Vasoconstrictors (Imidazole Derivatives)

Imidazole derivatives which act as sympathomimetics are usually derived from 2-imidazoline (dihydroimidazoles) which is the isomer of the nitrogen-containing heterocyclic derived from organic compound called imidazole. These imidazoline derivatives are biologically active and have characteristic substituent of aryl or alkyl group between the nitrogen centers. In ocular pharmacology, naphazoline, tetrahydrozoline, and oxymetazoline are being used as topical vasoconstrictors.

6.7.4.1 Naphazoline

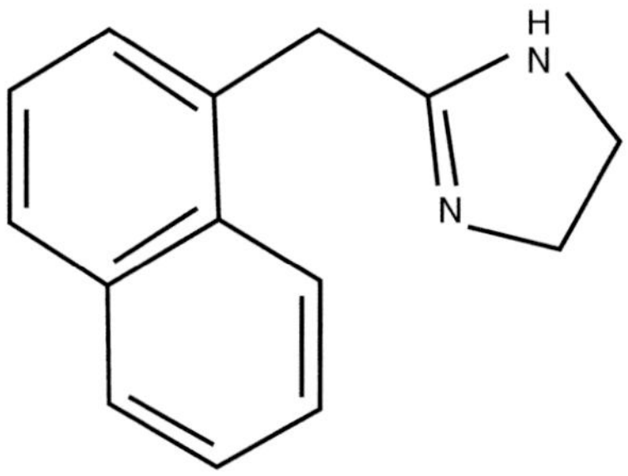

Naphazoline is the derivative of imidazoline, is an alpha adrenergic stimulant, and is used in ophthalmology as a topical vasoconstrictor.

Mechanism of Action and Therapeutic Use
Naphazoline is a sympathomimetic and it causes vasoconstriction by stimulating alpha adrenergic receptors. When applied topically it causes vasoconstriction of the arterioles of the conjunctiva and also produces mydriasis. Naphazoline is used for reducing the conjunctival congestion due to its course of mechanism.

Dosage
Naphazoline is used as ophthalmic decongestant and available in 0.012–0.1 % ophthalmic solutions.

Side Effects
Common ocular side effects of naphazoline include mydriasis, photosensitivity, conjunctival hyperemia, hypersensitivity, lacrimation, and increased intraocular pressure.

6.7.4.2 Tetrahydrozoline

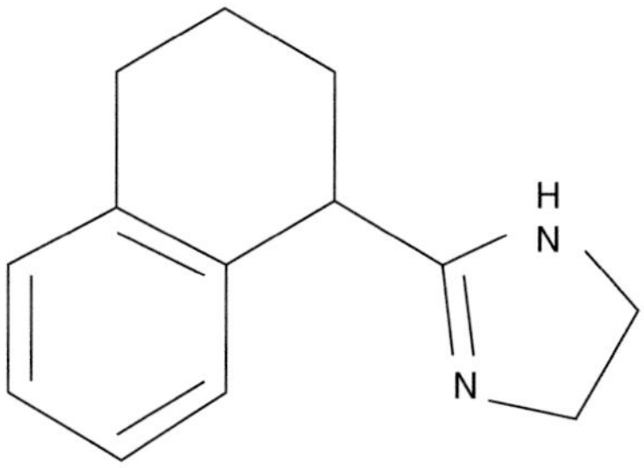

Tetrahydrozoline is also one of the derivatives of imidazoline and is used as conjunctival decongestant in ophthalmology.

Mechanism of Action and Therapeutic Use
Tetrahydrozoline is a sympathomimetic alpha adrenergic agonist which causes vasoconstriction. Tetrahydrozoline is also used as conjunctival decongestant like other imidazoline derivatives. It reduces the congestion by vasoconstricting the arterioles supplying to the conjunctiva.

Dosage
Tetrahydrozoline is available as 0.05 % solution for ophthalmic use for relieving the conjunctival hyperemia. Some dry eye ophthalmic preparation also contains 0.05 % of tetrahydrozoline. It is been advised to use 1–4 times a day according to the congestion status of the conjunctiva.

Side Effects
Tetrahydrozoline has almost similar side effects as other imidazoline derivatives such as burning, photosensitivity, hyperemia, and hypersensitivity.

6.7.4.3 Oxymetazoline

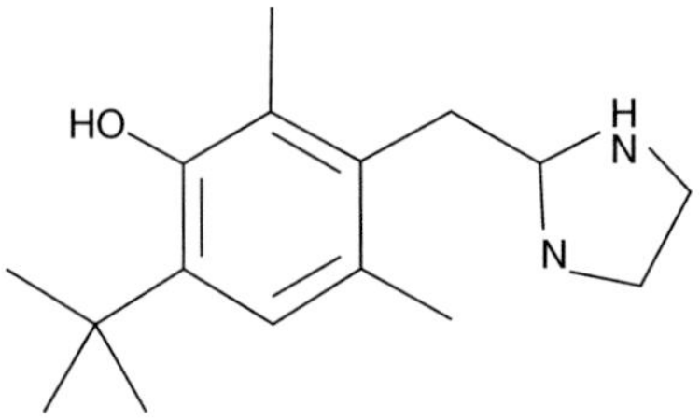

It was developed by Fruhstorfer in 1961 from xylometazoline. Oxymetazoline is a specific alpha-1 and partial alpha-2 agonist. Its specificity toward beta adrenergic receptors is not known.

Mechanism of Action and Therapeutic Use
Oxymetazoline is a sympathomimetic which selectively agonizes alpha-1 receptors and partially agonizes alpha-2 receptors. As vascular capillary beds are rich in alpha-1 receptors, after topical instillation, it acts on endothelial postsynaptic adrenergic receptors and causes vasoconstriction.

Usage
Oxymetazoline is available in 0.025 % of ophthalmic solution which is prescribed four times a day. As rebound hyperemia is one of the common side effects of this drug, it is not advised to be used for more than 72 h.

Side Effects
Oxymetazoline can cause severe burning, stinging, pain, and eye irritation. As it is specifically agonizes alpha-1 receptors in blood vessels, if absorbed systemically it can cause high blood pressure and tachycardia.

6.7.5 *Alpha-2 Adrenergic Receptor Agonist*

The α(2)-adrenergic receptors are predominantly present at the ciliary epithelium where aqueous humor production takes place. Involvement of these receptors is found to have an enormous importance in the treatment of ocular hypertension, glaucoma, uveitis, strabismus, and several diagnostic purposes.

6.7.5.1 Brimonidine

Brimonidine is used as a tartrate salt and it is a selective α(2)-adrenergic receptor agonist with potent vasoconstrictor activity. It is approved for the treatment of open-angle closure glaucoma and ocular hypertension. It has been found to have a neuro-protective role in the retinal ganglionic cells to prevent impairment of vision (Vidal-Sanz et al. 2001).

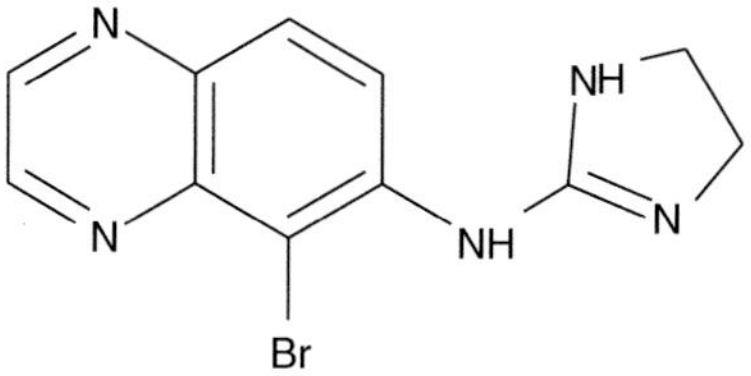

Mechanism of Action
Brimonidine activates membrane-bound G-protein-coupled receptors to inhibit adenylate cyclase which in turn reduces cAMP. Thus, it leads to constriction of smooth muscle and blood vessels. The primary site of action is the ciliary epithelium where brimonidine stimulates the receptor, in turn reducing the rate of aqueous humor production at the ciliary epithelium and at the same time increasing the uveoscleral outflow (Toris et al. 1995a). It is highly selective on α(2)-adrenergic receptor and accounts for 7–12-fold and 23–32-fold more than clonidine and apraclonidine respectively.

Therapeutic Uses
It is the drug of choice for the treatment of chronic open-angle glaucoma and ocular hypertension. It is considered as a major therapy in patients who are contraindicated to beta-blockers (Apatachioae and Chiseliţa 1999). Brimonidine (0.2 %) with brinzolamide (1 %) in fixed combination resulted in significantly greater IOP-lowering effect when compared to brimonidine or brinzolamide alone and exhibited a good safety profile (Aung et al. 2007).

It is commercially available as an ophthalmic solution at 0.15 %w/v and 0.2 %w/v. The topical solution is indicated to be instilled three times a day every 8 h apart. The peak effect of lowering ocular hypotension is observed after 2 h post dosing.

Side Effects
It has low incidences of ocular and peripheral side effects. Photosensitivity, ocular hyperemia, and hypersensitivity are the major side effects. Long-term use has been reported to cause anterior uveitis and allergic conjunctivitis (Becker et al. 2004). It is contraindicated in infants and children due to severe systemic side effects (Wright and Freedman 2009).

6.7.5.2 Apraclonidine

Apraclonidine, a para-amino derivative of clonidine, has shown low penetration across the blood-brain barrier, thus minimizing cardiovascular and systemic side effects. It stimulates α(2)-adrenergic receptors present on nonpigmented ciliary epithelium which in turn leads to reduction of IOP (Gharagozloo et al. 1988).

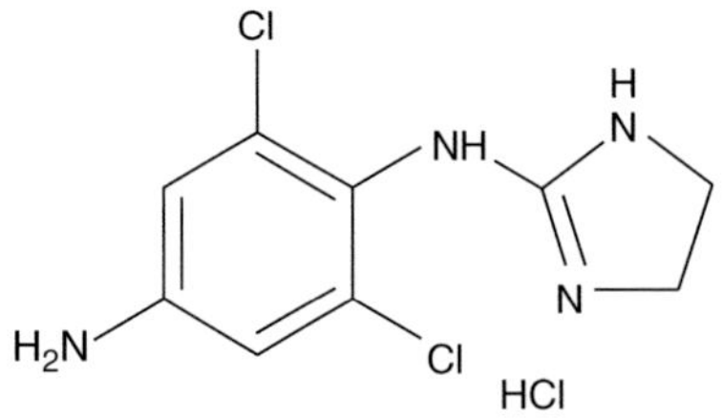

Mechanism of Action
Apraclonidine is a relatively selective agonist of prejunctional α(2)-adrenergic receptors present on nonpigmented ciliary epithelium. It causes inhibition of membrane-bound adenylate cyclase which in turn impairs the conversion of ATP to c-AMP, thereby reducing production of aqueous humor (Gharagozloo et al. 1988). Vasoconstriction of arterioles also resulted in less ciliary body blood flow, thus reducing aqueous production. It also influences the aqueous humor drainage pathway which includes mostly the uveoscleral outflow, and in less instances, conjunctival and episcleral vascular flow may also be involved (Hurvitz et al. 1991; Toris et al. 1995b).

Therapeutic Uses
Apraclonidine is approved for the treatment of elevated IOP in normotensive and glaucomatous human eyes by suppressing the rate of aqueous production (Yüksel et al. 1992). In a study, apraclonidine at 0.5 % was found to have better therapeutic efficacy than 1 % ophthalmic solution in reducing IOP (Rosenberg et al. 1995). It has been found useful as a short-term adjunctive therapy to timolol for the poorly controlled glaucoma (Morrison and Robin 1989; Stewart et al. 1995). It has been used as a diagnostic agent for Horner's syndrome (Chen et al. 2006). It has been reported that it is safe and effective as a single postoperative administration for reducing the elevated IOP after argon laser trabeculoplasty (Holmwood et al. 1992; Robin et al. 1987b), argon laser iridotomy (Hong et al. 1991; Robin

et al. 1987a), and Nd-YAG laser capsulotomy (Brown et al. 1988; Cullon and Schwartz 1993; Pollack et al. 1988).

Dosage
Apraclonidine is available commercially at 0.5 and 1 %w/v ophthalmic solution. It needs to be instilled one drop three times daily. Within 1 h post instillation, it produces 20 % reduction in IOP in the glaucomatous eye and maximum effect can be seen at 3–5 h. Its duration of action for IOP reduction stays for 5–8 h. It is commonly administered as an adjunctive therapy to timolol for reducing IOP. It is contraindicated in patients receiving monoamine oxidase (MAO) inhibitors or tricyclic antidepressants.

Side Effects
Ocular side effects include photosensitivity, transient lid retraction, mydriasis, and conjunctival blanching. Transitory Snellen acuity and allergic conjunctivitis are the other side effects.

6.7.6 β-Blockers

This class of drugs has become a major therapeutic option for the treatment of glaucoma and ocular hypertension. Due to their well tolerance and minimal side effects, β-blockers are the mainstay for the management of glaucoma classified as nonselective and selective β-blockers.

6.7.6.1 β-Blockers (Nonselective)

Timolol

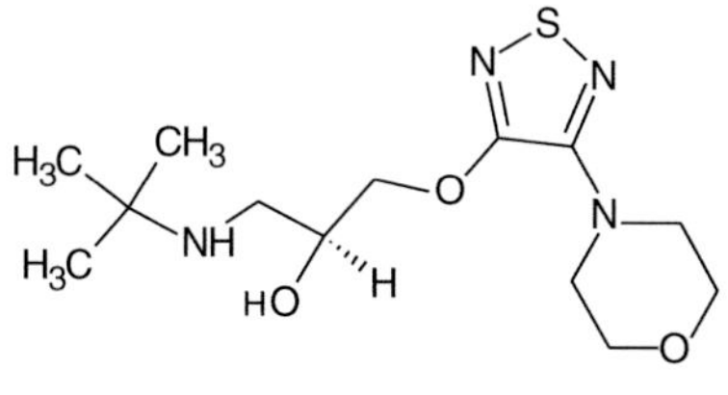

Timolol is a potent and standard nonselective β-adrenergic receptor blocker. It was the first beta-blocker introduced in 1978 for clinical use in ophthalmology after confirming its efficacy as an ocular hypotensive agent due to blocking effect at β(1)- and β(2)-adrenergic receptors. Currently it is a prototype drug against which all newly developed β-blockers are compared for the reduction in IOP in clinical trials of glaucoma. It does not have any significant intrinsic sympathomimetic, direct myocardial depressant, or local anesthetic (membrane-stabilizing) activity but does possess a relatively high degree of lipid solubility.

Mechanism of Action
Aqueous humor production governs by the stimulation of β-adrenergic receptor-mediated c-AMP-PKA pathway. Timolol acts by blocking both β(1)- and β(2)-adrenergic receptors present at ciliary processes and epithelium, resulting into a decrease in intracellular c-AMP, thus reducing aqueous humor formation. It does not inhibit the active transport system or prostaglandin biosynthesis. It also decreases ocular blood flow which in turn leads to a decrease in ultrafiltration responsible for aqueous production (Zimmerman and Kaufman 1977; Neufeld et al. 1983). It does not have any effect on aqueous outflow.

Therapeutic Uses
Timolol is used as a first-line agent found effective in reducing IOP (both on immediate and long-term basis) in ocular hypertension and glaucoma. It is effective in reducing IOP when compared to pilocarpine and epinephrine alone (Boger et al. 1978; Moss et al. 1978). Topical timolol when given in patients receiving oral beta-blockers for hypertension further reduces IOP (Maren et al. 1982). It has an additive effect when added to treatment regimen of miotics and carbonic anhydrase inhibitors (Boger et al. 1978; Sonty and Schwartz 1979).

Dosage
Timolol is available commercially at 0.25 and 0.5 % ophthalmic solution. It should be instilled one drop in each eye two times daily. The duration of action following topical instillation of a single drop persists at least 24 h. Its action is dose dependent and it has been shown that 0.5 % concentration gives maximum reduction in IOP.

Side Effects
Timolol is well tolerated with mild stinging or burning sensation, conjunctival hyperemia, and blurred vision.

Levobunolol

Levobunolol is a nonselective beta-adrenergic receptor antagonist. It was introduced as an alternative to timolol for the better management of glaucoma and ocular hypertension. Levobunolol has claimed to be as effective as timolol but having longer duration of action, resulting in better patient compliance after single topical application.

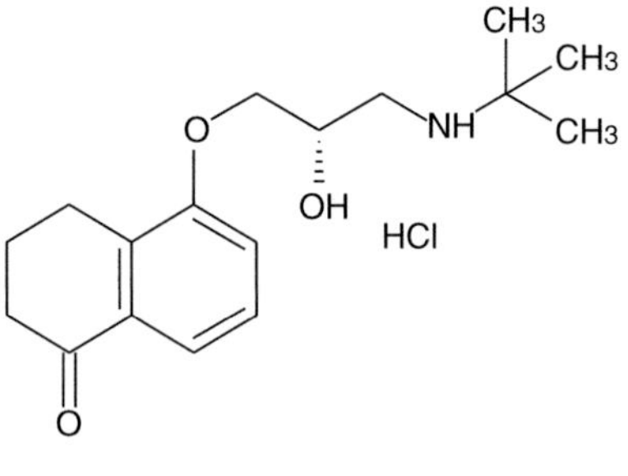

Mechanism of Action

Levobunolol shows the same mechanism of action as that of timolol. It suppresses aqueous humor production by blocking β(1)- and β(2)-adrenergic receptors. It also reduces the ocular blood flow due to blocking of β-receptor-mediated dilation of ciliary vessels. It does not have any significant intrinsic sympathomimetic, direct myocardial depressant, or local anesthetic (membrane-stabilizing) activity.

Therapeutic Uses

It is used in both short-term and long-term management of open-angle glaucoma and ocular hypertension. Its longer duration of action would allow single topical dosing per day (Rakofsky et al. 1989; Silverstone et al. 1991; Wandel et al. 1986). Its action on reducing IOP and ocular hypertension is roughly equivalent to that of timolol (Bensinger et al. 1985; Boozman et al. 1988; Silverstone et al. 1991).

Dosage

Levobunolol is available commercially as 0.5 % ophthalmic solution. It needs to be instilled one drop once a day in each eye. The peak reduction in IOP was found to occur within 1 h after single topical application. The duration of action following topical instillation of a single drop persists at least 24 h.

Side Effects

Mild stinging or burning sensation is noted after topical instillation.

Metipranolol

Metipranolol is a nonselective β-adrenoceptor blocker structurally similar to timolol, propranolol, and levobunolol. It is well tolerated and does not have any significant intrinsic sympathomimetic activities, direct myocardial depressant, or local anesthetic (membrane-stabilizing) activity.

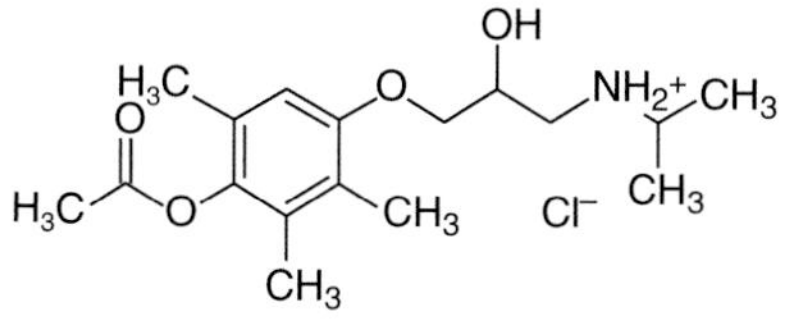

Mechanism of Action

Metipranolol reduces IOP in the glaucomatous eye and normal eye by the same mechanism of action as that of timolol. It suppresses aqueous humor production by blocking β(1)- and β(2)-adrenergic receptors. It also reduces the ocular blood flow due to blocking of β-receptor-mediated dilation of ciliary vessels. It does not affect aqueous outflow (Battershill and Sorkin 1988).

Therapeutic Uses

It is used in the treatment of open-angle glaucoma and ocular hypertension. Clinical significance of metipranolol with 0.1–0.5 % in glaucoma was found to have comparable to timolol, 0.25–0.5 % (Merte et al. 1983; Mills and Wright 1986), and levobunolol, 0.5–1 % (Krieglstein et al. 1987; Stryz and Merte 1985). Twice-daily administration of metipranolol (0.1 %) was found to be effective when compared to timolol 0.25 % and was associated with fewer side effects at lower concentration (Schmitz-Valckenberg et al. 1984).

Dosage

Metipranolol is available commercially as 0.3 % ophthalmic solution. It needs to be administered one drop two times a. The peak reduction in IOP was observed at 2 h. The duration of action after topical instillation persists for at least 24 h.

Side Effects

Mild stinging or burning sensation is noted after instillation. Bronchoconstriction, CNS effects and effect on blood pressure and heart rate have been also observed. It is contraindicated in patients with bradycardia, heart block, heart failure, chronic asthma, and other respiratory disorders. Its use in glaucoma is associated with development of granulomatous uveitis (Melles and Wong 1994; Akingbehin and Villada 1991) which further leads to increase in IOP.

Carteolol

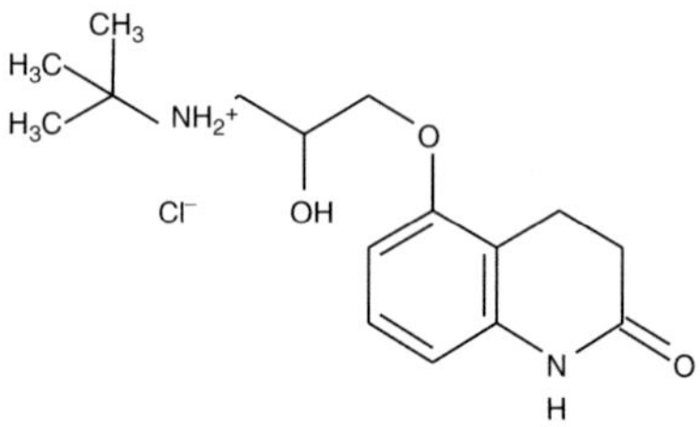

Carteolol is a nonselective β-adrenergic receptor antagonist with intrinsic sympathomimetic activity. Thus, this agent can be used safely in cardiac and asthmatic patients without precipitating systemic side effects such as bradycardia and bronchospasm, respectively (Henness et al. 2007). This drug is structurally similar to timolol and levobunolol. It is the second most topical drug prescribed worldwide in glaucoma.

Mechanism of Action

Carteolol shows same mechanism of action as that of timolol. It suppresses aqueous humor production by blocking β(1)- and β(2)-adrenergic receptors. It also reduces the ocular blood flow due to blocking of β-receptor-mediated dilation of ciliary vessels.

Therapeutic Uses

It is approved for the treatment of open-angle glaucoma and ocular hypertension. It possesses intrinsic sympathomimetic activity that produces minimal adrenergic agonistic activity which in turn causes fewer systemic side effects in patients suffering with cardiac and pulmonary diseases (Steward et al. 1991). In a crossover study, no significant difference was found in reduction of IOP in the glaucomatous eye between carteolol 1 and 2 % ophthalmic solutions (Duff 1987). In another study, carteolol 1 and 2 % topical solution administered twice daily for a month was compared with timolol 0.5 % and metipranolol 0.3 % and showed similar efficacy in reducing IOP in human patients (Scoville et al. 1988; Steward et al. 1991; Mirza et al. 2001). Carteolol has offered protection on visual function in addition to the treatment of glaucoma due to intrinsic sympathetic activity which reduces peripheral vascular resistance in ciliary vessels, thus improving perfusion of the optic nerve head measured by color Doppler imaging (Montanari et al. 2001).

Dosage

Carteolol is available commercially as 1 % ophthalmic solution. It needs to be administered one drop two times a day. The peak reduction in IOP was observed at 2 h post dosing. The duration of action of carteolol ophthalmic solution after topical instillation persists at least 12 h.

Side Effects

Transient irritation, burning, conjunctival hyperemia have been reported after topical application of carteolol.

Propranolol

Propranolol is a nonselective beta-adrenoceptor blocker agent found to decrease intraocular pressure (IOP) in early 1967, but due to its mild anesthetic properties, many investigators resisted themselves from using it as topical medication for glaucoma (Boger et al. 1978). In 2008, Christine Leaute-Labreze and colleagues reported that children with and without cardiac disease having capillary hemangiomas when given oral propranolol have shown a considerable amount of improvement within 24 h, further resolving the lesions with subsequent treatment without leading to any significant systemic side effects (Leaute-Labreze et al. 2008).

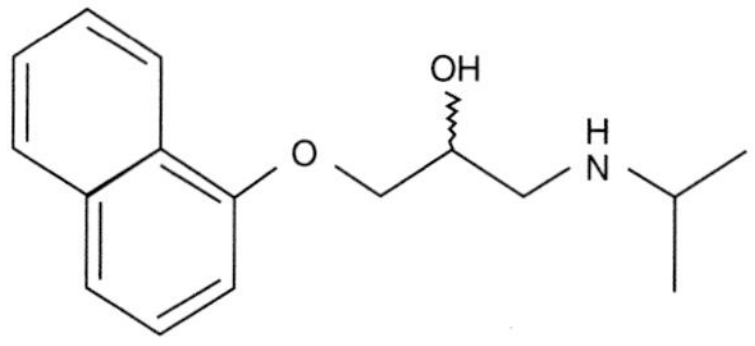

Mechanism and Therapeutic Uses

In general, propranolol is an orthosteric antagonist which binds to both β1- and β2-adrenergic receptors, thereby inhibiting further interaction of adrenaline and noradrenaline with the β-adrenergic receptors β1 or β2 (Benovic 2002). According to literature, VEGF-A is a critical factor for the growth of infantile hemangioma; its production in both normal and cancerous cells is enhanced by noradrenaline. Noradrenaline (NA) also upregulates HIF-1α protein in addition to VEGF through cAMP and PKA pathways (Park et al. 2011; Fredriksson et al. 2000). However, baseline VEGF-A production by the cells has not affected by propranolol, but it functions by the inhibition of catecholamine stimulation (Fredriksson et al. 2000; Thaker et al. 2006). Thus, either enhanced NA stimulation or enhanced sensitivity to NA in the tumor is a responsible factor which leads to VEGF-A production in the cells, and VEGF suppression could be a proposed mechanism of action.

Oral propranolol is used for the treatment of pediatric capillary hemangiomas (Hogeling 2012). It is used in the treatment of glaucoma and ocular hypertension but associated with side effects such as bradycardia and pulmonary dysfunction.

Dosage and Administration

Oral dose of 40 mg twice a day and 1 % ophthalmic solution and ointment are also used.

Side Effects

Stinging, irritation, and allergic reactions are the common side effects after topical instillation. It affects corneal sensitivity due to local anesthetic property of propranolol.

6.7.6.2 β-Blockers (Selective)

Betaxolol [β(1)-Adrenergic Receptor Antagonist]

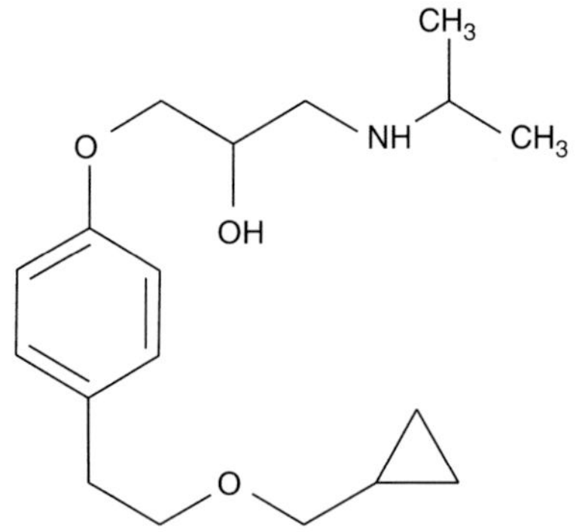

Betaxolol was first introduced in 1980 for clinical use and it was approved for the treatment of glaucoma in 1985 (Goldberg 1989). It reduces IOP by blocking of β(1)-adrenergic receptor with minimal effect on β(2)-adrenergic receptor.

Mechanism and Its Site of Action
Betaxolol is a relatively selective blocker of β(1)-adrenergic receptor present at the ciliary body in the human eye (Buckley et al. 1990; Reiss and Brubaker 1983). It produces reduction in aqueous humor production with no effect on aqueous outflow. Its activity of reducing IOP is shown to be dose dependent. It has no partial agonist activity and has no membrane-stabilizing effect; thus no corneal desensitization was noted after its ocular use (Boudot et al. 1979; Cavero and Lerevre-Borg 1983).

Therapeutic Uses
Betaxolol is used for the treatment of chronic open-angle glaucoma and ocular hypertension. It has low propensity to stimulate cardiac and pulmonary system due to selective β(1)-adrenergic receptor-blocking potential, thus representing a significant advantage over other ocular nonselective beta-adrenoceptor antagonists. The IOP lowering effect of betaxolol is roughly equivalent to that of timolol (Feghali et al. 1988). It has been reported that betaxolol has an additive effect when used with other hypotensive agents including miotics, viz., epinephrine, pilocarpine (Merte and Schnarr 1987; Rolle and Franzone 1987), and carbonic anhydrase inhibitors (Smith et al. 1984). Betaxolol was found to have neuroprotective effect to prevent damage to retinal ganglion cells due to elevated IOP. It is hypothesized that betaxolol is involved in the reduction of influx of sodium and calcium through the voltage-sensitive calcium and sodium channels (Wood et al. 2003).

Dosage
Betaxolol is available commercially for ocular use as a 0.5 % and 0.25 % ophthalmic solution. It is instilled one drop two times in each eye daily. The onset of action is within 30 min with maximal effect noted at 2 h after topical administration. Its duration of action persists at least for 12 h.

Side Effects
Transient local stinging, burning or irritation, pruritus, hyphema, vitreous separation, and blurred vision have been reported after topical administration of betaxolol.

6.8 Drugs Acting Through Parasympathetic System

Cholinergic agonists and antagonists are extensively used for diagnostic and therapeutic purposes in ophthalmology as mitotics and for the treatment of glaucoma. Acetylcholine (ACh) is an endogenous neurotransmitter for cholinergic receptors (muscarinic and nicotinic) present in the peripheral nervous system primarily on autonomic effector cells innervated by postganglionic parasympathetic nerves. It is mainly muscarinic receptors in various parts of eye tissues which are stimulated or blocked by muscarinic agonists and antagonists to produce their pharmacological effects. The distribution of muscarinic receptors in the eye is well described in Table 6.1. Cholinomimetic drugs act by mimicking the effects of acetylcholine. They either directly activate cholinergic receptors or indirectly through the inhibition of cholinesterase enzyme (AChE) that terminate the action of endogenous acetylcholine. They are classified as directly acting and indirectly acting cholinomimetics.

6.8.1 Directly Acting Cholinomimetics

6.8.1.1 Acetylcholine

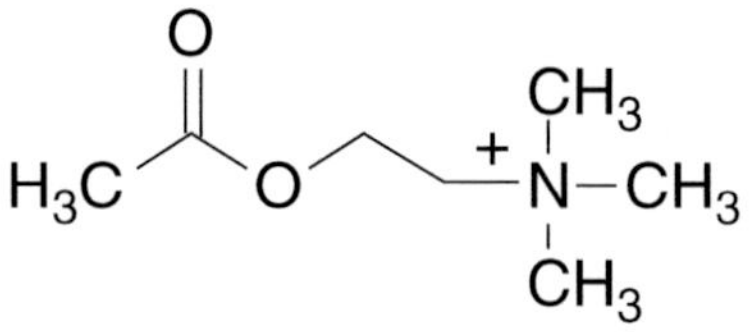

Acetylcholine (ACh) is an ester of acetic acid and choline with the IUPAC name 2-acetoxy-N,N,N-trimethylethanaminium. It was Henry Hallett Dale who first discovered ACh for its action in experimental heart tissues in 1915. Thereafter, Otto Loewi confirmed it as neurotransmitter and named it as Vagusstoff as it was released from the vagus nerve. Both received Nobel Prize for this work in physiology or medicine in 1936 (Vogt 1969; Halpern 1969).

Mechanism of Action

Acetylcholine acts either through muscarinic or nicotinic receptors. Five subgroups (M1-M5) have been identified, out of which M3 receptors are more abundant in different eye tissues such as circular muscle of the iris, ciliary muscle, and lacrimal gland (Kubo et al. 1986; Bonner 1989). M2 receptor was found in the lacrimal gland as well. However nicotinic receptors are not yet being found in the eye. Both M2 and M3 are G-protein-coupled receptors with 7 transmembrane amino acid sequences. M2 receptor acts by opening K+ channel and by inhibiting adenylyl cyclase, resulting in hyperpolarization. M3 receptors act by activating membrane-bound phospholipase C that finally in downstream pathway releases Ca2+, resulting in depolarization, glandular secretion, and constriction of smooth muscle (Gupta et al. 1994a, b; Kaufman 1984).

Therapeutic Use

Several clinical conditions get benefit from the increase in cholinergic tone in eye. In 1949, ACh was first time used in ophthalmic surgery. Injection of acetylcholine chloride solution (1 %) into the anterior chamber of the eye, resulting in contraction of circular muscle of the iris (miosis), is required during surgical procedures such as cataract extraction, keratoplasty, and iridectomy (Catford and Millis 1967; Harley and Mishler 1966). Acetylcholine causes contraction of ciliary muscle, resulting in spasm in accommodation, and increase in aqueous humor outflow facility, resulting in decrease in intraocular pressure especially in patients suffering from glaucoma. Acetylcholine is also useful in corneal grafting. Although ACh is abundant in corneal epithelium in most of the species, the function is still unknown (refer Table. 5.1, Chap. 4).

Side Effects

Since ACh is rapidly metabolized by acetylcholine esterase, frequency of side effects is relatively low. Side effects include hypotension, flushing, bradycardia, and sweating. Ocular side effects have rarely included corneal clouding, corneal decompensation, corneal edema, and transient cataract formation.

6.8.1.2 Methacholine

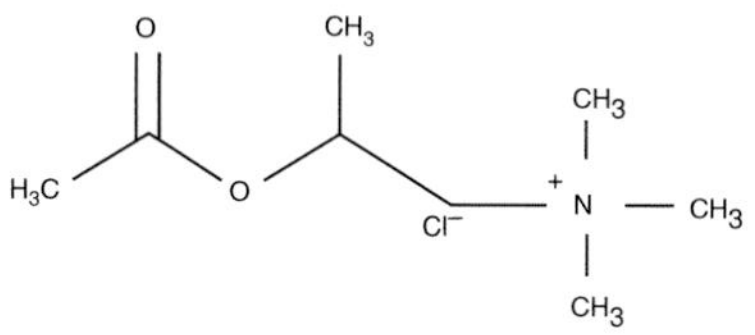

It is a synthetic choline ester formed with an addition of methyl group at the beta carbon atom. Like ACh, it stimulates the parasympathetic nervous system but has predominant effect on muscarinic receptors. It is more resistant to cholinesterase than acetylcholine. This results in longer duration of action with increased selectivity. Tonic pupil (Adie pupil) has been found to contract with 2.5 % methacholine instillation.

6.8.1.3 Carbachol

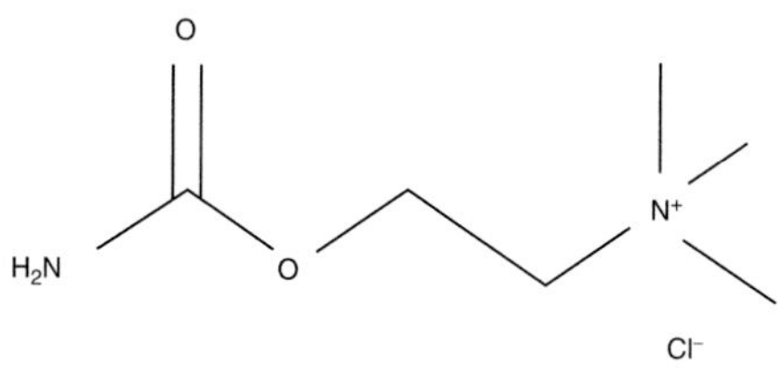

Mechanism of Action and Therapeutic Uses

Carbachol is a synthetic cholinomimetic drug containing a carbamino functional group and a positively charged quaternary ammonium compound instead of an acetyl group present in acetylcholine and methacholine. The pharmacological properties are similar to that of acetylcholine. It stimulates both muscarinic and nicotinic receptors and is highly resistant to hydrolysis by cholinesterase. Carbachol is rarely used therapeutically except in the eye because of its receptor nonselectivity, longer duration of action, and high potency.

Dosage
Carbachol at the concentration of 0.01–3 % used for the treatment of open-angle glaucoma and 0.1 % topical formulation is used after cataract surgery to produce miosis. It is commonly administered topically or through intraocular injection. In the eye it mainly causes miosis by contracting circular muscle of the iris and increases aqueous humor outflow through the trabecular meshwork by longitudinal ciliary muscle contraction. Onset of action for miosis is 10–20 min, whereas intra-ocular tension is reduced for 4–8 h.

Side Effects
Ocular side effects include corneal edema, diminished vision, miosis, brow ache, headache, temporary stinging sensation, cataract, and rarely retinal detachment.

6.8.1.4 Bethanechol

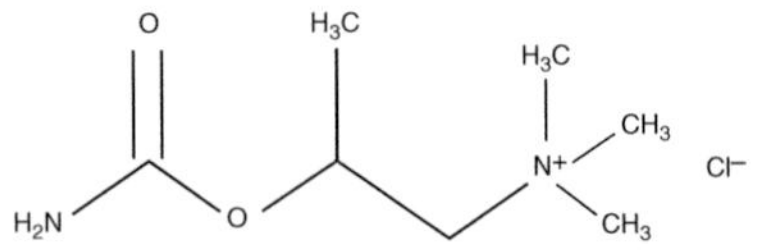

Bethanechol is a synthetic ester and is structurally unique than that of methacholine and carbachol. It contains beta methyl and carbamate functional groups that cause resistance to hydrolysis by cholinesterase and minor effect on nicotinic receptor. The effects are prolonged than that of acetylcholine. Bethanechol predominantly affects the smooth muscle of the urinary and GI tract. Therefore it is mainly indicated for the treatment of acute postoperative and postpartum nonobstructive (functional) urinary retention. It is no longer used in glaucoma because of its poor side effect profile in glaucoma patients.

6.8.1.5 Pilocarpine

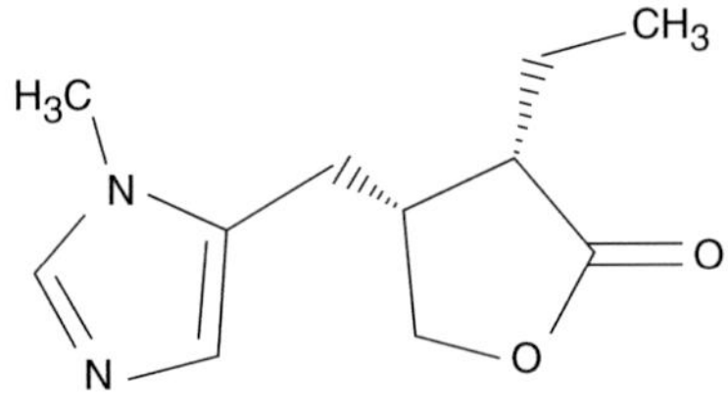

Mechanism of Action and Therapeutic Uses
Pilocarpine is an alkaloid derived from the leaves of *Pilocarpus microphyllus*. It is a nonselective muscarinic agonist which stimulates ganglia as well. In comparison to ACh and other derivatives, it is less potent and resistant to enzyme hydrolysis. It mainly acts on muscarinic receptor M3, and thus on topical application, it penetrates the cornea and produces acute miosis, ciliary muscle contraction, and finally

decrease in intraocular pressure. Pilocarpine is especially used for treatment of open-angle glaucoma where, by reducing iris diameter, it facilitates the flow of aqueous humor by the trabecular meshwork and canal of Schlemm. It is also used as a miotic agent postoperatively after the cataract surgery.

Dosage
Topical formulation of pilocarpine at the concentration of 0.5–6 % (2–6 times/day) is available for the treatment of glaucoma. The IOP reduction lasts for 4–8 h. It can be adjunctly given with other classes of antiglaucoma drugs. Pilocarpine-induced miosis persists for 3–24 h but the spasm of accommodation disappears within 2 h. Pilocarpine (2–5 %) is often used alternately with mydriatics to break the adhesion between the iris and the lens. Adie pupil contracts with 0.05–0.1 % pilocarpine. Pilocarpine can be slowly delivered (7 days) through ocular insert.

Side Effects
The frequent side effects of pilocarpine include the initial stinging sensation in the eye and painful spasm in accommodation. It also produces corneal edema, miosis, brow ache, diminished vision, and retinal detachment.

6.8.2 Cholinesterase Inhibitors

Acetylcholinesterase (AChE) enzyme terminates the action of ACh at various cholinergic nerve endings. Drugs that inhibit this enzyme are known as cholinesterase inhibitors. By preventing the hydrolysis of ACh, they potentiate the action of ACh by accumulating this cholinergic neurotransmitter at nerve terminals, resulting in stimulation of cholinergic receptors present in various effector organs including the eye. These agents can be classified into reversible and irreversible groups.

6.8.2.1 Reversible AChE Inhibitors

Physostigmine (Eserine)

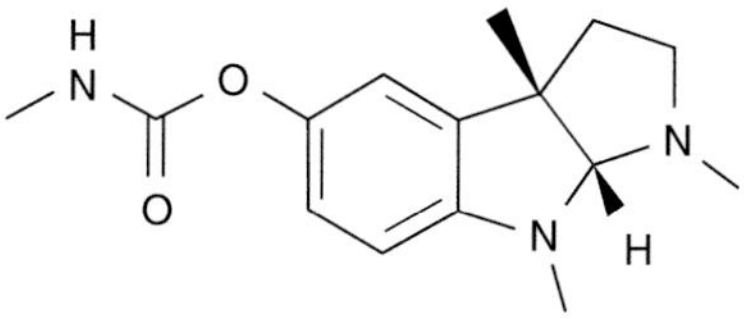

Mechanism of Action and Therapeutic Uses
Physostigmine is an alkaloid having nitrogenous carbamic acid ester with tertiary amine obtained from a natural source of Calabar bean, the dried ripe seed of an African woody climber *Physostigma venenosum*. It forms a carbamylated stable complex with acetylcholineesterase results in reversible inactivation of the enzyme. Physostigmine produces all cholinergic actions due to its effect on both muscarinic and nicotinic receptors.

Upon local application to the conjunctiva, it causes conjunctival hyperemia and constriction of circular (sphincter) muscle of the iris and ciliary muscle, resulting in miosis and block of accommodation reflex respectively. However, accommodation block is transient and may be recovered in a few hours. It also lowers the intraocular pressure by facilitating the outflow of aqueous humor.

Dosage
Physostigmine 0.25–0.5 % topical formulation or eye ointment is used for the eye to produce miosis or spasm of accommodation. Miosis occurs in a few minutes and is long lasting (hours to days). This is an intermediate-acting agent as the duration of action lasts for 2–4 h. Although it lowers IOP, but because of several side effects such blurring of far vision, limiting visual acuity restricts its use for open-angle glaucoma. It is only used when the patients become refractory to beta-blockers or carbonic anhydrase inhibitors. However, low concentration of physostigmine is used in Adie syndrome (tonic pupil) to decrease the blurred vision and associated pain in this condition.

Side Effects
Retinal detachment, miosis, cataract, pupillary block, iris cysts, brow ache, and punctual stenosis of the nasolacrimal system.

Neostigmine

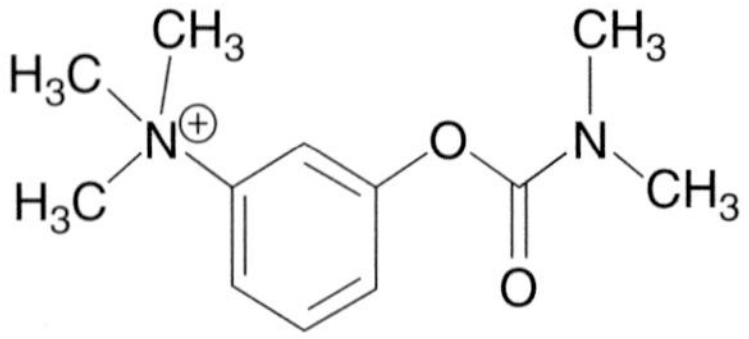

Neostigmine is a synthetic carbamic acid ester with quaternary ammonium. The pharmacological effects are similar to physostigmine. Unlike physostigmine it is more polar and less lipid soluble because of the presence of quaternary amine. Therefore the effective mitotic effect is not elicited and hence used occasionally as a mitotic agent. Like physostigmine, it is not the first-line therapy for open-angle glaucoma.

6.8.2.2 Irreversible AChE Inhibitors

Echothiophate (Phospholine Iodide)

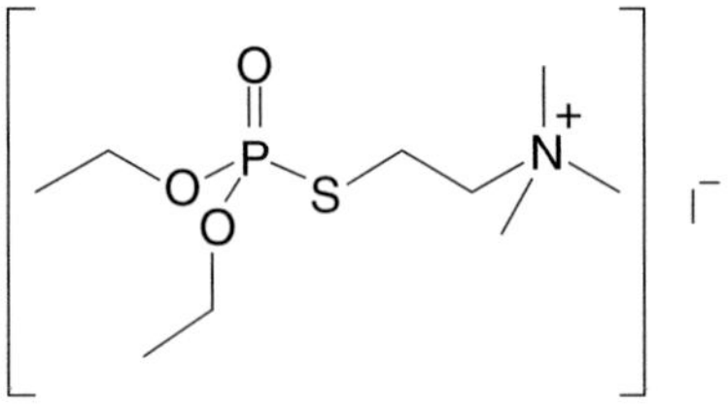

Mechanism of Action and Therapeutic Uses

Echothiophate is an indirectly acting cholinomimetic drug. It binds irreversibly to AChE, and since it gets hydrolyzed by the enzyme very slowly, its effect can last more than a week. Thus it is a strong and long-lasting miotic used mainly for the treatment of open-angle glaucoma. Echothiophate may be indicated in subacute or chronic angle-closure glaucoma when surgery is refused or contraindicated. It is also used to test certain eye conditions like accommodative esotropia.

Dosage

Echothiophate 0.125 % solution is available for patient application.

Side Effects

Ocular side effects include retinal detachment, miosis, cataract, papillary block, brow ache, iris cysts, and punctual stenosis of the nasolacrimal system.

Isoflurophate

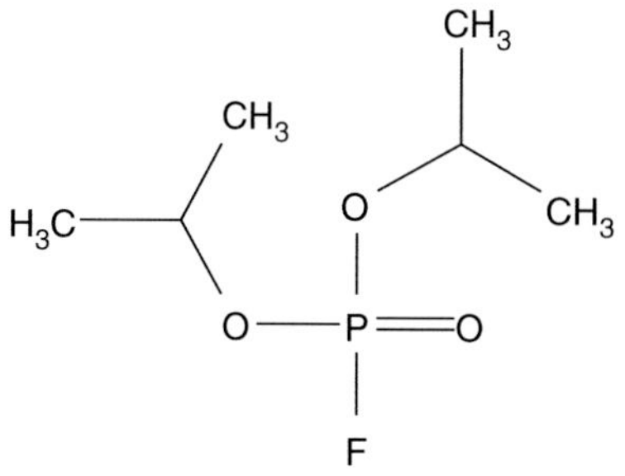

Mechanism of Action and Therapeutic Uses

Isoflurophate is a long-acting and effective mitotic. It is an indirectly acting parasympathomimetic agent acts by prolonging the ACh effect at the neuroeffector junction of parasympathetic postganglionic nerves by irreversibly inhibiting cholinesterase enzyme. It causes constriction of the iris circular (sphincter) muscle as well as ciliary muscle to produce miosis and to block the accommodation reflex with focusing to near vision respectively. It also facilitates the outflow of aqueous humor, thus reducing the intraocular pressure.

Dosage

Isoflurophate 0.1 % solution in peanut oil twice daily is used for open-angle glaucoma. It is also used to treat accommodative convergent strabismus.

Side Effects

Ocular side effects include iris cysts, headache, cataract, and retinal detachment.

6.8.3 Anticholinergics

6.8.3.1 Atropine

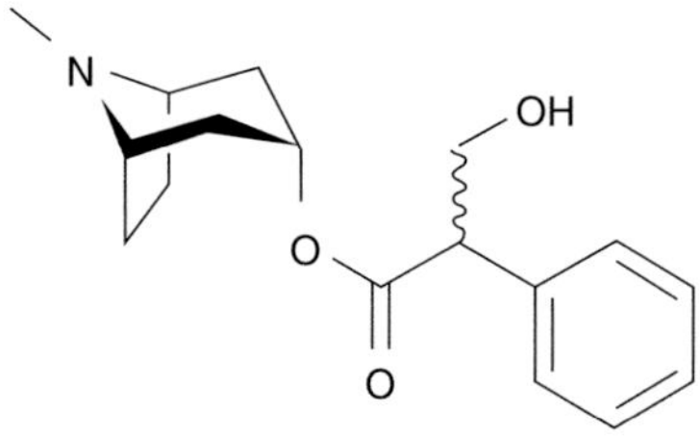

Mechanism of Action and Therapeutic Uses

Atropine inhibits cholinergic effect by blocking muscarinic receptors competitively and thus prevents ACh to bind to those sites. It is a natural alkaloid obtained from *Atropa belladonna*. Atropine inhibits M3 receptor present in circular muscle (sphincter) of the iris to remove the cholinergic tone, leading to relaxation of the circular muscle. This finally leads to the domination of adrenergic tone in radial muscle, causing mydriasis. Atropine blocks the cholinergic effect on ciliary muscle, controlling lens curvature and thus abolishing the effect of accommodation, causing the lens to fix for far vision. Thus atropine causes both mydriasis and cycloplegia (Spehlmann 1969; Mindel 1982; Rengstorff and Doughty 1982).

Atropine is specially used for cycloplegic refraction in younger patients. It actively accommodates children with accommodative esotropia. It is avoided in adults for causing prolonged accommodative paralysis. Atropine is also used for treating anterior uveal inflammation. Atropine does not alter IOP in the normal eye but it can increase IOP in patients with narrow-angle glaucoma. This is mainly due to the relaxation of the ciliary muscle and the crowding of the iris in the angle of the anterior chamber of the eye, causing interference in aqueous humor outflow. Atropine is also used for cycloplegic retinoscopy and dilated funduscopic examination.

Dosage

Atropine 0.5, 1, and 2 % solutions are mainly used for inducing cycloplegia and mydriasis. Topical application of 1 % atropine results in mydriasis in 30–60 min and the effect stays on up to 14 days and the cycloplegic effect lasts for 12 days. The longer duration of action is mainly attributed to the binding of atropine to the pigmented iris cells and subsequent release over a period of time onto the muscarinic receptors present in the iris and ciliary body. For pediatric use atropine is used as 1 % topical ointment to avoid systemic side effects.

Side Effects

Ocular side effects of atropine mainly include photosensitivity and blurring of vision. It can cause acute eye pain due to sudden increase in IOP in patients with narrow-angle glaucoma.

6.8.3.2 Homatropine

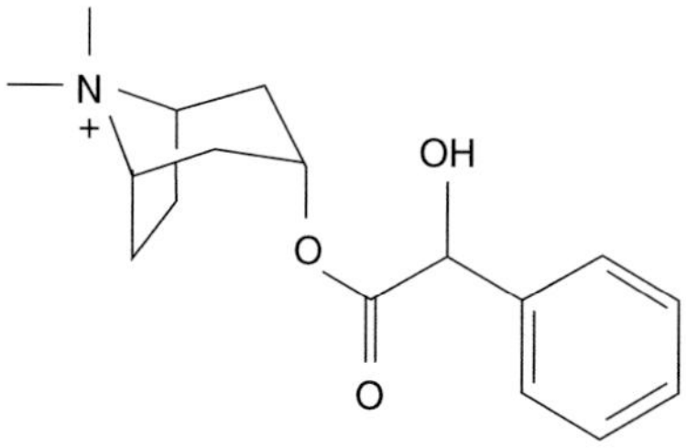

Mechanism of Action and Therapeutic Uses

Homatropine is derivative of tropane alkaloid having potency one tenth of atropine. Similar to atropine this also blocks the muscarinic effect on circular muscle of the iris, resulting in mydriasis, and causes relaxation of the ciliary muscle, resulting in paralysis in accommodation reflex (cycloplegia) (Marron 1940). It is used for various ophthalmic conditions. It is used as mydriatics in post- and preoperative conditions (Shutt and Bowes 1979). It is indicated for the measurement of refractive errors and treatment of uveitis. It causes pupillary dilatation and ciliary muscle relaxation that is desired during acute inflammation of the uveal tract. Homatropine is also used as an optical aid in some cases of axial lens opacities.

Dosage

Homatropine topical solution (2–5 %) is commercially available. Time to peak of mydriasis is 40–60 min. The duration of action is shorter than atropine and the effects last for 48 h with lesser side effects.

Side Effects

Mild itching, burning sensation, photosensitivity, and blurred vision are the side effects reported.

6.8.3.3 Tropicamide

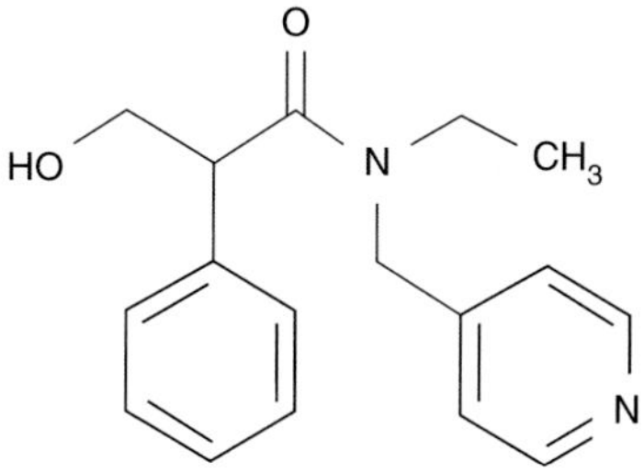

Mechanism of Action and Therapeutic Uses

Tropicamide mainly acts by blocking the cholinergic stimulation on circular muscle of the iris, resulting in mydriasis. It produces cycloplegia by paralyzing cilliary muscles leading to the loss of accommodation (Milder 1961). This is short and quick acting. This is a preferred agent for examination of the lens, retina, and vitreous humor (Merrill et al. 1960; Iribarren 2008). Due to its short duration of action, it is often used for fundus examination and also used before and after eye surgery. Cycloplegic drops are often also used for the treatment of uveitis as they reduce the risk of posterior synechiae and decrease the inflammation in the anterior chamber of the eye.

Dosage
It is available commercially in 0.5 and 1 % solution for ocular use. With 1 % topical solution (repeated in 5 min), mydriasis is apparent within 15 min and can last for 4–6 h (Siderov and Nurse 2005).

Side Effects
The ocular side effects of tropicamide include transient stinging sensation, blurring of vision, photophobia, and sudden rise in intraocular pressure. It may sometimes cause redness of the eye or conjunctivitis.

6.8.3.4 Scopolamine

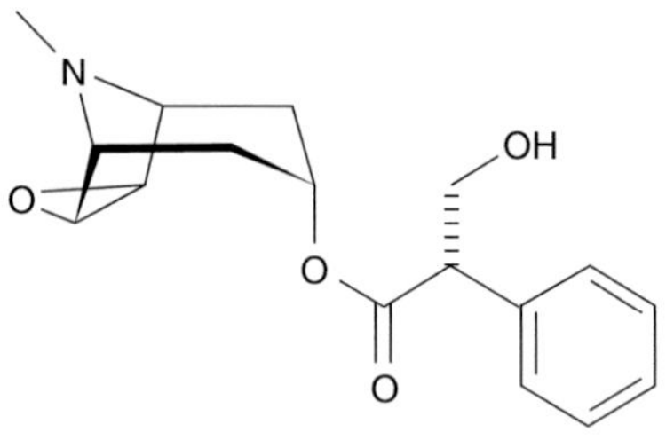

Mechanism of Action and Therapeutic Uses
Scopolamine is a tropane alkaloid that competitively blocks muscarinic receptors in the eye tissue. It is a more potent antimuscarinic agent than that of atropine with shorter duration of mydriatic and cycloplegic effect (Marron 1940). It is used for temporary dilation of the pupil and paralysis of certain parts of the eye for diagnostic procedures. Scopolamine is used to dilate the pupil for eye examination and may also be used before or after eye surgery to reduce pain and swelling in certain types of eye inflammation (iridocyclitis) by relaxing the eye muscles (Mindel 1982).

Dosage
It is commercially available in 0.25 and 0.5 % ophthalmic solution. Maximum pupillary dilation and cycloplegic effect occur at 20 min and 40 min, respectively, and lasted for at least 90 min.

Side Effects
The ocular side effects of scopolamine include blurred vision and burning and stinging sensation. It may also produce redness. CNS toxicity is also caused by the use of scopolamine eyedrops.

6.8.3.5 Cyclopentolate

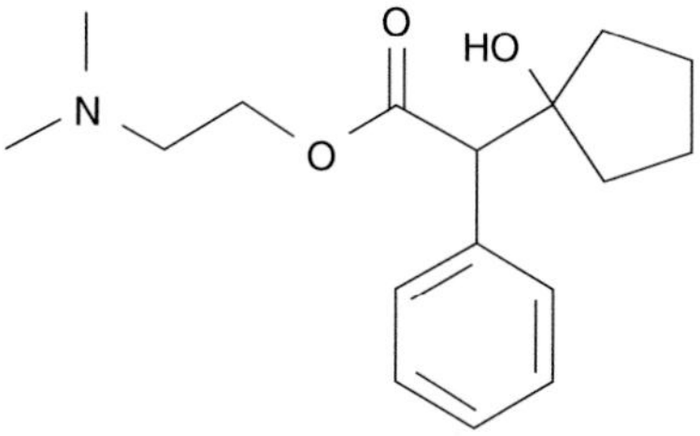

Mechanism and Therapeutic Uses

Cyclopentolate was introduced into clinical practices in 1951 (Priestly and Medine 1951). It is a stable water-soluble ester with anticholinergic property. It causes dilation of pupil (mydriatic) (Hancox et al. 2002) and loss of accommodation achieved by relaxing the ciliary muscle of the eye (cycloplegic) (Bagheri et al. 2007). It has a short duration of action and is useful in refraction in pediatric patients (Khurana et al. 1988). It is also prescribed for a condition of anterior uveitis. It is a painful condition due to the inflammation in the eye. Cyclopentolate reduces pain and relaxes the eye muscle. Clinically its cycloplegic effect is much better than that of homatropine and closely parallel to atropine (Gettes and Leopold 1953).

Dosage

Cyclopentolate 0.5, 1, and 5 % solution is available commercially. The onset of action is apparent in 20–30 min and lasts for 2–24 h.

Side Effects

Ocular side effects are rare that include burning and stinging sensation. Sometimes redness of the eye, eye irritation, conjunctival hyperemia, allergic blepharoconjunctivitis, and elevated intraocular pressure may occur.

6.9 Clinical Manifestations of Sympathetic Dysfunction

Sympathetic innervation to the eye consists of a 3-neuron arc. First-order central sympathetic fibers arise from the posterolateral hypothalamus, descend uncrossed through the midbrain and pons, and terminate in the intermediolateral cell column of the spinal cord at the level of C8–T2 (ciliospinal center of Budge). Second-order preganglionic pupillomotor fibers exit the spinal cord at the level of T1 and enter the cervical sympathetic chain, where they are in close proximity to the pulmonary apex and the subclavian artery (Fig. 6.1).

The fibers ascend through the sympathetic chain and synapse in the superior cervical ganglion at the level of the bifurcation of the common carotid artery (C3–C4). Postganglionic pupillomotor fibers exit the superior cervical ganglion and ascend along the internal carotid artery. Shortly after the postganglionic fibers leave the

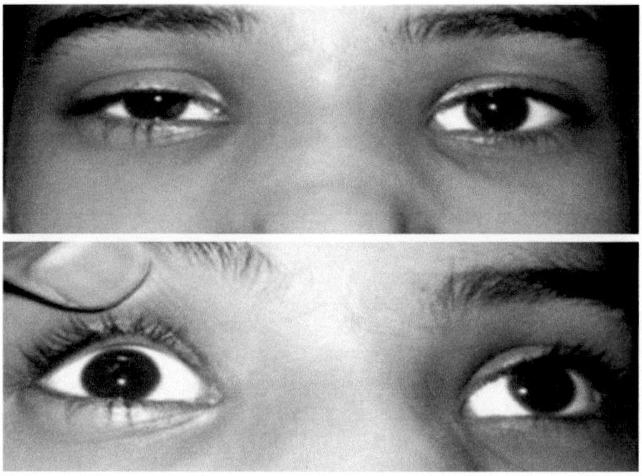

Fig. 6.3 A case of Horner syndrome showing ptosis and miosis

superior cervical ganglion, vasomotor and sudomotor fibers branch off, traveling along the external carotid artery to innervate the blood vessels and sweat glands of the face.

The third-order pupillomotor fibers ascending along the internal carotid artery enter the cavernous sinus. The fibers then leave the carotid plexus briefly to join the abducens nerve in the cavernous sinus and enter the orbit through the superior orbital fissure along with the ophthalmic branch of the trigeminal nerve via the long ciliary nerves. The long ciliary nerves then innervate the iris dilator and the Müller muscle.

The clinical features of oculosympathetic paresis is classically known as Horner's syndrome, which was first reported by Johann Friedrich Horner. Horner's syndrome includes the triad of miosis (pupillomotor fibers), ptosis (Muller's muscle), and anhidrosis (vasodilator fibers of the face) (Fig. 6.3). The other signs include mild elevation of the lower lid since sympathetic fibers innervated the smooth muscle of the lower lid as well, resulting in pseudo-enophthalmos, mild redness of the conjunctiva as a result of damage to vasoconstrictor fibers, and lower intraocular pressure. In the first year of life, sympathetic nerve fibers are important in supporting the normal melanization of ocular tissues, and so a congenital Horner may be associated with relative hypopigmentation of the iris ipsilateral to the lesion (heterochromia iridis). There is increase in accommodation amplitude on the ipsilateral side; however it is minor and clinically insignificant.

Obtaining a careful history is very helpful in the localization of lesions causing Horner's syndrome. First-order neuron lesions will present as hemisensory loss, dysarthria, dysphagia, ataxia, vertigo, and nystagmus. The second-order neuron lesions may have history of facial, neck, axillary, shoulder, or arm pain, cough, hemoptysis, previous thoracic or neck surgery, previous chest tube or central venous catheter placement, or neck swelling. The third-order neuron lesions may present as sixth nerve palsy, numbness in the distribution of the first or second division of the trigeminal nerve, and pain. Table 6.2 enlists the causes of Horner's syndrome (Kawasaki 2005).

Areas affected by anhidrosis may help in localizing the lesion. With central first-order neuron lesions, anhidrosis affects the ipsilateral side of the body. Lesions affecting second-order neurons may cause anhidrosis of the ipsilateral face. With

Table 6.2 Causes of Horner syndrome

First-order neuron	Second-order neuron	Third-order neuron
Arnold-Chiari malformation	Pancoast tumor	Internal carotid artery dissection (associated with sudden ipsilateral face or neck pain)
Basal meningitis (e.g., syphilis)	Birth trauma with injury to lower brachial plexus	Raeder syndrome (paratrigeminal syndrome) - oculosympathetic paresis and ipsilateral facial pain with variable involvement of the trigeminal and oculomotor nerves
Basal skull tumors	Aneurysm or dissection of the aorta	Carotid cavernous fistula
Cerebral vascular accident (CVA)/Wallenberg syndrome (lateral medullary syndrome)	Lesions of the subclavian or common carotid artery	Cluster or migraine headache
Lesions in the hypothalamus or medulla	Central venous catheterization	Herpes zoster
Intrapontine hemorrhage	Trauma or surgical injury (e.g., from radical neck dissection, thyroidectomy, carotid angiography, or coronary artery bypass grafting)	
	Lesions of the middle ear (e.g., acute otitis media)	

postganglionic lesions occurring after vasomotor and sudomotor fibers having branched off the sympathetic chain, anhidrosis is either absent or limited to an area above the ipsilateral brow; however in practice it may be difficult to make these distinctions. In patients with generalized dysautonomias who have bilateral sympathetic dysfunctions, it may be challenging to diagnose Horner's syndrome. Sometimes lesions of the peripheral sympathetic pathway may have partial damage of fibers, giving rise to incomplete or "partial" Horner's syndromes, which may present without ptosis or anhidrosis. In such cases pupillometric or pharmacological tests help in clinching the diagnosis.

6.10 Clinical Manifestations of Parasympathetic Dysfunction

The parasympathetic pathway is a two-neuron pathway. Presynaptic parasympathetic fibers originate in the Edinger-Westphal nucleus, the parasympathetic motor nucleus associated with the oculomotor nucleus in the brainstem. Axons from the Edinger-Westphal nucleus and the oculomotor nucleus run together in the brainstem and exit together as the oculomotor nerve. The oculomotor nerve passes through the lateral wall of the cavernous sinus and enters the orbit through the superior orbital fissure where it divides into superior and inferior branches. Parasympathetic fibers

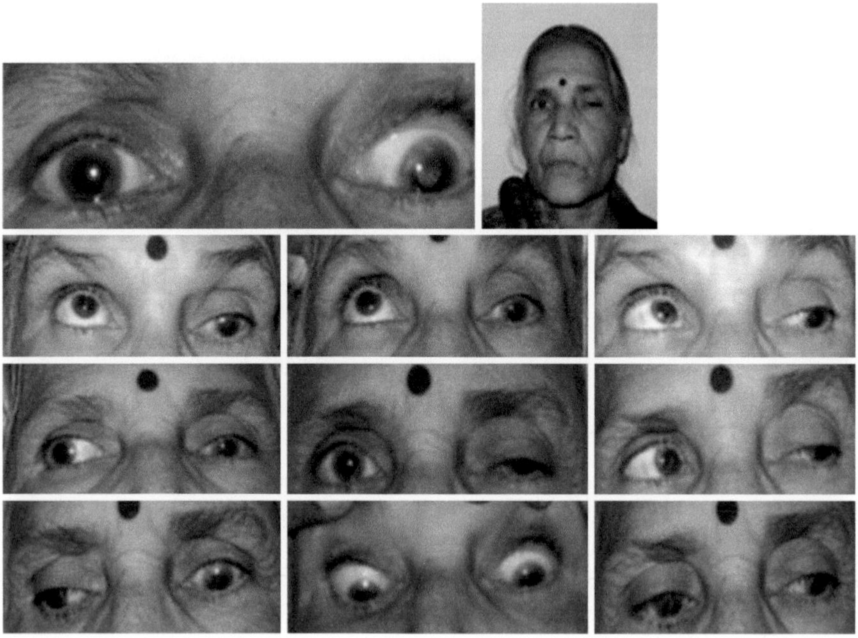

Fig. 6.4 A case of oculomotor nerve palsy showing ophthalmoplegia and ptosis with mydriasis

initially run in the inferior division of the oculomotor nerve. They exit as one or two short "motor roots" that synapse in the ciliary ganglion.

Postsynaptic parasympathetic fibers leave the ciliary ganglion in multiple (six to ten) short ciliary nerves. These nerves enter the posterior aspect of the eyeball to innervate the sphincter muscle of the pupil and ciliary body muscles.

The clinical signs of damage to this parasympathetic supply depend on whether the lesion is pre- or postganglionic. Since both pupillary and accommodative impulses originate and travel in same pathway, the accommodative paralysis frequently accompanies pupillary paralysis in lesions of the efferent parasympathetic pathway to the iris sphincter. This combination of iridoplegia and cycloplegia was called as internal ophthalmoplegia by Hutchinson.

Preganglionic lesions usually cause similar degrees of paresis in both ciliary and sphincter muscles, leading to weak or absent accommodation and a large nonreactive pupil. The pupil remains round and fails to constrict to light or an accommodative effort. Damage to the preganglionic portion of this pathway to the iris sphincter is caused by lesions involving the parasympathetic midbrain nuclei and the oculomotor nerve. Injury to Edinger-Westphal nucleus will invariably cause bilateral pupil defects, and since the oculomotor nerve nucleus is also closely related, the patient may present with ptosis and ophthalmoplegia.

In cases of infranuclear palsy of the oculomotor nerve, pupil defects are consistently accompanied by some degree of ptosis and/or ophthalmoplegia (Fig. 6.4). The causes of oculomotor nerve palsy are listed in Table 6.3.

Table 6.3 Causes of oculomotor nerve palsy

Location	Other symptoms and signs	Common causes
1. Nucleus	Complete IIIrd + C\L ptosis + C\L SR weakness	Vascular occlusion Hemorrhage, metastasis
2. Fascicles	C\L hemiparesis (Weber's), C\L tremor (Benedikt's), I\L ataxia (Nothnagel's)	Vascular occlusion Hemorrhage, neoplasm demyelination
3. Subarachnoid space	Typically isolated	Aneurysm, microvascular occlusion, neoplasm, meningitis Herniation, trauma
4. Cavernous sinus	IVth, VIth, V1, V2, oculosympathetic dysfunction; pain may be prominent	Neoplasm, inflammation, aneurysm, microvascular occlusion, thrombosis Arteriovenous fistula
5. Orbit	Proptosis, visual loss	Trauma, neoplasm, inflammation

In the subarachnoid part of the oculomotor nerve pathway, the pupillary fibers are superficially located which makes them particularly susceptible to direct compression, particularly aneurysm. And thus involvement of the pupil, particularly in a young patient, should warrant an imaging study to identify and localize the lesion. Cases of isolated internal ophthalmoplegia are extremely rare and are usually due to intrinsic lesion of the oculomotor nerve. Any lesion of the cavernous sinus can potentially compress and damage the oculomotor nerve and the pupil fibers. In such cases anisocoria may or may not be present depending on the disparity of involvement of both sympathetic and parasympathetic pathways present in this region.

In contrast, the postganglionic lesions will affect only the pupil and accommodation, sparing the extraocular muscles. The damage to the ciliary ganglion and short posterior ciliary nerves may be local. The common causes include localized injury, viral infections, inflammation of choroid, autoimmune diseases like sarcoidosis, rheumatoid arthritis, migraine, and primary or metastatic tumors of choroid and orbit.

The involvement of ciliary ganglion and short posterior ciliary nerves may be part of widespread generalized dysautonomia like in cases of syphilis, chronic alcoholism, diabetes mellitus, amyloidosis, systemic lupus erythematosus, Sjogren syndrome, some of the spinocerebellar degenerations, hereditary motor-sensory neuropathy (Charcot-Marie-Tooth disease), Landry-Guillain-Barre syndrome, Miller Fisher syndrome, and Shy-Drager and Ross syndrome.

6.11 Holmes-Adie Syndrome

Holmes-Adie syndrome is an uncommon, idiopathic condition that may develop in otherwise healthy persons and in patients with unrelated conditions. The pathophysiology of an Adie pupil is acute denervation followed by reinnervation of the ciliary body and iris sphincter (Corbett et al. 1998). The clinical findings depend on the stage of evolution in which the pupil is examined. In the acute phase, there is internal ophthalmoplegia, thus causing symptoms like photophobia and blurred vision. The pupil is large and dilated and may be confused with pharmacological mydriasis; a careful slit lamp examination reveals segmental contractions, called as "vermiform movements" of the pupil, as a result of sectoral palsy of the pupil in this condition (Kardon et al. 1998). With time, as the reinnervation occurs, the pupil becomes irregular and smaller in shape. The accommodation response is regained while the light response is still impaired. The pupil response to accommodation and then redilation is slow and sustained that earned its name as "tonic pupil."

The other associated features of this syndrome are areflexia of deep tendon reflex, decreased corneal sensation, and cholinergic denervation hypersensitivity of the pupil. Cholinergic supersensitivity develops in acute phase. About 80 % of tonic pupils demonstrate cholinergic supersensitivity and thus may help in diagnosing these cases.

6.11.1 Diagnosis of Autonomic Dysfunction

As it can be inferred from the above clinical manifestations, most patients with autonomic disorders show evidence of sympathetic or parasympathetic deficits in the pupil. In a recent systematic study of 150 consecutive patients with various types of dysautonomia referred for pupillometry, the overall prevalence of pupil abnormalities was found to be 66 % (Bremner and Smith 2006). Thus examination of the pupil is a simple, convenient, noninvasive technique for evaluating function in the autonomic nervous system (Bremner 2009). The examination entails determining the size of the pupil, measuring the pupil response to light and accommodation, and use of topical pharmacological agents to confirm as well as localize the lesions. These pupil signs in combination with other associated clinical signs help in clinching the diagnosis. Although the autonomic disturbance in the pupils may not correlate with autonomic function elsewhere, it may still help in discriminating between the various autonomic conditions.

The size and the tone of the pupil are determined by balance between the sympathetic and parasympathetic tone. A variety of instruments have been designed for measuring the pupil size, ranging from a simple handheld pupil gauge to infrared pupillometry (Wachler and Krueger 1999; Wilhelm and Wilhelm 2003).

The difference between the sizes of two pupils is termed as "anisocoria" and is an important clue to diagnose various conditions. Anisocoria up to 0.4 mm is seen in 20 % of normal population. While the amount of physiological anisocoria remains constant in all conditions, the pathological anisocoria may vary in different illumination conditions and thus provides critical evidence for diagnosis.

In cases of Horner's syndrome, the anisocoria is more in dark because of the paralysis of the dilator muscle of the affected pupil, also known as "dilatation lag." The initial redilatation is rapid and reflects withdrawal of the parasympathetic drive to the sphincter muscle, whereas the later phase is slower and is thought to be actively driven by the peripheral sympathetic supply to the dilator muscle. Damage to this peripheral sympathetic supply therefore delays the later phase, giving rise to 'redilatation lag'

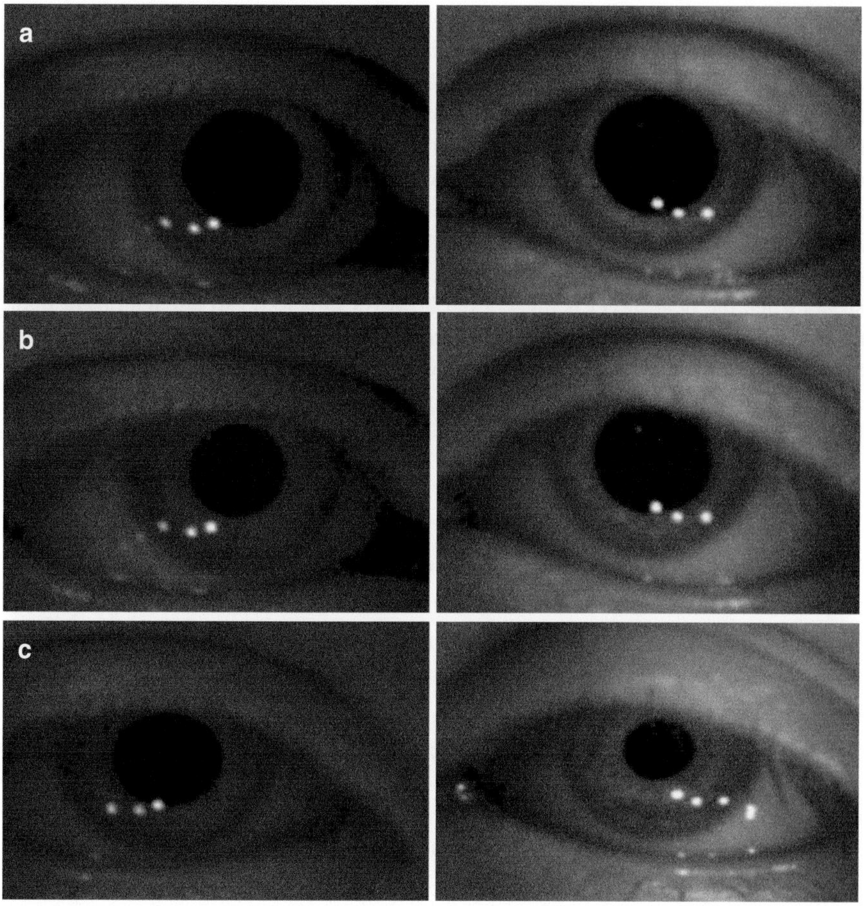

Fig. 6.5 A case of Adie syndrome; (**a**) anisocoria in light, (**b**) anisocoria in dark, (**c**) miosis after 0.1 % pilocarpine instillation

(Lowenstein and Loewenfeld 1950). Dilatation lag is detected by measuring the pupil size in very dim light after a bright room light has been turned off. Normal pupils return to their widest size within 12–15 s, with most of the dilation occurring in the first 5 s. Pupils that show dilation lag may take up to 25 s for complete dilatation (Digre 2005). In cases of unilateral Horner's syndrome redilatation lag may be readily detected both clinically (by directly comparing the time taken for the pupils to dilate after the room lights are turned out) and photographically (anisocoria measurements are greater at 5 s compared with 15 s after onset of darkness) (Pilley and Thompson 1975). However detection of bilateral sympathetic lesions requires an absolute measure of redilatation. Some studies have shown that the redilatation lag is the most sensitive test for the diagnosis of unilateral or bilateral Horner's syndrome. To further localize the site of the lesion, pharmacological tests are required.

The paralysis of parasympathetic pathway manifests as anisocoria which increases in bright light because of the paralysis of the sphincter muscle of the affected side

(Fig. 6.5b). The different causes of parasympathetic paralysis have been described above and can be differentiated on the basis of their associated clinical features. The damage to the preganglionic fibers in oculomotor nerve presents with internal ophthalmoplegia along with paralysis of extraocular muscles. The lesions of postganglionic parasympathetic pathway manifest as isolated internal ophthalmoplegia, which can be a part of generalized dysautonomia or can be due to local insult to ciliary body and short ciliary nerves. A careful slit lamp examination may reveal "vermiform movements" which are characteristic of Adie tonic pupil. One must also look for response to both light and near. In chronic cases of Adie tonic pupil, the pupil constricts when the near target is present but however fails to do so when a bright light is shone, thus seen as light-near dissociation. The accommodative response in such cases is quite slow and tonic. It can take over 10 s for peak miosis to be reached and even longer for the pupil to return to its original size. The pharmacological tests help in further differentiation and confirmation of diagnosis.

6.11.2 Pharmacological Tests for Pupil

The pharmacological tests are useful for the confirmation of the diagnosis as well as for the localization of the lesion. However they should be done in controlled environment and may also get affected by the patient's frame of mind.

Sympathetic Paralysis The most widely used confirmatory test for the diagnosis of Horner's syndrome is the cocaine 10 % eyedrop test. Cocaine blocks the reuptake of the norepinephrine that is released continuously from sympathetic nerve endings at the neuromuscular synapse, allowing norepinephrine to accumulate at the receptors of the effector cells. The failure of dilatation of the pupil indicates the presence of Horner's syndrome. It cannot differentiate between the central or peripheral Horner since cocaine has no direct affect on the receptors of the iris but just prevents the reuptake of norepinephrine at the local site. A lesion of the sympathetic pathway will prevent the presynaptic release of norepinephrine irrespective of its location, thus failure to dilate with cocaine. Kardon et al. analyzed photographs from a large number of cocaine tests in Horner patients and controls to establish the optimal diagnostic criteria; they concluded that an increase of anisocoria of 0.8 mm or more gives a mean odds ratio of 1050:1 (95 % lower limit 37:1) that the patient has a Horner (Kardon et al. 1990).

The 1 % hydroxyamphetamine test can be used to differentiate between a postganglionic and a preganglionic or central Horner's syndrome. Hydroxyamphetamine releases stored norepinephrine from the postganglionic adrenergic nerve endings (Cremer et al. 1990). Thus a lesion of the postganglionic neuron that results in loss of terminal nerve endings and their stores of norepinephrine will show no mydriatic effect even with hydroxyamphetamine, with lesions of the preganglionic or central neuron where the postganglionic nerve endings remain structurally intact. Thus, the pupil dilates fully and may even become larger than the opposite pupil from upregulation of the postsynaptic receptors on the dilator muscle. Hydroxyamphetamine

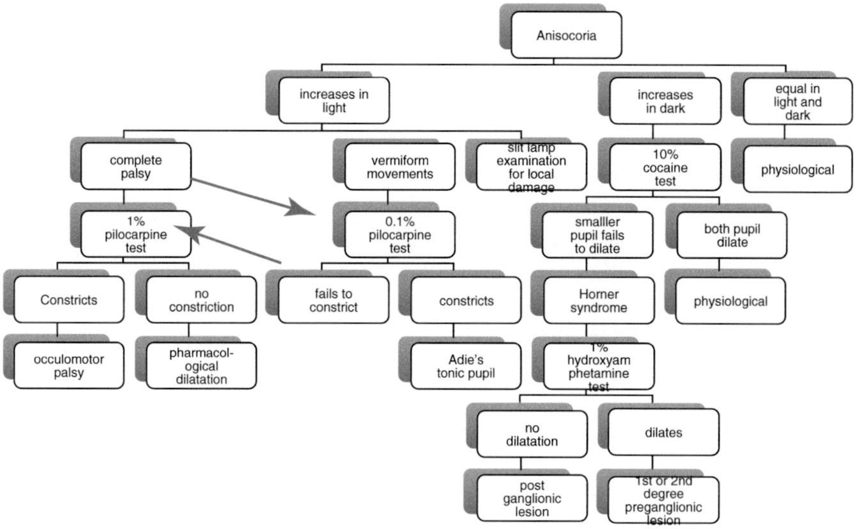

Fig. 6.6 A flowchart depicting the approach toward a case of anisocoria

testing is reported to localize the lesion in Horner's syndrome with a sensitivity of 93 % and specificity of 83 %. Thus a smaller pupil that fails to dilate to both cocaine and hydroxyamphetamine most likely has a lesion of the postganglionic fibers, while failure of dilatation with cocaine but exaggerated dilatation with hydroxyamphetamine is suggestive of postganglionic lesion.

Unfortunately nowadays it has become difficult to procure both cocaine and hydroxyamphetamine. In such cases diluted phenylephrine 1 % or any other alpha agonist can be used to diagnose Horner's syndrome. It based on the principle of deinnervational supersensitivity of adrenergic receptors of iris dilator muscle. Danesh-Meyer et al. have compared the pupillary responses to hydroxyamphetamine and 1 % phenylephrine in 3 pre- and 11 postganglionic Horner patients and found good concordance in the results between these two drugs (Danesh-Meyer et al. 2004).

Parasympathetic Paralysis The integrity of parasympathetic pathway tested by looking for evidence of denervation supersensitivity of the iris sphincter muscle receptors. The commonest drug used is 0.1 % pilocarpine (Jacobson 1990); this weak muscarinic agonist has little effect on the normal pupil but will produce an exaggerated miosis in any patient with a parasympathetic lesion (Fig. 6.5). This supersensitivity of iris cholinergic receptor is irrespective of site of lesion, pre- or postganglionic (Jacobson and Vierkant 1998). Figure 6.6 depicts the flow chart for the approach toward a patient of anisocoria.

The diagnosis of autonomic dysfunction appears to be simple and straightforward in presence of anisocoria. The pupillometric tests compare the pupil response to various stimuli, of one eye to the other; the pharmacological tests are based on the principle where the other eye serves as an internal control (Czarnecki et al. 1979). However in cases of generalized autonomic dysfunction, there is bilateral and symmetrical involvement of the pupil, which obscures the diagnosis (Smith and Smith

1999). In such cases the pharmacological tests become relatively insensitive, and clinical signs and pupillometric tests like redilatation lag and light-near dissociation may aid in diagnosing the condition.

The diagnosis turns out to be equally confounding in a rare case where both sympathetic and parasympathetic dysfunction coexists. In such a case presence of dysfunction of one system masks the clinical signs of dysfunction of the other. The pupillometric tests may not serve the purpose since both the iris sphincter and dilator muscles are affected. The pharmacological tests are positive only if there is asymmetric involvement or the dysfunction of one system predominates over the other. The comparison of this measure with the normal healthy population is the way to arrive at the conclusion.

References

Ackerknecht EH. The history of the discovery of the vegetative (autonomic) nervous system. Med Hist. 1974;18(1):1–8.

Akingbehin T, Villada JR. Metipranolol-associated granulomatous anterior uveitis. Br J Ophthalmol. 1991;75:519–23.

Alm A, Nilsson SF. Uveoscleral outflow – a review. Exp Eye Res. 2009;88(4):760–8.

Angenent WJ, Koelle GB. A possible enzymatic basis for the differential action of mydriatics on light and dark irides. J Physiol. 1953;119(1):102–17.

Apatachioae I, Chiseliţa D. Alpha-2 adrenergic agonists in the treatment of glaucoma. Oftalmologia. 1999;47(2):35–40.

Aung T, Laganovska G, Hernandez Paredes TJ, Branch JD, Tsorbatzoglou A, Goldberg I, Bagheri A, Givrad S, Yazdani S, Reza Mohebbi M. Optimal dosage of cyclopentolate 1% for complete cycloplegia: a randomized clinical trial. Eur J Ophthalmol. 2007;17(3):294–300.

Aung T, Laganovska G, Hernandez Paredes TJ, Branch JD, Tsorbatzoglou A, Goldberg I. Twice-daily brinzolamide/brimonidine fixed combination versus brinzolamide or brimonidine in open-angle glaucoma or ocular hypertension. Ophthalmology. 2014;121(12):2348–55.

Bagheri A, Givrad S, Yazdani S, Reza Mohebbi M. Optimal dosage of cyclopentolate 1% for complete cycloplegia: a randomized clinical trial. Eur J Ophthalmol. 2007;17(3):294–300.

Ballin N, Becker B, Goldman ML. Systemic effects of epinephrine applied topically to the eye. Invest Ophthalmol. 1966;125–129.

Bartlett JD, Classé JG. Dapiprazole: will it affect the standard of care for pupillary dilation? Optom Clin. 1992;2(4):113–20.

Battershill PE, Sorkin EM. Ocular metipranolol. Drugs. 1988;36(5):601–15.

Becker HI, Walton RC, Diamant JI, Zegans ME. Anterior uveitis and concurrent allergic conjunctivitis associated with long-term use of topical 0.2% brimonidine tartrate. Arch Ophthalmol. 2004;122(7):1063–6.

Benovic JL. Novel β2-adrenergic receptor signaling pathways. J Allergy Clin Immunol. 2002; 110:S229–35.

Bensinger RE, Keates EU, Gofman JD, Novack GO, Duzman E. Levobunolol: a three-month efficacy study in the treatment of glaucoma and ocular hypertension. Arch Ophthalmol. 1985;103: 375–8.

Boger WP, Steinert RF, Puliafito CA, Pavan-Langston D. Clinical trial comparing timolol ophthalmic solution to pilocarpine in open-angle glaucoma. Am J Ophthalmol. 1978;86:8–18.

Bonner TI. The molecular basis of muscarinic receptor diversity. Trends Neurosci. 1989;12: 148–51.

Boozman FW, Carriker R, Foerster R, Allen RC, Novack GO, et al. Long-term evaluation of 0.25% levobunolol and timolol for therapy for elevated intraocular pressure. Arch Ophthalmol. 1988;106:614–8.
Boudot JP, Cavero I, Fenard S, Lefevre-Borg F, Manoury P, et al. Preliminary studies on SL 75212, a new potent cardioselective β-adrenoceptor antagonist (Proceedings). Br J Pharmacol. 1979;66:445.
Bremner F. Pupil evaluation as a test for autonomic disorders. Clin Auton Res. 2009;19:88–101.
Bremner FD, Smith SE. Pupil findings in a consecutive series of 150 cases of generalized autonomic neuropathy. J Neurol Neurosurg Psychiatry. 2006;77:1163–8.
Brown RH, Stewart RH, Lynch MG, Crandall AS, Mandell AI, Wilensky JT, et al. ALO 2145 reduces the intraocular pressure elevation after anterior segment laser surgery. Ophthalmology. 1988;95:378–84.
Buckley MM, Goa KL, Clissold SP. Ocular betaxolol. A review of its pharmacological properties, and therapeutic efficacy in glaucoma and ocular hypertension. Drugs. 1990;40(1):75–90.
Casini G, Dal Monte M, Fornaciari I, Filippi L, Bagnoli P. The β-adrenergic system as a possible new target for pharmacologic treatment of neovascular retinal diseases. Prog Retin Eye Res. 2014;42:103–29.
Catford GV, Millis E. Clinical experience in the intra-ocular use of acetylcholine. Br J Ophthalmol. 1967;51:183–7.
Cavero I, Lefevre-Borg F. Antihypertensive activity of betaxolol in conscious spontaneously hypertensive rats (Proceedings). Br J Pharmacol. 1983;78:141.
Chen PL, Hsiao CH, Chen JT, Lu DW, Chen WY. Efficacy of apraclonidine 0.5% in the diagnosis of horner syndrome in pediatric patients under low or high illumination. Am J Ophthalmol. 2006;142:469–74.
Cremer SA, Thompson S, Digree KB, et al. Hydroxyamphetamine mydriasis in Horner's syndrome. Am J Ophthalmol. 1990;110:71–6.
Cullon Jr RD, Schwartz LW. The effect of apraclonidine on the intraocular pressure of glaucoma patients following Nd:YAG laser posterior capsulotomy. Ophthalmic Surg. 1993;24:623–6.
Czarnecki JSC, Pilley SFJ, Thompson HS. The analysis of anisocoria. Can J Ophthalmol. 1979; 14:297–302.
Danesh-Meyer HV, Savino P, Sergott R. The correlation of phenylephrine 1% and hydroxyamphetamine 1% in Horner's syndrome. Br J Ophthalmol. 2004;88:592–3.
Digre KB. Principles and techniques of examination of the pupils, accommodation, and lacrimation. In: Miller NR et al. editor. Walsh and Hoyt's clinical neuro-ophthalmology. 6th ed. Pennsylvania, USA: Lippincott Williams & Wilkins; 2005. p. 715–37.
Duff GR. A double-masked crossover study comparing the effects of carteolol 1% and 2% on intraocular pressure. Acta Ophthalmol. 1987;65(5):618–21.
Evans DW, Hosking SL, Gherghel D, Bartlett JD. Contrast sensitivity improves after brimonidine therapy in primary open angle glaucoma: a case for neuroprotection. Br J Ophthalmol. 2003; 87(12):1463–5.
Feghali JG, Kaufman PL, Radius RL, Mandell AI. A comparison of betaxolol and timolol in open angle glaucoma and ocular hypertension. Acta Ophthalmol (Copenh). 1988;66(2):180–6.
Filippi L, Dal Monte M, Casini G, Daniotti M, Sereni F, Bagnoli P. Infantile hemangiomas, retinopathy of prematurity and cancer: a common pathogenetic role of the β-adrenergic system. Med Res Rev. 2015;35(3):619–52.
Fredriksson JM, Lindquist JM, Bronnikov GE, Nedergaard J. Norepinephrine Induces vascular endothelial growth factor gene expression in brown adipocytes through a β-adrenoreceptor/cAMP/protein kinase a pathway involving Src but independently of Erk1/2. J Bioll Chem. 2000;275:13802–11.
Fujihara T, Murakami T, Fujita H, Nakamura M, Nakata K. Improvement of corneal barrier function by the P2Y(2) agonist INS365 in a rat dry eye model. Invest Ophthalmol Vis Sci. 2001; 42(1):96–100. German patent 1,117,588.
Gettes BD, Leopold IH. Evaluation of 5 new cycloplegic drugs. Arch Ophthalmol. 1953;49:24–7.
Gharagozloo NZ, Relf SJ, Brubaker RF. Aqueous flow is reduced by the alpha-adrenergic agonist, apraclonidine hydrochloride (ALO 2145). Ophthalmology. 1988;95(9):1217–20.

Goldberg I. Betaxolol. Aust N Z J Ophthalmol. 1989;17:9–13.
Gupta N, Drance SM, McAllister R, Prasad S, Rootman J, Cynader MS. Localisation of M3 muscarinic receptor subtype and mRNA in the human eye. Ophthalmic Res. 1994a;26:207–13.
Gupta N, McAllister R, Drance SM, Rootman J, Cynader MS. Muscarinic receptor Ml and M2 subtypes in the human eye: QNB, pirenzipine, oxotremorine, and AFDX-116 in vitro autoradiography. Br J Ophthalmol. 1994b;78:555–9.
Halpern B. Obituary notice: Henry Hallet dale. Rev Fr Allergol. 1969;9(2):117–9.
Hancox J, Murdoch I, Parmar D. Changes in intraocular pressure following diagnostic mydriasis with cyclopentolate 1%. Eye (Lond). 2002;16(5):562–6.
Harley RD, Mishler JE. Acetylcholine in cataract surgery. Br J Ophthalmol. 1966;50:429–33.
Henness S, Swainston Harrison T, Keating GM. Ocular carteolol: a review of its use in the management of glaucoma and ocular hypertension. Drugs Aging. 2007;24(6):509–28.
Hogeling M. Propranolol for infantile hemangiomas: a review. Curr Dermatol Rep. 2012;1(4):179–85.
Holmwood PC, Chase RD, Krupin T, Rosenberg LF, Ruderman JM, Tallman BA, et al. Apraclonidine and argon laser trabeculoplasty. Am J Ophthalmol. 1992;114:19–22.
Hong C, Song KY, Park WH, Sohn YH. Effect of apraclonidine hydrochloride on acute intraocular pressure rise after argon laser iridotomy. Korean J Ophthalmol. 1991;5:37–41.
Hurvitz LM, Kaufman PL, Robin AL, et al. New developments in the drug treatment of glaucoma. Drugs. 1991;41(4):514–32.
Iribarren R. Tropicamide and myopia progression. Ophthalmology. 2008;115(6):1103–4.
Jacobson DM. Pupillary response to dilute pilocarpine in pre-ganglionic 3rd nerve disorders. Neurology. 1990;40:804–8. PubMed.
Jacobson DM, Vierkant RA. Comparison of cholinergic supersensitivity in third nerve palsy and Adie's syndrome. J Neuro Ophthalmol. 1998;18:171–5.
Kalapesi FB, Coroneo MT, Hill MA. Human ganglion cells express the alpha-2 adrenergic receptor: relevance to neuroprotection. Br J Ophthalmol. 2005;89(6):758–63.
Kardon R. Anatomy and physiology of the autonomic nervous system. In: Miller NR et al. editor. Walsh and Hoyt's clinical neuro-ophthalmology. 6th ed. Pennsylvania, USA: Lippincott Williams & Wilkins; 2005. p. 649–714.
Kardon RH, Denison CE, Brown CK, et al. Critical evaluation of the cocaine test in the diagnosis of Horner's syndrome. Arch Ophthalmol. 1990;108:384–7.
Kardon RH, Corbett JJ, Thompson HS. Segmental denervation and reinnervation of the iris sphincter as shown by infrared videographic transillumination. Ophthalmology. 1998;105:313–21.
Kaufman PL. Mechanisms of actions of the cholinergic drugs in the eye. In: Drance SM, Neufeld AN, editors. Glaucoma. 1st ed. Orlando: Grune and Stratton; 1984. p. 295–327.
Kawasaki A. Disorders of pupillary function, accommodation, and lacrimation. In: Miller NR et al. editor. Walsh and Hoyt's clinical neuro-ophthalmology. 6th ed. Pennsylvania, USA: Lippincott Williams & Wilkins; 2005. p. 739–805.
Khurana AK, Ahluwalia BK, Rajan C. Status of cyclopentolate as a cycloplegic in children: a comparison with atropine and homatropine. Acta Ophthalmol (Copenh). 1988;66(6):721–4.
Krieglstein GK, Novack GO, Voepel E, Schwarzbach G, Lange U, et al. Levobunolol and metipranolol: comparative ocular hypotensive efficacy, safety, and comfort. Br J Ophthalmol. 1987;71:250–3.
Kubo T, Fukuda K, Mikami A, Maeda A, Takahashi H, Mishina M, et al. Cloning, sequencing and expression of complementary DNA encoding the muscarinic acetylcholine receptor. Nature. 1986;323:411–6.
Leaute-Labreze C, Dumas de la Roque E, Hubiche T, et al. Propranolol for severe hemangiomas of infancy. N Engl J Med. 2008;358:2649–51.
Lowenstein O, Loewenfeld IE. Mutual role of sympathetic and parasympathetic in shaping of the pupillary reflex to light: pupillographic studies. Arch Neurol Psychiatry. 1950;64:341–77.

Maren N, Alvan G, Calissendorff BM, et al. Additive intraocular pressure reducing effect of topical timolol during systemic beta- blockade. Acta Ophthalmol. 1982;60:16–23.

Marron J. Cycloplegia and mydriasis by use of atropine, scopolamine and homatropine-paredrine. Arch Ophthalmol. 1940;23:340–50.

McDougal DH, Gamlin PD. Autonomic control of the eye. Compr Physiol. 2015;5(1):439–73.

Melles RB, Wong IG. Metipranolol-associated granulomatous iritis. Am J Ophthalmol. 1994;118(6):712–5.

Merrill DL, Goldberg B, Zavell S. bis tropicamide. A new parasympatholytic. Curr Ther Res. 1960;2:43–50.

Merte HI, Schnarr KD. Ophthalmic betaxolol: a twelve-week study in glaucoma patients. New Trends Ophthalmol. 1987;2:98–108.

Merte H-J, Stryz JR, Mertz M. Comparative studies of initial pressure reduction using metipranolol 0.3% and timolol 0.25% in eyes with open-angle glaucoma. Klin Monbl Augenheilkd. 1983;182:286–9.

Milder B. Tropicamide as a cycloplegic agent. Arch Opthalmol. 1961;66:70–2.

Mills KB, Wright G. A blind randomised cross-over trial comparing metipranolol 0.3% with timolol 0.25% in open-angle glaucoma: a pilot study. Br J Ophthalmol. 1986;70:39–42.

Mindel JS. Cholinergic pharmacology, chap 26. In: Duane TD, Jaeger EA, editors. Biomedical foundations of ophthalmology, vol. 3. Philadelphia: Harpel & Row; 1982.

Mircheff AK. Lacrimal fluid and electrolyte secretion: a review. Curr Eye Res. 1989;8(6):607–17.

Mirza GE, Karakuçuk S, Temel E. Comparison of the effects of 0.5% timolol maleate, 2% carteolol hydrochloride, and 0.3% metipranolol on intraocular pressure and perimetry findings and evaluation of their ocular and systemic effects. J Glaucoma. 2001;9(1):45–50.

Montanari P, Marangoni P, Oldani A, Ratiglia R, Raiteri M, Berardinelli L. Color Doppler imaging study in patients with primary open-angle glaucoma treated with timolol 0.5% and carteolol 2%. Eur J Ophthalmol. 2001;11(3):240–4.

Mori A, Miwa T, Sakamoto K, Nakahara T, Ishii K. Pharmacological evidence for the presence of functional beta(3)-adrenoceptors in rat retinal blood vessels. Naunyn Schmiedebergs Arch Pharmacol. 2010;382(2):119–26.

Morrison JC, Robin AL. Adjunctive glaucoma therapy: a comparison of apraclonidine to dipivefrin when added to timolol maleate. Ophthalmology. 1989;96(1):3–7.

Moss AP, Ritch R, Hargett NA, et al. A comparison of the effects of timolol and epinephrine on intraocular pressure. Am J Ophthalmol. 1978;86:489–95.

Mundasad MV, Novack GD, Allgood VE, Evans RM, Gorden JC, Yerxa BR. Ocular safety of INS365 ophthalmic solution: a P2Y(2) agonist in healthy subjects. J Ocul Pharmacol Ther. 2001;17(2):173–9.

Murakami T, Fujihara T, Nakamura M, Nakata K. P2Y(2) receptor stimulation increases tear fluid secretion in rabbits. Curr Eye Res. 2000;21(4):782–7.

Neufeld AH, Bartels SP, Liu JHK. Laboratory and clinical studies on the mechanism of action of timolol. Surv Ophthalmol. 1983;28(1):286–90.

Neuhuber W, Schrödl F. Autonomic control of the eye and the iris. Auton Neurosci. 2011;165(1):67–79.

Nielsen CB, Nielsen PJ. Effect of alpha- and beta-receptor active drugs on corneal thickness. Acta Ophthalmol (Copenh). 1985;63(3):351–4.

Obianwu HO, Rand MJ. The relationship between the mydriatic action of ephedrine and the colour of the iris. Br J Ophthalmol. 1965;49:264.

Park SY, Kang JH, Jeong KJ, Lee J, Han JW, Choi WS, Kim YK, Kang J, Park CG, Lee HY. Norepinephrine induces VEGF expression and angiogenesis by a hypoxia-inducible factor-1α protein-dependent mechanism. Int J Cancer. 2011;128:2306–16.

Pilley S, Thompson HS. Pupillary 'dilatation lag' in Horner's syndrome. Br J Ophthalmol. 1975;59:731–5.

Pollack IP, Brown RH, Crandall AS, Robin AL, Stewart RH, White GL. Prevention of the rise in intraocular pressure following neodymium-YAG posterior capsulotomy using topical 1% apraclonidine. Arch Ophthalmol. 1988;106:754–7.

Priestly BS, Medine MM. A new mydriatic and cycloplegic drugs. Am J Opthalmol. 1951;34:572–5.

Rakofsky SI, Lazar M, Almog Y, LeBlanc RP, Mann C, Orr A, Lee PF, Friedland BR, Novack GD, Kelley EP. Efficacy and safety of once-daily levobunolol for glaucoma therapy. Can J Ophthalmol. 1989;24(1):2–6.

Reiss GR, Brubaker RF. The mechanism of betaxolol, a new ocular hypotensive agent. Ophthalmology. 1983;90:1369–72.

Rengstorff RH, Doughty CB. Mydriatic and cycloplegic drugs: a review of ocular and systemic complications. Am J Optom Physiol Opt. 1982;59(2):162–77. Review.

Robin AL, Pollack IP, deFaller JM. Effects of ALO 2145 (p-aminoclonidine hydrochloride) on the acute intraocular pressure rise after argon laser iridotomy. Arch Ophthalmol. 1987a;105:1208–11.

Robin AL, Pollack IP, House B, Enger C. Effects of ALO2145 on IOP following argon laser trabeculoplasty. Arch Ophthalmol. 1987b;105:646–50.

Rolle BB, Franzone M. Effects of topical betaxolol on ocular hypertensive or glaucomatous eyes. New Trends Ophthalmol. 1987;2:87–94.

Rosenberg LF, Krupin T, Ruderman J, McDaniel DL, Siegfried C, Karalekas DP, Grewal RK, Gieser DK, Williams R. Apraclonidine and anterior segment laser surgery. Comparison of 0.5% versus 1.0% Apraclonidine for prevention of postoperative intraocular pressure rise. Ophthalmology. 1995;102(9):1312–8.

Sanderson J, Dartt DA, Trinkaus-Randall V, et al. Purines in the eye: recent evidence for the physiological and pathological role of purines in the RPE, retinal neurons, astrocytes, Müller cells, lens, trabecular meshwork, cornea and lacrimal gland. Exp Eye Res. 2014;127:270–9.

Schmitz-Valckenberg P, Jonas J, Brambring DF. Reductions in pressure with metipranolol 0.1 %. Zeitschrift fur Praktische Augenheilkunde. 1984;5:171–5.

Scoville B, Mueller B, White BG, Krieglstein GK. A double-masked comparison of carteolol and timolol in ocular hypertension. Am J Ophthalmol. 1988;105(2):150–4.

Selvam S, Mircheff AK, Yiu SC. Diverse mediators modulate the chloride ion fluxes that drive lacrimal fluid production. Invest Ophthalmol Vis Sci. 2013;54(4):2927–33.

Sena DF, Lindsley K. Neuroprotection for treatment of glaucoma in adults. Cochrane Database Syst Rev. 2013;2, CD006539.

Shutt LE, Bowes JB. Atropine and hyoscine. Anesthesia. 1979;34:476–90.

Siderov J, Nurse S. The mydriatic effect of multiple doses of tropicamide. Optom Vis Sci. 2005;82(11):955–8.

Silverstone D, Zimmerman T, Choplin N, Mundorf T, Rose A, et al. Evaluation of once-daily levobunolol 0.25% and timolol 0.25% therapy for increased intraocular pressure. Am J Ophthalmol. 1991;112:56–60.

Smit DP. Pharmacological testing in Horner's syndrome – a new paradigm. S Afr Med J. 2010; 100:738–40.

Smith SA, Smith SE. Bilateral Horner's syndrome: detection and occurrence. J Neurol Neurosurg Psychiatry. 1999;66:48–51.

Smith JP, Weeks RH, Newland EF, Ward RL. Betaxolol and acetazolamide: combined ocular hypotensive effect. Arch Ophthalmol. 1984;102:1794–5.

Sneader W. The discovery and synthesis of epinephrine. Drug News Perspect. 2001;14(8):491–4.

Sonty S, Schwartz B. The additive effect of timolol on open angle glaucoma patients on maximal medical therapy. Surv Ophthalmol. 1979;23:381–8.

Spehlmann R. Acetylcholine facilitation, atropine block of synaptic excitation of cortical neurons. Science. 1969;165(3891):404–5.

Steward WC, Shields MB, Allen RC, Lewis RA, Cohen JS, Hoskins HD, Hetherington JN, Bahr RL, Noblin JE, Delehanty JT. A 3-month comparison of 1% and 2% carteolol and 0.5% timolol in open-angle glaucoma. Graefes Arch Clin Exp Ophthalmol. 1991;229(3):258–61.

Stewart WC, Ritch R, Shin DH, Lehmann RP, Shrader C, van Buskirk EM. The efficacy of apraclonidine as an adjunct to timolol therapy. Arch Ophthalmol. 1995;113:287–92.

Stryz JR, Merte H-J. Comparison of different i3-blockers in open angle glaucomas. In: Greve EL et al., editors. Second european glaucoma symposium, Helsinki, 1984. Dordrecht: Dr W. Junk Publishers; 1985. p. 119–23.

Thaker PH, Han LY, Kamat AA, Arevalo JM, Takahashi R, Lu C, Jennings NB, Armaiz-Pena G, Bankson JA, Ravoori M, et al. Chronic stress promotes tumor growth and angiogenesis in a mouse model of ovarian carcinoma. Nat Med. 2006;12:939–44.

Toda N, Toda M, Ayajiki K, Okamura T. Monkey central retinal artery is innervated by nitroxidergic vasodilator nerves. Invest Ophthalmol Vis Sci. 1996;37(11):2177–84.

Toris CB, Gleason ML, Camras CB, Yablonski ME. Effects of brimonidine on aqueous humor dynamics in human eyes. Arch Ophthalmol. 1995a;113(12):1514–7.

Toris CB, Tafoya ME, Camras CB, Yabloniski ME. Effects of apraclonidine on aqueous humor dynamics in human eyes. Ophthalmology. 1995b;102:456–61.

Vidal-Sanz M, Lafuente MP, Mayor S, de Imperial JM, Villegas-Pérez MP. Retinal ganglion cell death induced by retinal ischemia. neuroprotective effects of two alpha-2 agonists. Surv Ophthalmol. 2001;45 Suppl 3:S261–7; discussion S273–6.

Vogt M. Obituary. Sir Henry Hallett Dale, O.M., F.R.S. Int J Neuropharmacol. 1969;8(2):83–4.

Wachler BSB, Krueger RR. Agreement and repeatability of infrared pupillometry and the comparison method. Ophthalmology. 1999;106:319–23.

Wandel T, Charap AD, Lewis RA, Partamian L, Cobb S, et al. Glaucoma treated with once-daily levobunolol. Am J Ophthalmol. 1986;101:298–304.

Wilhelm H, Wilhelm B. Clinical applications of pupillography. J Neuro Ophthalmol. 2003;23: 42–9.

Wood JP, Schmidt KG, Melena J, Chidlow G, Allmeier H, Osborne NN. The beta-adrenoceptor antagonists metipranolol and timolol are retinal neuroprotectants: comparison with betaxolol. Exp Eye Res. 2003;76(4):505–16.

Wright TM, Freedman SF. Exposure to topical apraclonidine in children with glaucoma. J Glaucoma. 2009;18(5):395-8.

Yüksel N, Güler C, Çaglar Y, Elibol O. Apraclonidine and clonidine: a comparison of efficacy and side effects in normal and ocular hypertensive volunteers. International Ophthalmology. 1992;16(4):337–42.

Zimmerman TJ, Kaufman HE. Timolol. A beta-adrenergic blocking agent for the treatment of glaucoma. Arch Ophthalmol. 1977;95(4):601–4.

Chapter 7
Ocular Hypotensives and Neuroprotectants in Glaucoma

Tanuj Dada, Parul Ichhpujani, Srinivasan Senthilkumari, and Alain Bron

Abstract Glaucoma is the leading cause of blindness in the world. It is an optic neuropathy disease associated with elevated intraocular pressure. Glaucoma encompass a group of various clinical presentations that share the same anatomical feature, a progressive loss of retinal ganglion cells (RGCs) superior to the age-related loss. This chapter deals about the pharmacology of conventional antiglaucoma drugs and newer drugs/pathways which are under investigation. Medical management of glaucoma has been discussed with the concept of reaching target intraocular pressure ("Target IOP") using pharmacological agents. Newer concept of neuroprotectants for the management of glaucoma has also been included in the deliberations.

T. Dada, MD
Professor, Department of Ophthalmology,
Dr. Rajendra Prasad Center for Ophthalmic Sciences,
All India Institute of Medical Sciences, New Delhi, India

P. Ichhpujani, MD
Glaucoma and Neuro-ophthalmology Services,
Department of Ophthalmology,
Government Medical College and Hospital, Chandigarh, India

S. Senthilkumari, PhD (✉)
Department of Ocular Pharmacology,
Aravind Medical Research Foundation (AMRF),
Madurai, Tamil Nadu, India
e-mail: ss_kumari@aravind.org

A. Bron, MD
Department of Ophthalmology, University Hospital, Dijon, France

T. Velpandian (ed.), *Pharmacology of Ocular Therapeutics*,
DOI 10.1007/978-3-319-25498-2_7

7.1 Pharmacological agents in the medical management of glaucoma

7.1.1 Background

The glaucomas encompass a group of various clinical presentations that share the same anatomical feature, a progressive loss of retinal ganglion cells (RGCs) superior to the age-related loss. Glaucoma is still the first cause of irreversible blindness worldwide, and it has been estimated recently that the number of glaucoma cases will be 76 million in 2020 and about 112 million in 2040. Glaucoma is the second leading cause of blindness in the world. Primary open-angle glaucoma (POAG) is the most predominant form of glaucoma worldwide, accounting for 74 % of those affected (Kingman 2004). POAG is characterized by progressive retinal ganglion cell loss, optic nerve damage, and visual field loss leading to bilateral blindness in about 10 % of untreated individuals. Aqueous humor is a clear fluid which is secreted by the ciliary epithelium in the posterior chamber and travels to the anterior chamber wherein it nourishes the avascular tissues like the cornea and lens and drains into the episcleral vein through the trabecular meshwork (TM) (Fig. 7.1). Pharmacological management of glaucoma is achieved by either decreasing the aqueous production or by facilitating the aqueous outflow. Drugs with their target, mechanism of action in reducing IOP are shown in the Table 7.1. The goal of treatment of all patients with glaucoma and those suspected of having glaucoma is the same, specifically enhancing their quality of life, helping them celebrate life, and allowing them to be as healthy as they can.

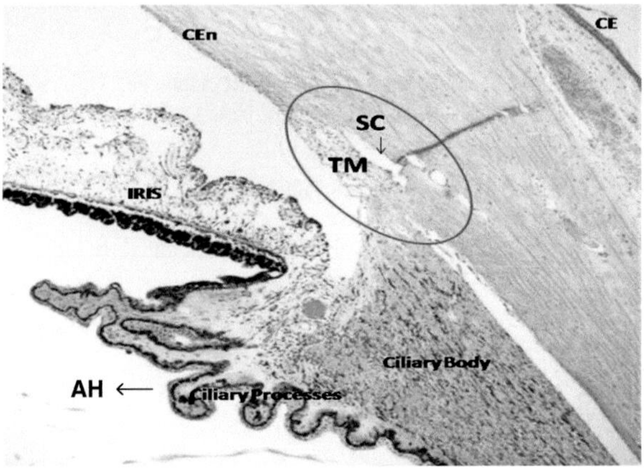

Fig. 7.1 Aqueous humor (AH) outflow pathway (*abbreviation*: *CE* corneal epithelium, *CEn* corneal endothelium, *SC* Schlemm's canal, *TM* trabecular meshwork)

Table 7.1 Classification of drugs, their target, and expected pharmacological effect used for the treatment of glaucoma

	Classification	Target	Pharmacological effect	Drugs
1.	*Beta-blockers*			
		β-1, β-2 blocker	Reduces aqueous humor (AH) production	Timolol, levobunolol, carteolol, and metoprolol
		β-1 selective blocker	Reduces AH production	Betaxolol
2.	*Alpha agonists*			
		α-1 receptor	Vasoconstriction-induced reduction in AH or enhanced outflow	Epinephrine and dipivefrin
		α-2 receptor (pre- and postsynaptic stimulation)	Decrease in sympathetic outflow and stimulation of Gi-mediated reduction of cAMP → decreased AH	Apraclonidine, brimonidine
3.	*Parasympathomimetics*			
		M_3 receptors	Facilitates aqueous outflow by producing traction on scleral spur or trabecular meshwork	Pilocarpine and carbachol
		Inhibition of cholinesterase	Indirectly facilitates stimulation of M_3	Echothiophate and physostigmine
4.	*Prostaglandin analogs*			
		Prostanoid FP receptor	Facilitates uveoscleral outflow	Latanoprost, bimatoprost, travoprost, tafluprost, and unoprostone
5.	*Carbonic anhydrase inhibitors*			
	Systemic	Carbonic anhydrase isoenzymes (II, IV, and XII) inhibition	Reduces the fluid transport by inhibiting bicarbonate ions	Acetazolamide, methazolamide, and dichlorphenamide
	Topical	Inhibition of carbonic anhydrase (higher affinity for type II)	Reduces the fluid transport by inhibiting bicarbonate ions	Dorzolamide and brinzolamide
6.	*Osmotic agents*			
		Plasma osmotic pressure	Increased osmotic pressure in plasma leading to shifting of water from eye → decreased IOP	Mannitol, glycerol

7.1.2 Concept of "Target IOP"

The concept of target intraocular pressure (IOP) arises from the fact that progression in advanced glaucoma, and occasionally in early glaucoma, may occur even at what is thought to be a "normal" intraocular pressure. The erstwhile magic figure of 21 mmHg or lower may not be low enough for many glaucomatous eyes to halt the progressive field damage.

Target IOP is defined as "*a range of acceptable IOP levels within which the progression of glaucomatous neuropathy will be halted /retarded.*" It is the specific level of pressure that, if achieved, will possibly prevent further optic nerve damage and is the IOP where the rate of loss of ganglion cell will equal the age-induced loss (Heijl et al. 2002; Feiner and Piltz-Seymour 2003; Hodapp et al. 1993; Jampel 1997). Further, this concept acknowledges that there may be pressure-independent factors, including aging, which may be superimposed upon the pressure-related process of glaucoma progression. This definition does not suggest that lowering IOP will completely halt progression of glaucomatous disease.

It can also be defined as the IOP at which the sum of the health-related quality of life (HRQ_OL) from preserved vision and the HRQ_OL from not having side effects from treatment is maximized.

7.1.3 Factors Influencing Target IOP

The target IOP is dependent on (Lichter et al. 2001):

(a) IOP level before treatment (the lower the untreated IOP levels, the lower the target IOP should be)
(b) Stage of glaucoma (the greater the preexisting glaucoma damage, the lower the target IOP should be)
(c) Rate of progression during follow-up
(d) Age and life expectancy (younger age requires lower target IOP)
(e) Presence of other risk factors, e.g., exfoliation syndrome
(f) Family history
(g) Systemic diseases (diabetes, HT, CAD, CVD)

The initial target pressure is an estimate toward the ultimate goal of protecting the optic nerve. The target pressure is different among patients, and even in the same patient it may require recalculation in the course of the disease.

When initiating therapy, it is assumed that the measured pretreatment pressure range resulted in optic nerve damage; so, the initial target pressure selected is at least 20 % lower than the pretreatment IOP

7.1.4 Setting Up Specific Target

The specific target IOP can be set by classifying the disease based on the severity of glaucomatous damage as follows:

Mild Glaucomatous optic nerve abnormalities with normal visual fields

- For 20 % IOP reduction from baseline values, keep IOP <18 mmHg.

Moderate Visual field abnormalities in one hemifield but not within 5° of fixation

- For 30 % IOP reduction, set IOP below 15 mmHg.

Severe Visual field abnormalities in either hemifield or field loss within 5° of fixation

- For 50 % IOP reduction, set IOP below 13 mmHg

In addition to setting the target IOP, it is important to keep watch on the *diurnal fluctuation of IOP*. The maximum IOP should always be kept below 18 mmHg at all follow-up visits (AGIS study data), and the fluctuation of IOP (both diurnal and long-term variations) should be below 4 mmHg.

The adequacy of the target IOP needs to be periodically reassessed by comparing optic nerve status (quantitative assessments of the disc and nerve fiber layer and visual field tests) with previous examinations. If progression occurs at the set target pressure, the target IOP should be lowered (Heijl et al. 2002; Feiner and Piltz-Seymour 2003; Hodapp et al. 1993; Jampel 1997; Lichter et al. 2001; AAO Glaucoma 2004–2005). The target IOP is just a guideline; it is better to use a range rather than a single number. Using a range of IOP prevents unnecessary aggressive therapy.

7.1.5 Medical Therapy

The ideal antiglaucoma medication is one that is effective, has minimal side effects, is cost-effective, and is easy to comply with.

Before we proceed further, it's important to understand that a *first-choice agent* is the drug chosen on medical grounds, whereas a *first-line agent* is selected on nonmedical (usually cost) grounds.

There are six classes of topical hypotensive medication: hypotensive lipids (prostaglandin analogues), beta-blockers, selective (alpha 2)-adrenergic agonists, carbonic anhydrase inhibitors (CAIs), cholinergics, and hyperosmotics (Table 7.1). Refer Chapter 6 for the detailed pharmacology of drugs acting through autonomic receptors.

7.1.5.1 Hypotensive Lipids

Hypotensive lipids fall into three subcategories: prostaglandin analogues (PGAs) which include latanoprost (Xalatan 0.005 %) and travoprost (Travatan and Travatan Z, both 0.004 %; Izba which is travoprost 0.003 %), prostamide which includes bimatoprost (Lumigan 0.03 % and 0.01 %), and the deconsanoid class which is represented by unoprostone isopropyl (Rescula 0.15 %). They are all derivatives of prostaglandin F2 alpha, based on pioneering work by Bito, Stjernschantz, and Camras (Bito 2001; Camras et al. 1989).

PGAs increase both trabecular meshwork and uveoscleral outflow (Lim et al. 2008) and are less affected by circadian variations in aqueous production than the beta-blockers (Walters et al. 2004). Although these drugs have dual mechanism of action, most of the increased outflow facility can be attributed to their effects on the pressure-independent uveoscleral outflow pathway.

Variations in the PGF2 alpha molecule result in changes in potency and side effects. Latanoprost was the first one to be developed commercially (by Pharmacia, now Pfizer). In order to reduce the hyperemia associated with PGF2 alpha, the unsaturated (double) bond between carbons 13 and 14 was saturated. This resulted in some loss of potency, but by reducing hyperemia made the drug cosmetically acceptable to patients. Because there is no major clinical difference in IOP-lowering efficacy whether this class of drugs is dosed daytime or nighttime, it has become customary to prescribe them at bedtime, so that the majority of the immediate hyperemia associated with drug dosing occurs while the patient is asleep. These drugs do have some "chronic" hyperemia that tends to subside over several months of use. Occasionally patients prefer morning dosing, which is acceptable from an efficacy perspective. Clinical IOP-lowering efficacy is better with OD dosing rather than BID dosing (Alm and Stjernschantz 1995). Systemic half-life of the drugs is brief (e.g., latanoprost 17 min). There is little effect of the drugs on the IOP of the contralateral eye when dosed unilaterally (Sjoquist and Stjernschantz 2002).

To improve efficacy, Alcon Laboratories modified the PGF2 alpha molecule to create travoprost by adding a CF3 on the unsaturated benzene ring. This allows for a tighter bonding of the travoprost free acid to the FP receptors (Sharif et al. 2003). This results in a longer-duration, clinically useful, IOP-lowering effect of both original travoprost and the BAK-free version, Travatan Z (Gross et al. 2008). This could be important in patients who occasionally miss doses.

Most of the hyperemia associated with the HLs results from dilated conjunctival vessels in response to direct activation of FP receptors found in the vasculature muscle walls. Bimatoprost has a six- to eightfold greater concentration than other hypotensive lipids. This may be related to the clinical observation that bimatoprost causes more red eye than the other two products (Stewart et al. 2003).

The three hypotensive lipids lower IOP on average between 25 and 30 %. These drugs have relatively flat IOP curves over 24 h, demonstrating both low circadian IOP fluctuation and, unlike the beta-blockers, effective diurnal and nocturnal IOP control (Konstas et al. 2005). They do not evidence short-term escape or long-term drift (Goldberg 2001; Cohen et al. 2004; Bayer et al. 2004).

Latanoprost is subject to deterioration when exposed to heat over 100 °F for longer than 8 days (Xalatan package insert, Pfizer, NY). The other hypotensive lipids seem to be somewhat more stable at temperatures likely to be found in most natural settings. All agents may deteriorate at an accelerated pace when exposed to direct sunlight.

7.1.5.2 Beta-Blockers

Topical beta-blockers were considered the gold standard initial treatment for open-angle glaucoma for nearly two decades, from 1978 to 1996, when the first prostaglandin analogue was granted approval by the FDA. Hypotensive lipids (prostaglandin analogues) are more potent IOP-lowering drugs than timolol and other beta-blockers. However, this fact does not mean that beta-blockers cannot be used as a first-line agent. This class of medication still remains efficacious, tolerated, and cost-effective.

Beta-blockers antagonize beta 1 and beta 2 receptors in the ciliary body's nonpigmented epithelium and thereby reduce secretion of the aqueous humor through an incompletely understood mechanism, which in turn lowers IOP. Action on the ciliary microvasculature may reduce the ultrafiltration component of aqueous secretion.

One drop of timolol maleate 0.25 or 0.50 % has its peak effect, 2 h following administration, and may last for 24 h. Some residual effect of timolol on IOP may be detected for as long as 2–3 weeks, and beta blockade can be detected up to 1 month after discontinuation of the drug.

Nonselective beta-blockers lower IOP 20–30 %. However, IOP reduction may be as high as 50 % and last greater than 24 h in some individuals. In up to 20 % of cases, the initial IOP reduction can be lost within 2–3 weeks. This has been called *short-term escape* and most likely reflects an upregulation in the number of ocular beta receptors after initial complete blockade (Boger 1983). For this reason, it is recommended to wait at least 4 weeks following initiation of therapy before assessing IOP effect.

Beta-blocker treatment can maintain control of IOP for years. However, in some patients IOP control may be lost after many years of therapy or even within 3 months (Gieser et al. 1996). This phenomenon is called *long-term drift* and may be the result of drug tolerance or progression of the trabecular meshwork outflow problems.

Selective beta 1 blockers are less potent at reducing IOP than their nonselective counterparts, which can make them less attractive in patients who need a bigger IOP reduction.

The advantage of selective beta 1 blockers is that they have less effect on the beta 2 receptors found predominantly in the pulmonary system, making them more tolerable in patients with the potential for bronchospasm. Among nonselective beta-blockers, there are no differences in terms of IOP-lowering efficacy.

Patients under treatment with systemic beta-blockers may experience a reduced effect of topical administration and increased side effects (Allingham et al. 2005).

There are ocular, cardiovascular, pulmonary, metabolic, and central nervous system side effects. In general, beta-blockers are well tolerated when applied topically; however, there are reports of ocular discomfort due to burning, hyperemia, toxic keratopathy, punctate keratopathy, periocular contact dermatitis, and dry eye (Dunham et al. 1994).

Chronic administration of benzalkonium chloride (BAK) used as preservative in most beta-blocker solutions may play a role in ocular toxicity. The use of preservative-free timolol may help identify preservative as the source of local side effects. Timolol is available as a solution and in a gel-forming preparation. Gel-forming preparations allow longer permanence on the ocular surface for a sustained effect, and the once-daily administration can lead to fewer side effects. Gel-forming solution is also less likely to reach the nasolacrimal duct, lessening the potential for systemic side effects.

Beta-blockers are absorbed via the nasolacrimal system by the nasal and oral mucosa, thus bypassing the first-pass effect in the liver (Sharif et al. 2003). Direct access to the blood stream explains many systemic side effects and contralateral IOP lowering. Systemic side effects must be thoroughly searched for by a careful medical history since patients often overlook their eyedrops as a potential cause of systemic symptoms.

Beta 1 receptor blockade lowers blood pressure and heart rate, which can cause severe bradycardia, especially in patients with advanced age or underlying medical conditions, such as greater than first-degree heart block (a contraindication for the use of beta-blockers). They also cause decrease myocardial contractility, which is a relative contraindication for beta-blockers in patients affected by heart insufficiency. Exercise-induced tachycardia may be blocked in healthy individuals.

Beta-2 receptor blockade may cause severe asthma attacks. Nonselective beta-blockers are contraindicated in asthmatic patients. They also may exacerbate airway disease in a previously controlled asthma patient or trigger airway disease in a previously undetected or asymptomatic patient. Betaxolol, a beta 1-receptor blocker, has been successfully used in patients with pulmonary disease, but it is not entirely free of potential side effects (Fechtner 1999). A trial of once-daily dosing at the lowest available concentration of an agent (preferably in one eye) would be a good way to start. Only then, if indicated, should the frequency and concentration be increased.

Beta-blockers have been observed to alter the blood lipid profile negatively and could increase the risk of coronary heart disease. They may also mask the symptoms of hypoglycemia, such as tachycardia, in diabetics.

Central nervous system side effects are often subjective in nature and rarely attributed to eyedrops by patients. It is prudent to directly question patients about symptoms of fatigue, lethargy, confusion, memory loss, sleep disturbance, and dizziness. If present, a lower dosage of beta-blocker or replacement with another class of drug should be discussed.

7.1.5.3 Alpha Agonists

The selective alpha-agonist agents used to treat glaucoma are modifications of the clonidine molecule (similar to the development of the hypotensive lipids that were derived from PGF2 alpha).

Two topical alpha-adrenergic agonists are available for glaucoma therapy, apraclonidine which is relatively nonselective for alpha 1 and alpha 2 receptors and brimonidine (Alphagan and generic) that is more selective for alpha 2 than alpha 1 receptors. These drugs work by preventing the release of norepinephrine at presynaptic terminals. They both decrease aqueous production, and they may have some effect on episcleral venous pressure as well as uveoscleral outflow (Reitsamer et al. 2006; Toris et al. 1999). Brimonidine may also affect conventional outflow in a positive manner. These drugs lower IOP between 20 and 25 %.

Apraclonidine (a) does not lower IOP in about 1/3 of patients, (b) has extreme tachyphylaxis (loss of effect) within about 90 days in about 1/3 of patients, and finally (c) causes blepharoconjunctivitis with red eyes, conjunctival follicles, pruritus, and periorbital dermatitis in about 1/3 of patients. Pupil dilation and lid retraction may also occur in a significant fraction of patients (Yuksel et al. 1992).

The newer lower concentrations of Alphagan-P, which contain the preservative purite instead of BAK, seem to be better tolerated, with a decreased incidence of allergy and almost as good intraocular pressure control as with the higher (0.2 %) concentration of the original drug (Whitson et al. 2006).

The pharmacokinetics of topically administered brimonidine requires that it be dosed three times per day, similar to the topical CAIs.

Brimonidine must be used with caution in neonates, young children, and the frail and elderly. With very young patients, brimonidine has resulted in apnea and coma (Mungan et al. 2003). Brimonidine can cause fatigue in elderly. Patients should specifically be queried about the presence of this important side effect. In these groups of patients, the drug seems to cross the blood–brain barrier in sufficient concentration to cause these severe side effects.

Alpha-adrenergic agonists should not be used in patients taking monoamine oxidase inhibitors (MAOIs) because they may precipitate a hypertensive crisis. They are also contraindicated in patients taking tricyclic antidepressants because of an increased risk of central nervous system (CNS)-mediated depression (Schuman 2002). These drugs cause symptoms of dry mouth (and dry nose) when drained through the nasolacrimal duct into the throat.

7.1.5.4 Carbonic Anhydrase Inhibitors (CAIs)

There are at least 14 known varieties of the alpha-carbonic anhydrases (a-CA) whose main function is the hydration of CO2 to bicarbonate (HCO–). Two of these enzymes are important for the production of the aqueous humor by the epithelium of the ciliary processes, cytoplasmic CA II and membrane-bound CA IV (Matsui et al. 1996). Part of aqueous production involving active secretion relies on the formation of bicarbonate by these enzymes to correct the imbalance caused by the ATPase-fueled transport of sodium into the space between the nonpigmented ciliary epithelial cells.

Patients should be specifically asked about breathing difficulties and skin reactions (Turtz and Turtz 1958), which are the most common form of allergic manifestations to sulfonamide antibiotics.

CAIs can be used topically or systemically. Topical CAIs are remarkably free from side effect and effective. They are the most effective class to use in combination with a prostaglandin analogue (Scozzafava and Supuran 2014). Systemic CAIs are also effective, but should be used with full knowledge of the frequency and severity of their side effects.

Topical CAIs

Approximately 80 % of the volume of topically administered eyedrops is absorbed systemically within 15–30 s of instillation. Topical dorzolamide is absorbed through the nasopharyngeal mucosa into the systemic circulation. Chronic administration of dorzolamide leads to its accumulation in erythrocytes. Hepatic metabolism of dorzolamide produces N-desmethyl metabolite which also binds to red blood cells but inhibits carbonic anhydrase I more than carbonic anhydrase II. Approximately 24–32 % of systemically absorbed dorzolamide is bound to plasma proteins. Urine is the major route of excretion for both parent and metabolite drugs. There is a rapid decline of dorzolamide from red blood cells, on discontinuation of the medication. This is followed by a gradual decline due to an elimination-phase half-life of approximately 4 months.

Brinzolamide 0.1 % (Azopt, Alcon Laboratories) is a suspension that allows buffering to a more neutral pH compared with dorzolamide. This seems to improve tolerance of the topical medication.

In 2013, Simbrinza (Alcon), a beta-blocker-free, fixed-combination therapy, was approved by the FDA. It combines brinzolamide 0.1 % and brimonidine tartrate 0.2 %.

CAIs have been reported to improve ocular blood flow profile by causing ocular vasodilation through metabolic acidosis via elevated carbon dioxide levels (Siesky et al. 2008).

Oral CAIs

Oral CAIs are powerful agents for lowering IOP (between 25 and 30 %) (Friedland et al. 1977) and may do very well when other medical therapies are unable to reach the target IOP in chronic glaucomas or to temporarily bring IOP to safe levels in acute emergent situations.

Paresthesias of the fingers, toes, and nose are common with oral CAIs, less so with methazolamide at lower doses. Paresthesias may diminish over time. Patients are less likely to be concerned about these symptoms if they are discussed before the drugs are prescribed.

Patients may suffer from abdominal cramps, nausea, and in some cases severe diarrhea. Symptoms may improve as time passes, but some patients need to discontinue oral CAIs because of the gastrointestinal intolerance. The oral CAIs cause a strange metallic taste with foods and carbonated beverages – patients should be warned this is likely to occur.

Patients taking oral CAIs, usually after several months, can have an unexpected onset of a malaise-syndrome complex involving (to varying degrees) tiredness, lack of appetite (with/without weight loss), and even severe depression (Alward 1998).

Salicylates interact with oral CAIs. Patients taking high-dose aspirin can get tinnitus, increased respiratory rate, and even confusion and coma (Sweeney et al. 1986).

CAIs in the kidney promote the absorption of bicarbonate through the renal tubules. CAIs cause alkalinization of the urine along with increased micturition, both day and night, and potassium excretion. Patients prescribed with chronic oral CAIs should have their electrolytes monitored, especially if taking other potassium-wasting drugs such as thiazide diuretics and oral corticosteroids (Bateson and Lant 1973).

One important feature of both topical and oral CAIs is that they work to suppress the aqueous and lower IOP throughout the 24-h day, both in the diurnal and nocturnal time periods.

The topical CAIs lower IOP about 20 % (similar to betaxolol) and the oral CAIs closer to 30 %. Further, patients receiving a full dose of oral CAIs are unlikely to see any additional pressure lowering by also using topical dorzolamide or brinzolamide.

Acetazolamide is the most commonly used and is supplied in 125- or 250-mg tablets or 500-mg sustained-release capsules. It may be dosed up to 250 mg four times daily or 500-mg SR capsules twice a day. CAIs are not the first-line choices for treatment, despite impressive IOP-lowering effects, due to their numerous adverse effects.

The use of oral CAIs is contraindicated in patients with a history of kidney stones or other renal disease, liver disease, cardiac disease, Addison's disease, and severe chronic obstructive pulmonary disease and in patients with sulfonamide allergy out of concern for sulfa cross-reactivity.

7.1.5.5 Miotics

The parasympathomimetic medications are the oldest form of eyedrops used to treat glaucoma. Since they all act on the iris sphincter muscle to make the pupil smaller, we shall use the simpler name "miotics" when referring to these agents. The miotics are subdivided into two classes based on mechanism of action, the *direct*-acting cholinergic agents like pilocarpine and carbachol and the *indirect*-acting anticholinesterase agents like echothiophate iodide.

Only ocular cholinergic agent used for therapeutic purpose these days is pilocarpine. It is available at 1–4 % solution for clinical use as nitrate or hydrochloride salt.

Pilocarpine lowers the IOP by constricting the ciliary body muscles that are connected to the scleral spur to open the trabecular meshwork mechanically and increase the outflow of the aqueous humor through the conventional drainage pathways. It has been demonstrated by Worthen that pilocarpine treatment reduces the diurnal variation of IOP of patients with glaucoma as well as lowers the mean IOP (Worthen 1976).

Pilocarpine penetrates the cornea well (Quigley and Pollack 1977). While the kinetics and distribution of pilocarpine within the eye have been studied, the exact mode by which the drug metabolizes is not fully understood. Enzymatic hydrolysis of pilocarpine, which occurs in the serum and liver, may not be an important factor in the eye. The relatively prolonged action of pilocarpine may be related to storage of the drug in ocular tissues. Van Hoose and Leaders have suggested that pilocarpine may be stored within the cornea, which may then serve as a drug reservoir (Van Hoose and Leaders 1974).

According to traditional teaching, pilocarpine needs to be instilled four times a day as its duration of action is 6 h, but a study has shown that even pilocarpine 2 % administered twice daily can lower IOP effectively in many patients with glaucoma.

Local side effects of these miotic agents include miosis, increased lacrimation, induced accommodation, and browache (Zimmerman and Wheeler 1982). Induced near accommodation (myopia) is particularly troublesome to young, phakic patients, especially with the waxing and waning of accommodation every 4–6 h given the normal QID dosing of drugs like pilocarpine. But miotics work fine in pseudophakes. Miotic agents can disrupt the blood–brain barrier and should not be used chronically in patients with ocular inflammation.

Although pilocarpine may be helpful for breaking an acute attack of angle-closure glaucoma, by causing miosis and pulling the mid-dilated pupil away from the lens it is blocking, stronger concentrations of pilocarpine may aggravate rather than help papillary block. The 4 % concentration of pilocarpine may move the lens–iris diaphragm too far forward.

It is better to use no more than 2 % pilocarpine when treating a patient with acute angle closure and pupillary block. Further, if IOP is over about 40 mmHg, the iris sphincter muscle is ischemic and hence cannot contract in response to pilocarpine. Thus, there is little benefit of this agent until the pressure can be reduced by topical beta-blockers, brimonidine, topical CAIs, oral CAIs, oral hyperosmotics, or emergent paracentesis.

Chronic use of any of the miotics may lead to the formation of posterior synechiae, leading in rare cases to an occluded pupil. Highly myopic patients may suffer retinal tears or detachments with the stronger concentrations of miotic agents (Pape and Forbes 1978).

Systemic side effects of the parasympathomimetic agents include crampy gastrointestinal upset, diarrhea, increased salivation, and increased secretion of stomach acid.

Because cholinesterase activity is suppressed by the indirect-acting miotics, succinylcholine should not be administered to patients undergoing anesthesia until at least 6 weeks after ceasing these glaucoma drugs (Eilderton et al. 1968). Today, miotic agents for glaucoma are used more as the exception (boutique use) rather than as the rule. They may be helpful in select patients when no other combination of medications can bring the patients' disease under control.

7.1.5.6 Hyperosmotic Agents

Hyperosmotic agents are generally used for short-term IOP control in emergency situations where other medications are unable to lower the IOP (Singh 2005). Intravenous (IV) mannitol and oral glycerins (or glycerol) are the most commonly used hyperosmotic agents. Both agents penetrate the blood–ocular barrier poorly, which is a definite advantage, since this fact creates a larger osmotic gradient for water to follow.

Mannitol

Mannitol can be given either as an IV infusion using a 20 % premixed solution (concentration of 200 mg/ml) at a dose of 1–2 g/kg of body weight.

Because of the limited solubility, storage at room temperature (25 °C) is recommended. Mannitol solutions commonly crystallize at low temperatures. If crystallization occurs, the solution should be warmed prior to use. Mannitol should not be administered if crystals are present.

Mannitol should be administered intravenously over 30–60 min. Too rapid an infusion of mannitol will cause a shift of intracellular water into the extracellular space, resulting in cellular dehydration with a high risk of hyponatremia, congestive heart failure, and pulmonary edema. Slow administration, over at least 20–30 min, may also avoid transient increases in cerebral blood flow that may exacerbate or increase intracranial bleeding in predisposed patients. Doses in excess of 200 g IV mannitol/day have been associated with acute renal failure.

Glycerin (or Glycerol)

Glycerol is usually used as a 50 % oral solution at a dose of 1–1.5 g/kg of body weight (McCurdy et al. 1966). Because of its unpleasantly sweet taste, it is often given with juice or over ice. The onset of effect can occur within 10 min, with a peak effect at approximately 1 h. The duration of action is 4–5 h. In elderly patients, the minimum dose (e.g., 1 g/kg) required to produce the desired effect should be used to avoid serious side effects.

Because hyperosmotic agents increase the extracellular space, they may precipitate pulmonary edema and cardiac failure in patients with compromised cardiac function.

7.2 Concept of Neuroprotection in Glaucoma

As glaucoma is characterized by a progressive optic neuropathy, it seems logical to try to find the "holy grail of neuroprotection" as do the neurologists for the neurodegenerative diseases of the brain and the nerves (Danesh-Meyer and Levin 2009; Chang and Goldberg 2012).

In our current management of glaucoma, we are only aiming to limit the impact of some risk factors that lead to the acceleration of RGC death. The most documented and most modifiable risk factor is IOP. Many studies in the last two decades have shown the effectiveness of decreasing IOP in several glaucoma types (Collaborative Normal-Tension Glaucoma study group 1998; AGIS 2000; Leske et al. 2003). Unfortunately some risk factors such as family history, aging, myopia, and ethnicity are not accessible to any treatment. Therefore it makes sense to concentrate on the final effect of these risk factors, namely, RGC loss (Osborne 2008).

Most of the attention of the researchers has been focused on neurons; however, neurons are strongly connected to their environment such as glia, vessels, and connective tissue, and all these components are potential targets for neuroprotection (Shih and Calkins 2012). Several pathogenic pathways are now clearly identified such as inflammation, immunity, neurotrophin deprivation, excitotoxicity, oxidative stress, mitochondrial dysfunction, etc. (Limb and Martin 2011).

There is a body of evidence to consider that neuroprotection in preclinical studies does work. Unfortunately we do not have a perfect animal model for glaucoma, and it is true that the models we are currently using do not mimic closely the human course of glaucoma (Quigley 2012). Therefore translational research from the lab to humans requires a lot of care and humility. More information on the pathogenesis of RGC death and preclinical studies can be found in several reviews (Baltmr et al. 2010; Osborne et al. 1999b). In this text we will only report two clinical trials in humans, one with a topical agent and one with a drug taken orally.

7.2.1 Brimonidine

Brimonidine has been evaluated as a neuroprotectant in three human clinical trials. In nonglaucomatous optic neuropathies, its efficacy was not demonstrated either in Leber hereditary optic neuropathy or in anterior ischemic optic neuropathy (Newman et al. 2005; Wilhelm et al. 2006).

The Low-Pressure Glaucoma Treatment Study (LoGTS), a multicenter double-masked randomized trial, evaluated the long-term visual field stability in patients with normal-tension glaucoma treated with brimonidine or timolol (Krupin et al. 2011). In the group treated with brimonidine, progression was less frequent than in the group receiving timolol. These results have been intensively discussed, and like in every clinical trial, some weaknesses were highlighted (Cordeiro and Levin 2011). Among the 178 analyzed patients, 9.1 % on brimonidine and 39.2 % on timolol progressed during a mean follow-up of 30 months. However many patients (20 %) discontinued the treatment in the brimonidine arm due to allergy, and the high rate of progressing patients on timolol could suggest that this beta-blocker is deleterious to retinal ganglion cells which has not been fully documented yet (Hare et al. 2004a, b). Anyway this study is probably the first trial showing a potential protective effect of a drug in a well-designed and conducted study.

7.2.2 *Memantine*

Memantine, an NMDA glutamate receptor antagonist, has shown some neuroprotective properties in laser-induced glaucoma in monkeys (Hare et al. 2004a, b; Reisberg et al. 2003). It was the first drug approved as a neuroprotective agent in moderate-to-severe Alzheimer's disease (Osborne 2009). Memantine, a widely available drug, has been evaluated in glaucoma patients, with a two parallel, double-masked, placebo-controlled three-armed phase III study. More than 1000 patients were recruited in 89 centers, and the primary end point progressive visual field loss was confirmed. There was a slower disease progression in patients receiving the higher memantine dose versus the lower dose and placebo. Unfortunately the results were never published in the scientific literature, and we are still wondering what can be taught from this study for the future (Osborne 2009; Sena and Lindsley 2010).

Neuroprotection is a fascinating area for research although a recent Cochrane review was not able to report any robust study showing the positive effect of a neuroprotective drug (Levin and Danesh-Meyer 2010). Researchers and companies have made tremendous efforts and spent a lot of money until now without practical and clinical results. Neville Osborne nicely defended the idea that although until now we have been disappointed by all the attempts to master and delay the degeneration of RGCs, it is not a good reason to abandon the fight against glaucoma-related blindness (Wang and Chang 2014). It is often taught in medical school that the first pioneer to operate cerebral tumors, Cushing, was faced with the death of his first ten patients. Hopefully for the future, he did not give up. So if we are not here yet with neuroprotection today, let's continue the fight against RGC degeneration, just keeping in mind that a major hurdle is the translation from basic research to clinical application (Wang and Chang 2014).

7.3 Newer Drug Classes

7.3.1 *Rho-Kinase and Glaucoma*

Rho-associated protein kinase (ROCK) plays an important physiological role in smooth muscle contraction and has been studied as a target for a variety of diseases. Substantial evidences with ex vivo, in vitro, and animal models showed that ROCK inhibition showed relaxation of tissues in the conventional outflow pathway and lower intraocular pressure and may represent a new treatment modality for POAG. Rho is a small GTPase that is involved in the regulation of many cell processes including contraction, cytoskeleton organization, adhesive interactions, trafficking, and permeability. Activation of the Rho/Rho-associated kinase (ROCK) pathway is activated via secreted bioactive molecules or via integrin activation after extracellular matrix binding. These lead to polymerization of actin stress fibers and formation of focal adhesions. This pathway has been demonstrated to increase the resistance to aqueous humor outflow through the trabecular meshwork pathway by inducing alterations in cell contraction, actomyosin assembly, cell adhesion, and ECM synthesis. Inhibition of ROCK pathway leads to decrease in flow resistance and increase in aqueous humor outflow and thus has a potential role in glaucoma therapy. The schematic representation for Rho-ROCK signaling is given below:

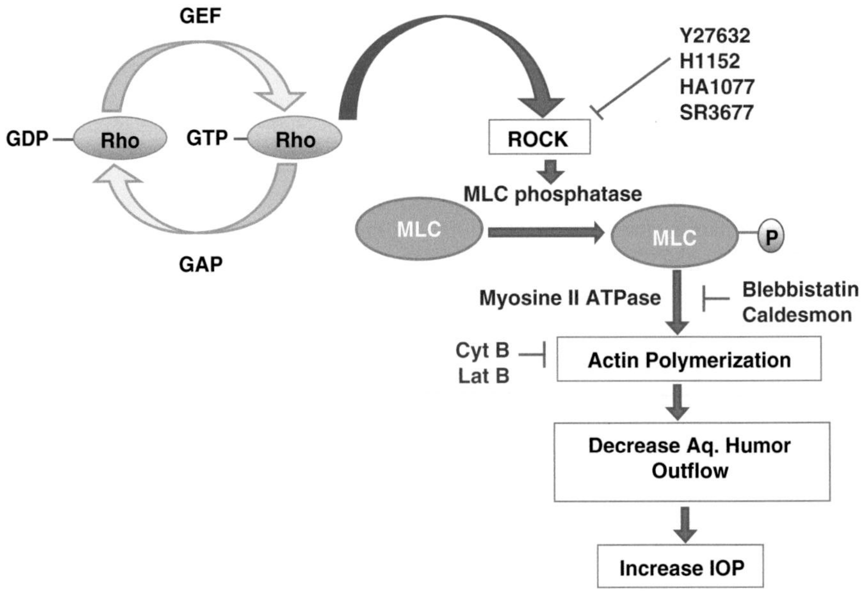

7.3.1.1 Rho-Kinase Inhibitors

Multiple studies have demonstrated that inhibition of ROCK and Rho GTPase would be an attractive strategy to increase aqueous humor drainage in TM tissues leading to reduction in IOP (Rao and Epstein 2007; Challa and Arnold 2014; Tanihara et al. 2008). These drugs reduce IOP by increasing aqueous humor outflow facility through actomyosin regulation. Several drugs have been developed over the past decade; however, only four drugs such as K-115, AR-13324, PG324, and AMA 0076 showed promising clinical efficacy in clinical trials. The only minor side effect with ROCK inhibitors is conjunctival hyperemia. On systemic level, ROCK inhibition is known to lower blood pressure and vascular resistance thus bearing potential consequences in case of unwanted systemic exposure (Hahmann and Schroeter 2010).

K-115: This compound is in the development by the Japanese company, Kowa Pharmaceuticals. In phase II randomized dose–response study, this compound lowered IOP by 3.1 mmHg 8 h after instillation which is comparable to prostaglandin analogues. This drug has now advanced to phase III trials, and it is anticipated that this drug will be used either as monotherapy or in combination with prostaglandins and beta-blockers. Conjunctival hyperemia, the most commonly reported adverse effect of ROCK inhibitors, occurred in 65.3% with the optimal dose.

ROCK inhibitors in the pipeline: Several Rho-kinase inhibitors are now in earlier stages of clinical testing.

AR-12286: Aerie Pharmaceuticals is developing a novel selective ROCK inhibitor which showed a statistically significant dose-dependent reduction in mean IOP with peak effects occurring 2–4 h after dosing in phase II trials with humans. The largest IOP reduction (−6.8 mmHg) was noted with 0.25 % w/v concentration of AR-12286 following twice-daily dosing. The 0.25 % w/v concentration produced trace to moderate conjunctival hyperemia that was transient and occurred in less than 10 % of patients with once-daily dosing.

The other compound of this series is **AR-13324** which is in phase IIb study in clinical trials. This molecule has been developed with a dual mechanism of action to lower IOP: one is to enhance the fluid outflow through trabecular pathway and the other is to decrease fluid inflow to the eye.

AMA0076: This compound has been developed by the Belgian company, Amakem Therapeutics, which showed to act on the trabecular meshwork where it relaxes the smooth muscle to widen the outflow channels. It has been designed to convert rapidly to inactive form to prevent off-target activity and reduce hyperemia.

7.3.2 *Nitric Oxide-Donating Latanoprost*

VESNEO™ (latanoprostene bunod; previously known as BOL-303259-X and NCX 116) is a novel nitric oxide-donating prostaglandin F2 alpha analogue licensed by Nicox to Bausch + Lomb. The pivotal phase 3 program includes two separate randomized, multicenter, double-masked, parallel-group clinical studies, APOLLO and LUNAR, designed to compare the efficacy and safety of VESNEO™ administered once daily (OD) against timolol maleate 0.5 % administered twice daily (BID) in lowering IOP in patients with open-angle glaucoma or ocular hypertension (Yang and Leffler 2013).

7.4 Newer Delivery Systems

Drug delivery systems currently being developed include conjunctival, subconjunctival, and intravitreal inserts, punctal plugs, and drug depots.

A hybrid dendrimer hydrogel/poly(lactic-co-glycolic acid) nanoparticle platform is being designed to release the drug slowly, and it is compatible with many of the currently used glaucoma drugs (Fulgencio et al. 2012).

A timolol maleate-loaded chitosan film has been recently found to be safe and efficient as an ocular drug delivery system in the treatment and prevention of glaucoma (Fulgencio et al. 2012). Chitosan is a cationic polysaccharide biopolymer with mucoadhesive properties.

Other alternatives used for extended drug release include particulate drug delivery systems or injectable formulations such as microspheres, liposomes, and nanospheres/nanoparticles (Manickavasagam and Oyewumi 2013). The drug is trapped in the nanocarrier matrix and delivered into the eye. After administration, the bioactive agent is released in a controlled fashion by diffusion through the matrix or by degradation of the polymer matrix. Additionally, once the nano/micro-carriers are injected, they can act as a reservoir system for drug release for a prolonged time period.

References

Kingman S. Glaucoma is second leading cause of blindness globally. Bull World Health Organ. 2004;82:887–8.

George R, Ve RS, Vijaya L. Glaucoma in India: estimated burden of disease. J Glaucoma. 2010;19:391–7.

Johnstone MA, Albert DM. Prostaglandin –induced hair growth. Surv Opthalmol. 2002;47 Suppl 1:S185–202.

Pfeiffer N, Thieme H. Prostaglandin analogues. In: Shaarawy T, Sherwood MB, Crowston JG, Hitchings RA, editors. Glaucoma-medical diagnosis and therapy. London. Elsveir Ltd; 2015. p. 543.

Tripathi KD. Essentials of Medical Pharmacology, New Delhi: Jaypee Brothers Medical Publishers. 2008 (5th ed), p.674.

Rao PV, Epstein DL. Rho GTPase/Rho kinase as a novel target for the treatment of glaucoma. BioDrugs. 2007;21:167–77.

Challa P, Arnold JJ. Rho-kinase inhibitors offer a new approach in the treatment of glaucoma. Expert Opin Investig Drugs. 2014;23(1):81–95.

Tanihara H, Inatani M, Honjo M, et al. Intraocular pressure-lowering effects and safety of topical administration of a selective ROCK inhibitor, SNJ-1656, in healthy volunteers. Arch Ophthalmol. 2008;126:309–15.

Hahmann C, Schroeter T. Rho-kinase inhibitors as therapeutics: from pan inhibition to isoform selectivity. Cell Mol Life Sci. 2010;67(2):171–7.

Heijl A, Leske MC, Bengtsson B, et al. Reduction of intraocular pressure and glaucoma progression: results from the early manifest glaucoma trial. Arch Ophthalmol. 2002;120:1268–79.

Feiner L, Piltz-Seymour JR. Collaborative Initial Glaucoma Treatment Study: a summary of results to date. Curr Opin Ophthalmol. 2003;14:106–11.

Hodapp E, Parrish 2nd RK, Anderson DR. Clinical decisions in glaucoma. St Louis: Mosby and Co; 1993. p. 63–92.

Jampel HD. Target pressure in glaucoma therapy. J Glaucoma. 1997;6:133–8.

Lichter PR, Musch DC, Gillespie BW, et al. Interim clinical outcomes in the Collaborative Initial Glaucoma Treatment Study comparing initial treatment randomized to medications or surgery. Ophthalmology. 2001;108:1943–53.

American academy of ophthalmology basic and clinical science course section 10. Glaucoma. 2004–2005.

Bito LZ. A new approach to the medical management of glaucoma, from the bench to the clinic, and beyond: the Proctor Lecture. Invest Ophthalmol Vis Sci. 2001;42(6):1126–33.

Camras CB, Siebold EC, Lustgarten JS, et al. Maintained reduction of intraocular pressure by prostaglandin F2 alpha-1-isopropyl ester applied in multiple doses in ocular hypertensive and glaucoma patients. Ophthalmology. 1989;96(9):1329–36; discussion 1336–27.

Lim KS, Nau CB, O'Byrne MM, et al. Mechanism of action of bimatoprost, latanoprost, and travoprost in healthy subjects. A crossover study. Ophthalmology. 2008;115(5):790–5 e794.

Walters TR, DuBiner HB, Carpenter SP, Khan B, VanDenburgh AM. 24-hour IOP control with once-daily bimatoprost, timolol gel-forming solution, or latanoprost: a 1-month, randomized, comparative clinical trial. Surv Ophthalmol. 2004;49 Suppl 1:S26–35.

Alm A, Stjernschantz J. Effects on intraocular pressure and side effects of 0.005% latanoprost applied once daily, evening or morning. A comparison with timolol. Scandinavian Latanoprost Study Group. Ophthalmology. 1995;102(12):1743–52.

Sjoquist B, Stjernschantz J. Ocular and systemic pharmacokinetics of latanoprost in humans. Surv Ophthalmol. 2002;47 Suppl 1:S6–12.

Sharif NA, Kelly CR, Crider JY, Williams GW, Xu SX. Ocular hypotensive FP prostaglandin (PG) analogs: PG receptor subtype binding affinities and selectivities, and agonist potencies at FP and other PG receptors in cultured cells. J Ocul Pharmacol Ther. 2003;19(6):501–15.

Gross RL, Peace JH, Smith SE, et al. Duration of IOP reduction with travoprost BAK-free solution. J Glaucoma. 2008;17(3):217–22.

Stewart WC, Kolker AE, Stewart JA, Leech J, Jackson AL. Conjunctival hyperemia in healthy subjects after short-term dosing with latanoprost, bimatoprost, and travoprost. Am J Ophthalmol. 2003;135(3):314–20.

Konstas AG, Katsimbris JM, Lallos N, Boukaras GP, Jenkins JN, Stewart WC. Latanoprost 0.005% versus bimatoprost 0.03% in primary open-angle glaucoma patients. Ophthalmology. 2005; 112(2):262–6.

Goldberg I. Comparison of tropical travoprost eye drops given once daily and timolol 0.5% given twice daily in patients with open-angle glaucoma or ocular hypertension. J Glaucoma. 2001; 10:414–22.

Cohen JS, Gross RL, Cheetham JK, VanDenburgh AM, Bernstein P, Whitcup SM. Two-year double-masked comparison of bimatoprost with timolol in patients with glaucoma or ocular hypertension. Surv Ophthalmol. 2004;49 Suppl 1:S45–52.

Bayer A, Weiler W, Oeverhaus U, Skrotzki FE, Stewart WC. Two year follow-up of latanoprost 0.005% monotherapy after changing from previous glaucoma therapies. J Ocul Pharmacol Ther. 2004;20(6):470–8.

Boger III WP. Short term "escape" and long term "drift": the dissipation effects of the beta adrenergic agents. Surv Ophthalmol. 1983;28(Suppl):235–42.

Gieser SC, Juzych M, Robin AL, et al. Clinical pharmacology of adrenergic drugs. In: Ritch R, Shields MB, Krupin T, editors. The glaucomas. St. Louis: Mosby; 1996.

Allingham RR, Damji K, Freedman S, et al. Adrenergic receptor antagonists. In: Shield's textbook of glaucoma. Philadelphia: Lippincott Williams and Wilkins; 2005.

Dunham CN, Spaide RF, Dunham G. The contralateral reduction of intraocular pressure by timolol. Br J Ophthalmol. 1994;78:38–40.

Fechtner RD. Beta blockers. In: Netland PA, Allen RC, editors. Glaucoma medical therapy principles and management. San Francisco: The Foundation of the American Academy of Ophthalmology; 1999.

Reitsamer HA, Posey M, Kiel JW. Effects of a topical alpha2 adrenergic agonist on ciliary blood flow and aqueous production in rabbits. Exp Eye Res. 2006;82(3):405–15.

Toris CB, Camras CB, Yablonski ME. Acute versus chronic effects of brimonidine on aqueous humor dynamics in ocular hypertensive patients. Am J Ophthalmol. 1999;128(1):8–14.

Yuksel N, Guler C, Caglar Y, Elibol O. Apraclonidine and clonidine: a comparison of efficacy and side effects in normal and ocular hypertensive volunteers. Int Ophthalmol. 1992;16(4–5): 337–42.

Whitson JT, Ochsner KI, Moster MR, et al. The safety and intraocular pressure-lowering efficacy of brimonidine tartrate 0.15% preserved with polyquaternium-1. Ophthalmology. 2006;113(8): 1333–9.

Mungan NK, Wilson TW, Nischal KK, Koren G, Levin AV. Hypotension and bradycardia in infants after the use of topical brimonidine and beta-blockers. J AAPOS. 2003;7(1):69–70.

Schuman JS. Short- and long-term safety of glaucoma drugs. Expert Opin Drug Saf. 2002; 1(2):181–94.

Matsui H, Murakami M, Wynns GC, et al. Membrane carbonic anhydrase (IV) and ciliary epithelium. Carbonic anhydrase activity is present in the basolateral membranes of the non-pigmented ciliary epithelium of rabbit eyes. Exp Eye Res. 1996;62(4):409–17.
Turtz CA, Turtz AI. Toxicity due to acetazolamide (diamox). AMA Arch Ophthalmol. 1958;60(1):130–1.
Michaud JE, Friren B, International Brinzolamide Adjunctive Study Group. Comparison of topical brinzolamide 1% and dorzolamide 2% eye drops given twice daily in addition to timolol 0.5% in patients with primary open-angle glaucoma or ocular hypertension. Am J Ophthalmol. 2001;132(2):235–43.
Siesky B, Harris A, Cantor LB, et al. A comparative study of the effects of brinzolamide and dorzolamide on retinal oxygen saturation and ocular microcirculation in patients with primary open-angle glaucoma. Br J Ophthalmol. 2008;92(4):500–4.
Friedland BR, Mallonee J, Anderson DR. Short-term dose response characteristics of acetazolamide in man. Arch Ophthalmol. 1977;95(10):1809–12.
Alward WL. Medical management of glaucoma. N Engl J Med. 1998;339(18):1298–307.
Sweeney KR, Chapron DJ, Brandt JL, Gomolin IH, Feig PU, Kramer PA. Toxic interaction between acetazolamide and salicylate: case reports and a pharmacokinetic explanation. Clin Pharmacol Ther. 1986;40(5):518–24.
Bateson MC, Lant AF. Dietary potassium and diuretic therapy. Lancet. 1973;2(7825):381–2.
Worthen DM. Effect of pilocarpine drops on the diurnal intraocular pressure variation in patients with glaucoma. Invest Ophthalmol. 1976;15:784–7.
Quigley HA, Pollack IP. Intraocular pressure control with twice daily pilocarpine in two vehicle solutions. Ann Ophthalmol. 1977;9:427–30.
Van Hoose MC, Leaders FE. The role of cornea in biological response to pilocarpine. Invest Ophthalmol. 1974;13:377–83.
Zimmerman TJ, Wheeler TM. Miotics: side effects and ways to avoid them. Ophthalmology. 1982;89(1):76–80.
Pape LG, Forbes M. Retinal detachment and miotic therapy. Am J Ophthalmol. 1978;85(4):558–66.
Eilderton TE, Farmati O, Zsigmond EK. Reduction in plasma cholinesterase levels after prolonged administration of echothiophate iodide eyedrops. Can Anaesth Soc J. 1968;15(3):291–6.
Singh A. Medical therapy of glaucoma. Ophthalmol Clin North Am. 2005;18:397–408.
McCurdy DK, Schneider B, Scheie HG. Oral glycerol: the mechanism of intraocular hypotension. Am J Ophthalmol. 1966;61:1244–9.
Danesh-Meyer HV, Levin LA. Neuroprotection: extrapolating from neurologic diseases to the eye. Am J Ophthalmol. 2009;148(2):186–91 e182.
Chang EE, Goldberg JL. Glaucoma 2.0: neuroprotection, neuroregeneration, neuroenhancement. Ophthalmology. 2012;119(5):979–86.
Comparison of glaucomatous progression between untreated patients with normal-tension glaucoma and patients with therapeutically reduced intraocular pressures. Collaborative Normal-Tension Glaucoma Study Group. Am J Ophthalmol. 1998;126(4):487–97.
The Advanced Glaucoma Intervention Study (AGIS): 7. The relationship between control of intraocular pressure and visual field deterioration. The AGIS investigators. Am J Ophthalmol. 2000;130(4):429–40.
Leske MC, Heijl A, Hussein M, Bengtsson B, Hyman L, Komaroff E. Factors for glaucoma progression and the effect of treatment: the early manifest glaucoma trial. Arch Ophthalmol. 2003;121(1):48–56.
Osborne NN. Pathogenesis of ganglion "cell death" in glaucoma and neuroprotection: focus on ganglion cell axonal mitochondria. Prog Brain Res. 2008;173:339–52.
Shih GC, Calkins DJ. Secondary neuroprotective effects of hypotensive drugs and potential mechanisms of action. Expert Rev Ophthalmol. 2012;7(2):161–75.
Limb GA, Martin KR. Current prospects in optic nerve protection and regeneration: sixth ARVO/Pfizer Ophthalmics Research Institute conference. Invest Ophthalmol Vis Sci. 2011;52(8):5941–54.

Quigley HA. Clinical trials for glaucoma neuroprotection are not impossible. Curr Opin Ophthalmol. 2012;23(2):144–54.

Baltmr A, Duggan J, Nizari S, Salt TE, Cordeiro MF. Neuroprotection in glaucoma – is there a future role? Exp Eye Res. 2010;91(5):554–66.

Osborne NN, Chidlow G, Nash MS, Wood JP. The potential of neuroprotection in glaucoma treatment. Curr Opin Ophthalmol. 1999a;10(2):82–92.

Osborne NN, Ugarte M, Chao M, et al. Neuroprotection in relation to retinal ischemia and relevance to glaucoma. Surv Ophthalmol. 1999b;43 Suppl 1:S102–28.

Newman NJ, Biousse V, David R, et al. Prophylaxis for second eye involvement in leber hereditary optic neuropathy: an open-labeled, nonrandomized multicenter trial of topical brimonidine purite. Am J Ophthalmol. 2005;140(3):407–15.

Wilhelm B, Ludtke H, Wilhelm H. Efficacy and tolerability of 0.2% brimonidine tartrate for the treatment of acute non-arteritic anterior ischemic optic neuropathy (NAION): a 3-month, double-masked, randomised, placebo-controlled trial. Graefes Arch Clin Exp Ophthalmol. 2006;244(5):551–8.

Krupin T, Liebmann JM, Greenfield DS, Ritch R, Gardiner S. A randomized trial of brimonidine versus timolol in preserving visual function: results from the Low-Pressure Glaucoma Treatment Study. Am J Ophthalmol. 2011;151(4):671–81.

Cordeiro MF, Levin LA. Clinical evidence for neuroprotection in glaucoma. Am J Ophthalmol. 2011;152(5):715–6.

Hare WA, WoldeMussie E, Lai RK, et al. Efficacy and safety of memantine treatment for reduction of changes associated with experimental glaucoma in monkey, I: functional measures. Invest Ophthalmol Vis Sci. 2004a;45(8):2625–39.

Hare WA, WoldeMussie E, Weinreb RN, et al. Efficacy and safety of memantine treatment for reduction of changes associated with experimental glaucoma in monkey, II: structural measures. Invest Ophthalmol Vis Sci. 2004b;45(8):2640–51.

Reisberg B, Doody R, Stoffler A, Schmitt F, Ferris S, Mobius HJ. Memantine in moderate-to-severe Alzheimer's disease. N Engl J Med. 2003;348(14):1333–41.

Osborne NN. Recent clinical findings with memantine should not mean that the idea of neuroprotection in glaucoma is abandoned. Acta Ophthalmol. 2009;87(4):450–4.

Sena DF, Lindsley K. Neuroprotection for treatment of glaucoma in adults. Cochrane Database Syst Rev. 2010;2:CD006539.

Scozzafava A, Supuran CT, Glaucoma and the applications of carbonic anhydrase inhibitors. Subcell Biochem. 2014;75:349–59.

Levin LA, Danesh-Meyer HV. Lost in translation: bumps in the road between bench and bedside. JAMA. 2010;303(15):1533–4.

Wang SK, Chang RT. An emerging treatment option for glaucoma: Rho kinase inhibitors. Clin Ophthalmol. 2014;8:883–90.

Bausch + Lomb and Nicox's Glaucoma Candidate VESNEO: http://ir.valeant.com/investor-relations/news-releases/news-release-details/2014/Bausch--Lomb-and-Nicoxs-Glaucoma-Candidate-VESNEO-latanoprostene-bunod-Meets-Primary-Endpoint-in-Phase-3-Studies/default.aspx

Yang H, Leffler CT. Hybrid dendrimer hydrogel/poly(lactic-co-glycolic acid) nanoparticle platform: an advanced vehicle for topical delivery of antiglaucoma drugs and a likely solution to improving compliance and adherence in glaucoma management. J Ocul Pharmacol Ther. 2013;29(2):166–72.

Fulgencio Gde O, Viana FA, Ribeiro RR, Yoshida MI, Faraco AG, Cunha-Junior Ada S. New mucoadhesive chitosan film for ophthalmic drug delivery of timolol maleate: in vivo evaluation. J Ocul Pharmacol Ther. 2012;28(4):350–8.

Manickavasagam D, Oyewumi MO. Critical assessment of implantable drug delivery devices in glaucoma management. J Drug Deliv. 2013;2013:895013.

Chapter 8
Steroidal and Nonsteroidal Anti-inflammatory Agents for Ocular Use

Rajani Mathur and Renu Agarwal

Abstract Multiple factors cause ocular inflammation in various anatomical regions of the eye. Such inflammations are usually tackled with limited symptomatic treatment modalities. The poor prognosis of or long-standing ocular inflammation can even culminate into permanent loss of vision. Ocular inflammation can be majorly divided into infections and non-infections conditions. This chapter deals with the various ocular anti-inflammatory agents used in conditions like uveitis, ocular manifestations of Behchets disease, diabetic retinopathy and allergic conditions leading to ocular surface inflammations.

8.1 Introduction

Ocular inflammation is a common condition, albeit multifactorial and originating in different anatomical regions of the eye, that is usually tackled with limited symptomatic modalities. The prognosis of long-standing ocular inflammation can even be permanent loss of vision.

One of the most common inflammatory eye diseases is uveitis. Uveitis can occur either as an autoimmune disorder or as a result of injury, infection, or exposure to toxins. The most common symptoms of uveitis are flares, redness,

---

R. Mathur, PhD (✉)
Department of Pharmacology, Delhi Institute of Pharmaceutical Sciences and Research (DIPSAR), New Delhi, India

University of Delhi, New Delhi, India
e-mail: mathurajani@yahoo.com; mathurajani@gmail.com

R. Agarwal, PhD
Faculty of Medicine, Universiti Teknologi MARA, Sungai Buloh, Selangor Darul Ehsan, Malaysia

T. Velpandian (ed.), *Pharmacology of Ocular Therapeutics*,
DOI 10.1007/978-3-319-25498-2_8

photophobia, floaters, blurred vision, and sometimes pain. Untreated uveitis can lead to serious sequelae such as permanent vision loss. It accounts for approximately 10 % of visual handicap in the Western World or 30,000 new cases of blindness at an incidence of 20–52 cases per 100,000 person-years (Larson et al. 2011).

The other noninfectious ocular inflammation is Behcet's disease (BD) that is chronic, relapsing, multisystem disorder characterized by ulcers of the oral and genital mucocutaneous tissue, skin lesions, and nonerosive arthritis.

Diabetic retinopathy, a complication of chronic long-standing diabetes mellitus, is also marked by inflammation of eye.

Diabetic retinopathy is characterized by appearance of microaneurysms, increased vascular permeability, capillary occlusion, and fibrous and neovascular proliferation.

The inflammatory processes play a considerable role in the pathogenesis and progression of DR (Kaštelan et al. 2013). Studies have shown marked presence of inflammatory factors in systemic as well as local (vitreous and aqueous fluid) areas with significant correlation to the development of impaired vision. The Early Treatment DR Study and the Dipyridamole Aspirin Microangiopathy of Diabetes Study have shown that the development of retinal microaneurysms is significantly minimized in patients with early stage of DR when treated with a high dose of aspirin (900 mg/day). Topical administration of COX-2 inhibitor was shown to reduce signs of DR similar to its systematic application without the side effects and holds promise for its therapeutic benefit.

Ocular inflammation is also common after ophthalmic surgery, particularly after surgical removal of cataracts combined with intraocular lens (IOL) implantation. The condition manifests as mild iritis, corneal edema, and flare in the anterior chamber of the eye, accompanied by hyperalgesia. If left untreated, postoperative inflammation can lead to suboptimal vision results or complications such as cystoid macular edema (CME).

Dry eye syndrome has been described as multifactorial disease of the tears and ocular surface that results in symptoms of discomfort, visual disturbance, and tear film instability with potential damage to the ocular surface that is accompanied by increased osmolarity of the tear film and inflammation of the ocular surface. It is most prevalent among the elderly and postmenopausal women. Chronic dryness of the surface of the eye can lead to neurogenic inflammation, activation of T cells, and release of inflammatory cytokines into the lacrimal glands, tear fluid, and conjunctiva. These inflammatory mediators are known to cause gradual dysfunction and destruction of the lacrimal glands and impairment of conjunctival epithelium.

Literature evidences that oxidative stress is the primary initiating event that leads to the inflammatory state of ocular surface. Thus, oxidative stress with associated inflammatory process can trigger severe injury of retina, cornea, conjunctiva, and lacrimal gland.

8.2 Steroidal and Nonsteroidal Anti-inflammatory Agents for Ocular Inflammation

Rajani Mathur

8.2.1 Corticosteroids

Corticosteroids have a broad mechanism of action. They inhibit phospholipase A2, an enzyme that converts membrane phospholipids to arachidonic acid. Thus, the inhibition of the cyclooxygenase and lipoxygenase pathways dramatically reduces the formation of all eicosanoids, which are the active mediators of inflammation. Corticosteroids effectively suppress both the early (capillary dilation, increased vascular permeability, recruitment of leukocytes) and late (deposition of fibrin, proliferation of inflammatory cells and chemokines) phases of inflammation.

Local corticosteroids may be used either topically (for anterior uveitis) or as periocular and intravitreal injections, or as implant devices (for inflammation of posterior segment) and remain the drugs of choice in management of ocular inflammation. Systemic corticosteroids are reserved for chronic uveitis involving the posterior segment, invariably affecting both eyes. However, chronic use of corticosteroid therapies is known to cause glaucoma, cataract, impaired glucose tolerance, hypertension, fluid retention, osteoporosis, mental disturbance, impaired wound healing, gastrointestinal bleeding and perforation, thromboembolic disorders, and weight gain. Of these, increased IOP is of most importance as it is understood to be due to structural and biochemical changes in the trabecular meshwork leading to rise in the resistance to aqueous humor outflow. The incidence of steroid-induced IOP elevation is quite high in as many as 18–36 % of users. Older corticosteroids, such as prednisolone and dexamethasone, are associated with a greater impact on IOP compared to newer corticosteroids. The limitations of chronic use of steroids, vis-a-vis lack of efficacy and need for reinjections, have led to the development of novel sustained-release intravitreal steroid delivery methods. These formulations have lower dose of corticosteroids and, therefore, less secondary side effects.

Multiple formulations like oral prednisone, intravenous methylprednisolone sodium succinate, topical prednisolone acetate or difluprednate, and intravitreal triamcinolone are preferentially used as they offer the benefit of avoiding systemic complications (Geltzer et al. 2013).

Recently, fluocinolone acetonide implant (Retisert) has been developed to deliver corticosteroid for up to 30 months for chronic noninfectious posterior uveitis. Dexamethasone implant for intravitreal use (Ozurdex) has also been approved by the FDA for the treatment of noninfectious posterior uveitis. It is available as 0.7 mg biodegradable implant that delivers extended release of dexamethasone through solid polymer delivery system. Although dexamethasone and prednisolone acetate offer good anti-inflammatory efficacy, their use suffers from clinically significant increase in IOP (up to 10 mmHg). In contrast, corticosteroids such as loteprednol etabonate, a novel C-20 ester-based derivative of prednisolone, offer potent anti-inflammatory efficacy, with limited adverse impact on IOP. Loteprednol etabonate (0.5 %) has been established as effective treatment of postoperative inflammation and resolving anterior chamber cells and flare (Amon and Busin 2012).

Another prednisolone derivative, difluprednate with structural modifications that include the addition of fluorine atoms at C-6 and C-9 positions, a butyrate ester at the C-17 position, and acetate ester at the C-21 and C-20 ketone moiety, is significantly effective in controlling secondary events of ocular inflammation like photophobia, chemosis, and corneal edema. The incidence of clinically significant increase in IOP is low.

The efficacy of loteprednol etabonate, rimexolone, and difluprednate in resolving ocular inflammation is similar. The difference lies in the degree of side effect like corticosteroid-induced ocular hypertension and is often the determining factor in clinical use.

8.2.2 Antimetabolites

Antimetabolites refer to a class or drugs which inhibit nucleic acid synthesis to inhibit cell proliferation. Drugs belong to this class include methotrexate, azathioprine, and mycophenolate mofetil.

Methotrexate was first introduced in 1948 as an antineoplastic agent. It is a folate analogue that acts by inhibiting dihydrofolate reductase. It interferes with the synthesis of thymidylate and purine nucleotide, to inhibit the growth of rapidly dividing cells. The most serious side effects of methotrexate include hepatotoxicity, cytopenias, and interstitial pneumonitis. Monitoring of liver function tests is required during treatment. It is teratogenic and thus contraindicated in pregnancy.

Azathioprine is widely used in organ transplantation, inflammatory bowel disease, systemic lupus erythematosus, and other autoimmune conditions. It is a prodrug of 6-mercaptopurine, a purine nucleoside analogue that interferes with DNA replication and RNA transcription. It also inhibits actively dividing immune cells to restrain inflammatory process.

Mycophenolate mofetil (MMF) is commonly used in management of organ transplant rejection and other autoimmune conditions. Its mechanism of action is selective inhibition of inosine-5-monophosphate dehydrogenase in the de novo purine synthesis pathway. As B and T lymphocytes depend on the de novo pathway for proliferation, its selective inhibition effectively curtails inflammatory state. MMF has been shown to be effective in combination with steroids or another immunomodulatory treatment as well as monotherapy.

8.2.3 T-Cell Inhibitors

This class of agents includes cyclosporine, tacrolimus, and sirolimus.

Cyclosporine is an 11 amino acid peptide derived from fungus. Cyclosporine acts by forming a complex with cyclophilin which binds calcineurin that then inhibits the cytosolic translocation of nuclear factors. Consequently, there is preferential inhibition of antigen-triggered signal transduction of T lymphocytes. It is available in two formulations, as oil-based gelatin capsules (Sandimmune, Novartis Pharmaceuticals) and a microemulsion (Neoral, Novartis Pharmaceuticals). Cyclosporine has been used safely in children with severe, sight-threatening uveitis. The adverse effects of cyclosporine therapy include gastrointestinal upset, metabolic abnormalities, paresthesias, tremor, gingival hyperplasia, and hirsutism.

Voclosporin is a calcineurin inhibitor that has been developed for the treatment of uveitis. It has been shown to be more potent and less toxic than cyclosporine. In extensive placebo-controlled clinical studies, voclosporin has been reported to improve vitreous haze that is part of active posterior disease. It significantly reduced eye inflammation but failed to meet the primary endpoint of all-cause therapeutic failure. In the condition of anterior inflammation, voclosporin failed to establish itself from placebo.

Tacrolimus or FK506 is a macrolide isolated from the soil fungus *Streptomyces tsukubaensis* that was originally used in solid organ transplantation. It has a similar mechanism of action to cyclosporine and binds to an intracellular binding protein, FK-binding protein, that associates with calcineurin and thus inhibits activation of T cells and production of cytokines.

Sirolimus (Rapamune) is another immunosuppressive drug. Its binds to FK-binding protein-12 (FKBP-12) to form a complex that binds to and inhibits the activation of the mammalian target of sirolimus (mTOR) to suppress cytokine-driven T-cell proliferation.

8.2.4 Alkylating Agents

Cyclophosphamide and chlorambucil belong to the class of drugs called alkylating agents as they act by alkylating DNA leading to DNA cross-linking and inhibition of DNA synthesis. Although they were originally developed for the treatment of cancers, they are now widely being used for management of rheumatologic conditions. Owing to their serious, life-threatening side effects, their use is limited to severe, sight-threatening uveitis.

Cyclophosphamide, a mustard gas derivative, alkylates the purines of DNA and RNA resulting in cross-linking and impaired cell division. Thus, the number of inflammatory cells like T and B lymphocytes is reduced.

8.2.5 Biologic Agents

Conventional therapy with corticosteroids and immunosuppressive agents may not be sufficient to control ocular inflammation or prevent non-ophthalmic complications in refractory patients. Off-label use of biologic response modifiers has been studied as primary and secondary line of therapy and reported to be very useful in such conditions. Strategies for biologics employ formulating new drugs that target specific receptors, cytokines, or signaling pathways (Pasadhika and Rosenbaum 2014).

8.2.5.1 Anti-Tumor Necrosis Factor-α (TNF-α)

TNF-α is a well-known proinflammatory cytokine that has been shown to play a key role in pathogenesis of inflammatory diseases. Thus, inhibiting TNF-α with antibodies has been a well-accepted strategy to suppress autoimmune uveitis (Karampetsou et al. 2010). TNF-α inhibitors include infliximab, a chimeric mAb, and adalimumab, a fully humanized IgG1 mAb, against TNF-α (Verma et al 2013). Certolizumab pegol and golimumab have only been recently introduced and there is limited clinical experience with them. Other agents such as abatacept, canakinumab, gevokizumab, tocilizumab, and alemtuzumab hold promise for the treatment of uveitis in the future. Systemic administration of anti-TNF-α agents has shown encouraging preliminary results in uveitic and diabetic cystoid macular edema and age-related macular degeneration.

Infliximab (Remicade) is a 149 kDa chimeric IgG1 monoclonal antibody composed of human constant region of IgG1 and murine variable binding site for TNF-α. It has been approved for use in rheumatoid arthritis, ankylosing spondylitis, psoriatic arthritis, and plaque psoriasis and Crohn's disease. It is well accepted for management of various subtypes of refractory uveitis and retinal vasculitis, especially Behcet's disease-related eye conditions and the uveitis associated with juvenile idiopathic arthritis. Infliximab in BD-associated uveitis is advocated as an add-on therapy to DMARDs. The combination significantly reduced the frequency of uveitis flares compared to administration of DMARDs alone.

Etanercept (Enbrel) is a fusion protein consisting of the binding part of the human type II receptor of TNF-α linked to the Fc portion of IgG1a. It is a blocker of soluble TNF-α receptor that has also been investigated as subcutaneous injection (25 mg/week). But it has been found to be less effective than infliximab or adalimumab in the treatment of uveitis. In retrospective study, when infliximab was compared to etanercept, the number of recurrences and ocular inflammation was improved with former as compared to latter.

Apremilast, a selective cytokine inhibitory drug, inhibits phosphodiesterase IV and TNF-α production to suppress the immune response. It is currently in phase II clinical trials for Behcet's disease. As the drug is projected for oral administration, the need for injection is circumvented and reduces cost considerably.

ESBA-105 is a topical anti-TNF-α single-chain antibody and possesses good anterior and posterior intraocular penetration. It is under development for the treatment of ocular conditions including uveitis and diabetic retinopathy.

8.2.5.2 Cytokine Receptor Antibodies

Daclizumab is a humanized monoclonal antibody directed against the alpha subunit of the interleukin-2 receptor (CD25) present on activated T cells. The drug is also approved for management of renal allograft rejection and autoimmune diseases such as multiple sclerosis and human T-cell leukemia virus-1-associated T-cell leukemia. The drug can be administered as 1–2 mg/kg infusions every 2–4 weeks. Side effects include rashes, edema, granulomatous reactions, viral respiratory infections, elevated liver enzymes, and leukopenia.

Rituximab, a chimeric monoclonal antibody against CD20, a B-cell marker, results in depletion of B cells. It was originally developed for the treatment of B-cell lymphomas and now finding application in ocular inflammation.

MM-093, a recombinant human alpha-fetoprotein, has recently completed phase II study for sarcoid or birdshot uveitis.

8.2.6 Antiangiogenic Therapy

Vascular endothelial growth factor (VEGF) is a potent vasoactive cytokine that is involved in the breakdown of blood-retinal barrier and angiogenesis in the ischemic retina. The VEGF levels are significantly elevated in patients with DME and its intravitreal concentration increases with the progression of DR. Antiangiogenic therapy acts to reduce vascular permeability, reduce the breakdown of the blood-retinal barrier, inhibit leukocyte adhesion to vascular walls, and inhibit VEGF gene transcription and translation and therefore finds use in ocular inflammatory conditions (Geltzer et al. 2013).

Bevacizumab (Avastin) and ranibizumab (Lucentis) are also monoclonal antibodies to vascular endothelial growth factor (VEGF). Ranibizumab was designed specifically for ocular use and received FDA approval for the treatment of choroidal neovascularization in age-related macular degeneration. Bevacizumab is increasingly finding off-label use for ocular diseases.

Ranibizumab (Lucentis), a recombinant humanized antibody fragment, is active against all isoforms of VEGF-A and approved for the treatment of exudative AMD and DME.

8.2.7 Blocking Oxidative Stress

As a key mediator in inflammation, oxidative stress serves as an important target for anti-inflammatory therapy. The etiology of ocular inflammation involves free radical-mediated oxidative damage, hypoxia, decreased blood supply to ocular tissues, angiogenesis, increased vascular permeability, and leakage of vascular contents.

Flavonoids have been attributed with multi-thronged action including antioxidant, antiangiogenic, reducing fluid retention, and strengthening capillary walls that together contribute to anti-inflammatory activities. Bioflavonoids have been found effective in the prevention and treatment of diabetic retinopathy, macular degeneration, and cataract (Majumdar and Srirangam 2010). Some of the common bioflavanoids that have been documented for their anti-inflammatory action are quercetin, apigenin, hesperidin, hesperetin, luteolin, epigallocatechin gallate, epicatechin gallate, rutin, cyanidin, naringenin, myricetin, chrysin, eriodictyol, and kaempferol.

Flavanoids are hypothesized to act as antioxidant through various actions such as:

(a) By scavenging the free radicals directly—Flavanoids are also known as "quenchers" due to their low redox potential or high reactivity that may be attributable to the presence of hydroxyl groups. Flavonoids are capable of reducing the highly oxidizing free radicals (e.g., superoxide, peroxyl, alkoxyl, and hydroxyl) to form stable, less-reactive radicals.
(b) By inhibiting the nitric oxide production—Nitric oxide (NO) is produced by several types of cells including endothelial cells and macrophages. The inducible nitric oxide synthase (iNOS) is understood to be responsible for the production of high concentrations of NO during oxidative damage. Further, NO reacts with free radicals to generate the highly reactive and damaging peroxynitrite. Flavonoids through their free radical-scavenging properties can prevent the generation of peroxynitrite. They also inhibit iNOS directly and thereby decrease production of NO.
(c) By inhibiting certain enzymes—Flavonoids can inhibit the enzymes such as xanthine oxidase and protein kinase C that are responsible for the production of superoxide anions. They are also capable of inhibiting other enzymes involved in ROS generation such as cyclooxygenase, lipoxygenase, microsomal monooxygenase, glutathione S-transferase, mitochondrial succinoxidase, and NADH oxidase.
(d) By chelating trace elements—Flavonoids are good chelaters of trace elements, like free iron and copper, that are potential enhancers of ROS generation and important in oxygen metabolism.

The major pharmacokinetic limitation of flavonoids is their poor oral bioavailability due to poor intrinsic transmembrane diffusion characteristics, poor solubility, and intestinal and hepatic metabolism. The ocular bioavailability of the flavonoids depends on the formulation and on the route of administration. When administered by the oral route, diffusion of the hydrophilic metabolites from the plasma into the neural retina is severely restricted by the blood-retinal barriers.

Curcumin is also reported for anti-inflammatory properties that are linked to its ability to downregulate the expression of the IκBα gene; cyclooxygenase-2 gene (COX-2); prostaglandin E2 (PGE2); interleukin-1, interleukin-6, and interleukin-8 (IL-1, IL-6, IL-8); and tumor necrosis factor-α (TNF-α). Curcumin also exhibits antioxidant properties and was found useful in chronic anterior uveitis, diabetic retinopathy, glaucoma, age-related macular degeneration, and dry eye syndrome (Pescosolido et al 2014).

8.2.8 Newer Strategies

Renin-angiotensin system (RAS) is well established in the pathogenesis of diabetes and hypertension-induced retinal inflammation. Further, it also activates pathways leading to oxidative stress and AGEs. Hence, blocking RAS is fast emerging as promising target in the management of diabetic retinopathy. Specifically, blockade of AT1R (losartan, candesartan) and angiotensin-converting enzyme inhibitor (Enalapril) has been shown to prevent oxidative stress, inflammation, and vascular damage in diabetic retinopathy. Further studies are ongoing to evaluate the clinical benefits of blocking RAS in ocular inflammation.

8.3 Ocular Allergy and Its Pharmacotherapy

Renu Agarwal

8.3.1 Introduction

Allergic disorders of ocular surface are a group of immune-mediated inflammatory reactions that generally involve conjunctiva, lids, lid margins and lacrimal system. The cornea is relatively protected due to its anatomical, physiological, and immunological properties. Various clinical forms of ocular allergy include seasonal allergic conjunctivitis (SAC), perennial allergic conjunctivitis (PAC), vernal keratoconjunctivitis (VAC), atopic keratoconjunctivitis (AKC), giant papillary conjunctivitis, and drug-induced or contact dermatoconjunctivitis. The acute forms of allergic conjunctivitis, SAC and PAC, involve type I hypersensitivity reaction. On the other hand, more chronic conditions such as VAC and AKC involve type IV hypersensitivity reactions.

The allergic reactions typically develop through 3 phases. The first phase of "sensitization" begins upon exposure of ocular surface to allergens. The antigen-presenting cells (APCs) in conjunctival epithelium such as dendritic cells phagocytize the allergen. After processing within APCs, the peptide fragments of allergen are expressed on the cell surface in association with major histocompatibility complex (MHC) class II molecule. The allergen-MHC complex interacts with T-helper (Th) cells causing their maturation to Th type 1 (Th1) or Th type 2 (Th2) cells, of which Th2 cells, in particular, play a significant role in allergic response. APC-Th2 interaction results in production of cytokines, which interact with naive B cells stimulating production of immunoglobulin E (IgE)-type antibodies. IgE binds to its high-affinity receptors on the surface of basophils and mast cells. Upon subsequent exposure to same allergen, its interaction with IgE on mast cells and basophils results in increased membrane permeability to calcium ions (Ca^{++}) and subsequently, there is mobilization of Ca^{++} from intracellular stores. Significant amount of IgE-antigen interaction, hence, leads to degranulation of mast cells and basophils releasing inflammatory mediators such as histamine, serotonin, leukotriene C4, prostaglandin D2, platelet-activating factor, tryptase, chymase, cathepsin G, and other eosinophil and neutrophil chemoattractants. These mediators lead to "early-phase reaction" often characterized by redness, itching, and tearing. Exposure to large doses of allergen leads to more persistent "late-phase reaction." This reaction is associated with significant recruitment of inflammatory cells, particularly the eosinophils. In the chronic form of ocular allergy, mast cells also relocate from the substantia propria to the epithelial surface of conjunctiva and play a significant role in the development of allergic reactions. In both the early- and late-phase reactions, mast cells and basophils release histamine, which is the major inflammatory mediator in ocular allergic reaction.

8.3.2 Histamine and Histamine Receptors

Histamine is a biologically active endogenous amine that affects the activity of a variety of cells. Histamine exerts its biological effects through specific G-protein-coupled cell surface receptors that are of 4 types. H1 histamine receptors are ubiquitous in distribution and play a central role in immune and inflammatory responses. Stimulation of H1 receptors results in smooth muscle contraction except in vessels where they cause vasodilation. In the eye, they have significant impact on sensory signaling (Abelson and Schaefer 1993). H2 histamine receptors are predominantly present in gastrointestinal mucosa. To a lesser extent, they are also present in the blood vessels, myocardium, mast cells, and brain. In the eye, H2 receptors are almost exclusively located in association with blood vessels and, hence, have a greater impact on the redness rather than the itching associated with conjunctivitis (Abelson and Udell 1981). H3 histamine receptor is expressed throughout the central nervous system and acts primarily to modulate the function of other signaling molecules such as GABA, serotonin, and dopamine (Esbenshade et al. 2008). It has also been found in nasal mucosa and may play a role in rhinoconjunctivitis (Yokota et al. 2008). H4 histamine receptor is expressed primarily in immune cells such as mast cells and leukocytes and is involved in inflammation and allergy. It has been shown to play a role in chemotaxis and cytokine production during inflammatory reactions (Leite-de-Moraes et al. 2009). It is also expressed by some T cells, including CD4+ T cells (Saravanan et al. 2011). In the eye, H4 receptors are co-localized with H1 receptors and may be as important as H1 receptors in mediating ocular allergic responses (Thurmond et al. 2008).

8.3.3 Treatment of Ocular Allergies

Aim of the treatment in ocular allergies is to provide symptomatic relief, to alleviate the underlying cause and to treat complications in severe forms of allergy. Patients are advised to avoid contact with allergen, if it is known. Cold compresses help in relieving pruritus. Patients are also advised to keep the topical medications refrigerated as the cold drops provide symptomatic relief. Tear substitutes are prescribed as they provide relief by diluting and/or washing out the allergen and inflammatory mediators from ocular surface.

Several groups of drugs are used in the treatment of ocular allergies. Use of topical NSAIDs and corticosteroids has previously been discussed. Ocular decongestants are used to whiten the eye and provide rapid relief. Considering the role of mast cells, basophils, and histamine in ocular allergy, antihistamines, mast cell stabilizers, and drugs with dual action form the mainstay of treatment.

8.3.3.1 Ocular Decongestants

Topical sympathomimetics are used as ocular decongestants. They relieve hyperemia, watering, and irritation by causing local vasoconstriction. The commonly used drugs in this class are phenylephrine and imidazole derivatives.

Phenylephrine

Phenylephrine is a direct-acting α-adrenoreceptor agonist (refer Chap. 6 for detailed pharmacology). The ophthalmic preparations of phenylephrine are available in the concentration range of 0.12–10 %. Concentrations greater than 0.125 % cause mydriasis and are used for dilating the pupil. At 0.125 and 0.12 % concentration, phenylephrine produces little or no effect on pupil (Kubo et al. 1975) but does produce vasoconstriction of the conjunctival vessels. Hence, at this concentration, it is used as ocular decongestant. It can also be added to other medications such as antihistamines and antibiotics. Use of phenylephrine requires caution, particularly in those with angle-closure glaucoma.

The ophthalmic solution of phenylephrine is clear and colorless; however, it turns darker with time upon exposure to air, light, and heat due to oxidation. Such oxidized solutions should not be used. It is also important to follow manufacturer's instructions regarding expiry dates as the solution may lose activity even before any visible color change.

The topical side effects such as pain, stinging, and lacrimation are more common at higher concentrations of phenylephrine. It can cause rebound conjunctival congestion. Systemic absorption of significant amount of phenylephrine can cause hypertension, headache, tachycardia or reflex bradycardia and blanching of skin. It has also been reported to cause dermatoconjunctivitis.

Imidazole Derivatives

Imidazole derivatives include naphazoline, tetrahydrozoline, and oxymetazoline. They cause constriction of conjunctival vessels due to α-adrenoreceptor agonistic action and hence are used as ocular decongestants. Naphazoline 0.1 % causes constriction of superficial conjunctival vessels without significantly affecting deeper scleral vessels. It may slightly dilate the pupil but does not affect the accommodation. Oxymetazoline 0.25 % has been shown to relieve the symptoms of allergic conjunctivitis effectively (Duzman et al. 1986) and the relief may last for 6 h. Tetrahydrozoline 0.1 and 0.05 % also provides rapid relief of symptoms without affecting the pupil size and intraocular pressure (Grossmann and Lehman 1956; Menger 1959).

Few studies have compared the effects of different decongestants. In one of the studies involving 20 patients with nonspecific allergic conjunctivitis, 0.01 % oxymetazoline was found to be superior to 0.01 % naphazoline in relieving the symptoms of conjunctivitis (Nayak et al. 1987). However, naphazoline 0.2 % produced greater conjunctival blanching compared to tetrahydrozoline 0.05 % and phenylephrine 0.12 % (Abelson et al. 1980). A significant difference favoring oxymetazoline was also observed for the duration of action (Rybiczka and Mauracher 1983).

The topical application of the above agents has been reported to cause significant systemic adverse effects such as change in heart rate or blood pressure. Ocular side effects such as pupillary dilation and increase in intraocular pressure may occur with naphazoline. Prolonged and repeated use of these agents may cause ocular xerosis. Rebound congestion with the use of these agents has not been reported.

8.3.3.2 Antihistamines

H1 antihistamines are particularly useful in the treatment of ocular allergies. H1 antihistamines are now considered to act as inverse agonists and not, as previously thought, as antagonists of histamine. Stimulation of the H1 receptor, a Gq/11-coupled GPCR, classically activates inositol phospholipid signaling pathways resulting in formation of inositol triphosphate and diacylglycerol which leads to an increase in intracellular calcium. H1 antihistamines prevent the effects of H1 receptor stimulation by inhibiting activation of the intracellular signaling pathways. They also modulate the activity of transcription factor NF-κB, inhibit intracellular adhesion molecule-1 (ICAM-1) expression and the effects of bradykinin (Leurs et al. 2002).

H1 antihistamines are grouped into two classes: first-generation (older) drugs and second-generation (newer) drugs. The major differentiating property of the two groups of H1 antihistamines is their ability to cross blood-brain barrier (BBB). First-generation drugs easily cross BBB and hence cause CNS-related adverse effects. Second-generation drugs are largely devoid of CNS-related adverse effects as they do not cross BBB. Additionally, first-generation drugs also block other autonomic receptors and hence cause a range of other adverse effects. The topical route is the preferred choice for the treatment of ocular allergies as it directly delivers the drugs to target site, shortening the onset of action. Additionally, smaller concentrations of drugs are required compared to systemic administration.

Topical Antihistamines

The most widely used first-generation topical antihistamines are antazoline (0.5 %) and pheniramine (0.3 %). Levocabastine (0.05 %) and emedastine (0.05 %) are the second-generation antihistamines available for topical use. Often, they are used in combination with sympathomimetics. After topical application, they spread in the precorneal tear film and get distributed to conjunctiva and cornea. They may be absorbed systemically through conjunctival vessels and through nasal and oropharyngeal mucosa.

These agents effectively control hyperemia and itching. The efficacy of emedastine and levocabastine in the prevention and treatment of allergic conjunctivitis has been assessed. It was observed that both drugs are significantly more effective than placebo and emedastine was more effective than levocabastine (Verin et al. 2001).

Topical antihistamines are generally well tolerated. They may cause transient burning or stinging upon instillation, eyelid edema, and ocular irritation. They may also cause bad taste, blurred vision, corneal infiltrates, corneal staining, dermatitis, dry eye, foreign body sensation, hyperemia, keratitis, pruritus, rhinitis, sinusitis, and tearing. Systemic adverse effects after local application are not common; however, indiscriminate use may result in the adverse effects as seen with the administration of oral antihistamines.

Oral Antihistamines

Several oral antihistamines, both first and second generation, are available for treatment of ocular allergies; however, due to unfavorable therapeutic index of first-generation agents, second-generation antihistamines are the preferred class (del Cuvillo et al. 2006). The second-generation antihistamines that have commonly been used include levocetirizine, desloratadine, rupatadine, ebastine, cetirizine, loratadine, fexofenadine, and mizolastine.

Oral antihistamines are well absorbed from gastrointestinal tract. They are widely distributed and achieve the peak plasma concentration in 1–2 h. Symptomatic relief may appear in 30 min–1 h and the effect generally lasts for 12 h or more. The effects of first-generation agents are short lasting. First-generation agents cross the BBB, whereas second-generation agents do not cross BBB due to their poor lipophilicity and also because they are substrates of P-glycoprotein reverse transporter in BBB. They are metabolized by cytochrome P450 enzymes and the metabolites are excreted in urine within 24 h. Metabolites of some agents, like hydroxyzine, terfenadine, and loratadine, retain the activity of parent compounds.

Oral antihistamines may be particularly useful in patients with rhinoconjunctivitis. Although topical antihistamines administered to ocular surface may also be used, oral antihistamines more effectively relieve the nasal symptoms (Spangler et al. 2003; Crampton 2003). All of them have been shown to effectively relieve the symptoms of perennial and seasonal rhinoconjunctivitis. Ebastine was shown to be more effective than loratadine in relieving symptoms of seasonal allergic rhinoconjunctivitis (Ratner et al. 2005). The safety of desloratadine, rupatadine, ebastine, and mizolastine in children is not established.

The adverse effect profile of second-generation antihistamines is considerably better than first-generation agents. As the second-generation agents do not cross BBB, hence, sedation is not a common adverse effect. Antimuscarinic side effects such as dry mouth, blurred vision, constipation, and retention of urine are also less likely with second-generation agents. However, elderly and those with benign hypertrophy of prostate may require caution due to the risk of urinary retention. Generally, second-generation agents are devoid of troublesome adverse effects.

8.3.3.3 Mast Cell Stabilizer

Mast cell stabilizers act by stabilizing the mast cell membrane and preventing release of histamine and slow-reacting substance of anaphylaxis (SRS-A). These agents bind with the calcium transporter on the surface of mast cells and inhibit binding of calcium with this transporter which is essential for the release of histamine and other mediators after antigen-antibody interaction. There may also be additional mechanisms of action of mast cell stabilizers such as phosphorylation of membrane proteins essential for degranulation and release of mediators.

Disodium cromoglycate was the first mast cell stabilizer used in clinical practice. It is not absorbed from gastrointestinal tract after oral administration and hence is administered topically as 4 % eyedrops. It is well distributed in the precorneal tear film and also penetrates the conjunctival epithelium and substantia propria. Systemic absorption following repeated instillation is negligible. Other mast cell stabilizers that are used in clinical practice include nedocromil sodium (2 %), lodoxamide (0.1 %), and pemirolast (0.1 %). Their mechanism of action is similar to disodium cromoglycate.

Since mast cell stabilizers inhibit the release of histamine even upon exposure of sensitized cells to antigens, they are primarily used for prophylaxis. Disodium cromoglycate 4 % requires administration of 1–2 drops four to six times daily. Lodoxamide (0.1 %) and pemirolast (0.1 %) are administered as 1–2 drops four times daily, whereas nedocromil sodium (2 %) is administered twice daily.

Systemic adverse effects of mast cell stabilizers are uncommon because they are not absorbed systemically. Headache, however, may occur especially with pemirolast. They may cause local adverse effects such as mild and transient irritation, redness, and ocular and periocular itching. Mast cell stabilizers are contraindicated in patients who are allergic to drug or any other constituent of the topical preparation.

8.3.3.4 Dual-Action Agents

Introduction of dual-action drugs was an important step forward in the treatment of ocular allergies. Since the dual-action drugs combine the histamine receptor-blocking and mast cell-stabilizing effects, they not only relieve the symptoms but can also prevent the further occurrence of allergic episodes. The drugs available from this class for topical use include azelastine 0.05 %, epinastine 0.05 %, ketotifen 0.025 %, and olopatadine 0.1 %. Among all, ketotifen is the only drug available as unit dose without preservatives and hence is most suitable for contact lens wearers, although olopatadine has also been successfully used to treat allergic conjunctivitis in contact lens wearers (Brodsky et al. 2003).

Emedastine and ketotifen were found to be equally effective in relieving itching (Verin et al. 2001; D'Arienzo et al. 2002) and the efficacy of both of them has been shown to outperform levocabastine (Kidd et al. 2003). Olopatadine was found to be more effective than azelastine for relief of itching (Spangler et al. 2001). However, when compared to ketotifen, olopatadine showed no significant differences (Avunduk et al. 2005) but patient preferences were found to be in favor of olopatadine due to convenience of dosing (Leonardi and Zafirakis 2004). When compared with epinastine and levocabastine, olopatadine was found to have higher efficacy in relieving the redness and itching (Lanier et al. 2004; Abelson and Greiner 2004).

Headache, burning, and irritation are common side effects of dual-action drugs. They may also cause foreign body sensation, dry eyes and itching in and around the eyes. Systemic adverse effects are not seen with these drugs as the systemic absorption is minimal.

References

Abelson MB, Greiner JV. Comparative efficacy of olopatadine 0.1% ophthalmic solution versus levocabastine 0.05% ophthalmic suspension using the conjunctival allergen challenge model. Curr Med Res Opin. 2004;20:1953–8.

Abelson MB, Schaefer K. Conjunctivitis of allergic origin: Immunologic mechanisms and current approaches to therapy. Surv Ophthalmol. 1993;38:S115–32.

Abelson MB, Udell IJ. H2-receptors in the human ocular surface. Arch Ophthalmol. 1981;99:302.

Abelson MB, Yamamoto GK, Allansmith MR. Effects of ocular decongestants. Arch Ophthalmol. 1980;98(5):856–8.

Amon M, Busin M. Loteprednol etabonate ophthalmic suspension 0.5 %: efficacy and safety for postoperative anti-inflammatory use. Int Ophthalmol. 2012;32:507–17.

Avunduk AM, Tekelioglu Y, Turk A, Akyol N. Comparison of the effects of ketotifen fumarate 0.025% and olopatadine HCl 0.1% ophthalmic solutions in seasonal allergic conjunctivitis: a 30-day, randomized, double-masked, artificial tear substitute controlled trial. Clin Ther. 2005;27:1392–402.

Brodsky M, Berger WE, Butrus S, Epstein AB, Irkec M. Evaluation of comfort using olopatadine hydrochloride 0.1% ophthalmic solution in the treatment of allergic conjunctivitis in contact lens wearers compared to placebo using the conjunctival allergen challenge model. Eye Contact Lens. 2003;29:113–6.

Crampton HJ. Comparison of ketotifen fumarate ophthalmic solution alone, desloratadine alone, and their combination for inhibition of the signs and symptoms of seasonal allergic rhinoconjunctivitis in the conjunctival allergen challenge model: a double-masked, placebo- and active-controlled trial. Clin Ther. 2003;25:1975–87.

D'Arienzo PA, Leonardi A, Bensch G. Randomized, doublemasked, placebo-controlled comparison of the efficacy of emedastine difumarate 0.05% ophthalmic solution and ketotifen fumarate 0.025% ophthalmic solution in the human conjunctival allergen challenge model. Clin Ther. 2002;24:409–16.

del Cuvillo A, Mullol J, Bartra J, Davila I, Jauregui I, Montoro J, Sastre J, Valero AL. Comparative pharmacology of the H1 antihistamines. J Investig Allergol Clin Immunol. 2006;16 Suppl 1:3–12.

Duzman E, Warman A, Warman R. Efficacy and safety of topical oxymetazoline in treating allergic and environmental conjunctivitis. Ann Ophthalmol. 1986;18(1):28–31.

Esbenshade TA, Browman KE, Bitner RS, Strakhova M, Cowart MD, Brioni JD. The histamine H3 receptor: an attractive target for the treatment of cognitive disorders. Br J Pharmacol. 2008;154:1166–81.

Geltzer A, Turalba A, Vedula SS. Surgical implantation of steroids with antiangiogenic characteristics for treating neovascular age-related macular degeneration. Cochrane Database Syst Rev. 2013;1: CD005022. doi:10.1002/14651858.CD005022.pub3.

Grossmann EE, Lehman RH. Ophthalmic use of tyzine; a clinical study of this new vasoconstrictor. Am J Ophthalmol. 1956;42(1):121–3.

Karampetsou MP, Liossis SN, Sfikakis PP. TNF-a antagonists beyond approved indications: stories of success and prospects for the future. Q J Med. 2010;103:917–28.

Kaštelan S, Tomi MT, Gverovic Antunica A, Salopek Rabati J, Ljubi S. Inflammation and pharmacological treatment in diabetic retinopathy. Mediators Inflamm. 2013:Article ID 213130, 8.

Kidd M, McKenzie SH, Steven I, Cooper C, Lanz R. Efficacy and safety of ketotifen eye drops in the treatment of seasonal allergic conjunctivitis. Br J Ophthalmol. 2003;87:1206–11.

Kubo DJ, Wing TW, Polse KA, Jauregui MJ. Mydriatic effects using low concentrations of phenylephrine hydrochloride. J Am Optom Assoc. 1975;46(8):817–22.

Lanier BQ, Finegold I, D'Arienzo P, Granet D, Epstein AB, Ledgerwood GL. Clinical efficacy of olopatadine vs epinastine ophthalmic solution in the conjunctival allergen challenge model. Curr Med Res Opin. 2004;20:1227–33.

Larson T, Nussenblatt RB, Sen HN. Emerging drugs for uveitis. Expert Opin Emerg Drugs. 2011;16(2):309–22.

Leite-de-Moraes MC, Diem S, Michel ML, Ohtsu H, Thurmond RL, Schneider E, Dy M. Cutting edge: histamine receptor H4 activation positively regulates in vivo IL-4 and IFN-gamma production by invariant NKT cells. J Immunol. 2009;182:1233–6.

Leonardi A, Zafirakis P. Efficacy and comfort of olopatadine versus ketotifen ophthalmic solutions: a double-masked, environmental study of patient preference. Curr Med Res Opin. 2004;20:1167–73.

Leurs R, Church MK, Taglialatela M. H1-antihistamines: inverse agonism, anti-inflammatory actions and cardiac effects. Clin Exp Allergy. 2002;32:489–98.

Majumdar S, Srirangam R. Potential of the bioflavonoids in the prevention/treatment of ocular disorders. J Pharm Pharmacol. 2010;62(8):951–65.

Menger HC. New ophthalmic decongestant, tetrahydrozoline hydrochloride; clinical use in 1,156 patients with conjunctival irritation. J Am Med Assoc. 1959;170(2):178–9.

Nayak BK, Kishore K, Gupta SK. Evaluation of oxymetazoline and naphazoline in benign red eyes: a double blind comparative clinical trial. Indian J Ophthalmol. 1987;35(4):190–3.

Pasadhika S, Rosenbaum JT. Update on the use of systemic biologic agents in the treatment of noninfectious uveitis. Biologics: Targets and Therapy. 2014;8:67–81.

Pescosolido N, Giannotti R, Plateroti AM, Pascarella A, Nebbioso M. Curcumin: therapeutical potential in ophthalmology. Planta Med. 2014;80:249–54.

Ratner P, Falques M, Chuecos F, Esbri R, Gispert J, Peris F, Luria X, Rosales MJ. Meta-analysis of the efficacy of ebastine 20 mg compared to loratadine 10 mg and placebo in the symptomatic treatment of seasonal allergic rhinitis. Int Arch Allergy Immunol. 2005;138:312–8.

Rybiczka R, Mauracher E. Oxymetazoline ophthalmic solution versus naphazoline solution in non-infectious conjunctivitis. Pharmatherapeutica. 1983;3(6):376–81.

Saravanan C, Bharti SK, Jaggi S, Singh SK. Histamine H(4) receptor: a novel target for inflammation therapy. Mini Rev Med Chem. 2011;11(2):143–58.

Spangler DL, Bensch G, Berdy GJ. Evaluation of the efficacy of olopatadine hydrochloride 0.1% ophthalmic solution and azelastine hydrochloride 0.05% ophthalmic solution in the conjunctival allergen challenge model. Clin Ther. 2001;23:1272–80.

Spangler DL, Abelson MB, Ober A, Gotnes PJ. Randomized, double-masked comparison of olopatadine ophthalmic solution, mometasone furoate monohydrate nasal spray, and fexofenadine hydrochloride tablets using the conjunctival and nasal allergen challenge models. Clin Ther. 2003;25:2245–67.

Thurmond RL, Gelfand EW, Dunford PJ. The role of histamine H1 and H4 receptors in allergic inflammation: the search for new antihistamines. Nat Rev Drug Discov. 2008;7:41–53.

Verin P, Easty DL, Secchi A, Ciprandi G, Partouche P, Nemeth-Wasmer G, Brancato R, Harrisberg CJ, Estivin-Ebrardt C, Coster DJ, Apel AJ, Coroneo MT, Knorr M, Carmichael TR, Kent-Smith BT, Abrantes P, Leonardi A, Cerqueti PM, Modorati G, Martinez M. Clinical evaluation of twice-daily emedastine 0.05% eye drops (Emadine eye drops) versus levocabastine 0.05% eye drops in patients with allergic conjunctivitis. Am J Ophthalmol. 2001;131:691–8.

Verma S, Kroeker KI, Fedorak RN. Adalimumab for orbital myositis in a patient with Crohn's disease who discontinued infliximab: a case report and review of the literature. BMC Gastroenterol. 2013;13:59.

Yokota E, Kuyama S, Sugimoto Y, Ogawa M, Kamei C. Participation of histamine H3 receptors in experimental allergic rhinitis of mice. J Pharmacol Sci. 2008;108:206–11.

Chapter 9
Antiangiogenic Agents and Photodynamic Therapy

Atul Kumar, S.N. Mohanraj, Kavitha Duraipandi, and Anuradha V. Pai

Abstract Diabetic retinopathy, Age Related Macular Degeneration (ARMD) and Retinopathy of Prematurity(ROP), are few of the many pathological conditions which are vision threatening. Their classical feature is neovascularization. Angiogenic factors such as VEGF, PEDF, Tyrosine Kinase etc., have a significant role in the causation of angiogenesis in the hypoxic areas of the ocular tissues. This chapter covers the causative factors of ocular angiogenesis and the possible pharmacological intervention to inhibit these factors in order to improve the vision of the patients. This chapter also deals with the possible benefits of the photodynamic therapy in the ocular neovascularisation.

A. Kumar, MD, FAMS (✉)
Vitreous-Retina Service, Dr. Rajendra Prasad Center for Ophthalmic Sciences,
All India Institute of Medical Sciences, New Delhi, India
e-mail: atul56kumar@gmail.com

S.N. Mohanraj, MD
Vitreoretina Unit, Nethradhama Superspeciality Eye Hospital, Bangalore, India

K. Duraipandi, MD, FICO, DNB
Department of Ophthalmology, Dr. Rajendra Prasad Center for Ophthalmic Sciences,
All India Institute of Medical Sciences, New Delhi, India

A.V. Pai, PhD
Ocular Pharmacology and Pharmacy, Dr. Rajendra Prasad Center for Ophthalmic Sciences,
All India Institute of Medical Sciences, New Delhi, India

T. Velpandian (ed.), *Pharmacology of Ocular Therapeutics*,
DOI 10.1007/978-3-319-25498-2_9

9.1 Antiangiogenic Agents

Atul Kumar, S.N. Mohanraj, Kavitha Duraipandi

9.1.1 Introduction

Angiogenesis is the formation of new blood vessels from preexisting vessels. It is a normal process in growth and development as well as in wound healing. However, this process can occur in pathological conditions such as in transition of tumors from dormant to malignant state. The process of angiogenesis is tightly regulated by balance of two sets of counteracting cellular signaling molecules: angiogenic activators and inhibitors. Vascular Endothelial Growth Factor (VEGF) is one of the principal molecules among a large number of proangiogenic growth factors that induce migration, proliferation, and formation of tubes by endothelial cells of the basal lamina.

Ocular angiogenesis is the hallmark of many ocular diseases like diabetic retinopathy (DR), vascular occlusions, age-related macular degeneration (ARMD), and retinopathy of prematurity (Campochiaro and Hackett 2003; Gariano 2003; Gariano and Gardner 2005; Witmer et al. 2003). The major trigger for angiogenesis in these conditions is tissue hypoxia which arises due to compromised vascular supply that cannot cope up to high metabolic demand of associated neuronal tissue. This condition is further aggravated by oxidative stress and inflammatory mediators.

As in generalized angiogenesis, vascular endothelial growth factor (VEGF) plays a major role in the process of retinal neovascularization (Blaauwgeers et al. 1999; Gariano and Gardner 2005; Witmer et al. 2003). VEGF is mainly released by Muller cells, the retinal pigment epithelium (RPE), astrocytes, ganglion cells, and endothelial cells. Muller cells and astrocytes are the largest sources of VEGF in hypoxic conditions (Gerhardt et al. 2003; Gogat et al. 2004; Patan 2000).

Angiogenesis is known to occur in a series of stages with immediate early events caused due to growth factors and signaling, followed by early events that comprise of change in genetic programming of vascular cells, followed by invasive angiogenesis culminating in a resolution stage wherein cells revert to their quiescent stage. The process of angiogenesis is an orderly set of events as follows (Cheresh and Stupack 2008):

1. The blood vessels providing nutrients and oxygen throughout the body are composed of an inner lining of endothelial cells that completely encircle the lumen. The basal lamina surrounds the endothelial cells and pericytes (Hynes 1992). Pericytes are responsible for regulating endothelial cell proliferation, survival, migration, differentiation, and vascular branching via selective inhibition of endothelial cell growth (Hellstrom et al. 2001). The basal lamina provides mechanical support for cell attachment, serves as a substrate for cell migration, separates adjacent tissue, and acts as a barrier for the passage of macromolecules (Hynes 1992).

2. In healthy adults, a balance of growth factor signaling keeps endothelial cells in a quiescent or resting state to monitor and supply sufficient amounts of oxygen to surrounding tissues. To achieve this, blood vessels have receptors for sensing oxygen and hypoxia that allow minute-to-minute readjustment of vessel diameter (to adjust the blood flow) to keep pace with oxygen demand.
3. Hypoxia or endogenous signals induce the release of signaling factors (such as VEGF, bFGF, Ang-2, and chemokines) to promote endothelial cell migration (Rousseau et al. 2000).
4. As a result, there is disruption of endothelial cell junctions leading to vascular permeability. As a result, various plasma-borne components leak into local interstitial tissues (Lamalice et al. 2007).
5. Consequently, pericytes detach from the vessel (Ang-2 signaling), and as the vessel dilates, endothelial cells lose their contact with the basal lamina.
6. This is followed by coordinated cytoskeletal remodeling and disruption of cell-cell junctions: this is assisted by signaling factors such as neuropilin, VGEF/VGEFR, NOTCH/DLL4, and JAGGED1 which release matrix metalloproteases (MT1-MMP) to degrade the basement membrane and remodel the extracellular matrix.
7. New focal contacts (tip cells) are formed which extend numerous filopodia (via semaphorin, ephrin, and integrin guidance signals) toward angiogenic stimuli (VEGF gradient).
8. Stalk cells follow the tip cell and proliferate and extend the sprout. Proliferating stalk cells establish junctions with neighboring endothelial cells and release molecules such as EGFL7 (an endothelial cell chemoattractant expressed by proliferating endothelial cells) that bind to extracellular membrane components and regulate vascular lumen formation.
9. Fusion of neighboring branches occurs when two tip cells encounter each other, establish EC-EC junctions (VE-cadherin, Ang-1), and form a continuous lumen. Extracellular matrix is deposited to establish a new basement membrane (TIMPs), endothelial cell proliferation ceases, and pericytes are recruited to stabilize the new vessel (PDGFR/PDGF-B, Ang-1).
10. Once blood flow is established, the perfusion of oxygen and nutrient reduces angiogenic stimuli (VEGF expression) and inactivates endothelial cell oxygen sensors, reestablishing the quiescent state of the blood vessel (Cheresh and Stupack 2008).

9.1.2 *Factors that Modulate Angiogenesis*

Angiogenesis is controlled by a number of growth factors and inhibitors. Some of the well-known angiogenic (stimulatory) growth factors are angiogenin, angiopoietin-1, Del-1, and fibroblast growth factors: acidic (aFGF) and basic (bFGF), follistatin, granulocyte colony-stimulating factor (G-CSF), hepatocyte growth factor

(HGF)/scatter factor (SF), interleukin-8 (IL-8), leptin, midkine, placental growth factor, platelet-derived endothelial cell growth factor (PD-ECGF), platelet-derived growth factor-BB (PDGF-BB), pleiotrophin (PTN), progranulin, proliferin, transforming growth factor-alpha (TGF-alpha), transforming growth factor-beta (TGF-beta), tumor necrosis factor-alpha (TNF-alpha), and vascular endothelial growth factor (VEGF)/vascular permeability factor (VPF).

Angiogenic inhibitors are angioarrestin, angiostatin (plasminogen fragment), antiangiogenic antithrombin III, arrestin, chondromodulin, canstatin, cartilage-derived inhibitor (CDI), CD59 complement fragment, endostatin (collagen XVIII fragment), endorepellin, fibronectin fragment, fibronectin fragment (anastellin), Gro-beta, heparinases, heparin hexasaccharide fragment, human chorionic gonadotropin (hCG), interferon alpha/gamma, interferon-inducible protein (IP-10), interleukin-12, kringle 5 (plasminogen fragment), metalloproteinase inhibitors (TIMPs), 2-Methoxyestradiol, PEX, pigment epithelium-derived factor (PEDF), placental ribonuclease inhibitor, plasminogen activator inhibitor, platelet factor-4 (PF4), prolactin 16kD fragment, proliferin-related protein (PRP), prothrombin kringle 2, retinoids, soluble Fms-like tyrosine kinase-1 (S-Flt-1), targeting fibronectin-binding integrins, tetrahydrocortisol-S, thrombospondin-1 (TSP-1) and −2, transforming growth factor-beta (TGF-b), troponin I, tumstatin, vasculostatin, and vasostatin (calreticulin fragment)

9.1.3 Angiogenesis in Disease

In various disease conditions, dysregulated angiogenesis has been seen. Angiogenesis-dependent diseases result when new blood vessels either grow excessively or insufficiently. Excessive angiogenesis occurs in diseases such as cancer, ischemic heart or limbs, rheumatoid arthritis, psoriasis, peptic ulcers, bowel atresias, vascular malformations, hemangiomas, diabetic blindness, age-related macular degeneration, and more than 70 other conditions. As a result, diseased cells and tissue produce abnormal amounts of angiogenic growth factors, overwhelming the effects of natural angiogenesis inhibitors. New blood vessels grow and feed diseased tissues; new vessels are abnormal and leaky and can destroy normal tissues. In the case of cancer, the abnormal vessels allow tumor cells to escape into the circulation and lodge in other organs (tumor metastases). Antiangiogenic therapies, aimed at halting new blood vessel growth, are used to treat these conditions. Insufficient angiogenesis occurs in diseases such as coronary artery disease, stroke, and chronic wounds. In these conditions, blood vessel growth is inadequate, and circulation is not properly restored, leading to the risk of tissue death. Insufficient angiogenesis occurs when tissues do not produce adequate amounts of angiogenic growth factors. Therapeutic angiogenesis therapies, aimed at stimulating new blood vessel growth with growth factors, are being developed to treat these conditions.

9.1.4 Types of Pathological Angiogenesis

Pathological ocular angiogenesis is classified into two major forms: preretinal angiogenesis, arising from the retinal vessels, and subretinal (or choroidal neovascularization) angiogenesis, arising from the choriocapillaris.

Preretinal angiogenesis generally develops during vascular occlusion (where there is capillary non-perfusion along with ischemia) in conditions like diabetic retinopathy wherein VEGF is secreted by the RPE, Muller cells, and astrocytes. During this condition, abnormal vessels breech the internal limiting membrane of the retina and breakthrough into the vitreous cavity. These vessels in the vitreous cavity acquire fibrous component and form fibrovascular membrane that bleed leading to severe vision loss. Fibrovascular membranes also cause tractional retinal detachment when not treated adequately by retinal photocoagulation. When the retinal ischemia is global, angiogenesis and scarring occur in the anterior chamber angle of the iris and cause neovascular glaucoma which responds poorly to antiglaucoma medications.

Subretinal neovascularization is associated with pathological changes in the retinal pigment epithelium, Bruch's membrane, and the choriocapillaris. Any breech in the Bruch's membrane triggers the healing response in the form of neovascularization. Oxidative stress, local inflammatory mediators, and hypoxia also play an important role in the sequence of events. The exact role of each of these contributory factors is yet to be ascertained. Subretinal neovascularization can develop either between the retinal pigment epithelium and Bruch's membrane (occult choroidal neovascularization), or between the retinal pigment epithelium and the neurosensory retina (classic choroidal neovascularization).

Subretinal neovascularization can regress, leaving an area of retinal atrophy, or can progress to be ultimately replaced by fibrotic scar over a period of time. Neovascular membranes can also bleed producing massive subretinal hemorrhage which can break through the internal limiting membrane into the vitreous cavity. Ultimately, the overlying neuroretina will degenerate, leading to loss of central vision, contrast sensitivity, and color vision.

In this chapter, we discuss various antiangiogenic agents which inhibit the vasculogenesis cascade at different steps. These include the ones which have been approved for clinical use, the ones which are used off label, and the ones still undergoing trials.

9.1.5 Tyrosine Kinase Inhibitors

The PI3K/AKT/MTOR (phosphoinositide 3 kinase/Akt/mammalian target of rapamycin) pathway is an intracellular signaling pathway important in regulating cell cycle. Second-generation inhibitors of PI3K/Akt/mTOR pathway have been found to be efficacious in managing various stages of disease progression in DR thus presenting a unique opportunity for the management of neovascularization.

During early stages of neovascularization, mTOR inhibitors suppress HIF-1α and VEGF thus preventing leakage and breakdown of the blood-retinal barrier. These inhibitors impart a pronounced inhibitory effect on inflammation (which is an early component with diverse ramifications) influencing the progression of DR. mTOR inhibitors suppress IKK and NF-κB along with downstream inflammatory cytokines, chemokines, and adhesion molecules. These inhibitors also suppress several growth factors that play pivotal roles in the induction of pathological angiogenesis (Jorge and David 2011).

Inhibition of the PI3K/Akt/mTOR pathway that disrupts the Akt-RhoB interaction is postulated to promote endothelial cell death based on experimental evidence (Adini et al. 2003). Prevention of endothelial cell proliferation and enhancement of endothelial cell apoptosis could serve as a treatment modality to delay or prevent progression of vasculopathies as observed in diabetic retinopathy since enhanced migration of endothelial cells is a requirement for neovascularization to occur.

Sirolimus (MacuSight, Union City, Calif, USA) and Palomid 529 (Paloma Pharmaceuticals, Inc. Jamaica Plain, Mass, USA) and everolimus (Novartis) are currently being evaluated in NIH-sponsored trials for ocular indications. Sirolimus is in phase II trial to treat diabetic macular edema and advanced ARMD. Palomid 529 is being evaluated for ARMD (Clinical Trial 2008; Sherris 2007). Everolimus in combination with ranibizumab is in phase II trial for patients with wet ARMD. However, several adverse events have been reported with the tyrosine kinase inhibitors particularly in diabetics such as gastrointestinal effects (Soefje et al. 2011), hematological (Sofroniadou and Goldsmith 2011), decreased glucose tolerance, hyperglycemia, and hypertriglyceridemia (Majewski et al. 2004). Cutaneous and oral ulceration with delayed wound healing (Mills et al. 2008), renal toxicity (Letavernier and Legendre 2008), and infertility (Boobes et al. 2010) have also been reported. However, these adverse events have been found to be reversible and medically manageable.

9.1.6 *Small Interfering RNA (siRNA)*

Small interfering RNA (siRNA) is another approach that is used to inhibit VEGF expression. PF-655 is a synthetic siRNA known to inhibit the expression of DNA damage-inducible transcript 4 protein (DDIT4; also known as RTP801) associated with pathological retinal neovascularization in animal models (Brafman et al. 2004). Expression of RTP801 is rapidly upregulated in response to ischemia, hypoxia, and/or oxidative stress. The mechanism of action of PF-655 is different from that of different types of VEGF inhibitors (Shoshani et al. 2002). Intravitreal injection of PF-655 in preclinical animal models of laser-induced choroidal neovascularization (CNV) has been found to inhibit RTP801 expression and induce expression of anti-angiogenic and neurotrophic factors leading to subsequent reduction of CNV volume, vessel leakage, and infiltration of inflammatory cells into the choroid. It is currently in phase II trials for diabetic macular edema and wet ARMD (clinical trial).

Bevasiranib is a naked, 21-nucleotide-long siRNA that specifically targets VEGF. Upon introduction into the cell, this siRNA binds to and activates the RNA-induced silencing complex (RISC). The RISC in turn targets and degrades mRNA molecules that are complementary to the introduced siRNA. A single activated RISC complex can bind to and destroy hundreds of mRNAs, thus preventing translation and protein synthesis (Liu et al. 2010).

Bevasiranib is known to downregulate VEGF-A mRNA. However, this drug has failed to achieve the expected endpoint of "stabilization of vision" in treated individuals. This could be because siRNAs need to be formulated to achieve cell permeation in order to cause bona fide RNA interference. They also need to be modified to avoid off-target effects and recognition of their nucleotide structure by the innate immune system (Hornung et al. 2005; Kleinman et al. 2008; Sledz et al. 2003).

9.1.7 Pigment Epithelium-Derived Factor (PEDF)

PEDF is one of the most potent known antiangiogenic proteins found in humans. Ad(GV)PEDF.11D, is an E1-, partial E3-, E4-deleted replication-deficient, adenovirus serotype 5, gene transfer vector. The transgene in this vector is cDNA for human pigment epithelium-derived factor (PEDF). While Ad(GV)PEDF.11D is able to transduce many somatic cell types, the natural barrier to other tissues created by the retina limits the ability of Ad(GV)PEDF.11D to affect tissues other than in the eye.

Intravitreal administration of Ad(GV)PEDF.11D provides a convenient means of delivering PEDF to the relevant cells within the eye that is likely to result in a more prolonged duration of effect than administration of the PEDF protein alone (Rasmussen et al. 2001). Pigment epithelium-derived factor (PEDF) has an antagonistic effect on endothelial cell proliferation and migration, and its levels are decreased in ARMD (Bhutto et al. 2008; Dawson et al. 1999; Holekamp et al. 2002). A phase I clinical trial has been initiated using an adenoviral vector (AdGVPEDF.11D) to deliver PEDF via intravitreal injections.

9.1.8 Anti-VEGF Agents

Vascular endothelial growth factor (VEGF), also known as vascular permeability factor (VPF), is a signal protein produced by cells under normal as well as pathological conditions like hypoxia, ischemia, and neoplasia. VEGF stimulates vasculogenesis and angiogenesis. It is a part of the system that attempts to restore the oxygen supply to tissues under hypoxic and ischemic conditions. Serum concentration of VEGF has been found to be high in bronchial asthma and diabetes mellitus (Cooper et al. 1999).

The VEGF family in mammals comprises of five different molecules, namely, VEGF-A, placenta growth factor 1 and 2 (PGF- 1 and 2), VEGF-B, VEGF-C, and

VEGF-D. VEGF-A acts mostly on cells of the vascular endothelium. It also has effects on a number of other cell types like monocytes and macrophages stimulating their migration in neurons, cancer cells, and kidney epithelial cells. In vitro, VEGF-A has been shown to stimulate endothelial cell mitogenesis and cell migration. VEGF-A is also vasodilator and increases microvascular permeability and was originally referred to as vascular permeability factor. There are several isoforms of VEGF-A, including VEGF-A121, VEGF-A145, VEGF-A148, VEGF-A183, VEGF-A189, and VEGF-A206; the best characterized proangiogenic isoform of VEGF is VEGF-A165 (Harper and Bates 2008; Nowak et al. 2010).

Monoclonal antibodies against VEGF were first developed as an intravenous treatment for metastatic colorectal cancer (Homsi and Daud 2007; Los et al. 2007). The three available anti-VEGF agents for intravitreal use are bevacizumab (Avastin) and ranibizumab (lucentis) and pegaptanib. Ranibizumab is a shorter 48-kDa antibody fragment (κ isotype) that binds to the receptors of biologically active VEGF-A, including VEGF-110. It blocks the binding of VEGF-A to VEGR receptors, VEGFR1 and VEGFR2 receptors on endothelial cells (Patan 2000). Bevacizumab, however, is a larger whole antibody of 149 kDa and possesses two antigen-binding domains for its receptors Flt-1 and KDR. It binds to all isoforms of VEGF7. Pegaptanib sodium is a 50-kDa aptamer, a pegylated modified oligonucleotide that adopts a specific 3D configuration and has a high affinity for extracellular VEGF-165, the isoform of VEGF-A implicated in ocular angiogenesis (Eyetech Study Group 2002).

The difference in molecular weights of these molecules may determine their potential difference in efficacy and their duration of action. Detailed safety profiles and risks of adverse effects are now available for these agents as they have been used extensively in patients for the treatment of ARMD, diabetic macular edema, and retinal vascular occlusions (Tolentino 2011). Furthermore, the incidence of raised IOP and development of lens opacity with anti-VEGF agents is negligible when compared with intravitreal steroid injections (Jager et al. 2004; Sampat and Garg 2010).

9.1.9 VEGF Trap

It's a fusion protein comprised of segments of the extracellular domains of human vascular endothelial growth factor receptors 1 (VEGFR1) and 2 (VEGFR2) fused to the constant region (Fc) of human immunoglobulin G1 (IgG1) with potential anti-angiogenic activity. Aflibercept acts as a soluble decoy receptor, binds to proangiogenic vascular endothelial growth factors (VEGFs), thereby preventing VEGFs from binding to their cell receptors.

Aflibercept binds to circulating VEGFs and acts like a "VEGF trap" (Stewart 2012). It thereby inhibits the activity of the vascular endothelial growth factor subtypes VEGF-A and VEGF-B, as well as to placental growth factor (PGF), inhibiting the growth of new blood vessels in the choriocapillaris (Saishin et al. 2003). VEGF trap has been found to be beneficial in ARMD (Cho et al. 2013) and diabetic macular edema (Korobelnik et al. 2014). Aflibercept has been approved by the FDA for the management of ARMD since Nov 2011 and DME from July 2014 (FDA-approved aflibercept for diabetic retinopathy in patients with diabetic macular edema in March 2015).

9.1.10 VEGF Inhibitors: AAV2-sFLT01

AAV2-sFLT01 is an adeno-associated virus (AAV) (Maclachlan et al. 2011) that expresses a modified soluble Flt1 receptor designed to neutralize the proangiogenic activities of vascular endothelial growth factor (Maclachlan et al. 2011; Takahashi et al. 2009) (VEGF) AAV2-sFLT01 which produces a soluble VEGFR1 that can bind to free VEGF (Ambati et al. 2006; Kendall and Thomas 1993) to interrupt VEGF signaling. VEGF-A binds primarily to VEGFR1 and VEGFR2, both of which are tyrosine kinases (Ferrara et al. 2003). It is under phase I trial in the management of wet ARMD via an intravitreal injection (clinical trial).

9.1.11 Chemokine CC Motif Receptor 3 Blockers

Another approach that is currently undergoing testing involves the blockade of chemokine CC motif receptor 3, which mediates angiogenic signaling initiated by eotaxins (Takeda et al. 2009). Takeda et al. (2009) demonstrated that the eosinophil/mast cell chemokine receptor CCR3 is specifically expressed in choroidal neovascular endothelial cells in humans with ARMD and that despite the expression of its ligands eotaxin-1, eotaxin-2, and eotaxin-3, neither eosinophils nor mast cells are present in human choroidal neovascularization (CNV). Genetic or pharmacologic targeting of CCR3 or eotaxins has been found to inhibit injury-induced CNV in mice. CNV suppression by CCR3 blockade has been found to be due to direct inhibition of endothelial cell proliferation (and was uncoupled from inflammation, since it occurred in mice lacking eosinophils or mast cells) and to be independent of macrophage and neutrophil recruitment. CCR3 blockade has been more effective at reducing CNV than VEGF-A neutralization when used in the treatment of ARMD and, unlike VEGF-A blockade, is not toxic to the mouse retina. In vivo imaging with CCR3-targeting quantum dots located spontaneous CNV in mice where diagnosis with fluorscein angiography was not possible. Takeda et al. (2009) concluded that CCR3 targeting might reduce vision loss due to ARMD through early detection and therapeutic angioinhibition (Takeda et al. 2009).

9.1.12 Other Tyrosine Kinase Inhibitors

Pazopanib is a tyrosine kinase inhibitor that inhibits VEGFR1, VEGFR2, VEGFR3, PDGFR, c-KIT, and FGFR1 (Kumar et al. 2007). Pazopanib is effective in preclinical models of CNV (Takahashi et al. 2009). Pazopanib, formulated as eye drops, is under investigation for the treatment of neovascular ARMD as a self-administered, potentially lower burden therapy (clinical trial). Pazopanib inhibits the same pathway that has been clinically validated in ARMD with anti-VEGF therapies, but with inhibition at the tyrosine kinase receptor level. Additional benefit may come from inhibition of the proangiogenic platelet-derived growth factor pathway. Inhibition of PDGFR-α and PDGFR-β, in combination with inhibition of the VEGF pathway, may lead to regression of aberrant blood vessels (Jo et al. 2006; Takahashi et al. 2009).

Vatalanib (PTK787 or PTK/ZK) is a small molecule protein kinase inhibitor that is orally administrated and inhibits angiogenesis. Oral administration of vatalanib blocks phosphorylation of VEGF and PDGF receptors and provides inhibition of retinal neovascularization. There is no effect on mature retinal vessels. Vatalanib has been tested previously as a treatment for CNV in phase I and phase II clinical studies (clinical trial).

AL39324 is an intravitreally administered tyrosine kinase inhibitor that is in a phase II clinical trial in combination with ranibizumab (clinical trial).

TG100801 is a tyrosine kinase inhibitor that binds and inhibits VEGFR and PDGFR. It is administered as an eye drop and has been found to suppress CNV and retinal edema (Palanki et al. 2008). A phase I trial was completed successfully, but a phase II trial was discontinued because of corneal toxicity.

9.1.13 Nicotinic Acetylcholine Receptor (nAChR) Pathway Inhibitors: Mecamylamine

VEGF inhibition can also be achieved by preventing the activation of the nicotinic acetylcholine receptor (nAChR) pathway in the vasculature, which inhibits VEGF-induced angiogenesis in endothelial cells (Heeschen et al. 2002). ATG-3 is an eye drop formulation of mecamylamine, an antagonist of the nAChR pathway (Kiuchi et al. 2008). It is the first antiangiogenic eye drop that has been studied in humans. ATG-3 has successfully completed two phase II clinical trials, one in patients with diabetic macular edema (Campochiaro et al. 2010) and the other in patients with wet ARMD who were receiving anti-VEGF treatments.

9.1.13.1 Anti-Sphingosine-1-Phosphate (S1P) Monoclonal Antibody

Sphingosine-1-phosphate (S1P) is the extracellular ligand for S1P receptor 1 (also known as EDG1), a G protein-coupled lysophospholipid receptor, and it is a proangiogenic and profibrotic mediator (Ozaki et al. 2003; Watterson et al. 2007). Intravitreous injection of an anti-S1P monoclonal antibody inhibited CNV formation and subretinal collagen deposition in a preclinical model of laser-induced CNV and in a preclinical model of diabetic retinopathy (Caballero et al. 2009; Xie et al. 2009). A humanized S1P monoclonal antibody (iSONEP) is under clinical trial in patients with wet ARMD (clinical trial). iSONEP was well tolerated, and no drug-related serious adverse events were observed in any of the patients. iSONEP also exhibited positive biological effects (including lesion regression, reduction of retinal thickness, and resolution of pigment epithelium detachment). The mechanisms responsible for the positive effects exerted by S1P appear to be independent to those of anti-VEGF agents, indicating the potential of S1P antibodies to serve as a monotherapy (or an adjunct therapy to anti-VEGF agents) for the treatment of neovascular ARMD and polypoidal choroidal vasculopathy.

9.1.13.2 Anti-α5β1 Integrin Monoclonal Antibody

Endothelial cell migration involves interactions between integrins (transmembrane heterodimeric proteins) and extracellular matrix ligands. α5β1 integrin is expressed on the surface of vascular endothelial cells and mediates cell migration (Orecchia et al. 2003). Intravitreal JSM6427 (Jerini Inc) is a potent and selective inhibitor of integrin α5β1. Its potency as an inhibitor of angiogenesis has been demonstrated in animal models of CNVM blocking angiogenesis through inhibition of integrin-mediated signaling and has the potential to inhibit the cellular responses to growth factors, cytokines, and other inflammatory mediators.

Intravitreal administration of volociximab has resulted in strong inhibition of rabbit and primate retinal neovascularization. In monkeys with laser-induced choroidal neovascularization (CNV), volociximab significantly inhibited CNV proliferation and reduced the degree of lesion formation. In a rabbit model, volociximab administered either intravenously or intravitreally prior to the onset of neovascularization significantly reduced angiogenesis as compared to control.

Thus, JSM6427 and volociximab both bind to α5β1 integrin and block the migration of endothelial cells. Both agents have been shown to inhibit CNV formation in preclinical models (Zahn et al. 2009). They are in phase I trial for the treatment of ARMD (clinical trial).

9.1.13.3 Fosbretabulin (Combretastatin A-4 Phosphate)

Fosbretabulin is a vascular disrupting agent, and its active metabolite is combretastatin A4 (CA4) (Pettit et al. 1995). The active metabolite CA4 binds to tubulin and prevents microtubule polymerization in proliferating endothelial cells, thus inducing vessel regression (Dark et al. 1997). In animal models, CA4 has been demonstrated to inhibit retinal neovascularization and suppress the development of CNV (Griggs et al. 2002; Nambu et al. 2003). Currently phase II trials are underway to evaluate the safety and efficacy of fosbretabulin in patients with myopic CNVM (clinical trial).

9.1.13.4 E10030: A Pegylated Aptamer

E10030 (Ophthotech), an antiplatelet-derived growth factor (anti-PDGF-B) aptamer, strongly binds to PDGF-β. Platelet-derived growth factor-B plays a key role in recruiting the pericytes that envelop the new vessels and make them more resistant to the anti-VEGF attack. Pericyte recruitment is a crucial step in vascular maturation and stabilization. PDGF has a key role in this process (Benjamin et al. 1998; Jo et al. 2006).

With this in mind, E10030—a pegylated aptamer that inhibits PDGF-β—was developed. Inhibition of PDGF results in the stripping of pericytes from endothelial cells, which increases the sensitivity of mature CNV to VEGF inhibition. PDGF inhibition may therefore synergize with VEGF inhibition in CNV treatment. In a phase I dose-escalating study, some CNV regression was observed in over 90 % of patients receiving the combination therapy of E10030 and ranibizumab, compared to about 10 % of patients receiving ranibizumab alone (Boyer and Ophthotech Anti-PDGF in AMD Study Group 2009). A phase II study is currently underway.

9.2 Photodynamic Therapy

Anuradha V. Pai

9.2.1 Introduction/Definition

Also known as photochemotherapy, it is a form of phototherapy using a photosensitizer (a nontoxic light-sensitive chemical which when selectively exposed to light becomes toxic) and causes damage to target malignant and other diseased cells. This method is used for both disease diagnosis and treatment (Jia and Jia 2012).

The spectrum of possible applications of PDT encompasses the entire range of infectious (viral, bacterial, fungal, protozoal) disorders, epidermal and dermal inflammatory diseases, tumors of lymphocytes, adnexal diseases, and premature skin aging due to sun exposure. With PDT, it is possible to eradicate pathogens in simple locations such as oral cavities as well as in deep-seated bone marrow. Nowadays' PDT is being explored as a new line of antimicrobial therapy in order to eradicate drug-resistant pathogens.

Photodynamic therapy (PDT) has also recently grown as a proven method of treatment for various types of cancers with a proven potential to target even HIV and MRSA (methicillin-resistant *Staphylococcus aureus*). Another key indication is for small areas of cancer that are unsuitable for or have persisted or recurred after conventional management. It can be applied in areas already exposed to the maximum safe dose of radiotherapy. Photodynamic therapy (PDT) is of particular value for precancer and early cancers of the skin and mouth because of good cosmetic and functional results.

PDT also has considerable potential in arterial diseases for preventing restenosis after balloon angioplasty and in the treatment of infectious diseases, where the responsible organisms are accessible to both the photosensitizer and light. New developments on the horizon include techniques for increasing the selectivity for cancers, such as coupling photosensitizers to antibodies, and for stimulating immunological responses, but many further preclinical and clinical studies are needed to establish PDT's role in routine clinical practice (Bown 2013).

9.2.2 *Photodynamic Therapy Process*

Most PDT applications involve three key components: a photosensitizer, a light source, and tissue oxygen. A photosensitizer is a chemical compound that gets converted to an excited state upon absorption of light and forms free radicals which react with oxygen to produce a highly reactive state of oxygen (reactive oxygen species (ROS)) known as singlet oxygen. Exposure of cell to light energy wavelengths is typically in the visible region. ROS produces cell inactivation and death through modification of intracellular components thus becoming highly cytotoxic within few microseconds of activation. Generally, the photosensitizer is applied locally to target area or the photosensitive targets are locally excited with light. In the localized treatment of internal tissues and cancers, photosensitizers are administered intravenously and light is delivered through endoscopes or fiber-optic catheters. Once the photosensitizer is localized to the intended area (tissue/organ), an appropriate wavelength of light is chosen in order to excite the photosensitizer.

9.2.2.1 Mechanism of Photodynamic Therapy

Photodynamic process begins when photosensitizer absorbs a photon and gets converted into an excited (singlet) state. This singlet state of photosensitizer undergoes simultaneous or sequential decay resulting in intramolecular energy transfer reactions which are of three types. Type I reaction involves photooxidation by radicals, type II reaction involves photooxidation by singlet oxygen, and in type III reaction, photoreaction does not involve oxygen. Photosensitizer in excited singlet state readily decays back to the ground state with the emission of light (fluorescence) or heat. Sometimes it goes into a "triplet state." In addition, excited molecules also undergo type III reactions. Photosensitizer in triplet state reacts with ground state oxygen to produce singlet state oxygen, then decay to ground state by phosphorescence, or undergo type I and III reactions. Singlet oxygen generated during the process is a highly reactive form of oxygen and is highly damaging species with the potential to cause blood flow stasis, vascular collapse, and/or vascular leakage ultimately leading to tumor ablation. PDT has also been demonstrated to induce apoptosis causing orderly elimination of unwanted cells (Sibata et al. 2000).

9.2.2.2 Light Used

The light source for PDT can range from an ordinary light bulb to a diode array (emitting a broad band incoherent spectrum) or a laser. Broad-spectrum light sources such as xenon arc lamps or slide projectors equipped with red filters (to eliminate short wavelengths) are used for in vitro and preclinical in vivo studies of tumors. Lasers are standard light sources for PDT as they are monochromatic, have high power output, and can be easily coupled to fiber optics for endoscopic light delivery to localized areas in body cavity. The most common lasers are tunable dye lasers

(Sibata et al. 2000). Argon lasers have been employed for the treatment of human corneal neovascularization (Sheppard et al. 2006) and neovascular maculopathy (Barbara et al. 1991). Copper-pumped dye laser, a double laser consisting of KTP (potassium titanyl phosphate/YAG (yttrium aluminum garnet)) medium, has been used in dermatology and in facial telangiectasias (Cassuto et al. 2000), while LED (light-emitting diode) has been used in treatment of viral warts (Ohtsuki et al. 2009).

9.2.2.3 Dyes Used

Photofrin was the first US FDA-approved photosensitizer for treatment of cancer. Thereafter, a variety of dye sensitizers have been developed and approved for PDT treatment of skin and organ diseases ranging from simple bacterial infections (acne vulgaris) to more serious cancers. Some of the very common dyes used in the treatment of photodynamic therapy are listed as follows:

(i) Psoralen compounds in conjunction with UVA (300–400 nm) radiation are used in the treatment of psoriasis, atopic dermatitis, seborrheic dermatoses, histiocytosis, lichen planus, mycosis fungoides, polymorphous light eruption, pityriasis lichenoides, lymphomatoid papulosis, prurigo, palmar and plantar pustulosis, and vitiligo. Examples of psoralen photosensitizers include 5-methoxypsoralen, 8-methoxypsoralen, and trioxsalen.
(ii) Porphyrinoid photosensitizers porphyrin, chlorin, bacteriochlorin, pheophorbide, bacteriopheophorbide, texaphyrin, porphycene, and phthalocyanine.
(iii) Non-porphyrin dyes are anthraquinones, phenothiazines, xanthenes, cyanines, and curcuminoids.

9.2.2.4 Molecules Used

Photofrin is the only photosensitizer approved by US FDA for palliation of various types of cancer such as cancer of the esophagus and Barrett esophagus, endobronchial cancer, certain skin cancers such as basal cell carcinoma and squamous cell carcinoma, and some tumors of the vagina, vulva, and cervix that can be reached by activating light. Aminolevulinic acid has been approved for the treatment of actinic keratosis of face or scalp. Methyl ester of ALA has been approved by US FDA in July 2004 for treatment of some types of actinic keratoses of face and scalp. Verteporfin (Visudyne) had been approved for treatment of pathologic myopia, ocular histoplasmosis, and for age-related macular degeneration.

9.2.2.5 Side Effects

Photofrin comes with the side effects of accumulation. Also skin and eyes of the patient become photosensitive with Photofrin treatment. Application of aminolevulinic acid causes redness and tingling or burning sensation to skin. Photosensitivity reactions can also be observed with methyl ester of ALA, and therefore, this drug is not recommended for people whose skin is sensitive to light, in immunosuppressed individuals, and those with peanut or almond allergy.

Some of the other general adverse effects include burns, swelling, pain, and scarring of surrounding tissues (Dolmans et al. 2003). Skin and eyes become sensitive to light. Stenosis and perforation of hollow organs have also been observed in some cases (Wittmann et al. 2014). PDT has also been reported to cause damage to DNA such as strand breaks, degradation, DNA-protein cross-links, and chromosomal aberrations and mutations. Other shortcomings include limitation of treatment depth due to ineffective penetration of light. Revascularization of treated areas is one of the biggest adverse effects that pose threat to benefits of PDT. In some cases, damage to vascular endothelium leading to increased vascular permeability, platelet aggregation, blood flow stasis, vasoconstriction, and ultimately vascular occlusion has been observed. Vascular damage further leads to hypoxia-related re-angiogenesis necessitating re-treatment (Verteporfin in Photodynamic Therapy Study Group 2001).

9.2.2.6 Advantages of PDT

(i) It has no long-term side effects when used properly.
(ii) It is less invasive than surgery.
(iii) It usually takes only a short time and is most often done as an outpatient.
(iv) It can be targeted very precisely.
(v) It can be used to treat one lesion at a time.
(vi) Unlike radiation, PDT can be repeated many times at the same site if needed.
(vii) Since this therapy uses nonionizing radiation, there is relatively rapid recovery.
(viii) There is little or no scarring after the site heals.
(ix) It often costs less than other cancer treatments.
(x) It can also be used in combination with other therapies so as to achieve synergistic effects.

Calculations for doses applied/based on body surface area: Successful treatment with PDT is highly dependent upon the light dose delivered to the target tissue. The unit of total energy of light is joule (J) and is determined by watt (W) multiplied by time (s). The number of photons (N) in a joule depends on the wavelength (λ) of light. If two different wavelengths of light are used, the number of photons per joule varies as the inverse ratio of the wavelength (hc/λ, where $h = 6.623 \times 10–34$ J is Planck's constant and $c = 2.998 \times 108$ m/s is the speed of light). Another factor that needs to be considered is fluence rate (i.e., rate of light delivered; fluence rate= W/area). Fluence rate, and thus treatment time, depends on the light source used. It the light is delivered at a high rate, significant heating of the tissue and its surrounding may take place. Generally, fluence rates less than 200 mW/cm^2 (for microlens) or 400 mW/cm (for cylindrical diffusers) should be used in order to avoid thermal damage to the normal tissues (Sibata et al. 2000).

9.2.2.7 Photodynamic Therapy in Ophthalmic Disorders

PDT finds widespread use in treatment of ocular diseases. In ophthalmology, PDT is used to treat ARMD and malignant cancers. This is because maintaining the mechanical integrity of hollow organs is easy with PDT therapy since its biological effect is different from surgery, radiotherapy, and chemotherapy as connective tissues like collagen are largely unaffected. In ophthalmology, it is established for all types of ARMD such as nonexudative, exudative, dry, and wet ARMD. PDT with verteporfin along with laser photocoagulation and administration of pegaptanib sodium is known to reduce the risk of vision loss in selected cases of neovascular ARMD as well as wet ARMD (55–56). PDT with verteporfin causes stabilization or improvement of visual acuity in patients suffering from chorioretinal anastomosis (Silva et al. 2004).

Some of the other applications of PDT are in treatment of ocular herpes using antimetabolites ara A and F3T (Pavan-Langston and Langston 1975), to reduce subretinal fluid in choroidal nevus with serous macular detachment (Garcia-Arumi et al. 2012), to induce closure of superficial vasculature of pigmented choroidal melanoma with verteporfin (Tuncer et al. 2012) and with bevacizumab (Canal-Fontcuberta et al. 2012), for the treatment of progressive keratoconus using collagen cross-linking by the photosensitizer riboflavin and UVA light (Wollensak 2006), for the treatment of chronic cases of central serous chorioretinopathy with verteporfin (64–66), for the treatment of polypoidal choroidal vasculopathy [using ICGA-guided photodynamic therapy (PDT) with verteporfin, combined PDT, and antivascular endothelial growth factor (VEGF) therapy (anti-VEGF therapy)] (Wong and Lai 2013). PDT with intravitreal bevacizumab has also shown good visual improvements in cases of polypoidal choroidal vasculopathy (Fan et al. 2014). Preoperative PDT has also been useful in reducing the potential of bleeding at the time of tissue biopsy (Canal-Fontcuberta et al. 2012).

9.2.3 Photodynamic Therapy in Angiogenesis

PDT is clinically approved for the treatment of angiogenic disorders, including certain forms of cancer and neovascular eye diseases. PDT for ocular angiogenesis is generally a two-step process, consisting initially of an intravenous (within the vein) injection of photosensitizer followed by laser treatment to the targeted sites of neovascularization in the retina after 15 min. The laser treatment is intended to selectively damage the vascular endothelium. In case choroidal neovascularization persists, patients are re-treated. In some cases, PDT is combined with angiostatic agents intended to target various parts of angiogenic pathway: mRNA, VGEFs, endothelial cell proliferation, migration, and proteolysis. Some of the angiostatic agents under study are verteporfin, pegaptanib, ranibizumab, bevacizumab, anecortave acetate, squalamine, vatalanib, and triamcinolone acetonide. Some of the typical cases of angiogenesis treated with PDT are:

(i) *Subfoveal and juxtafoveal choroidal neovascularization*: Choroidal neovascularization is the most common vision-threatening complication of high myopia. In this disease, new vessels grow under the retina distorting vision and leading to scarring. Photodynamic therapy (PDT) is a new experiment treatment for CNV that combines the application of low-intensity light with a photosensitizing agent in the presence of oxygen to produce tissue effects. It uses the noninvasive potential of the laser light to cause a nonthermal localized chemotoxic reaction and obtain highly selective occlusion of the neovascular channels while sparing the overlying photoreceptors (Donati et al. 1999). Verteporfin photodynamic therapy is used in these cases due to its angio-occlusive mechanism of action that reduces visual acuity loss and underlying leakage associated with lesions. Verteporfin PDT has also been associated with encouraging treatment outcomes in case studies involving patients with choroidal vascular disorders such as polypoidal choroidal vasculopathy, central serous chorioretinopathy, choroidal hemangioma, angioid streaks, and inflammatory CNV (Chan et al. 2010). Verteporfin photodynamic therapy has also been found to be beneficial as a part of triple therapy for neovascular ARMD (Ehmann and Garcia 2010). PDT therapy has been found to effectively induce tumor regression and resolution of exudative subretinal fluid, improving or stabilizing vision in circumscribed choroidal hemangioma (Elizalde et al. 2012). Visudyne has already been approved by US FDA for the treatment of subfoveal choroidal neovascularization (Rivellese and Baumal 2000) and juxtafoveal neovascularization (Blair et al. 2004).

(ii) *Corneal neovascularization* (*CNV*): It is excessive ingrowth of blood vessels from the limbal vascular plexus into the cornea as a result of oxygen deprivation. CNV causes significant visual loss because of the scarring and lipid deposition that frequently accompany it and is generally induced by nonspecific inflammatory stimuli mediated primarily by polymorphonuclear neutrophils. CNV can also be caused due to specific corneal immune reactions such as herpes simplex keratitis. Photodynamic therapy with argon laser following intravenous injection of hematoporphyrin derivative or purified dihematoporphyrin ether (DHE) has been used to suppress tumor growth and blood vessel growth in the eye (Epstein et al. 1987; Sheppard et al. 2006). Currently, verteporfin in conjunction with photodynamic therapy has been reported to be effective against CNV (Al-Torbak 2012).

9.2.3.1 Mechanism of Action of Molecules Used for PDT in Angiogenesis

(i) Verteporfin: it is composed of two semisynthetic porphyrin isomers and is four times more powerful as compared to porphyrin sensitizers when used alone. It is a chlorin-type molecule and an efficient generator of singlet oxygen. It has a maximum absorption in the UVA range with an additional absorption peak between 680 and 695 nm. Therefore, it can be activated with a low-power light that can penetrate blood, melanin, and fibrotic tissue. It binds with LDL to form a complex within abnormally proliferating cells. Thereafter, it becomes bound to intracellular or membrane components and, when activated through light, causes cellular damage (Schmidt-Erfurth and Hasan 2000).

(ii) Pegaptanib: it is a pegylated anti-VGEF aptamer (single strand of nucleic acid that binds with a particular target). It is a selective antagonist of 165 isoform of VGEF. As a result, growth of blood vessels is curtailed to control leakage and swelling in angiogenesis (Ng et al. 2006).

(iii) Bevacizumab: it is the first monoclonal antibody synthesized for treatment of angiogenesis in cancer. It is a recombinant monoclonal antibody that blocks VGEF-A, which is an angiogenesis stimulator. It finds application in treatment of certain metastatic cancers such as colon cancer, ovarian cancer, and renal cancer. In eye diseases, it is used in the treatment of diabetic retinopathy (Agarwal et al. 2014), neovascular glaucoma (Jiang et al. 2014), diabetic macular edema (Stewart 2014), and retinopathy of prematurity.

(iv) Ranibizumab: it is a monoclonal antibody fragment similar to bevacizumab with similar effectiveness and clinical applications (Agarwal et al. 2014; Jiang et al. 2014; Stewart 2014).

(v) Anecortave acetate: it is a unique angiostatic agent derived from glucocorticoid cortisol acetate and is a nonselective inhibitor of different angiogenic factors. It is useful in the treatment of iatrogenic glaucoma (Razeghinejad and Katz 2012) and wet ARMD (Augustin 2006) and shows promise in the treatment of choroidal neovascularization (Slakter 2006).

(vi) Squalamine: it is an aminosterol compound obtained from dogfish shark. It has potent antimicrobial activity. It is a cationic peptide that binds to phospholipid membranes and interacts with plasma membranes of infective bacteria to prevent their function. It shows promise in the treatment of neovascular ARMD (Emerson and Lauer 2007) and exudative ARMD (Connolly et al. 2006).

(vii) Vatalanib: it is a VEGF substrate that inhibits tyrosine kinase receptor that is an important enzyme contributing to formation of new blood vessels. It has been found to be useful in treatment of neovascular ARMD (Emerson and Lauer 2007) and wet ARMD (Ni and Hui 2009).

(viii) Triamcinolone acetonide: it is a synthetic fluorinated corticosteroid and is about eight times more potent as compared to prednisone. It possesses good anti-inflammatory action and therefore used in the management of ocular inflammatory disease. Its use is being explored in the treatment of diabetic macular edema (Ciulla et al. 2014).

Recently, the concept of angiostatic targeted therapy is under rapid development. It involves use of clinically effective angiogenesis inhibitors in combination with PDT (Weiss et al. 2012). However, this therapy has not got a full-fledged entrance into the clinical management of cancer mainly because of secondary complications such as inflammation and neoangiogenesis.

The recent development of anti-VEGF substances for use in clinical routine has markedly improved the prognosis of patients with neovascular ARMD. Intravitreal treatment with substances targeting all isotypes of vascular endothelial growth factor (VEGF), for the first time in the history of ARMD treatments, results in a significant increase in visual acuity in patients with neovascular ARMD. Overall, antiangiogenic approaches provide vision maintenance in over 90 % and substantial improvement in 25–40 % of patients. The combination with occlusive therapies like photodynamic therapy (PDT) potentially offers a reduction of re-treatment frequency and long-term maintenance of the treatment benefit.

9.3 Summary

Photodynamic therapy is a unique treatment modality wherein a photosensitizer localized to specific tissue/organ is activated by use of light of specific wavelength. This method has revolutionized therapeutic strategies for the treatment of several infectious as well as angiogenic diseases. It also finds promising applications in several malignant as well as nonmalignant conditions of the ocular system.

References

Adini I, Rabinovitz I, Sun JF, Prendergast GC, Benjamin LE. RhoB controls Akt trafficking and stage-specific survival of endothelial cells during vascular development. Genes Dev. 2003;17:2721–32.

Agarwal P, Jindal A, Saini VK, Jindal S. Advances in diabetic retinopathy. Indian J Endocrinol Metab. 2014;18:772–7. doi:10.4103/2230-8210.140225.

Al-Torbak AA. Photodynamic therapy with verteporfin for corneal neovascularization. Middle East Afr J Ophthalmol. 2012;19:185–9. doi:10.4103/0974-9233.95246.

Ambati BK, et al. Corneal avascularity is due to soluble VEGF receptor-1. Nature. 2006; 443:993–7.

Augustin A. Anecortave acetate in the treatment of age-related macular degeneration. Clin Interv Aging. 2006;1:237–46.

Barbara SH, Blackhurst DW, Schachat AP, Olk J, Novak MA, Maguire MG. Argon laser photocoagulation for neovascular maculopathy: five-year results from randomized clinical trials. Arch Ophthalmol. 1991;109:1109–14.

Benjamin LE, Hemo I, Keshet E. A plasticity window for blood vessel remodelling is defined by pericyte coverage of the preformed endothelial network and is regulated by PDGF-B and VEGF. Development. 1998;125:1591–8.

Bhutto IA, Uno K, Merges C, Zhang L, McLeod DS, Lutty GA. Reduction of endogenous angiogenesis inhibitors in Bruch's membrane of the submacular region in eyes with age-related macular degeneration. Arch Ophthalmol. 2008;126:670–8.

Blaauwgeers HG, et al. Polarized vascular endothelial growth factor secretion by human retinal pigment epithelium and localization of vascular endothelial growth factor receptors on the inner choriocapillaris. Evidence for a trophic paracrine relation. Am J Pathol. 1999;155: 421–8.

Blair MP, Apte RS, Miskala PH, Bressler SB, Goldberg MF, Schachat AP, Bressler NM. Retrospective case series of juxtafoveal choroidal neovascularization treated with photodynamic therapy with verteporfin. Retina. 2004;24:501–6.

Boobes Y, Bernieh B, Saadi H, Raafat Al Hakim M, Abouchacra S. Gonadal dysfunction and infertility in kidney transplant patients receiving sirolimus. Int Urol Nephrol. 2010;42: 493–8.

Bown SG. Photodynamic therapy for photochemists. Philos Trans A Math Phys Eng Sci. 2013; 371:28. doi:10.1098/rsta.2012.0371.

Boyer DS, Ophthotech Anti-PDGF in AMD Study Group. Combined inhibition of platelet derived (PDGF) and vascular endothelial (VEGF) growth factors for the treatment of neovascular age-related macular degeneration (NV-AMD)—results of a Phase 1 study. Invest Ophthalmol Vis Sci. 2009;50.

Brafman A, et al. Inhibition of oxygen-induced retinopathy in RTP801-deficient mice. Invest Ophthalmol Vis Sci. 2004;45:3796–805.

Caballero S, et al. Anti-sphingosine-1-phosphate monoclonal antibodies inhibit angiogenesis and sub-retinal fibrosis in a murine model of laser-induced choroidal neovascularization. Exp Eye Res. 2009;88:367–77.

Campochiaro PA, Hackett SF. Ocular neovascularization: a valuable model system. Oncogene. 2003;22:6537–48.

Campochiaro PA, et al. Topical mecamylamine for diabetic macular edema. Am J Ophthalmol. 2010;149:839–51.

Canal-Fontcuberta I, Salomao DR, Robertson D, Cantrill HL, Koozekanani D, Rath PP, Pulido JS. Clinical and histopathologic findings after photodynamic therapy of choroidal melanoma. Retina. 2012;32:942–8.

Cassuto DA, Deborah MA, Guglielmo E. Treatment of facial telangiectasias with a diode-pumped Nd:YAG laser at 532 nm. J Cutan Laser Ther. 2000;2:141–6.

Chan WM, Lim TH, Pece A, Silva R, Yoshimura N. Verteporfin PDT for non-standard indications--a review of current literature. Graefes Arch Clin Exp Ophthalmol. 2010;248:613–26.

Cheresh DA, Stupack DG. Regulation of angiogenesis: apoptotic cues from the ECM. Oncogene. 2008;27:6285–98.

Cho H, Shah CP, Weber M, Heier JS. Aflibercept for exudative AMD with persistent fluid on ranibizumab and/or bevacizumab. Br J Ophthalmol. 2013;97:1032–5.

Ciulla TA, Harris A, McIntyre N, Jonescu-Cuypers C. Treatment of diabetic macular edema with sustained-release glucocorticoids: intravitreal triamcinolone acetonide, dexamethasone implant, and fluocinolone acetonide implant. Expert Opin Pharmacother. 2014;15:953–9.

Connolly B, Desai A, Garcia CA, Thomas E, Gast MJ. Squalamine lactate for exudative age-related macular degeneration. Ophthalmol Clin North Am. 2006;19:381–91.

Cooper ME, et al. Increased renal expression of vascular endothelial growth factor (VEGF) and its receptor VEGFR-2 in experimental diabetes. Diabetes. 1999;48:2229–39.

Dark GG, Hill SA, Prise VE, Tozer GM, Pettit GR, Chaplin DJ. Combretastatin A-4, an agent that displays potent and selective toxicity toward tumor vasculature. Cancer Res. 1997;57:1829–34.

Dawson DW, Volpert OV, Gillis P, Crawford SE, Xu H, Benedict W, Bouck NP. Pigment epithelium-derived factor: a potent inhibitor of angiogenesis. Science. 1999;285:245–8.

Dolmans DE, Fukumura D, Jain RK. Photodynamic therapy for cancer. Nat Rev Cancer. 2003; 3:380–7.

Donati G, Kapetanios AD, Pournaras CJ. Principles of treatment of choroidal neovascularization with photodynamic therapy in age-related macular degeneration. Semin Ophthalmol. 1999;14:2–10.

Ehmann D, Garcia R. Triple therapy for neovascular age-related macular degeneration (verteporfin photodynamic therapy, intravitreal dexamethasone, and intravitreal bevacizumab). Can J Ophthalmol. 2010;45:36–40.

Elizalde J, Vasquez L, Iyo F, Abengoechea S. Photodynamic therapy in the management of circumscribed choroidal hemangioma. Can J Ophthalmol. 2012;47:16–20.

Emerson MV, Lauer AK. Emerging therapies for the treatment of neovascular age-related macular degeneration and diabetic macular edema. BioDrugs. 2007;21:245–57.
Epstein RJ, Stulting RD, Hendricks RL, Harris DM. Corneal neovascularization. Pathogenesis and inhibition. Cornea. 1987;6:250–7.
Eyetech Study Group. Preclinical and phase 1A clinical evaluation of an anti-VEGF pegylated aptamer (EYE001) for the treatment of exudative age-related macular degeneration. Retina. 2002;22:143–52.
Fan NW, Lau LI, Chen SJ, Yang CS, Lee FL. Comparison of the effect of reduced-fluence photodynamic therapy with intravitreal bevacizumab and standard-fluence alone for polypoidal choroidal vasculopathy. J Chin Med Assoc. 2014;77:101–7.
Ferrara N, Gerber HP, LeCouter J. The biology of VEGF and its receptors. Nat Med. 2003;9:669–76.
Garcia-Arumi J, et al. Photodynamic therapy for symptomatic subretinal fluid related to choroidal nevus. Retina. 2012;32:936–41.
Gariano RF. Cellular mechanisms in retinal vascular development. Prog Retin Eye Res. 2003;22: 295–306.
Gariano RF, Gardner TW. Retinal angiogenesis in development and disease. Nature. 2005; 438:960–6.
Gerhardt H, et al. VEGF guides angiogenic sprouting utilizing endothelial tip cell filopodia. J Cell Biol. 2003;161:1163–77.
Gogat K, et al. VEGF and KDR gene expression during human embryonic and fetal eye development. Invest Ophthalmol Vis Sci. 2004;45:7–14.
Griggs J, Skepper JN, Smith GA, Brindle KM, Metcalfe JC, Hesketh R. Inhibition of proliferative retinopathy by the anti-vascular agent combretastatin-A4. Am J Pathol. 2002;160:1097–103.
Verteporfin in Photodynamic Therapy Study Group. Verteporfin therapy of subfoveal choroidal neovascularization in age-related macular degeneration: two-year results of a randomized clinical trial including lesions with occult with no classic choroidal neovascularization – verteporfin in photodynamic therapy report 2. Am J Ophthalmol. 2001;131:541–60. http://dx.doi.org/10.1016/S0002-9394(01)00967-9.
Harper SJ, Bates DO. VEGF-A splicing: the key to anti-angiogenic therapeutics? Nat Rev Cancer. 2008;8:880–7.
Heeschen C, Weis M, Aicher A, Dimmeler S, Cooke JP. A novel angiogenic pathway mediated by non-neuronal nicotinic acetylcholine receptors. J Clin Invest. 2002;110:527–36.
Hellstrom M, Gerhardt H, Kalen M, Li X, Eriksson U, Wolburg H, Betsholtz C. Lack of pericytes leads to endothelial hyperplasia and abnormal vascular morphogenesis. J Cell Biol. 2001;153:543–54. doi:10.1083/jcb.153.3.543.
Holekamp NM, Bouck N, Volpert O. Pigment epithelium-derived factor is deficient in the vitreous of patients with choroidal neovascularization due to age-related macular degeneration. Am J Ophthalmol. 2002;134:220–7.
Homsi J, Daud AI. Spectrum of activity and mechanism of action of VEGF/PDGF inhibitors. Cancer Control. 2007;14:285–94.
Hornung V, et al. Sequence-specific potent induction of IFN-alpha by short interfering RNA in plasmacytoid dendritic cells through TLR7. Nat Med. 2005;11:263–70.
Hynes RO. Integrins: versatility, modulation, and signaling in cell adhesion. Cell. 1992;69: 11–25.
Jager RD, Aiello LP, Patel SC, Cunningham Jr ET. Risks of intravitreous injection: a comprehensive review. Retina. 2004;24:676–98.
Jia X, Jia L. Nanoparticles improve biological functions of phthalocyanine photosensitizers used for photodynamic therapy. Curr Drug Metab. 2012;13:1119–22.
Jiang S, Park C, Barner JC. Ranibizumab for age-related macular degeneration: a meta-analysis of dose effects and comparison with no anti-VEGF treatment and bevacizumab. J Clin Pharm Ther. 2014;39:234–9. doi:10.1111/jcpt.12146.
Jo N, et al. Inhibition of platelet-derived growth factor B signaling enhances the efficacy of anti-vascular endothelial growth factor therapy in multiple models of ocular neovascularization. Am J Pathol. 2006;168:2036–53.

Jorge JL, David S. Potential therapeutic roles for inhibition of the PI3K/Akt/mTOR pathway in the pathophysiology of diabetic retinopathy. J Ophthalmol. 2011;2011:19. doi:10.1155/2011/589813.

Kendall RL, Thomas KA. Inhibition of vascular endothelial cell growth factor activity by an endogenously encoded soluble receptor. Proc Natl Acad Sci U S A. 1993;90:10705–9.

Kiuchi K, et al. Mecamylamine suppresses basal and nicotine-stimulated choroidal neovascularization. Invest Ophthalmol Vis Sci. 2008;49:1705–11.

Kleinman ME, et al. Sequence- and target-independent angiogenesis suppression by siRNA via TLR3. Nature. 2008;452:591–7.

Korobelnik JF, et al. Intravitreal aflibercept for diabetic macular edema. Ophthalmology. 2014;121:2247–54.

Kumar R, et al. Pharmacokinetic-pharmacodynamic correlation from mouse to human with pazopanib, a multikinase angiogenesis inhibitor with potent antitumor and antiangiogenic activity. Mol Cancer Ther. 2007;6:2012–21.

Lamalice L, Le Boeuf F, Huot J. Endothelial cell migration during angiogenesis. Circ Res. 2007;100:782–94. doi:10.1161/01.RES.0000259593.07661.1e.

Letavernier E, Legendre C. mToR inhibitors-induced proteinuria: mechanisms, significance, and management. Transplant Rev. 2008;22:125–30.

Liu Q, Xu Q, Zheng VW, Xue H, Cao Z, Yang Q. Multi-task learning for cross-platform siRNA efficacy prediction: an in-silico study. BMC Bioinformatics. 2010;11:1471–2105.

Los M, Roodhart JM, Voest EE. Target practice: lessons from phase III trials with bevacizumab and vatalanib in the treatment of advanced colorectal cancer. Oncologist. 2007;12:443–50.

Maclachlan TK, et al. Preclinical safety evaluation of AAV2-sFLT01- a gene therapy for age-related macular degeneration. Mol Ther. 2011;19:326–34.

Majewski N, et al. Hexokinase-mitochondria interaction mediated by Akt is required to inhibit apoptosis in the presence or absence of Bax and Bak. Mol Cell. 2004;16:819–30.

Mills RE, Taylor KR, Podshivalova K, McKay DB, Jameson JM. Defects in skin gamma delta T cell function contribute to delayed wound repair in rapamycin-treated mice. J Immunol. 2008;181:3974–83. doi:10.4049/jimmunol.181.6.3974.

Nambu H, Nambu R, Melia M, Campochiaro PA. Combretastatin A-4 phosphate suppresses development and induces regression of choroidal neovascularization. Invest Ophthalmol Vis Sci. 2003;44:3650–5.

Ng EW, Shima DT, Calias P, Cunningham ET, Guyer DR, Adamis AP. Pegaptanib, a targeted anti-VEGF aptamer for ocular vascular disease. Nat Rev Drug Discov. 2006;5:123–32.

Ni Z, Hui P. Emerging pharmacologic therapies for wet age-related macular degeneration. Ophthalmologica. 2009;223:401–10.

Nowak DG, et al. Regulation of vascular endothelial growth factor (VEGF) splicing from pro-angiogenic to anti-angiogenic isoforms: a novel therapeutic strategy for angiogenesis. J Biol Chem. 2010;285:5532–40.

Ohtsuki A, Hasegawa T, Hirasawa Y, Tsuchihashi H, Ikeda S. Photodynamic therapy using light-emitting diodes for the treatment of viral warts. J Dermatol. 2009;36:525–8.

Orecchia A, Lacal PM, Schietroma C, Morea V, Zambruno G, Failla CM. Vascular endothelial growth factor receptor-1 is deposited in the extracellular matrix by endothelial cells and is a ligand for the alpha 5 beta 1 integrin. J Cell Sci. 2003;116:3479–89. doi:10.1242/jcs.00673.

Ozaki H, Hla T, Lee MJ. Sphingosine-1-phosphate signaling in endothelial activation. J Atheroscler Thromb. 2003;10:125–31.

Palanki MS, et al. Development of prodrug 4-chloro-3-(5-methyl-3-{[4-(2-pyrrolidin-1-ylethoxy) phenyl]amino}-1,2,4-benzotria zin-7-yl)phenyl benzoate (TG100801): a topically administered therapeutic candidate in clinical trials for the treatment of age-related macular degeneration. J Med Chem. 2008;51:1546–59.

Patan S. Vasculogenesis and angiogenesis as mechanisms of vascular network formation, growth and remodeling. J Neurooncol. 2000;50:1–15.

Pavan-Langston D, Langston RH. Recent advances in antiviral therapy. Int Ophthalmol Clin. 1975;15:89–100.

Pettit GR, et al. Antineoplastic agents 322. Synthesis of combretastatin A-4 prodrugs. Anticancer Drug Des. 1995;10:299–309.

Rasmussen H, et al. Clinical protocol. An open-label, phase I, single administration, dose-escalation study of ADGVPEDF.11D (ADPEDF) in neovascular age-related macular degeneration (AMD). Hum Gene Ther. 2001;12:2029–32.

Razeghinejad MR, Katz LJ. Steroid-induced iatrogenic glaucoma. Ophthalmic Res. 2012;47: 66–80. doi:10.1159/000328630.

Rivellese MJ, Baumal CR. Photodynamic therapy of eye diseases. J Ophthalmic Nurs Technol. 2000;19:134–41.

Rousseau S, Houle FO, Huot J. Integrating the VEGF signals leading to actin-based motility in vascular endothelial cells. Trends Cardiovasc Med. 2000;10:321–7. http://dx.doi.org/10.1016/S1050-1738(01)00072-X.

Saishin Y, Takahashi K, Lima e Silva R, Hylton D, Rudge JS, Wiegand SJ, Campochiaro PA. VEGF-TRAP(R1R2) suppresses choroidal neovascularization and VEGF-induced breakdown of the blood-retinal barrier. J Cell Physiol. 2003;195:241–8.

Sampat KM, Garg SJ. Complications of intravitreal injections. Curr Opin Ophthalmol. 2010;21:178–83.

Schmidt-Erfurth U, Hasan T. Mechanisms of action of photodynamic therapy with verteporfin for the treatment of age-related macular degeneration. Surv Ophthalmol. 2000;45:195–214. http://dx.doi.org/10.1016/S0039-6257(00)00158-2.

Sheppard Jr JD, Epstein RJ, Lattanzio Jr FA, Marcantonio D, Williams PB. Argon laser photodynamic therapy of human corneal neovascularization after intravenous administration of dihematoporphyrin ether. Am J Ophthalmol. 2006;141:524–9.

Sherris D. Ocular drug development--future directions. Angiogenesis. 2007;10:71–6.

Shoshani T, et al. Identification of a novel hypoxia-inducible factor 1-responsive gene, RTP801, involved in apoptosis. Mol Cell Biol. 2002;22:2283–93.

Sibata CH, Colussi VC, Oleinick NL, Kinsella TJ. Photodynamic therapy: a new concept in medical treatment. Braz J Med Biol Res. 2000;33:869–80. doi:10.1590/S0100-879X2000000800002.

Silva RM, Faria de Abreu JR, Travassos A, Cunha-Vaz JG. Stabilization of visual acuity with photodynamic therapy in eyes with chorioretinal anastomoses. Graefes Arch Clin Exp Ophthalmol. 2004;242:368–76.

Slakter JS. Anecortave acetate for treating or preventing choroidal neovascularization. Ophthalmol Clin North Am. 2006;19:373–80.

Sledz CA, Holko M, de Veer MJ, Silverman RH, Williams BR. Activation of the interferon system by short-interfering RNAs. Nat Cell Biol. 2003;5:834–9.

Soefje SA, Karnad A, Brenner AJ. Common toxicities of mammalian target of rapamycin inhibitors. Target Oncol. 2011;6:125–9. doi:10.1007/s11523-011-0174-9.

Sofroniadou S, Goldsmith D. Mammalian target of rapamycin (mTOR) inhibitors: potential uses and a review of haematological adverse effects. Drug Saf. 2011;34:97–115. doi:10.2165/11585040-000000000-00000.

Stewart MW. Aflibercept (VEGF Trap-eye): the newest anti-VEGF drug. Br J Ophthalmol. 2012;96:1157–8.

Stewart MW. Anti-VEGF therapy for diabetic macular edema. Curr Diab Rep. 2014;14:510. doi:10.1007/s11892-014-0510-4.

Takahashi K, Saishin Y, King AG, Levin R, Campochiaro PA. Suppression and regression of choroidal neovascularization by the multitargeted kinase inhibitor pazopanib. Arch Ophthalmol. 2009;127:494–9.

Takeda A, et al. CCR3 is a target for age-related macular degeneration diagnosis and therapy. Nature. 2009;460:225–30.

Tolentino M. Systemic and ocular safety of intravitreal anti-VEGF therapies for ocular neovascular disease. Surv Ophthalmol. 2011;56:95–113.

Tuncer S, Kir N, Shields CL. Dramatic regression of amelanotic choroidal melanoma with PDT following poor response to brachytherapy. Ophthalmic Surg Lasers Imaging. 2012;43: 15428877–20120426.

Watterson KR, Lanning DA, Diegelmann RF, Spiegel S. Regulation of fibroblast functions by lysophospholipid mediators: potential roles in wound healing. Wound Repair Regen. 2007; 15:607–16.

Weiss A, den Bergh H, Griffioen AW, Nowak-Sliwinska P. Angiogenesis inhibition for the improvement of photodynamic therapy: the revival of a promising idea. Biochim Biophys Acta. 2012; 1826:53–70.

Witmer AN, Vrensen GF, Van Noorden CJ, Schlingemann RO. Vascular endothelial growth factors and angiogenesis in eye disease. Prog Retin Eye Res. 2003;22:1–29.

Wittmann J, Huggett MT, Bown SG, Pereira SP. Safety study of photodynamic therapy using talaporfin sodium in the pancreas and surrounding tissues in the syrian golden hamster. Int J Photoenergy. 2014;2014:7. doi:10.1155/2014/483750.

Wollensak G. Crosslinking treatment of progressive keratoconus: new hope. Curr Opin Ophthalmol. 2006;17:356–60.

Wong RL, Lai TY. Polypoidal choroidal vasculopathy: an update on therapeutic approaches. J Ophthalmic Vis Res. 2013;8:359–71.

Xie B, Shen J, Dong A, Rashid A, Stoller G, Campochiaro PA. Blockade of sphingosine-1-phosphate reduces macrophage influx and retinal and choroidal neovascularization. J Cell Physiol. 2009;218:192–8.

Zahn G, Vossmeyer D, Stragies R, Wills M, Wong CG, Loffler KU. Preclinical evaluation of the novel small molecule integrin α5β1 inhibitor JSM6427 in monkey and rabbit models of choroidal neovascularization. Arch Ophthalmol. 2009;127:1329–35. doi:10.1001/archophthalmol.2009.265.

Chapter 10
Mucoadhesive Polymers and Ocular Lubricants

Thirumurthy Velpandian and Laxmi Moksha

Abstract Dry Eye Disease (DED) is defined as a multifactorial condition that results in discomfort, visual disturbance, tear film instability and damage to the ocular surface. It is characterized by the increased osmolarity of the tear film and inflammation of the ocular surface. Tear film stability is maintained by the coordinated functions of the outer lipid monolayer with its critical composition and the contents of aqueous interface. This chapter discusses the structure and function attributing to tear film integrity, mucoadhesive polymers used in tear substitutes/lubricants, tear secretagogues agents, anti-inflammatory immunosuppressants, and use of autologous serum, umbilical cord serum for the management of dry eye.

10.1 Introduction

The conditions of tear film formation and stability are governed by the surface chemical characteristics of the tear film system and proper functioning of the lacrimal apparatus. The tear film has to remain continuous between blinks in order to fulfill its function. Dry eye is a multifactorial disease of the tears and the ocular surface that manifests in a wide variety of signs and symptoms. It is prevalent in about 33 % of the population worldwide. The presence of an abnormal tear film results in dry eye states that can be detrimental to vision (Holly and Lemp 1977). Dry eye syndrome (DES) is a common ocular disorder affecting 5–6 % of population characterized by decreased production of tear or its increased evaporation. In Latin it is called as keratoconjunctivitis sicca (KCS), indicating the inflammation induced by dryness. Although it is a multifactorial disease, the end result of ocular surface damage is due to the lack of tear film stability in terms of its volume and

T. Velpandian, BPharm, MS(Pharmacol), PhD (✉) • L. Moksha, M. Pharm
Ocular Pharmacology and Pharmacy, Dr. Rajendra Prasad Centre for Ophthalmic Sciences, All India Institute of Medical Sciences, New Delhi, India
e-mail: tvelpandian@hotmail.com

T. Velpandian (ed.), *Pharmacology of Ocular Therapeutics*,
DOI 10.1007/978-3-319-25498-2_10

composition. In either case corneal epithelial drying is accompanied by increased tear osmolarity due to water evaporation, causing hyperosmotic stress on epithelial cells. This osmotic effect is capable of dehydrating the corneal epithelium and precipitating foreign body sensation, itching, and irritation leading toward inflammation. Therefore, ultimately replenishing precorneal tear film, stimulating or improving tear secretion, and stabilizing the tear film are the current methods being adopted for its management.

Dry eye could be due to ocular surface disorders, surface surgeries (LASIK surgery), surface disturbances (contact lens usage), hormonal changes (postmenopausal and androgen deficiency), and secondary side effect of systemically administered drugs having anti-muscarnic activity (antihistaminics, antipsychotics, etc.). In most of the aforesaid cases, administration of tear substitutes have been found to be beneficial. Sjögren's syndrome is a chronic systemic autoimmune disease characterized by lymphocytic infiltration of exocrine glands causing poor lacrimal gland function. Sjögren's syndrome (SS) is the second most common autoimmune rheumatic disease. However, differential diagnosis remains confusing due to the high prevalence of vague symptoms of dryness, fatigue, and myalgias in the general population (Fox et al. 2000).

After overlapping "general" and "operational" definitions of dry eye, the definition and classification subcommittee of the International Dry Eye Workshop (2007) redefined it as, "Dry eye is a multifactorial disease of the tears and ocular surface that results in symptoms of discomfort, visual disturbance, and tear film instability with potential damage to the ocular surface. It is accompanied by increased osmolarity of the tear film and inflammation of the ocular surface" (2007).

10.2 Structure and Functions Attributing to Tear Film Stability

Human tear film consists of a monolipid layer in the air-tears interface followed by soluble mucin-containing aqueous layer resting on the glycocalyx matrix on the corneal epithelium. The lipid layer is an essential component of the tear film, providing a smooth optical surface for the cornea and retarding evaporation from the eye (Fig. 10.1). The composition of meibomian lipids are well adapted for this purpose. They form a thin, smooth film containing lower amphiphilic phospholipids having their polar heads oriented toward aqueous film and hydrophobic tails giving interface for hydrophobic cholesteryl esters, wax esters, [O-acyl]-ω-hydroxy fatty acid, triglyceride, etc. (McCulley and Shine 2004). It has been reported that the thickness and composition of this layer influence the rate of evaporation (Bron et al. 2004). The protein and electrolyte composition of the aqueous part of the tears are derived from the lacrimal gland, as well as the accessory secretions of other glands and the conjunctiva.

Mucins are large, extracellular glycoproteins with molecular weights ranging from 0.5 to 20 MDa and belong to the family having O-linked carbohydrates. They

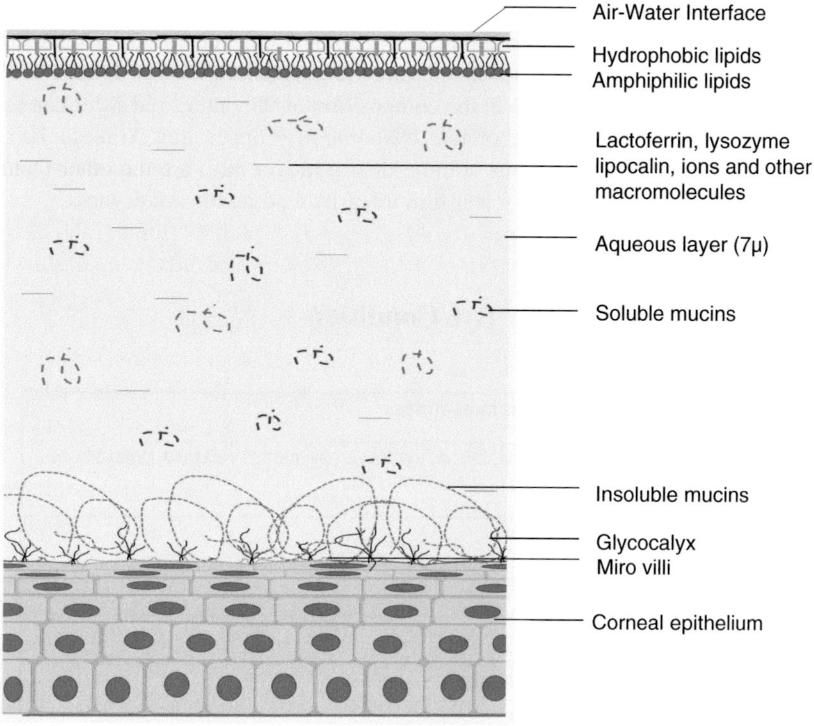

Fig 10.1 Human tear film comprise of the lipid layer followed by the aqueous layer resting on the glycocalyx matrix of mucin layer on the corneal epithelium

are classified as transmembrane or secretory mucins. Secreted mucins can be further subclassified as gel forming or soluble, based on their ability to form polymers. They are highly glycosylated, containing 80 % of carbohydrates, primarily N-acetylgalactosamine, N-acetylglucosamine, fucose, galactose, and sialic acid (N-acetylneuraminic acid), and traces of mannose and sulfate. Both secreted and membrane bound forms of mucins share many common features (Bansil and Turner 2006). Mucins that have been detected in the eye are MUC1, MUC2, MUC4, MUC5AC, MUC7, MUC13, MUC15, MUC16, and MUC17 (Johnson and Murphy 2004). Transmembrane mucins contain hydrophobic, membrane-spanning domains in their carboxyl-terminal region, which anchor them to the apical surface of conjunctival and corneal epithelial cells, facilitating formation of the ocular surface glycocalyx (Johnson and Murphy 2004; Tiffany 2008). MUC5AC, the major gel-forming mucin of tears, is secreted by conjunctival goblet cells. This complex macromolecule gives interface for holding moisture on the biological membrane due to various non-covalent interactions.

The primary function of tear film includes providing nutrition to the epithelium of the cornea, lubricating ocular surface, and removal of debris from the precorneal area along with the factors for antimicrobial and immune functions. Tear film stability is achieved by the coordinated functions of lipid monolayer with its critical composition and the contents of aqueous interface. Tear instability causes dry eye due to various factors; any disturbance in the composition of the outer lipid layer can lead to the loss of primary defense of tear evaporation (Gipson and Argüeso 2003). Deficiency in mucin and aqueous volume (tear turnover rate) are the other factors responsible for destabilization of tear film integrity leading toward dryness.

10.3 Drugs Used in Dry Eye Condition

Mucoadhesive polymers in tear substitutes
Methyl cellulose, carboxymethyl cellulose, hydroxypropyl methyl cellulose, poloxomer, Hyaluronic acid
Ocular anti-inflammatory agents
Topical cyclosporine and tacrolimus
Secretagogue agents
Tear stimulants: Pilocarpine, cemeviline
Mucin and secretors: Rebamipide and diquafosol sodium
Miscellaneous
Topical sex steroids, androgens, estrogens, and phytoestrogens

10.3.1 Mucoadhesive Polymers for Ocular Surface

Conjunctival goblet cells in the eye secrete mucin which coats the epithelial cells to convert the hydrophobic epithelium to hold water against gravity which in turn maintains tear integrity. Goblet cells intercalated within the stratified epithelium of the conjunctiva secrete the large gel-forming mucin MUC5AC, and lacrimal gland epithelia secrete the small soluble mucin MUC7. Apical cells of the stratified epithelium of both corneal and conjunctival epithelium express at least three membrane-associated mucins (MUCs 1, 4, and 16), which extend from their apical surface to form the thick glycocalyx at the epithelium-tear film interface (Johnson and Murphy 2004). This interface is responsible for the conversion of the property of hydrophobic corneal epithelium into hydrophilic layer to hold tear of 7 μm thickness upon the cornea against gravity. In the inadequacy of the function of mucin, mechanical forces during blinking can result in inflammation of the ocular surface (Itakura et al.

2013). Therefore, efforts were made to constitute artificial tear solutions with mucoadhesive polymers, extracellular cations with a suitable pH and osmolarity for the management of dry eye syndrome.

Mucoadhesion is the property of some of the natural or synthetic macromolecules which can adhere to a biological surface and retain their presence for a prolonged duration. Polyvinylpyrrolidone (PVP), polyvinyl alcohol (PVA), methyl cellulose, hydroxypropyl methyl cellulose (HPMC), carboxymethyl cellulose, hyaluronic acid, polyethylene glycols, etc., are some of the polymers regularly used in most of the topical tear substitutes. However, mucoadhesive polymers such as thiolated poly(acrylic acid), poloxamer, celluloseacetophthalate, methyl cellulose, hydroxy ethyl cellulose, poly(amidoamine) dendrimers, poly(dimethyl siloxane), and poly(vinyl pyrrolidone) are also used for increasing the precorneal drug residence time in ocular drug delivery approaches (Wagh et al. 2008).

These bioadhesive polymers used in topical tear substitutes are known to have numerous hydroxyl or carboxyl functional groups having the capability of making hydrogen bond with water molecules in the precorneal area. In ophthalmic products, bioadhesive pre-swollen polymers in water are used in a concentration to exhibit low viscosity. In the swollen state the interdistance between their chains leading to polymer flexibility causes uniform spreading upon the cornea and conjunctiva. Occurrence of polymer-mucin force of interaction has been reported when mucoadhesive polymers interact with corneal epithelium. Using in vitro and in vivo visometric data, mucoadhesive polymer interaction has been defined as polymer-cumin force of interaction in precorneal area. Depleting precorneal mucin by treatment with N-acetylcysteine reduced this interaction significantly (Saettone et al. 1994).

10.3.1.1 Tear Substitutes

Cellulose derivatives such as HPMC, methyl cellulose, and hyaluronic acid all share a common finding of having an –OH group to make hydrogen bonding and hydrophobic methyl groups (Fig. 10.2). The amphiphilic nature of these polymers would be having required hydrophobicity to bind toward hydrophobic epithelium and get entangled in the glycocalyx matrix, thereby giving a required polyhydric hydroxyl groups, creating hydrogen bonding with water molecules. This function makes them as a substitute for mucin in artificial tears. Solutions of hydroxypropyl methylcellulose (HPMC) and polyvinyl alcohol (PVA) are widely used as artificial tears. However, their usefulness is limited by the short duration of their effect. Dilute sodium hyaluronate solutions exhibit non-Newtonian rheology with high viscosities at low shear rates, which would be expected to enhance their ocular surface residence time (Snibson et al. 1992). Although several combinations are available worldwide either with single or more than one polymer, so far they are not studied for their compositional variation to make it more suitable for its use in tear substitute.

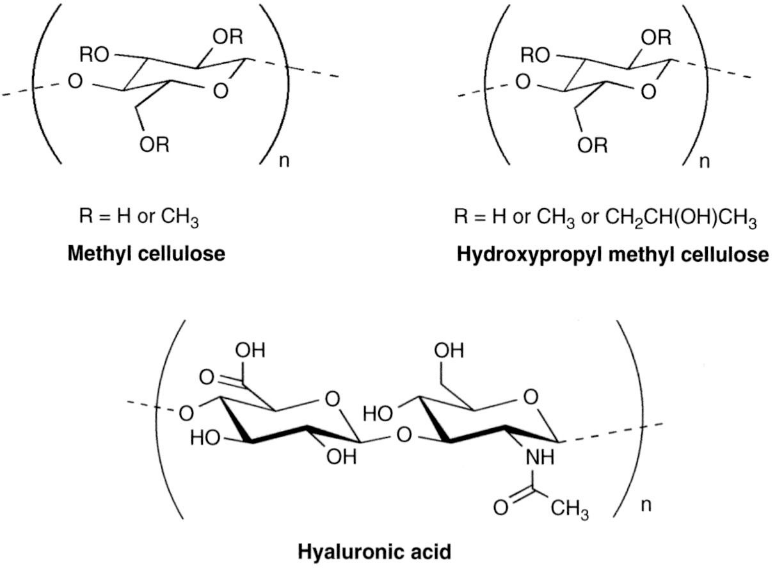

Fig 10.2 Tear Substitutes-Cellulose derivatives used in dry eye disease; HPMC, methyl cellulose, and hyaluronic acid

Throughout the world several compositions of artificial tear are being used and studied in different settings for dry eye. A meta-analysis reviewed 51 of such studies and reported that nearly all formulations of artificial tears provided significant benefit to patients with dysfunctional tear syndrome, but some proved superior to others (Moshirfar et al. 2014). This shows that artificial tear holds a prime position in the management of dry eye syndrome.

Although artificial tear solutions are mostly preferred for dry eye syndrome, at times ophthalmic ointments are used for prolonged management during ocular surgery or enabling nighttime applications. Changing refractive index between the tears and ointment causes blurring of vision and has been considered as one of the major disadvantages of ointments.

10.3.1.2 Other Ophthalmic Uses of Mucoadhesive Polymers

Mucoadhesive polymers are extensively used in ophthalmology during surgical procedures. Sodium hyaluronate (1 %) is very commonly used as one of the ophthalmic viscoelastic substance during capsulorhexis and intraocular lens (IOL) implantation in phacoemulsification surgery. Sodium hyaluronate, chondroitin, and hydroxypropyl methylcellulose are placed in the anterior chamber to prevent corneal endothelial damage during phacoemulsification and are removed after the completion of the procedure (Hutz et al. 1996). Intracameral injection of 2 % HPMC during trabeculectomy has been reported to maintain anterior chamber depth and reduces incidence of complications related to shallow anterior chamber depth following trabeculectomy (Agarwal et al. 2005).

Extensively, mucoadhesive polymers were studied for their activity to enhance the contact time of drugs on the precorneal area (Bucolo et al. 2011); they are also reported to reduce the ocular irritation of drugs when applied topically.

The conditioning properties of the multipurpose contact lens solution with polymers such as HPMC showed improved wetting of lenses and enhanced lens wearing comfort. Moreover, it has also been suggested that binding of HPMC to the lens surface and subsequent time-release is the probable mechanism for these benefits (Simmons et al. 2001).

10.3.2 Secretagogue Agents (Tear Stimulants and Mucin Inducers)

10.3.2.1 Tear stimulants

Lacrimal glands having M3 muscarinic receptors are the prime targets for increasing the tear secretion rate. Pilocarpine and cevimeline are the muscarinic agents approved for the treatment of symptoms of xerostomia in Sjögren's syndrome.

Pilocarpine

Pilocarpine is a well-known muscarinic agonist used for decades for inducing lacrimation. It is an alkaloid isolated from the plant Pilocarpus jaborandi. Being a muscarinic agonist on all muscarinic receptors, its systemic side effects are bothersome. Administration of 5-mg pilocarpine tablets 4 times daily (20 mg/day) was well tolerated and produced significant improvement in symptoms of dry mouth and dry eyes and other xeroses in patients (Vivino et al. 1999).

Cevimeline

Cevimeline is a synthetic compound, chemically ((±)-cis-2-methylspiro [1,3- oxathiolane-5, 3′-quinuclidine]), available as monohydrochloride reported to be an agonist on M1 and M3 receptors. Cevimeline at a dosage of 30 mg 3 times daily resulted in substantive improvement by increasing the rate of saliva and tear flow in patients with Sjögren's syndrome, as well as improving subjective symptoms of dry mouth, dry eyes, and overall dryness (Petrone et al. 2002). Frequently reported adverse events included headache, increased sweating, abdominal pain, and nausea. Increasing the dose to 60 mg TID increased higher gastrointestinal side effects.

However, at the dose of 20 mg three times daily, it has showed significant improvements in the subjective symptoms, tear dynamics, condition of the corneoconjunctival epithelium, and global improvement rating with lesser side effects (Ono et al. 2004)

10.3.2.2 Mucin inducers

Conjunctival epithelial and goblet cell P2Y2 nucleotide receptors regulate ion transport and glycoprotein release onto the ocular surface to promote tear and mucin secretion via elevated intracellular Ca^{2+} concentrations. Diquafosol tetrasodium (INS-365), a second-generation uridine nucleotide analog reported to act through P2Y2 receptor, induces the secretion of aqueous tear components from conjunctival epithelial cells and secretion of mucin from conjunctival goblet cells, thereby improving corneal epithelial integrity and stabilizing the tear film (Terakado et al. 2014). Diquafosol ophthalmic solution (3 %) is currently approved in Japan and South Korea for the treatment of dry eye.

In patients with dry eye, topical therapy with diquafosol significantly improved fluorescein and rose bengal staining scores as compared with placebo. Topical solution of 3 %, one drop, four times a day, was reported as noninferior to sodium hyaluronate ophthalmic solution 0.1 % (Keating 2015). Based on the published randomized clinical trial data on the use of diquafosol (3 % topical) in the management of dry eye, it has been suggested that topical therapy consistently improved tear film volume and stability (Lau et al. 2014). Whereas it was not accompanied with major improvement in symptoms related to dry eye disease. This could be due to the complex nature of dry eye disease having multiple etiologies. In most of the cases, the treatment period required was also long (6 months) to get subjective and objective improvement in aqueous-deficient dry eye, whereas topical diquafosol therapy was effective for patients with obstructive meibomian gland dysfunction (Arita et al. 2013). Diquafosol ophthalmic solution 3 % was generally well tolerated in patients with dry eye, with eye irritation the most commonly reported adverse event (Keating 2015).

10.3.2.3 Rebamipide

Rebamipide is initially developed as a gastroprotective compound capable of inducing mucin secretion through prostaglandin generation in the gastric mucosa. This compound has been selected from over 500 amino acid analogs of 2(1H)-quinolinone tested for gastroprotective action and for efficacy to heal experimental gastric ulcers (Arakawa et al. 1998) and nonsteroidal anti-inflammatory drug-induced gastric ulcers. MUC5AC has been identified as a major secretory mucin of conjunctival goblet cells and precorneal tear film. It has been found to decrease significantly in patients suffering from dry eye (Zhao et al. 2001). In vitro studies showed that rebamipide stimulated proliferation of conjunctival goblet cells in primary culture (Rios et al. 2006). Oral administration of rebamipide represents a new therapeutic modality in the treatment of Sjogren syndrome (Kohashi et al. 2008). It has been reported to stimulate EGF receptor (EGFR) and p44/p42 mitogen-activated protein kinase (MAPK) to cause mucin secretion from conjunctival goblet cells (Ríos et al. 2008). Rebamipide promoted glycol conjugate, which has a property as a mucin-like glycoprotein, in human corneal epithelial cells. The increased production was mediated by MUC1 and MUC4 gene expression (Takeji et al. 2012).

Being a suspension, it has been reported to affect optical quality by ocular higher-order aberrations and forward light scatter upon its use in patients (Koh et al. 2013)

Clinically, rebamipide ophthalmic suspensions were tested and reported to be effective in restoring tear stability in patients with dry eye. Topical rebamipide has also been shown to be effective in treating other ocular surface disorders such as lagophthalmos, lid wiper epitheliopathy, and persistent corneal erosion Kashima et al. (2015). Oral rebamipide administration for the period of 3 months showed significant levels of rebamipide in the tear film, indicating potential value in management of mucin-deficient tear film dysfunction (Tandon et al. 2012).

10.3.3 Anti-inflammatories and Immunosuppressants

10.3.3.1 Topical Cyclosporine

Cyclosporine-A (CsA) is a lipophilic cyclic undecapeptide, produced by the fungus *Beauveria nivea*. CsA suppresses humoral immunity and T-cell-dependent immune mechanisms which are responsible for transplant rejection and forms autoimmunity. Systemically administered CsA is metabolized by CYP3A4 and showed severe systemic toxicity such as renal dysfunction, tremor, hirsutism, hypertension, hyperlipidemia, and gum hyperplasia.

The mechanism involved in chronic immune inflammation during dry eye disease has been defined as a sequence of primary insult of various etiologies. An acute corneal inflammation caused by the irritation of the ocular surface (viral, bacterial, and environmental) leads to rapid vascular endothelial selectin expression and diapedesis of non-primed (non-targeted) T cells into the conjunctiva. When this condition gets into chronic phase, its challenge to the ocular surface (over time) leads to activation and drainage of antigen-presenting (including dendritic) cells to lymphoid organs permitting T cells to be primed and capable of targeting the ocular surface. These symptoms correlate primarily with corneal epithelial damage, thought to be due to cumulative damage mediated by cytotoxic effects of inflammatory and pro-apoptotic stimuli and hyperosmolarity. This cascade proceeded on to epithelial loss/devitalization is the stimulation for corneal nociceptive nerve endings (McDermott et al. 2005)

Although topical cyclosporine in vegetable oils (olive and arachis oil) at higher concentrations (1–2 %) was attempted for immunosuppression in corneal graft survival, its anti-inflammatory role, predominately T cells, made it to be used in ocular surface inflammation. For this purpose it was approved at the concentration of 0.05 % in keratoconjunctivitis sicca. Lack of systemic toxicity upon topical administration of CsA due to its low/undetectable levels in the blood paved the way for its safer use in dry eye (Pfau et al. 1995). A recent meta-analysis included 12 randomized clinical trials comparing topical CSA with placebo involving 3034 eyes of 1660 participants with dry eye syndrome. This study showed that statistically significant improvements on scores of breakup time (Zhou and Wei 2014).

10.3.3.2 Tacrolimus

Tacrolimus, formerly known as FK506, is a macrolide antibiotic with immunosuppressive properties. It belongs to the class of immunosuppressants but structurally unrelated to cyclosporine A (CsA); it principally acts through the impairment of gene expression in target cells. Tacrolimus bonds to an immunophilin, FK506-binding protein (FKBP). This complex inhibits calcineurin phosphatase. The drug inhibits calcium-dependent events, such as interleukin-2 gene transcription, nitric oxide synthase activation, cell degranulation, and apoptosis (Thomson et al. 1995). Recently, a double-blind randomized study showed that topical 0.03 % tacrolimus eye drop (vegetable oil based) instilled one drop every 12 hours has been reported to improve tear stability and ocular surface status in cases of inflammatory or Sjögren-related dry eye (Moscovici et al. 2015).

10.3.4 Autologous Serum and Umbilical Cord Serum Eye Drops for Dry Eye

Autologous serum is usually prepared from the patients and diluted to 20 % by saline. The detailed protocol to prepare autologous serum is given in the chapter of extemporaneous formulations (Chapter 15). The use of blood derivatives represents an alternative therapeutic approach that is gaining interest in regenerative medicine due to its potential to stimulate and accelerate tissue healing (Anitua et al. 2015). Autologous serum is rich in several plasma-driven growth factors which are reported to increase the tissue repair and rejuvenation of cells.

Epitheliotropic effect of serum eye drops is attributed to the number of bioactive factors such as fibronectin, EGF, TGF beta-1, HGF, vitamin A, and antiproteases.

As this formulation is expected to contain approximately 1 % albumin, it serves as a natural polymer; with this it improves the signs and symptoms of dry eye. Umbilical cord serum eye drops were more effective in decreasing symptoms and keratoepitheliopathy in severe dry eye syndrome and increasing goblet cell density in Sjögren's syndrome compared with autologous serum eye drops (Yoon et al. 2007).

Autologous serum eye drops are safe if they are compounded in sterile form and used with proper care of not contaminating it. Moreover, such eye drops must be stored in frozen or refrigerated conditions to improve the shelf life. Autologous serum is used in the conditions like keratoconjunctivitis sicca, superior limbal keratoconjunctivitis, recurrent erosion syndrome, persistent epithelial defects, etc. However, it may not be useful in secondary Sjögren's syndrome due to the elevation of proinflammatory cytokine levels in the serum.

10.3.5 Miscellaneous Agents

In Sjögren's syndrome, oral prednisone or hydroxychloroquine showed limited benefits in a few clinical trials. However their benefits are not clearly elucidated (Ramos-Casals et al. 2010). Gefarnate, a water-insoluble terpene fatty acid, has been reported to contribute to restoring mucins on the ocular surface. Similarly, the mucolytic drug bromhexine has also been reported to induce mucin production in the tears. There are studies attempted to evaluate the role of male/female sex (Piwkumsribonruang et al. 2010) hormones, their combination (Scott et al. 2005), metabolic precursor (dehydroepiandrostenedione), and phytoestrogens (Scuderi et al. 2012) for postmenopausal dry eye. However, their therapeutic role still remains uncertain.

10.4 Treatment for Dry Eye

As there is no definitive diagnostic test, it is often difficult to segregate patients to rationalize drug treatment. Therefore, treatment strategies are decided based on the severity of the symptoms. Mild intermittent bouts of symptoms can be solely managed by ophthalmic lubricants. If symptoms remain unresolved on lubricant therapy and ocular irritation persists, one can opt for topical anti-inflammatory therapy including short-term corticosteroids, topical cyclosporine A emulsion, oral tetracycline therapy, oral omega-3 fatty acid supplements, and autologous serum eye drops. In case of moderate conditions, topical secretagogue agents such as rebamipide or diquafosol can be attempted.

Physical measures (punctal plugs, moisture-retaining eye wear) are implemented for those with moderate-to-severe symptoms. Autologous serum tears, scleral contact lenses, and surgery are reserved for patients with severe symptoms who have an unsatisfactory response to anti-inflammatory medications.

Sjögren's syndrome is a systemic autoimmune disease characterized by dry eyes and dry mouth. In primary disease, Sjogren's syndrome is a solitary process, whereas in secondary cases it accompanies another autoimmune disease, most often rheumatoid arthritis. The recommended treatments include topical lubricants, topical anti-inflammatory therapy, and tear-conserving strategies and orally administered secretagogues; however, they seem to be of greater value in the treatment of oral dryness than ocular dryness (Akpek et al. 2011). Surprisingly, systemic TNF-alpha antagonists did not show any significant use in this condition.

Diquafosol

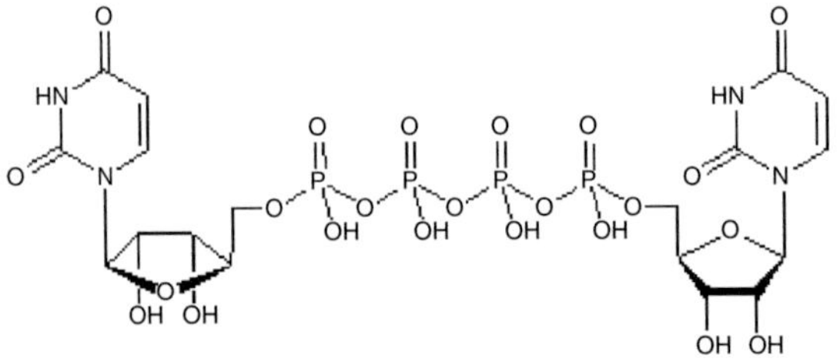

Rebamipide

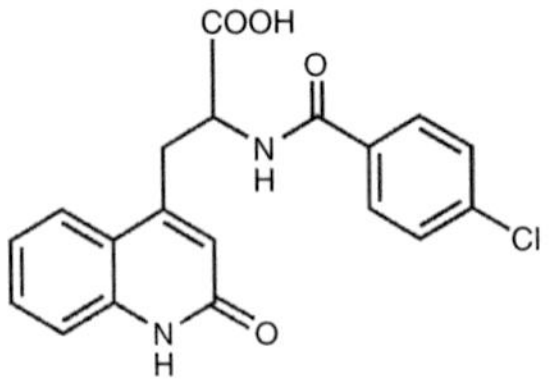

Cyclosporine

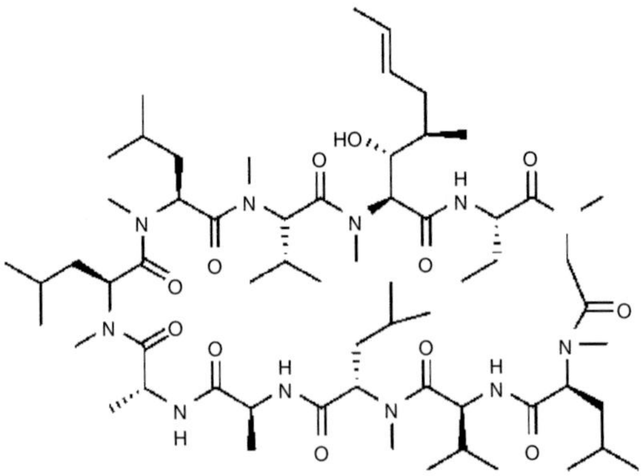

Cevimiline

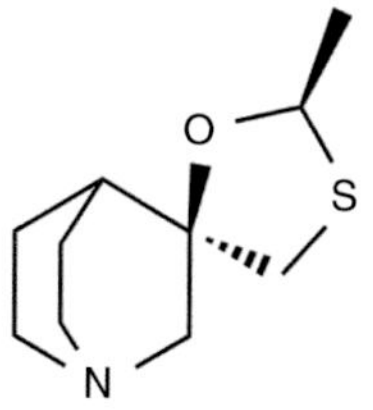

Pilocarpine

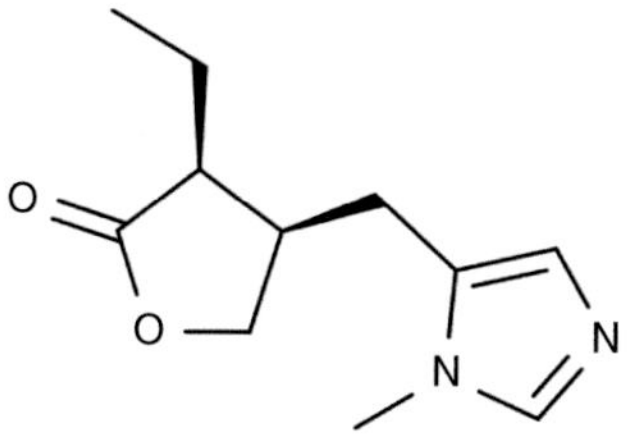

Tacrolimus

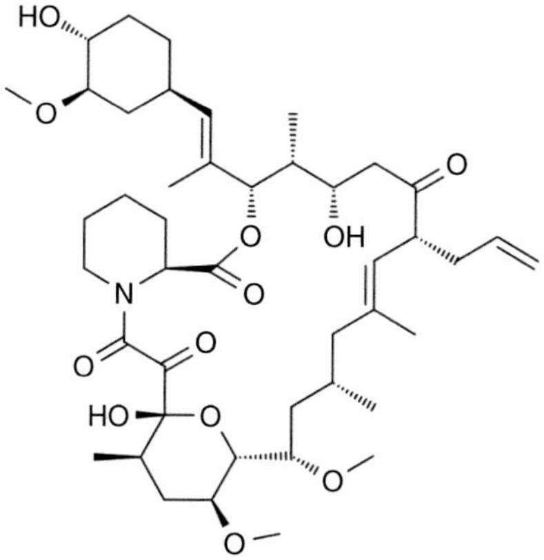

References

Agarwal HC, Anuradha VK, Titiyal JS, Gupta V. Effect of intraoperative intracameral 2% hydroxypropyl methylcellulose viscoelastic during trabeculectomy. Ophthalmic Surg Lasers Imaging. 2005;36(4):280–5.

Akpek EK, Lindsley KB, Adyanthaya RS, Swamy R, Baer AN, McDonnell PJ. Treatment of Sjögren's syndrome-associated dry eye an evidence-based review. Ophthalmology. 2011; 118(7):1242–52.

Anitua E, Muruzabal F, Tayebba A, Riestra A, Perez VL, Merayo-Lloves J, Orive G. Autologous serum and plasma rich in growth factors in ophthalmology: preclinical and clinical studies. Acta Ophthalmol. 2015. doi:10.1111/aos.12710 [Epub ahead of print].

Arakawa T, Kobayashi K, Yoshikawa T, Tarnawski A. Rebamipide: overview of its mechanisms of action and efficacy in mucosal protection and ulcer healing. Dig Dis Sci. 1998;43(9 Suppl):5S–13.

Arita R, Suehiro J, Haraguchi T, Maeda S, Maeda K, Tokoro H, Amano S. Topical diquafosol for patients with obstructive meibomian gland dysfunction. Br J Ophthalmol. 2013;97(6):725–9. doi:10.1136/bjophthalmol-2012-302668.

Bansil R, Turner BS. Mucin structure, aggregation, physiological functions and biomedical applications. Curr Opin Colloid Interface Sci. 2006;11:164–70.

Bron AJ, Tiffany JM, Gouveia SM, Yokoi N, Voon LW. Functional aspects of the tear film lipid layer. Exp Eye Res. 2004;78(3):347–60.

Bucolo C, Melilli B, Piazza C, Zurria M, Drago F. Ocular pharmacokinetics profile of different indomethacin topical formulations. J Ocul Pharmacol Ther. 2011;27(6):571–6.

Fox RI, Stern M, Michelson P. Update in Sjögren syndrome. Curr Opin Rheumatol. 2000; 12(5):391–8.

Gipson IK, Argüeso P. Role of mucins in the function of the corneal and conjunctival epithelia. Int Rev Cytol. 2003;231:1–49.

Holly FJ, Lemp MA. Tear physiology and dry eyes. Surv Ophthalmol. 1977;22(2):69–87.

Hütz WW, Eckhardt HB, Kohnen T. Comparison of viscoelastic substances used in phacoemulsification. J Cataract Refract Surg. 1996;22(7):955–9.

IDEW-2007. The definition and classification of dry eye disease: report of the Definition and Classification Subcommittee of the International Dry Eye WorkShop (2007). Ocul Surf. 2007;5(2):75–92.

Itakura H, Kashima T, Itakura M, Akiyama H, Kishi S. Topical rebamipide improves lid wiper epitheliopathy. Clin Ophthalmol. 2013;7:2137–41. doi:10.2147/OPTH.S5451. Epub 2013 Oct 31.

Johnson ME, Murphy PJ. Changes in the tear film and ocular surface from dry eye syndrome. Prog Retin Eye Res. 2004;23:449–74.

Kashima T, Itakura H, Akiyama H, Kishi S. Rebamipide ophthalmic suspension for the treatment of dry eye syndrome: a critical appraisal. Clin Ophthalmol. 2014;8:1003–10. doi:10.2147/OPTH.S40798. eCollection 2014.

Keating GM. Diquafosol Ophthalmic Solution 3%: A Review of Its Use in Dry Eye. Drugs. 2015;75(8):911–22.

Koh S, Maeda N, Ikeda C, Takai Y, Fujimoto H, Oie Y, Soma T, Tsujikawa M, Nishida K. Effect of instillation of eyedrops for dry eye on optical quality. Invest Ophthalmol Vis Sci. 2013; 54(7):4927–33. doi:10.1167/iovs.13-12409.

Kohashi M, Ishimaru N, Arakaki R, Hayashi Y. Effective treatment with oral administration of rebamipide in a mouse model of Sjögren's syndrome. Arthritis Rheum. 2008;58(2):389–400. doi:10.1002/art.23163.

Lau OC, Samarawickrama C, Skalicky SE. P2Y2 receptor agonists for the treatment of dry eye disease: a review. Clin Ophthalmol. 2014;8:327–34.

McCulley JP, Shine WE. The lipid layer of tears: dependent on meibomian gland function. Exp Eye Res. 2004;78(3):361–5.

McDermott AM, et al. Pathways of corneal and ocular surface inflammation: a perspective from the Cullen Symposium. Ocul Surf. 2005;3(4):S131–8.

Moscovici BK, Holzchuh R, Sakassegawa-Naves FE, Hoshino-Ruiz DR, Albers MB, Santo RM, Hida RY. Treatment of Sjögren's syndrome dry eye using 0.03% tacrolimus eye drop: prospective double-blind randomized study. Cont Lens Anterior Eye. 2015;38(5):373–8. doi:10.1016/j.clae.2015.04.004. Epub 2015 May 5.

Moshirfar M, Pierson K, Hanamaikai K, Santiago-Caban L, Muthappan V, Passi SF. Artificial tears potpourri: a literature review. Clin Ophthalmol. 2014;8:1419–33.

Ono M, Takamura E, Shinozaki K, Tsumura T, Hamano T, Yagi Y, Tsubota K. Therapeutic effect of cevimeline on dry eye in patients with Sjögren's syndrome: a randomized, double-blind clinical study. Am J Ophthalmol. 2004;138(1):6–17.

Petrone D, Condemi JJ, Fife R, Gluck O, Cohen S, Dalgin P. A double-blind, randomized, placebo-controlled study of cevimeline in Sjögren's syndrome patients with xerostomia and keratoconjunctivitis sicca. Arthritis Rheum. 2002;46(3):748–54.

Piwkumsribonruang N, Somboonporn W, Luanratanakorn P, Kaewrudee S, Tharnprisan P, Soontrapa S. Effectiveness of hormone therapy for treating dry eye syndrome in postmenopausal women: a randomized trial. J Med Assoc Thai. 2010;93(6):647–52.

Pfau B, Kruse FE, Rohrschneider K, Zorn M, Fiehn W, Burk RO, Völcker HE. Comparison between local and systemic administration of cyclosporin A on the effective level in conjunctiva, aqueous humor and serum. Ophthalmologe. 1995;92(6):833–9.

Ramos-Casals M, Tzioufas AG, Stone JH, Sisó A, Bosch X. Treatment of primary Sjögren syndrome: a systematic review. JAMA. 2010;304(4):452–60. doi:10.1001/jama.2010.1014.

Ríos JD, Shatos M, Urashima H, Tran H, Dartt DA. OPC-12759 increases proliferation of cultured rat conjunctival goblet cells. Cornea. 2006;25(5):573–81.

Ríos JD, Shatos MA, Urashima H, Dartt DA. Effect of OPC-12759 on EGF receptor activation, p44/p42 MAPK activity, and secretion in conjunctival goblet cells. Exp Eye Res. 2008;86(4):629–36.

Saettone MF, Monti D, Torracca MT, Chetoni P. Mucoadhesive ophthalmic vehicles: evaluation of polymeric low-viscosity formulations. J Ocul Pharmacol. 1994;10(1):83–92.

Scott G, Yiu SC, Wasilewski D, Song J, Smith RE. Combined esterified estrogen and methyltestosterone treatment for dry eye syndrome in postmenopausal women. Am J Ophthalmol. 2005;139(6):1109–10.

Scuderi G, Contestabile MT, Gagliano C, Iacovello D, Scuderi L, Avitabile T. Effects of phytoestrogen supplementation in postmenopausal women with dry eye syndrome: a randomized clinical trial. Can J Ophthalmol. 2012;47(6):489–92.

Simmons PA, Donshik PC, Kelly WF, Vehige JG. Conditioning of hydrogel lenses by a multipurpose solution containing an ocular lubricant. CLAO J. 2001;27(4):192–4.

Snibson GR, Greaves JL, Soper ND, Tiffany JM, Wilson CG, Bron A. Ocular surface residence times of artificial tear solutions. Cornea. 1992;11(4):288–93.

Takeji Y, Urashima H, Aoki A, Shinohara H. Rebamipide increases the mucin-like glycoprotein production in corneal epithelial cells. J Ocul Pharmacol Ther. 2012;28(3):259–63.

Tandon R, Shiva P. Gantyala A, Velpandian T, et al. Study of ocular bioavailability of oral rebamipide to determine its potential value in the management of dry eye. Proceedings of ARVO. 2012.

Terakado K, Yogo T, Kohara Y, Soeta S, Nezu Y, Harada Y, Hara Y, Amasaki H, Tagawa M. Conjunctival expression of the P2Y2 receptor and the effects of 3% diquafosol ophthalmic solution in dogs. Vet J. 2014;202(1):48–52. doi:10.1016/j.tvjl.2014.05.022. Epub 2014 May 22.

Thomson AW, Bonham CA, Zeevi A. Mode of action of tacrolimus (FK506): molecular and cellular mechanisms. Ther Drug Monit. 1995;17(6):584–91.

Tiffany JM. The normal tear film. Dev Ophthalmol. 2008;41:1–20. doi:10.1159/000131066.

Vivino FB, Al-Hashimi I, Khan Z, LeVeque FG, Salisbury 3rd PL, Tran-Johnson TK, Muscoplat CC, Trivedi M, Goldlust B, Gallagher SC. Pilocarpine tablets for the treatment of dry mouth and dry eye symptoms in patients with Sjögren syndrome: a randomized, placebo-controlled, fixed-dose, multicenter trial. P92-01 Study Group. Arch Intern Med. 1999;159(2):174–81.

Wagh VD, Inamdar B, Samanta MK. Polymers used in ocular dosage form and drug delivery systems. Asian J Pharm. 2008;2:12–7.

Yoon KC, Heo H, Im SK, You IC, Kim YH, Park YG. Comparison of autologous serum and umbilical cord serum eye drops for dry eye syndrome. Am J Ophthalmol. 2007;144(1):86–92. Epub 2007 May 9.

Zhao H, Jumblatt JE, Wood TO, Jumblatt MM. Quantification of MUC5AC protein in human tears. Cornea. 2001;20(8):873–7.

Zhou XQ, Wei RL. Topical cyclosporine A in the treatment of dry eye: a systematic review and meta-analysis. Cornea. 2014;33(7):760–7.

Chapter 11
Antimicrobial Agents for Ocular Use: Bacterial, Fungal, Viral, and Protozoal Infections

Namrata Sharma, Neelima Aron, Tushar Agarwal, and Charu Sharma

Abstract Ocular microbial infections are one of the leading causes of avoidable visual impairment in the world with higher prevalence in developing countries. The incidence and organism responsible for ocular infections are attributed to indiscriminate use of antibiotics, corticosteroids, poor sanitary conditions, rising trend of the use of contact lens etc. A wide variety of microorganisms; bacterial, fungal, viral and protozoal in origin are reported to be involved in ocular infections. These ocular infections include conjunctivitis, blepharitis, endophthalmitis and corneal ulcers which are vision threatening if not treated in time. This chapter dwells with the type of antibiotics/antimicrobial agents used for bacterial, fungal, viral and protozoal ocular infections and provides the insight for the judicious use of antibiotics/antimicrobial agents in treating these infections.

11.1 Antifungal Agents for Ocular Use

Infectious keratitis is one of the leading causes of corneal blindness in the world with a higher prevalence in developing countries. Infections caused by fungal organisms have been on a rise especially in developing countries where 50 % of

N. Sharma, MD • N. Aron • T. Agarwal
Cornea Services, Dr. Rajendra Prasad Center for Ophthalmic Sciences,
All India Institute of Medical Sciences, New Delhi, India
e-mail: namrata103@hotmail.com

C. Sharma, PhD (✉)
Department of Internal Medicine, College of Medicine and Health Sciences,
UAE University, Al-Ain, UAE
e-mail: shree.charu@gmail.com

T. Velpandian (ed.), *Pharmacology of Ocular Therapeutics*,
DOI 10.1007/978-3-319-25498-2_11

the cases are due to fungal organisms. The implicated factors in its causation are indiscriminate use of antibiotics and corticosteroids leading to ocular compromise. Despite the emergence of newer drugs, the cure still remains difficult in view of poor ocular penetration of the drugs.

The common antifungals used for fungal keratitis are classified as follows:

1. Polyenes
   (i) Large polyenes: Nystatin and amphotericin B
   (ii) Small polyenes: Natamycin
2. Azoles
   (i) Imidazoles: Miconazole, ketoconazole, and clotrimazole
   (ii) Triazoles: Fluconazole, itraconazole, voriconazole, and posaconazole
3. Pyrimidines

   Flucytosine
4. Echinocandins

   Caspofungin and micafungin

11.1.1 Polyenes

This class of drugs includes amphotericin B (AMB), natamycin, and nystatin. Nystatin is not used routinely to treat ocular infection due to its low intraocular penetration, toxicity, and resistance to the drug. However, natamycin and amphotericin B are the most commonly used drugs in cases of fungal keratitis.

11.1.1.1 Amphotericin B

AMB was the first broad-spectrum antifungal agent to be discovered. It is produced by the actinomycete *Streptomyces nodosus*. It was approved by the FDA in the 1960s due to its great efficiency in controlling disseminated fungal infections.

Mechanism of Action AMB works by creating pores in the cell wall by binding to ergosterol, allowing small ions such as potassium to leak out causing imbalances in the osmotic gradient and eventually cell lysis. Its action is primarily fungistatic, with fungicidal action depending on the concentration reached in the target tissue (Khoo et al. 1994).

AMB acts on both yeast and filamentous fungi. It has an excellent spectrum, being effective against *Candida* species, *Aspergillus* species, *Penicillium marneffei*, *Cryptococcus* species, and the causative agents of mucormycosis. It is also effective, to a lesser extent, against *Fusarium*.

Systemic administration of AMB produces little penetration into the ocular tissues and does not reach therapeutic levels in the cornea and aqueous or vitreous humor (Kaur et al. 2008 and O'Day et al. 1985). Also, the multiple side effects preclude its systemic administration. Ocular administration therefore is the commonly used form of treatment. It is one of the few drugs which can be used through the subconjunctival, topical, intrastromal, intracameral, and intravitreal routes.

Dosage AMB is prepared from the intravenous formulation diluted in distilled water. It is used at a concentration of 1.5–5 mg/ml and administered at one-hour intervals at the beginning of treatment and then every 4 h once the therapeutic response is observed. Periodic debridement of the corneal epithelium is recommended since the drug has a poor penetration in an intact epithelium (O'Day et al. 1984).

Subconjunctival administration is used in patients not compliant to topical therapy; however, it is not preferred in view of reports of conjunctival necrosis, scleral thinning, and scleral melt (O'Day 1987). Intrastromal administration of AMB at a concentration of 5–10 μg is administered for deep infections affecting the stroma that do not respond well to topical and systemic treatment. The interval between two doses should be at least 72 h. Intracameral administration of the drug is suggested for infection penetrating the Descemet's membrane affecting the anterior chamber. Yoon et al. compared 14 eyes who were administered intracameral AMB versus 17 eyes who were on conventional antifungal therapy. It was noted that eyes that received intracameral AMB had an early disappearance of hypopyon and final improvement in comparison to eyes on conventional therapy (Yoon et al. 2007).

In keratitis associated with fungal endophthalmitis, intravitreal administration of AMB is recommended in a dose of 5–10 μg and may be repeated within 48–72 h.

Side Effects The main reason for the side effects of AMB is its binding to cholesterol which is present in the cell wall of the host cells. Systemic administration via infusion can lead to fever, chills, hyperventilation, hypotension, nausea and vomiting, and tubular injury. Intrastromal and intracameral administration of the drug may lead to pain, endothelial cell loss, iritis, and persistent corneal edema in doses greater than 15–20 μg. Intravitreal injections in higher doses can lead to retinal necrosis and toxicity.

11.1.1.2 Natamycin

Similar to amphotericin B, natamycin is a polyene antifungal and is the drug of choice for the treatment of keratitis caused by filamentous fungi.

Mechanism of Action Natamycin binds to ergosterol in the cell wall of the fungi, forming blisters and causing lysis of the cells. This action is not concentration dependent unlike AMB.

It is used in a concentration of 5 % (50 mg/ml) and is well tolerated when used topically. Epithelial debridement is recommended as an adjuvant therapy so that higher concentrations can be achieved in the corneal stroma. For deeper infections, natamycin should be combined with other antifungals for the treatment.

Natamycin is a broad-spectrum antifungal. Although it also works against *Candida* infection, AMB remains the drug of choice for yeast infections. The dosing interval is similar to AMB. The drug is administered at 1-h interval until the signs of resolution are visible. Once the therapeutic response is seen, the dosing interval can be increased to one drop administered every 4 h. Natamycin is effective against *Fusarium,* and it has been observed that it has a lower minimum inhibitory concentration than AMB against both *Aspergillus* and *Fusarium* (Lalitha et al. 2007).

Subconjunctival injections can be given but are not recommended in view of risk of scleritis and melt. There are no reports of administration of NTM through other routes (intracameral, intravitreal, intrastromal, or systemic).

The Mycotic Ulcer Treatment Trial (MUTT) has been conducted to compare topical natamycin versus voriconazole in the treatment of filamentous fungal keratitis. It was a multicenter trial which randomized 368 patients of fungal keratitis to natamycin 5 % or voriconazole 1 %. It was found that the natamycin treatment was associated with significantly better clinical and microbiological outcomes than voriconazole treatment for smear-positive filamentous fungal keratitis, with much of the difference attributable to improved results in Fusarium cases (Prajna et al. 2013).

Another study was conducted comparing natamycin versus VZ in 120 patients with fungal keratitis in which there was no significant difference in visual acuity, scar size, and perforations between voriconazole- and natamycin-treated patients (Prajna et al. 2010).

11.1.2 Azoles

This class of drugs has a broader spectrum of activity as compared to AMB and fewer side effects. They are divided into two classes: imidazoles which were first to be introduced in the market, and followed by triazoles. The imidazoles used more often include miconazole (MCZ), econazole (ECZ), and ketoconazole (KCZ). Among the first-generation triazoles, the most often used are itraconazole (ICZ) and fluconazole. Second-generation triazoles were introduced into clinical practice in the past decade and include voriconazole and posaconazole (PCZ). Azoles act on cytochrome P450 enzymes and block the synthesis of ergosterol in the plasma membrane, thus inhibiting fungal growth.

11.1.2.1 Imidazoles

The imidazoles have various mechanisms of action for their antifungal activity. At low concentrations, they affect the formation of ergosterol present in the cell membranes. At higher concentrations, they can disrupt lysosomes, causing direct damage. Also, most imidazoles inhibit catalase and cytochrome C peroxidase intracellularly, causing accumulation of hydrogen peroxide leading to cell death.

11.1.2.2 Miconazole

It is a broad-spectrum antifungal with activity against *Cryptococcus*, *Fusarium*, *Aspergillus*, *Curvularia*, *Candida,* and *Trichophyton*. It not only acts on the synthesis of ergosterol but also leads to inhibition of peroxidases, resulting in the accumulation of free radicals in the fungal cytoplasm which leads to cell death (Kobayashi et al. 2002). Topical use at a dose of 10 mg/ml or a 1 % solution is effective especially if associated with epithelial scraping. Compared to polyenes, MCZ is less effective but provides better penetration into ocular tissues (Foster and Stefanyszyn 1979).

11.1.2.3 Econazole

Econazole is primarily used in the treatment of superficial mycosis and not used routinely for the treatment of ocular infections. In a clinical trial, 116 eyes with fungal keratitis were randomized to either econazole 2 % or natamycin 5 %, and it was found that econazole is as efficacious as natamycin for the treatment of fungal keratitis (Prajna et al. 2010). However, the drug is not commercially available for ocular administration which prevents its ophthalmic use.

11.1.2.4 Ketoconazole

KCZ was the first systemic imidazole to be used successfully for the treatment of fungal infections. It is available in 200 mg tablets with a recommended dose of 200–400 mg daily. Its oral absorption depends on the gastric pH ($pH<3$); therefore, it should be taken on empty stomach and without gastric acid suppressives. KCZ is available in a topical formulation of 1–5 % concentration, but other drugs have been shown to be superior in comparative studies (Torres et al. 1985).

Currently, systemic KCZ is indicated only for the adjuvant treatment of deep fungal keratitis. The indications of oral ketoconazole are fungal corneal ulcers >6 mm in size, >2/3rd in depth, perforated ulcer, impending perforation, and limbal and scleral involvement. Recently, a randomized controlled trial was carried out to assess the role of additive oral antifungal therapy in deep keratitis caused by filamentous fungi. All patients with corneal ulcer size measuring 2–6 mm and involving >50 % depth were randomized to topical natamycin 5 % alone or topical natamycin plus oral ketoconazole 200 mg twice a day. It was found that there was no statistically significant difference in the ulcer healing rates between the two groups. Hence, the study showed that oral KCZ did not add significant benefit to topical natamycin therapy in treating deep fungal keratitis (Torres et al. 1985).

The systemic side effects include pruritus, nausea, vomiting, diarrhea, cramps, reversible gynecomastia, and elevation in liver enzymes.

11.1.2.5 Triazoles

Itraconazole

ICZ is used in a dose of 400 mg/day in the treatment of infections by *Candida* spp. (Klotz et al. 1996). However, when administered orally, it exhibits lower bioavailability, solubility, and penetration into ocular tissues than other azoles (Rajaraman et al. 1987). However, ICZ has not been found to be very effective against *Fusarium*.

In a randomized controlled trial involving 100 patients, topical itraconazole 1 % was found to be inferior when compared to natamycin 5 % (Kalavathy et al. 2005). The study concluded that when natamycin is unavailable, topical itraconazole therapy could be used, particularly if the infections are due to *Aspergillus* or *Curvularia* spp. The MIC of ICZ is higher than both AMB and KCZ; hence, systemic use should be limited only to the adjuvant treatment of eye infections by yeasts.

Fluconazole

Oral use at 200–400 mg per day is effective in the treatment of eye infections, with or without topical NTM (Urbak and Degn 1994). Unlike KCZ and ICZ, FCZ shows excellent absorption from the gastrointestinal tract unaffected by gastric acidity. Its penetration into the ocular tissue is effective and reaches aqueous concentration similar to that of plasma (O'Day et al. 1990). FCZ achieves good intracorneal levels at a dose of 2 mg/ml with penetration being better after epithelial scraping. However, it is less effective in the treatment of fungal endophthalmitis.

The ocular penetration of FCZ has been shown to be superior to KCZ. However, the antifungal spectrum of FCZ is narrow. In many studies, it has shown to be effective against yeasts like *Candida,* whereas filamentous fungi like *Aspergillus* and *Fusarium* have shown to exhibit marked resistance to it (Li et al. 2008).

Topical FCZ 2 % was found to be effective in six eyes with microbiologically proven *Candida* keratitis with abscess formation. The average duration of healing was found to be 22.6 ± 2.3 days (Panda et al. 1996).

Voriconazole

VCZ is the next generation of triazoles with a similar mechanism of action but is more effective in blocking the synthesis of ergosterol. It has a lower MIC as compared to first triazoles which increases its efficacy against the filamentous fungi (Martinez 2006). VCZ is commercially available for oral and parenteral administration. It is given orally at a dose of 200 mg at 12-hour intervals reaching peak plasma concentrations after 2–3 h.

It is metabolized by the liver; therefore, liver enzymes should be monitored during the therapy. The side effects include visual disorders (blurred vision, change in color perception, and photophobia), which are present in about 30 % of patients using the drug and are usually reversible.

Topical VCZ has been used extensively in a concentration of 1 mg/ml for the treatment of fungal keratitis, both caused by *Candida* and filamentous fungi. Its advantages compared to polyenes include its greater stability to light and temperature, remaining effective for up to 30 days (Dupuis et al. 2009).

Intrastromal and intracameral VCZ has been used in cases with deep stromal involvement and anterior chamber penetration unresponsive to topical therapy. The dose of VCZ used is 50–100 μg/0.1 ml which can be repeated every 72 h (Prakash et al. 2008). Intravitreal VCZ has been shown to be safe in animal models with no changes in electroretinogram (Gao et al. 2003).

Three eyes of three patients with deep stromal recalcitrant fungal keratitis not responding to topical antifungal medications were subjected to intrastromal injection of voriconazole 50 μg/0.1 ml as an adjunct to topical therapy. A faster reduction in the size of corneal infiltration was documented, and a complete resolution of the ulcers was seen within 3 weeks in all cases after the injection (Prakash et al. 2008).

Another study was conducted in 40 eyes comparing topical versus intrastromal voriconazole as an adjunct to natamycin in recalcitrant fungal keratitis. It was found that topical voriconazole was a useful adjunct to natamycin in fungal keratitis not responding to topical natamycin. Intrastromal injections did not offer any beneficial effect over topical therapy (Sharma et al. 2013a, b).

In another prospective randomized controlled trial, 118 patients with fungal keratitis were treated with either voriconazole 1 % or natamycin 5 %. Again, natamycin was found to be more effective than voriconazole in the treatment of fungal keratitis, especially *Fusarium* (Sharma et al. 2013a, b).

Posaconazole

Similar to VCZ, PCZ is a second-generation triazole introduced recently in medical practice. It is primarily indicated for the treatment of invasive fungal infections in onco-hematological patients. It is available in an oral preparation which is administered 200 mg four times a day or 400 mg twice a day. Only adverse effects reported until date include gastrointestinal side effects.

PCZ has been shown to have a broad spectrum of activity against both yeasts and filamentous fungi including Fusarium. It was shown to be effective in the treatment of recalcitrant fungal keratitis unresponsive to conventional therapy (fluconazole, amphotericin, natamycin, and voriconazole) (Altun et al. 2014).

11.1.3 Pyrimidines

They are represented by 5-fluorocytosine which is the only antifungal drug with intracellular action. After being absorbed by the fungus, it gets converted to 5-fluorouracil which acts as an antimetabolite and inhibits fungal DNA synthesis (Vermes et al. 2000).

It is not routinely used in the treatment of fungal keratitis in view of narrow antifungal spectrum and poor ocular penetration which makes it ineffective in comparison to the new triazoles and polyenes (Morris and Villmann 2006). It is effective against *Candida* and has varied action against *Aspergillus* species, whereas it is ineffective against *Fusarium*. It should be administered along with AMB due to its potentiating effect and to prevent the development of resistance to 5-FC.

11.1.4 Echinocandins

They are semisynthetic lipopeptides that inhibit the synthesis of glucan in the fungal cell wall through noncompetitive inhibition of 1,3-α-glucan synthase, causing osmotic imbalance and cell lysis. This class of drugs includes caspofungin and micafungin. They have fungicidal action against *Candida* species but not against other yeast cells. It has fungistatic action against *Aspergillus* but is ineffective against *Fusarium*.

Topical CFG is used in a concentration of 1.5–5 mg/ml and was found to be as effective as AMB in an animal model against *Candida* (Goldblum et al. 2005). Also, few case reports suggest successful topical application of caspofungin in the treatment of candida keratitis refractory to voriconazole (Hurtado-Sarrió et al. 2010).

11.1.5 Combination Therapy

In order to broaden the antifungal spectrum and increase the efficacy of treatment, two or more drugs are often combined in the treatment of fungal keratitis. Azoles are often combined with NTM or AMB. However, several studies showed an antagonistic effect between these drugs. The introduction of an azole decreases the synthesis of ergosterol in the cell membrane, a binding site for polyenes, whose action is therefore decreased. However, polyenes such as natamycin and triazoles such as voriconazole are often combined in the treatment of filamentous fungi and have shown a synergistic effect. The combination of two drugs of the same class is often discouraged such as NTM and AMB since it increases local and systemic toxicity and fails to increase therapeutic efficacy (Lin et al. 2005).

Table 11.1 depicts the dosing and indication of use of the various antifungal drugs available in the market.

11.1.6 Conclusion

To conclude, a variety of antifungal drugs are available in the market for topical and systemic use, the choice of which depends upon the causative organism, the location, and the extent of infection. Standard therapy with polyenes remains the first choice of treatment for fungal keratitis. New-generation triazoles act as an add-on therapy in cases of poor responsiveness to the former. Studies until date lack the demonstration of superiority of the newer-generation triazoles over the conventional therapy with polyenes.

Table 11.1 Antifungal agents and their indications

Drug	Route	Dosing	Indication
Amphotericin B	Topical	1.5–5 mg/ml	First choice in keratitis by yeasts
	Intrastromal	5–10 μg/0.1 ml	Deep keratitis with partial response to topical treatment
	Intracameral	5–10 μg/0.1 ml	Keratitis affecting anterior chamber/lens
	Intravitreal	1–10 μg/0.1 ml	First choice in fungal endophthalmitis (yeast/filamentous fungi)
Natamycin	Topical	50 mg/ml	First choice in filamentous fungi
Miconazole	Subconjunctival	1.2–10 mg/1 ml	Associated with topical therapy in low adherence to treatment
Econazole	Topical	20 mg/ml	Alternative to NTM for filamentous fungi
Ketoconazole	Oral	100–400 mg every 12 h	Deep keratitis along with topical therapy
Itraconazole	Oral	400 mg/day	Deep keratitis by yeasts
Fluconazole	Topical	2 mg/ml	Alternative to polyenes in Candida keratitis
	Subconjunctival	2 mg/1 ml	Associated with topical therapy in low adherence to treatment
	Oral	200–400 mg/day	Deep keratitis
Voriconazole	Topical	1 mg/ml	Fungal keratitis resistant to polyenes and first-line triazoles
	Intrastromal	50 μg/0.1 ml	Deep keratitis with partial response to topical therapy
	Intracameral	50 μg/0.1 ml	Deep keratitis affecting anterior chamber/lens
	Intravitreal	50 μg/0.1 ml	Alternative to AMB in fungal endophthalmitis
	Oral	200 mg every 12 h	Deep keratitis
Posaconazole	Topical	100 mg/ml	Fungal keratitis resistant to polyenes or first-line triazoles
	Oral	200 mg every 6 h or 400 mg every 12 h	Deep keratitis or endophthalmitis
Flucytosine	Topical	10 mg/ml	Association with topical AMB in Candida keratitis
Caspofungin	Topical	1.5–5 mg/ml	Fungal keratitis by yeasts resistant to polyenes or first-line triazoles
Micafungin	Topical	1 mg/ml	Fungal keratitis by yeasts resistant to polyenes or first-line triazoles

11.2 Antiviral Drugs for Ocular Use

Neelima Aron, Tushar Agarwal, Neelima Sharma,

Viruses are intracellular microorganisms which replicate inside the host cell. The development of antiviral therapy involves the identification of drugs which only attack the virus without affecting the host cells. The recognition of viral enzymes and proteins that can serve as molecular targets for drugs has revolutionized the treatment of viral infections.

Topical antiviral therapy has been available since the past 50 years, but it is only with the advent of acyclovir that a safe and effective therapy has been established for the treatment of herpetic keratitis.

Table 11.1 enumerates the various topical antiviral drugs that are available in the market as of today.

Drug	Preparation	Dosage
Trifluridine	1 % solution	Initially, 1 drop every 2 h. On healing, treatment should be continued for 7 days at a dose of 1 drop every 4 h during day time
Vidarabine	3 % ointment	Applied daily at 4-h intervals. On healing, treatment should be continued for 7 days at a twice daily dose
Idoxuridine	0.1 % solution	One drop every 2 h during the day and every 4 h at night. Treatment should be continued for 3–5 days after healing is complete
	0.5 % ointment	Applied every 4 h during daytime. Treatment should be continued for 3–5 days on healing
Acyclovir	3 % ointment	Applied five times daily at 3–4-h intervals and continued for at least 3 days after complete healing
Ganciclovir	0.15 % ointment	Applied five times a day at 3–4-h intervals and continued for at least 3 days after epithelial healing

11.2.1 Idoxuridine

It was the first topical antiviral to be used for the treatment of herpetic epithelial keratitis (Kaufman et al. 1962a, b). However, it was later replaced by its thymidine analogue, trifluridine.

Mechanism of Action IDU owes its antiviral activity to the conversion into a triphosphate form, which mimics thymidine triphosphate and becomes incorporated into viral DNA which results in faulty transcription of viral proteins and inhibition of viral replication.

Indication IDU has been used in the treatment of herpetic epithelial keratitis. Owing to its lower intraocular penetration, it is ineffective in the treatment of herpetic stromal keratitis or uveitis. It is formulated as a 0.1 % solution and a 0.5 % ointment. The recommended regimen is one hourly during the day and 2 hourly at night and tapered once healing starts to take place (Kaufman et al. 1962a, b).

IDU has been replaced by trifluridine, and it is no longer commercially available for the treatment of viral keratitis.

Toxicity IDU gets incorporated into the mammalian DNA along with viral DNA and hence is toxic to replication of normal host cells. This results in a low therapeutic ratio and accounts for systemic toxicity (Boston Inter-Hospital Viral Study Group 1975). Its use has been associated with chronic follicular conjunctivitis, conjunctival scarring, punctate keratopathy, pseudodendrites, corneal edema and opacities, indolent ulceration, punctal and canalicular stenosis, narrowing of meibomian gland orifices, and contact dermatitis of the lids (Wilson 1979).

11.2.2 Trifluridine

Trifluridine, like IDU, is a thymidine analogue which is far more potent and has less ocular and systemic toxicity.

Mechanism of Action Trifluridine, like IDU, gets converted into a triphosphate form and gets incorporated into the viral DNA leading to inhibition of transcription and viral protein synthesis. Though it also gets incorporated into the host DNA, however, viral DNA polymerase utilizes trifluridine triphosphate more efficiently than does host cell DNA polymerase. Hence, it has a more selective antiviral activity with lower ocular toxicity as compared to IDU (Prusoff et al. 1985).

Indication Trifluridine is active in vitro and in vivo against HSV-1, HSV-2 (Kaufman and Heidelberger 1964), and vaccinia and in vitro against CMV and some strains of adenovirus. It is more potent than IDU against HSV. It is available as a 1 % solution. Though its penetration is better than IDU, however, it is not very efficient in iridocyclitis or stromal keratitis. The recommended dosage is one drop every 2 h until healing is complete. This is followed by one drop every 4 h for 7 days to prevent reactivation of disease (Coster et al. 1976).

In a study, it was found that trifluridine was at least as effective as topical vidarabine ointment in the treatment of superficial herpetic dendritic keratitis with insignificant difference in the efficacy of the two drugs (Travers and Patterson 1978).

Toxicity Toxic side effects in the eye are similar to those of IDU and include punctate keratopathy, filamentary keratopathy, epithelial and stromal edema, punctal narrowing, and contact blepharodermatitis. It is too toxic for systemic use (Wilson 1979).

11.2.3 Vidarabine

Vidarabine was the second agent approved for the topical treatment of herpetic epithelial keratitis. It was also the first antiviral agent approved for systemic use; however, recently it has been replaced with acyclovir.

Mechanism of Action Vidarabine is obtained from fermentation cultures of *Streptomyces antibioticus* (Lee et al. 1960). It is a purine nucleoside analogue that resembles deoxyadenosine. It gets converted into its triphosphate form which gets incorporated into the viral DNA. Unlike IDU, trifluridine, or acyclovir, vidarabine does not require viral thymidine kinase for its phosphorylation. Therefore, it might be expected to have high activity against thymidine kinase-deficient mutants of HSV (Larder and Darby 1986).

Indication It is highly effective in the treatment of herpetic epithelial keratitis. In a study comparing trifluridine and vidarabine in 66 patients with herpetic dendritic keratitis, no difference was noted in the antiviral activity of the two drugs (Van Bijsterveld and Post 1980). A meta-analysis concluded that vidarabine was superior to IDU and equivalent to topical acyclovir and trifluridine in relative efficacy for dendritic epithelial keratitis (Wilhelmus 2000). Similar to IDU and trifluridine, it is not effective in herpetic stromal keratitis and uveitis. It is available as a 3 % ophthalmic ointment to be applied 5 times daily. Therapy should not be continued for more than 21 days.

Toxicity It is less toxic than IDU to the regenerating corneal epithelium. Clinically, the ocular toxicity is similar to IDU. The major systemic side effects include gastrointestinal upset, elevation in liver enzymes (Nicholson 1984), and neurotoxicity (Sacks et al. 1982) when administered in patients with renal dysfunction.

11.2.4 Acyclovir

The development of acyclovir revolutionized the treatment of herpetic keratitis with its better efficacy and safety profile.

Mechanism of Action It is an acyclic analogue of guanosine which is activated by viral thymidine kinase and becomes a potent inhibitor of viral DNA polymerase. It gets converted into the triphosphate form and is found in HSV-infected cells in a concentration which is 40–100 times higher than uninfected cells (Elion 1982). It has a greater affinity of viral DNA polymerase as compared to cellular DNA polymerase.

Indications The drug inhibits HSV-1 and HSV-2, VZV, Epstein-Barr virus (EBV), human herpesvirus 6 (HHV-6), and CMV (Wagstaff et al. 1994). It can be administered topically, orally, and intravenously. Topical acyclovir 3 % ophthalmic ointment has the best corneal penetration of any topical antiviral drug. It penetrates intact corneal epithelium to achieve aqueous levels well within the therapeutic range for HSV-1 and HSV-2. Hence, it is effective in the treatment of herpetic stromal keratitis and iridocyclitis.

Significant intraocular levels of the drug are also present after oral and intravenous administration. The oral dose is 400 mg five times a day (5 mg/kg body weight) for HSV and 800 mg five times a day (10 mg/kg body weight) for VZV (Biron and Elion 1980).

Prophylactic antiviral therapy is indicated in patients post-keratoplasty to prevent reactivation of the virus while patients are on topical corticosteroids. The drug is given in a dose of 400 mg twice a day for 1 year.

The Herpetic Eye Disease Studies were carried out in order to determine the role of acyclovir in the treatment of herpetic keratitis. HEDS I and HEDS II consisted of three randomized, placebo-controlled trials. It was found that compared with placebo, corticosteroid therapy reduced the risk of persistent or progressive stromal keratouveitis by 68 % with faster resolution of the ulcer. It determined that there is no clinical benefit of adjunctive oral acyclovir for treating HSV stromal keratitis in patients receiving concomitant topical corticosteroids and trifluridine (Barron et al. 1994). For the treatment of HSV iridocyclitis, there was a strong suggestion of clinical benefit from the addition of oral acyclovir 400 mg 5 times daily as an adjunct to topical corticosteroids and trifluridine (50 % treatment failures with acyclovir vs. 68 % with placebo) (the Herpetic Eye Disease Study Group, 1996). The addition of a 3-week course of oral acyclovir to topical trifluridine treatment of acute HSV epithelial keratitis did not prevent the subsequent development of stromal keratitis or iritis over the following year (the Epithelial Keratitis Trial, 1997). There is, however, a clear-cut benefit from long-term suppressive oral acyclovir in preventing recurrent HSV epithelial keratitis and stromal keratitis. The cumulative recurrence rate of any ocular HSV was significantly reduced from 32 to 19 % by acyclovir (Herpetic Eye Disease Study Group, 1998).

Toxicity It has not been shown to have a detrimental effect on the regenerating corneal epithelium. Superficial punctate keratopathy has been noted; however, the frequency is less than that seen with IDU. Other less common side effects include burning or stinging, tearing, follicular conjunctivitis, palpebral allergy, and punctal stenosis.

Oral acyclovir causes gastrointestinal side effects such as nausea, vomiting, and diarrhea. Liver function tests should be monitored every 2 weeks. Intravenous infusion of acyclovir can cause renal shutdown especially in patients with preexisting renal dysfunction.

11.2.5 Resistance

There are three mechanisms by which the virus can become resistant to acyclovir therapy. The most common mutation is loss of synthesis of viral thymidine kinase so that acyclovir is not phosphorylated to its active form (Wagstaff et al. 1994). A second type of mutation induces thymidine kinase with altered substrate specificity that phosphorylates thymidine but not acyclovir. Finally, a mutation of the viral DNA polymerase gene induces altered DNA polymerase that is not sensitive to inhibition by acyclovir triphosphate.

11.2.6 Ganciclovir

Ganciclovir is another antiviral agent that has been developed recently for ophthalmic use. It was the first drug to be approved by the Food and Drug Administration (FDA) for use in the treatment of CMV retinitis in immunocompromised patients.

Mechanism of Action Ganciclovir is a nucleoside analogue that is selectively phosphorylated by virus-encoded thymidine kinase and is subsequently phosphorylated by cellular enzymes. Similar to acyclovir, it is converted into ganciclovir triphosphate which inhibits herpesvirus DNA polymerase and arrests HSV replication (Davies et al. 1987).

Indication Following topical application of ganciclovir, it has been shown that the drug can penetrate the corneal stroma and can reach the aqueous humor in therapeutic levels. Corneal penetration of ganciclovir was due to the small size of the ganciclovir molecule, its high lipophilicity, and its high cellular affinity. It is available as an ophthalmic gel in a concentration of 0.15 % five times daily. Compared to acyclovir 0.3 % ointment, ganciclovir 0.15 % gel has been shown to be better tolerated and no less effective in several phase II and III trials. Randomized multicenter clinical trials demonstrated that ganciclovir ophthalmic gel 0.15 % is as effective as acyclovir in the treatment of acute epithelial herpetic keratitis. Also, ganciclovir is available in a gel form which induces lower blurring following its ophthalmic administration as compared to acyclovir which is available in an ointment form.

Ganciclovir 0.15 % gel may also help in the prevention of recurrences of herpetic keratitis in patients undergoing corneal transplantation. It is given in a dose of four times a day along with topical corticosteroids.

Toxicity The most frequent adverse effects clinically have been hematological, primarily neutropenia (40 % of patients) and thrombocytopenia (20 %) after systemic administration of the drug. No ocular toxicity has been noted after ophthalmic use.

11.2.7 Other Drugs

11.2.7.1 Valacyclovir

Valacyclovir, the L-valyl ester of acyclovir, is a prodrug that is rapidly and nearly completely converted to acyclovir after oral administration. Its excellent bioavailability results in serum acyclovir levels comparable to intravenous acyclovir but requiring less frequent dosing than oral acyclovir. Therefore, it has much the same antiviral indications and safety as oral acyclovir with the advantage of simpler dosing. For herpetic epithelial keratitis or iritis, it is used in a dose of 1000 mg twice or thrice a day which has been shown to be as effective as acyclovir 400 mg 5 times a day. For prophylaxis, it is used in a dose of 1000 mg once daily. A large multicentered randomized double-blind trial of herpes zoster was carried out which compared valacyclovir 1000 mg 3 times daily with acyclovir 800 mg 5 times daily. There was no significant difference between the drugs in the resolution of HZO. Valacyclovir, therefore, is a reasonable alternative to oral acyclovir for the treatment of HZO in immunocompetent patients at a dosage of 1000 mg 3 times daily for 7 days.

11.2.7.2 Famciclovir/Penciclovir

Famciclovir is the diacetyl-6-deoxyester prodrug of the acyclic guanosine analogue penciclovir which is similar in efficacy to acyclovir. Similar to valacyclovir, it is as effective as oral acyclovir with a less frequent dosing requirement. It is used in a dose of 250 mg three times daily for HSV and 500 mg three times daily for VZV. Tyring and associates performed a multicenter randomized study comparing famciclovir 500 mg 3 times daily with oral acyclovir 800 mg 5 times daily for 7 days in 454 immunocompetent patients with HZO. The efficacy of the two drugs was similar, with no significant difference in the percentage of patients who experienced ocular manifestations.

11.2.7.3 Valganciclovir

Valganciclovir is a valyl ester prodrug of ganciclovir that is well absorbed orally and rapidly metabolized to ganciclovir. It provides blood levels similar to that seen after intravenous infusion of ganciclovir and has been FDA approved for the induction and maintenance treatment of CMV retinitis. It is used in a dose of 900 mg twice daily for 3 weeks for induction followed by 900 mg once daily for chronic maintenance.

11.2.7.4 Foscarnet

Foscarnet has also been used for the treatment of CMV retinitis in AIDS patients. It is used in patients who are unresponsive to or intolerant to ganciclovir and in the treatment of acyclovir-resistant herpetic infections. Oral absorption is very poor; hence, the drug is administered intravenously. It is also given intravitreally for the treatment of CMV retinitis.

11.2.7.5 Cidofovir

Cidofovir has been approved only for intravenous therapy of CMV retinitis in AIDS patients. It is given in a dosage of 5 mg/kg once a week for 2 weeks induction and then every 2 weeks for maintenance therapy. Intravitreal injections have also been given for the same.

11.2.7.6 Fomivirsen

It belongs to a new class of drugs of antisense nucleotides to be used clinically. It is administered only via intravitreal injections and is a second-line drug in the treatment of CMV retinitis.[33]

11.2.8 Conclusion

A variety of antiviral drugs have been identified for the treatment of herpetic and other eye infections. The advent of acyclovir and its prodrugs has revolutionized the treatment of herpetic eye infections. The search for newer drugs with better efficacy and an enhanced safety profile is still on.

11.3 Antibacterial Agents in Ocular Infections

Antibiotics are the substances produced by microorganisms which selectively inhibit the growth of microorganisms (bacteriostatic drugs) or kill the microorganisms (bactericidal drugs). When bacteriostatic drugs are used to treat ocular infection, the host defense mechanisms are ultimately responsible for clearing and eradicating the infective organism (Leeming 1999). In bacterial keratitis, the infection develops in the avascular cornea, and in endophthalmitis it develops in the fluid-filled aqueous or vitreous cavity (Ryan and Durand 2011). In either case, the immune system may be unable to control the microorganism fast enough to prevent the sight-threatening sequelae. Within the first 24 h, pathogens may multiply and release toxins and degradative enzymes that destroy the function and integrity of ocular tissues (Snyder and Glasser 1994).

Therefore, the bactericidal drugs are preferred for the treatment of severe ocular infections. Sometime, for severe systemic infections involve ocular components, systemic antibiotics are instituted with adjunctive topical therapy (Andreoli et al. 2004). Systemic antibiotics have poor penetration into the anterior chamber of the eye, and thus, both systemic and topical aminoglycoside antibiotics, and occasionally subconjunctival injections, are required for effective treatment.

11.3.1 General Classification of Antibacterial Agents

The antibiotics are classified on the basis of the following:

- Chemical structure (sulfonamides, diaminopyrimidines, quinolones, β-lactam antibiotics, tetracyclines, nitrobenzene derivatives, macrolides, lincosamides, glycopeptides, oxazolidinones, polypeptides, nitrofuran derivatives, nitroimidazoles, azoles, and nicotinic acid derivatives)
- Mechanism of action (inhibit cell wall synthesis, disrupt cell membrane, inhibit protein synthesis, inhibit DNA topoisomerase, interfere with DNA function or synthesis, and interfere with intermediary metabolism)
- Spectrum of activity (narrow spectrum and broad spectrum)
- Type of action (bacteriostatic and bactericidal), origin (from bacteria, actinomycetes, and fungi)

- Type of organism against which they are primarily active (antibacterial, antifungal, antiviral, antiprotozoal, and anthelmintic).
- Site of action (usually target against cell wall, cytoplasmic membrane, intermediate metabolites, and DNA synthesis in microorganisms)

11.3.2 Factors Affecting the Choice of Antibacterial Agent

The choice of an antibacterial is based on considerations of pharmacodynamic, pharmacokinetic, and bacteriological characteristics, risk of selecting resistant mutants, and cost. The bioavailability of an antibacterial agent depends on the target bacterial species, the site of infection, and the integrity of the hemato-aqueous barrier (Leeming 1999). The bactericidal agents like Penicillins, cephalosporins, aminoglycosides and fluoroquinolones are used to treat ocular infections. Whereas, bacteriostatic agents like tetracyclines, erythromycin, chloramphenicol and sulfonamides are often used for less severe infections or for specific benefit such as tetracycline in the treatment of ocular rosacea.

Some agents (fusidic acid, quinolones) penetrate the cornea, passing into the anterior chamber of normal eyes at therapeutic concentrations, whereas others (polymyxin B, bacitracin) have no penetrating powers and remain at the surface of the eye. Toxicity is mostly manifested by allergic reactions to excipients or active ingredients in topical antibacterial preparations. A few cases of hematological toxicity have brought suspicion on topical chloramphenicol, but the link has yet to be proven. Erythromycin and polymyxin B are good to use as topical applications in pregnant women and nursing mothers (Robert and Adenis 2001; Leeming 1999).

The ophthalmic antibacterial preparations are frequently used topically either as eye drop or eye ointment in the treatment of patients with superficial ocular infections, including conjunctivitis, blepharitis, and corneal ulcers. In addition, these are also used to augment treatment for intraocular infection administered systemically or by local instillation. Topically administered antibiotics are appropriate for external ocular infections, including the conjunctiva and cornea. The addition of subconjunctival antibiotic administration is indicated for serious corneal as well as anterior segment infections. Intravitreal antibiotic administration is potentially hazardous but indicated for bacterial endophthalmitis. Some cataract surgeons incorporate antibiotics into infusion fluid during phacoemulsification. The knowledge of the pharmacokinetics of topically applied agents is useful in guiding treatment regimens, particularly in serious corneal infections (Robert and Adenis 2001).

Systemic ceftazidime can be used for many Gram-negative bacteria, but intravitreal injection is recommended for better coverage, especially for more-potent organisms. Systemic moxifloxacin can be considered for most Gram-positive and Gram-negative infections due to its excellent intraocular penetration and broad coverage, but the patient's previous history of its topical use and increasing resistance patterns must be considered (Ahmed et al. 2014). Intracameral cefuroxime is significantly more effective than not using prophylaxis or the use of a topical antibiotic.

The economic evaluation comparing different prophylaxis regimens had also shown that intracameral cefuroxime has best cost-effectiveness ratio (Linertová et al. 2014).

Costs of treatment must be evaluated as a whole (regimen, drug associations) as the prices for a bottle of eye drops or the ointments may vary severalfolds. The cheapest drugs include chloramphenicol, polymyxin B, and gentamicin, the most expensive being fusidic acid and the quinolones (Robert and Adenis 2001). Intravitreal antibiotic penetration of systemic antibiotics with or without penetrating ocular injury varies depending on the antibiotic. For prevention or treatment of Gram-positive bacteria-causing endophthalmitis, intravitreal vancomycin is necessary and provides the most reliable coverage.

The widespread use of an antibacterial increases risks of selecting resistance to it. Acquired resistance is well documented for fusidic acid and several cephalosporins and newly described fluoroquinolones. The details of each antibiotics class divided based on mechanism of action used in ocular preparation or ophthalmic usages are described below.

11.3.2.1 Cell Wall Synthesis Inhibitors

Penicillins, cephalosporins, glycopeptide, and polypeptide are the class of antibiotics known to target cell wall synthesis machinery.

Penicillins

The penicillins structurally consist of a thiazolidine ring with a β-lactam ring connected to a side chain. Several of the penicillins are used in ophthalmic preparations. These are as follows: penicillin G, penicillin V (acid-resistant penicillin), methicillin, cloxacillin (penicillinase-resistant penicillins), carbenicillin, mezlocillin, piperacillin, and ticarcillin (extended-spectrum penicillins).

Spectrum of Activity Penicillins have higher susceptibility against Gram-positive bacteria. Extended-spectrum penicillins have significant activity against Pseudomonas aeruginosa and certain Proteus, Enterobacter, and Acinetobacter spp. that are not susceptible to most other penicillins.

Mechanism of Action Penicillins act by interfering with synthesis of bacterial cell wall. They inhibit the transpeptidases so that cross-linking (which maintains the close knit structures of the cell wall) does not occur.

Indications Topical use of penicillins for treatment of eye disease is limited by their narrow spectrum and high incidence of allergic reaction to these drugs. Penicillin G has a narrow spectrum of activity though used for the treatment of patients with keratitis caused by susceptible *Streptococcus pneumoniae*. A 14-day course of high-dose intravenous penicillin G is first-line therapy for all stages of ocular syphilis and chorioretinitis (Benson et al. 2015). Oral penicillin is used in the treatment of poststreptococcal syndrome uveitis (PSU), a newly recognized immune-mediated response to group A β-hemolytic streptococcus infection (Tinley et al. 2012).

Ticarcillin and piperacillin are used with an aminoglycoside antibiotic topically and subconjunctivally for the treatment of bacterial corneal ulcers caused by Pseudomonas and other Gram-negative rods. Carbenicillin is useful in corneal ulcer caused by the opportunistic organism Achromobacter xylosoxidans which developed during chronic topical steroid treatment of an eye with neovascular glaucoma (Newman et al. 1984). Topical piperacillin/tazobactam is used as an option for the treatment of therapy-resistant P. aeruginosa keratitis (Chew et al. 2010). Also, methicillin is preferred in combination with aminoglycoside for the treatment of keratitis.

Cephalosporins

Cephalosporins are semisynthetic antibiotics derived from a fungus, cephalosporium. It shares its pharmacology with penicillins in structure and mechanism of action. The compounds are commonly classified from first to fifth generation based on their clinical uses and varying spectrum of activity. The cephalosporins that belong to each generation used in ophthalmic preparations are the following: first-generation cephalosporins (cefazolin, cephalexin, and cefadroxil), second-generation cephalosporins (cefamandole, cefaclor, cefprozil, cefoxitin, and cefuroxime), third-generation cephalosporins (ceftriaxone, cefixime, cefoperazone, ceftazidime, ceftibuten, cefdinir, and cefepime), and fourth-generation cephalosporins (cefepime and cefpirome) appear more active against Gram-negative organisms and appear more active against Gram-negative enteric bacteria. All are effective against Gram-positive bacteria, but their activity against Gram-negative bacteria is relatively modest. The activity of cephalosporins increased toward Gram-negative bacteria along with generations.

Spectrum of Activity Second-generation cephalosporins appear more active against Gram-negative enteric bacteria. Third-generation cephalosporins are more active against Gram-negative organisms.

Mechanism of Action All cephalosporins are bactericidal and inhibit bacterial cell wall synthesis, similar to the penicillins, but bind to other proteins than penicillin.

Indications Cefazolin is used to treat bacterial corneal ulcers as part of a broad-spectrum approach in combination with an aminoglycoside or fluoroquinolone such as ciprofloxacin. It is used due to its activity against Gram-positive cocci, including penicillin-resistant Staphylococci. The clinical response is variable in infections caused by the viridans group of Streptococci. Cefazolin is not available as an ophthalmic preparation so it is administered topically as a specially prepared solution or subconjunctivally. It is found to be highly active against Gram-positive bacteria, a common cause of bacterial keratitis (Rautaraya et al. 2014). Cefazolin and cefuroxime are resistant to staphylococcal β-lactamases and used in combination with aminoglycosides in the empirical treatment of keratitis. Cefazolin and cefuroxime intracameral injection are used to decrease the risk of endophthalmitis at the end of cataract surgery (Vazirani and Basu 2013; Kessel et al. 2015).

Second-generation cephalosporins have limited use in ophthalmic practice. Ceftazidime shows excellent activity against Gram-negative bacteria including Pseudomonas aeruginosa and remains the most popular mode of antibiotic prophylaxis in cataract surgery patients for prophylaxis from endophthalmitis (Sridhar et al. 2015). Ceftazidime is also suggested as an alternative for intravitreal amikacin in the treatment of endophthalmitis (Mehta et al. 2011). It possesses high therapeutic index with a lower risk of retinal toxicity than amikacin.

Polypeptide Antibiotic

Bacitracin, gramicidin, and colistin are the polypeptide antibiotics used in ophthalmic topical formulations.

Bacitracin

Spectrum of Activity It is active against Gram-positive bacteria, including Streptococci and Staphylococci.

Mechanism of Action It inhibits cell wall synthesis of bacteria by a different mechanism than do the β-lactam antibiotics.

Indications Because of its systemic renal toxicity, it is used topically alone and in fixed combination products. It is unstable in solution, thus available only as an ointment in combination with neomycin, effective against Gram-negative bacteria and polymyxin B. The inclusion of bacitracin produces broad antibacterial spectra against most common ocular pathogens. Bacitracin appears useful to clear corneal wound infection caused by Gram-positive organisms after phacoemulsification is a serious complication of cataract surgery (Cosar et al. 2001). Bacitracin or trimethoprim-polymyxin B sulfate is found useful for perioperative antibiotic prophylaxis (Ritterband et al. 2003).

Vancomycin

It is a glycopeptide antibiotic first isolated in 1953 from a soil bacterium *Amycolatopsis orientalis* (formerly known as *Nocardia orientalis*).

Spectrum of Activity It possesses broad-spectrum activity against Gram-positive bacteria including methicillin- and cephalosporin-resistant Staphylococci. Also, it shows activity against coagulase-negative Staphylococcus, Gram-positive cocci, including Streptococcus, Staphylococcus, Clostridium, and Corynebacterium (Suemori et al. 2010).

Mechanism of Action It acts by inhibiting cell wall synthesis by binding to the two D-ala residues on the end of the peptide chain bound to the peptide chains prevents them from interacting properly with the cell wall cross-linking enzyme and cross-links are not formed and the cell wall falls apart.

Indications It is reserved for serious infections for which less toxic antibiotics are not indicated, not effective, or not tolerated. It is an excellent empiric antibiotic for treating endophthalmitis and an alternative to penicillins or cephalosporins for serious infections (Gentile et al. 2014). It is used as the final choice in serious cases of methicillin-resistant Staphylococcus aureus (MRSA) or methicillin-resistant Staphylococcus epidermidis (MRSE) keratitis. It is recommended as intravitreal, topical, or subconjunctival for treatment of bacterial endophthalmitis (Mehta et al. 2011).

11.3.2.2 Cytoplasmic Membrane Inhibitors

Polymyxin B and gramicidin are the antibiotics known to impair the bacterial cytoplasmic membrane.

Polymyxin B

Spectrum of Activity It is active against Gram-negative bacteria except Proteus, Serratia, and Neisseria. It is also active against Pseudomonas, Salmonella, and Shigella.

Mechanism of Action It is surfactant in nature that disrupts the osmotic integrity of bacterial cell membranes.

Indications Currently, it used as a last resort antibiotic for the treatment of infections caused by Gram-negative bacteria. Topical neomycin/polymyxin B is found effective in reducing the conjunctival bacterial load given before cataract surgery (Li et al. 2015). The combination of topical trimethoprim/polymyxin B and topical moxifloxacin is found to effectively control the corneal ulcer in keratitis caused by Elizabethkingia meningosepticum (Erdem et al. 2013). Polymyxin B and trimethoprim are found useful in infectious keratitis after photorefractive keratectomy (Donnenfeld et al. 2003). Topical therapy with gentamicin 1.3 %, cefazolin 5 %, chlorhexidine 0.02 %, propamidine 0.1 %, polymyxin B 30,000 IU eye drops, and neosporin (neomycin, bacitracin, polymyxin) eye ointment is used for the treatment of coinfection with Acanthamoeba and Pseudomonas aeruginosa in patients with contact lens-associated keratitis (Sharma et al. 2013a, b). Polymyxin

B-trimethoprim continues to be an effective treatment for acute conjunctivitis and bacterial keratitis and may combine with chloramphenicol and gentamicin (Williams et al. 2013). Polymyxin B may be used for multidrug-resistant Pseudomonas spp. It is available in combination with various other agents such as bacitracin (ointment), trimethoprim (eye drops and ointment), and neomycin plus gramicidin (eye drops).

Colistin

Spectrum of Activity It is active against the multidrug-resistant (MDR) Gram-negative organisms except Proteus, Serratia, and Neisseria. It is also active against Pseudomonas, Salmonella, and Shigella.

Mechanism of Action Its rapidly acting bactericidal agent exhibits a surfactant-like action on the cell membrane and causes distortion or pseudopor formation.

Indications Topical colistin 0.19 % found a safe and effective alternative in the management of multidrug-resistant P. aeruginosa bacterial keratitis (Jain et al. 2014).

Gramicidin

Spectrum of Activity It is active against Gram-positive bacteria, except for the Gram-positive bacilli, and against select Gram-negative organisms, such as *Neisseria.*

Mechanism of Action It is bactericidal and causes cell membrane leakage and uncouples oxidative phosphorylation in the microorganisms.

Indications It replaces bacitracin in some fixed combination formulations used topically for eye infections. It is used in therapeutics in the name of tyrothricin which is a mixture of gramicidin (20 %) and tyrocidine (80 %). Its use is limited to topical application only, as it is very toxic on systemic use.

Fusidic Acid

Spectrum of Activity It is a narrow-spectrum antibiotic effective against Streptococci, Haemophilus, and methicillin-susceptible Staphylococcus aureus.

Mechanism of Action It inhibits protein synthesis in bacteria.

Indications It achieves high concentrations at the surface of the eye. It is available as 1 % viscous drops which liquefy in contact with the eye and results in a relatively better half-life in the tear film, therefore reducing the frequency of application compared to other formulations (Mason et al. 2003).

11.3.2.3 Protein Synthesis Inhibitors

Aminoglycosides, tetracyclines, and macrolide antibiotics as well as the individual drugs clindamycin and chloramphenicol inhibit the protein synthesis in bacteria.

Aminoglycosides

Gentamicin, neomycin, netilmicin, tobramycin, and amikacin are the aminoglycoside antibiotics used in ocular preparations. Gentamicin was discovered in 1963 and was introduced into parenteral usage in 1971. Since then, it has been widely used in medicinal applications including eye diseases (Chen et al. 2014).

Spectrum of Activity These are effective against most Gram-negative bacteria and Staphylococci with lesser activity against Streptococci. Aminoglycosides showed differences in the type and doses associated with toxic reactions; thereby, the following order of toxicity can be described (from most toxic to least toxic): gentamicin > netilmicin = tobramycin > amikacin = kanamycin (Penha et al. 2010). Aminoglycosides display concentration-dependent bactericidal activity and are the cornerstone of therapy against serious Gram-negative bacterial infections.

Mechanism of Action These inhibit protein synthesis by binding to 30S bacterial ribosomes and cause inaccurate mRNA translation and so inhibit the biosynthesis of proteins preceded by inhibition of ribosomal translocation, i.e., movement of the peptidyl-tRNA from the A to the P site.

Indications Gentamicin and tobramycin are more active than neomycin and framycetin, particularly against P. aeruginosa. The rapid bactericidal action of gentamicin and tobramycin and their potential activity against P. aeruginosa make them useful in the treatment of bacterial keratitis. They do not penetrate the cornea well; therefore, they are generally used at fortified concentrations until the condition of the cornea improves. Marked irritation can be experienced its use (McDonald et al. 2014).

Gentamicin is used to treat many bacterial infections such as conjunctivitis, blepharitis, and dacryocystitis. It is also used for the initial treatment of bacterial corneal ulcers or prophylaxis of endophthalmitis after cataract surgery by intracameral antibiotics or subconjunctival injection (Katibeh et al. 2015), though it is considered inadequate for the initial treatment of serious bacterial keratitis. The solutions containing fortified concentrations are prepared from sterile products to be intended for parenteral use. The fortified gentamicin or tobramycin solution is combined with a penicillinase-resistant cephalosporin and considered a useful initial empiric treatment for serious bacterial keratitis. The initial loading dose of fortified aminoglycosides is given to increase the antibiotic concentrations in the cornea, followed by regular applications.

Neomycin is most commonly administered topically in combination with other antibiotics or corticosteroids. Topical application frequently results in sensitization to the drug; therefore, long-term use should be avoided. Netilmicin appears the most effective antibiotic tested against both MRSA and MRSE and may curtail the emergence, spreading, and persistence of antibiotic-resistant bacteria (Blanco et al. 2013). Netilmicin appears a safe and broad-spectrum antibiotic comparable with that of ciprofloxacin, ofloxacin, norfloxacin, and gentamicin that can be used as first-line therapy for the treatment of acute bacterial conjunctivitis (Papa et al. 2002).

Tobramycin is used similar to gentamicin; however, Staphylococci are generally susceptible to tobramycin, whereas Streptococci are not susceptible to tobramycin (Donnenfeld et al. 2003). Cross-resistance between gentamicin and tobramycin is common. Amikacin is usually effective for most strains of Klebsiella, Enterobacter, E. coli, and Serratia. However, for bacterial keratitis, tobramycin is often preferred in combination with ticarcillin. Dual therapy with a β-lactam agent is recommended for empirical therapy to cover streptococcal infection and improve activity against Staphylococci. The aminoglycosides are slowly inactivated in the presence of some β-lactams; thus, they should be administered separately, preferably at least 5 min apart.

Tobramycin 1.4 % topical is found useful in mycobacterial keratitis after laser in situ keratomileusis (LASIK) (Freitas et al. 2003) and infectious keratitis after photorefractive keratectomy (Donnenfeld et al. 2003). Tobramycin also may be useful as prophylactic topical antibiotics for preventing secondary corneal infections or recurrent corneal erosion syndrome (Park et al. 2015).

Amikacin, the first semisynthetic aminoglycoside, has been chemically modified to be protected from aminoglycoside-inactivating enzymes. It is popular as a primary antibiotic for intravitreal injection along with vancomycin for the treatment of bacterial endophthalmitis due to its broad spectrum against resistant Gram-negative organisms and reduced toxicity.

Tetracyclines

Tetracyclines were first acknowledged in 1948 as the natural fermentation product of the soil bacterium *Streptomyces aureofaciens* and, 6 years later, were chemically purified for the first time. Tetracycline analogues are classified as short-, intermediate-, and long-acting based on duration of action. Analogues in each category have generally similar patterns of bacterial susceptibility and resistance.

Spectrum of Activity Tetracyclines are the broad-spectrum antibiotics, active against Gram-positive, Gram-negative, aerobic, and anaerobic bacteria as well as Spirochetes, Mycoplasma, Rickettsia, Chlamydophila, Brucella, Bartonella, and a few protozoa.

Mechanism of Action Primarily these are bacteriostatic in action, inhibit protein synthesis by binding to 30S ribosomes, and interfere with attachment of aminoacyl-tRNA to the mRNA-ribosome complex and inhibition of growth of peptide chain required for protein synthesis.

Indications Tetracyclines also interact with matrix metalloproteinases (MMP), tissue inhibitors of MMPs, growth factors, and cytokines; therefore, tetracyclines are capable of affecting inflammation, immunomodulation, cell proliferation, and angiogenesis. Slow-release doxycycline 40 mg given daily appears an effective and safe therapy of ocular rosacea (Sobolewska et al. 2014). Oral minocycline or doxycycline can provide clinical benefits in treating moderate and severe meibomian gland dysfunction by reducing inflammatory cytokine levels.

Oral doxycycline is also used with topical amikacin, oral ketoconazole in the treatment of keratitis caused by Nocardia organisms. (TRichet et al. 2011). Oral doxycycline and topical corticosteroid are used in the treatment of recurrent corneal erosion syndrome (Wang et al. 2008). Tetracycline and chlortetracycline both are available in the ophthalmic preparations and indicated for the treatment of chlamydial (TRIC) infections. Several ocular surface infections caused by susceptible organisms respond satisfactorily to topical tetracyclines.

Macrolides

These antibiotics have macrocyclic lactone ring attached with sugar. Erythromycin, clarithromycin, and azithromycin are the popular macrolide antibiotics used in ocular preparations.

Spectrum of Activity It is narrow spectrum and active mainly against Gram-positive cocci, Streptococcus, Staphylococcus, Gram-positive rods, and a few Gram-negative bacteria. It is also effective against Mycoplasma, Rickettsia, and Chlamydophila.

Mechanism of Action These are primarily bacteriostatic at low concentration but become bactericidal at high concentration. They act by inhibiting protein synthesis through binding to the bacterial 50S ribosomal subunit and interfering with translocation in protein synthesis.

Indications The first-generation macrolide, erythromycin, is a widely used macrolide antibiotic for human external ocular infections because of its lack of toxicity and good activity against microorganisms. Erythromycin decreases the risk of gonococcal ophthalmia neonatorum in newborns (Darling and McDonald 2010). The American Academy of Pediatrics recommends a 14-day course of systemic erythromycin (50 mg/kg/day, divided in 4 doses).

The second-generation macrolide, azithromycin, is available as a 1.5 % ophthalmic solution for use in the treatment of bacterial or trachomatous conjunctivitis (Garnock-Jones 2012). Azithromycin 1.5 % ophthalmic solution for 3 days (1 drop twice daily) is found non-inferior to tobramycin 0.3 % ophthalmic solution for 7 days (1 drop every 2 h) in pediatric and adult patients with purulent bacterial conjunctivitis, with regard to clinical cure and bacteriological resolution. Azithromycin administered orally is rapidly absorbed and widely distributed. A single oral dose of azithromycin can eliminate trachoma infection, but cannot be used in infants under 6 months old, and needs to be given every few years in communities with a high prevalence of disease (Baneke 2012).

Azithromycin 1 % ophthalmic solution is also used in the treatment of blepharitis and blepharitis-associated ocular dryness (Veldman and Colby 2011). Azithromycin 1.5 % ophthalmic solution was found effective in bacterial or trachomatous conjunctivitis and appears well tolerated (Garnock-Jones 2012). Topical azithromycin is also used in meibomian gland dysfunction, a common problem associated with evaporative dry eye disease (Foulks et al. 2013).

Mass azithromycin treatments are highly effective for the ocular strains of chlamydia causing trachoma (Keenan et al. 2012). Several extra-label dosage regimens have been anecdotally recommended (e.g., 5 mg/kg once daily for 2 doses and then every third day for 5 doses, 5 mg/kg once daily for 5 doses followed by the same dose every 3 days for 5 doses). A short course of oral azithromycin (20 mg/kg once daily for 3 days) appears an effective treatment alternative for Chlamydia trachomatis.

Macrolides are considered bacteriostatic, but clarithromycin may provide a bactericidal effect against non-tuberculous mycobacteria keratitis if used at a high concentration. Clarithromycin 1 % topical is found useful in mycobacterial keratitis after laser in situ keratomileusis (LASIK) (Freitas et al. 2003).

Chloramphenicol

It was first obtained from *Streptomyces venezuelae* in 1947.

Spectrum of Activity It is a broad-spectrum antibiotic and active against most Gram-positive and Gram-negative bacteria, Rickettsia, Chlamydophila, Spirochetes, and Mycoplasma except P. aeruginosa or Chlamydia trachomatis. It is effective against Haemophilus influenzae and Haemophilus parainfluenzae, Legionella pneumophila, Moraxella catarrhalis, Neisseria meningitidis, Pasteurella multocida, and Streptococcus pneumonia (Cagini et al. 2013).

Mechanism of Action It binds to 30S bacterial ribosomes and hinders the access of aminoacyl-tRNA to the acceptor site for amino acid incorporation and inhibits protein synthesis. Primarily, it is bacteriostatic in action.

Indications It is one of the oldest and commonest antibiotics, available over the counter and considered least expensive. It is used for the treatment of methicillin-resistant Staphylococcus aureus ocular surface infections and bacterial conjunctivitis and available as 0.5 % drops and 1 % ointments (Fukuda et al. 2002). A high incidence of resistance was reported, and even topical use also may cause bone marrow toxicity and aplastic anemia.

11.3.2.4 Intermediary Metabolism Inhibitors

The sulfonamides are the first antimicrobial agents and considered derivative of sulfanilamide. Several sulfonamides were developed and used extensively, but the emergence of resistance and availability of safer and effective agents currently limited the clinical usage. Currently they are used mainly in combination with pyrimethamine and trimethoprim.

Spectrum of Activity Sulfonamides are broad-spectrum drugs found effective against Gram-positive and Gram-negative bacteria as well as Chlamydophila, Actinomyces, Plasmodia, and Toxoplasma. They generally exert bacteriostatic effect; therefore, cellular and humoral immune mechanisms are potentially more important for eradicating bacterial infections when they are used than for some other antibiotic agents.

Mechanism of Action Mechanistically, sulfonamides inhibit synthesis of folic acid which is required for synthesis of nucleic acid and protein in bacteria. This inhibition can be reversed by several antagonists, i.e., para-aminobenzoic acid (PABA). Antibacterial action of sulfonamides is also inhibited by tissue breakdown products, blood and pus. Thus, sulfonamide treatment is contraindicated for infections with marked suppuration. Pyrimethamine and trimethoprim are chemically 4-diaminapyrimidine derivatives which inhibit folic acid synthesis. They appear synergistic when used in combination with the sulfonamides. The sulfonamides inhibit an early step in the synthesis of folic acid, and pyrimethamine or trimethoprim inhibits a later step in the pathway.

Indications Sulfonamides have been used to treat chlamydial diseases, but other antibiotics are now the first choice and in wide use due to availability of more effective and less irritant agents. Topical ophthalmic preparations of sulfonamides include 10 % sulfacetamide and sulfasoxasole as well as the former in combination with prednisolone. Sulfacetamide administered topically achieves high concentration aqueous humor and anterior segment. Intravitreal injection of vancomycin combined with ceftazidime following intravenous penicillin G and topical sulfacetamide sodium is found to be effective in endogenous endophthalmitis caused by Actinomyces neuii (Graffi et al. 2012). Sulfacetamide sodium in combination with betamethasone is found useful in patients with meibomian gland dysfunction (Akyol-Salman et al. 2012).

Pyrimethamine in combination with sulfadiazine is an effective therapy for the treatment of toxoplasmic encephalitis, whereas trimethoprim + sulfamethoxazole and pyrimethamine + clindamycin are possible alternatives. Treatment with either oral or intravitreal antibiotics seems reasonable for ocular toxoplasmosis (Rajapakse et al. 2013).

Trimethoprim in combination with polymyxin B is available as a topical ophthalmic solution used against Gram-negative bacteria including Pseudomonas. The combination of trimethoprim-sulfamethoxazole is found to clear corneal wound infection caused by Gram-positive organisms after phacoemulsification is a serious complication of cataract surgery (Cosar et al. 2001).

11.3.2.5 Bacterial DNA Synthesis Inhibitors

Fluoroquinolones antibiotics have quinolone moiety with one or more fluorine substitutions. These are divided into generations based on their antibacterial spectrum. Most of the quinolone including nalidixic acid belongs to first generation. Second-generation fluoroquinolones include ciprofloxacin, ofloxacin, norfloxacin, lomefloxacin, nadifloxacin, and pefloxacin. Third-generation fluoroquinolones include balofloxacin, levofloxacin, grepafloxacin, and sparfloxacin. Fourth-generation fluoroquinolones include gatifloxacin, moxifloxacin, gemifloxacin, and trovafloxacin.

Spectrum of Activity They are active against the majority of ocular pathogens, including Staphylococci, Haemophilus spp., Chlamydia trachomatis, Neisseria gonorrhoeae, Enterobacteriaceae, Listeria, Legionella, Brucella, Shigella, Proteus, Klebsiella, Bacillus anthracis, and Pseudomonas aeruginosa, but modest activity against Streptococci. These drugs have bactericidal action and relatively confer higher potency against Gram-positive bacteria. Most of the fluoroquinolone drugs penetrate corneal stroma and exhibit MICs against Gram-positive and Gram-negative bacteria. Fluoroquinolones have greater efficacy and a broader spectrum of activity than some other antibacterial drugs, including bacitracin, erythromycin, tobramycin, and gentamicin against ocular pathogens (Smith et al. 2001).

Mechanism of Action The fluoroquinolones inhibit the bacterial enzyme DNA gyrase, which required for nicking double-stranded DNA and introducing the negative supercoils.

Indications Quinolones, such as ciprofloxacin, ofloxacin, norfloxacin, levofloxacin, gatifloxacin, and moxifloxacin, are available as topical ophthalmic solution, and application remains the most popular mode of antibiotic prophylaxis in cataract surgery patients for prophylaxis from endophthalmitis (Vazirani and Basu 2013; Sridhar et al. 2015). They are also effective agents for non-tuberculous mycobacterial keratitis. They are well tolerated and effective in the treatment of patients with superficial eye infection.

Monotherapy of bacterial keratitis with ciprofloxacin or ofloxacin eye drops is found superior over conventional regimens of multiple fortified agents. Topical ciprofloxacin is effective for bacterial conjunctivitis and is also used to treat bacterial keratitis caused by a variety of pathogens. It is found effective in perioperative prophylaxis for endophthalmitis after cataract surgery (Katibeh et al. 2015). Ciprofloxacin is also available as an ointment too.

Ciprofloxacin may be useful as prophylactic topical antibiotics for preventing secondary corneal infections or recurrent corneal erosion syndrome (Park et al. 2015). Topical formulation with intravenous ofloxacin achieves aqueous and vitreous levels that inhibit many common pathogens and hold promise for treating intraocular infections. The empiric use of second-generation fluoroquinolones (ciprofloxacin and ofloxacin) seems to be contraindicated in the treatment of MRSA keratitis (Chang et al. 2015).

Norfloxacin is indicated for the treatment of bacterial conjunctivitis but is not useful for bacterial keratitis due to lesser penetration of the cornea thanofloxacin.

Levofloxacin recently became available as a 0.5 % ophthalmic solution. It exhibits high solubility in comparison with ciprofloxacin. It possesses greater activity against Streptococcus species than ciprofloxacin or ofloxacin.

Moxifloxacin has an impressive spectrum of coverage, and this pharmacokinetic study reinforces its potential as a prophylactic drug against intraocular infections, given the high aqueous level post topical administration (Sharma et al. 2015). Intravitreal moxifloxacin is found useful for the treatment of bacterial endophthalmitis (Mehta et al. 2011). Topical moxifloxacin with tobramycin is found effective in postoperative prophylaxis against infectious keratitis after laser in situ keratomileusis (LASIK) and surface ablation (Ortega-Usobiaga et al. 2015). Intracameral moxifloxacin appears most suitable for the prevention of endophthalmitis (Kessel et al. 2015).

Topical besifloxacin seems to be a useful adjunct agent in the treatment of nontuberculous mycobacterial keratitis by Mycobacterium chelonae and may be viable for use as a first-line agent in cases of nodular conjunctivitis by Mycobacterium chelonae (Nguyen et al. 2015). Besifloxacin 0.6 % produces similar antibacterial and clinical efficacy as that with moxifloxacin 0.5 % in the treatment of bacterial conjunctivitis (Garg et al. 2015).

Gatifloxacin is found effective against Gram-negative bacteria, a common cause of bacterial keratitis (Rautaraya et al. 2014). Gatifloxacin 0.5 % ophthalmic solution is found safe and effective for the treatment of acute bacterial conjunctivitis with twice-daily administration for 5 days in patients 1 year of age or older (Heller et al. 2014).

Sparfloxacin 0.3 % is a broad-spectrum fluoroquinolone antibiotic commonly used for various bacterial corneal infections (Agarwal et al. 2014). Topical fluoroquinolone therapy may be an adjunct to the innate immune response in eradicating less fulminant keratomycosis (Munir et al. 2007).

Topical use of fluoroquinolones is considered to be safe leading to their widespread use. Common indications include blepharitis, conjunctivitis, and corneal ulcers. However, unsupervised prolonged use is associated with deposition of crystalline material in the epithelial and anterior stromal layers of the cornea. Several fluoroquinolones which were not promoted for systemic use are currently under evaluation (including grepafloxacin and moxifloxacin) for their favorable activity against Gram-positive cocci.

11.3.3 Topical Drug Therapy for Resistant Microbial Infections

11.3.3.1 MRSA

With the early discovery of antibiotics, adaptation of bacteria to resist against the antibiotics has become a growing concern. Methicillin-resistant *Staphylococcus aureus* (MRSA) infections are the nosocomial infection, where the *S. aureus* bacteria have developed immunity against the methicillin, penicillin, and beta lactam antibiotics including third- and fourth-generation fluoroquinolones. The important aspect of these bacteria is they often colonize in the nose and skin of the patients, and that might be a precipitating factor of hospital-based infections and contamination of postsurgical wounds (Mamalis 2014). MRSA infections have been observed in high prevalence rate in ophthalmic setup following routine ophthalmic surgery, like cataract, laser in situ keratomileusis, and photorefractive keratectomy, and MRSA wound infections have been reported with clear corneal phacoemulsification wounds, penetrating keratoplasty, lamellar keratoplasty, and following ex vivo epithelial transplantation associated with amniotic membrane grafts. MRSA infection is also prevalent in patients wearing therapeutic contact lenses following corneal corrective surgeries (Koh et al. 2012 and Khalil and Sonbol 2014).

Treatment Modalities

Cefazolin and other fourth-generation fluoroquinolones are used to treat MRSA infection. Vancomycin, which is sensitive to Gram-positive pathogen, has reported to be beneficial in treating MRSA ophthalmic infection (Nick Mamalis 2014). Beside vancomycin, chloramphenicol, ciprofloxacin, clindamycin, gentamicin, and sulfamethoxazole/trimethoprim have shown effectiveness in controlling MRSA infection (Donald et al. 2012) .

11.3.3.2 VRSA

MRSA is a resistant nosocomial infection, which is very difficult to treat and accounts for nosocomial infection-related death worldwide. Vancomycin is an effective bactericidal against MRSA; however, this species has developed resistance to vancomycin, and since 2002, a number of case have been reported for the vancomycin-resistant Staphylococcus aureus (VRSA) (Kos et al. 2012).

Treatment Modalities

Ceftobiprole, linezolid, and trimethoprim/sulfamethoxazole are common treatment options to treat VRSA infection.

11.4 Antimicrobial Agents for Ocular Use: Protozoal Infections

The Protozoans are considered to be a subkingdom of the kingdom Protista, although in the classical system, they were placed in the kingdom Animalia. They are free-living organisms found almost in every possible habitat. All humans have exposure to protozoa in their life, as some are considered commensals, i.e., normally not harmful, whereas others are pathogenic and may produce disease. The diseases range from very mild to life-threatening specifically in immunosuppressed patients with acquired immune deficiency syndrome (AIDS).

The Protozoans known for their disease capabilities are Pneumocystis carinii (pneumonia), Toxoplasma gondii (fatal toxoplasmic encephalitis), Cryptosporidium and Microsporidiosis in AIDS patients, and Acanthamoeba species (keratitis), specifically in contact lens users through contaminated lens cleaning solutions. The lack of effective vaccines, the scarcity of reliable drugs, and other problems, including difficulties of vector control, prompted the World Health Organization to target these protozoal diseases.

The pharmacological agents used in the treatment of these protozoal diseases and their basis of pharmacological basis of inclusion in therapeutics are presented further in next paragraphs.

11.4.1 Acanthamoeba Keratitis

Acanthamoeba keratitis (AK) is a debilitating eye disease that requires effective topical alone or followed by oral drug therapy. Acanthamoeba spp. (Acanthamoeba polyphaga, A. castellanii, and A. hatchetti) are small, free-living Protozoans that cause AK.

Pharmacological agents in treatment: The susceptibility tests of isolates are needed to choose the most appropriate agent, and our results can be a guideline for choosing the most appropriate agent for immediate empirical treatment of AK (Sunada et al. 2014). *Acanthamoeba* cysts are most susceptible to topical natamycin (5.0 %), povidone-iodine (1.0 %), benzalkonium chloride (0.05 %), chlorhexidine gluconate (0.02 %), hexamidine diisethioonate (0.1 %), propamidine isethionate (0.1 %), polyhexamethylene biguanide (PHMB, 0.02 %), voriconazole (1.0 %), clotrimazole (1 %), and paromomycin (0.1 %) or propamidine isethionate (Kowalski et al. 2013; Lin et al. 2009).

Pharmacological basis of therapeutics and indications:

Natamycin and povidone-iodine had excellent cystic-static (or cysticidal) effects (Sunada et al. 2014). Intracameral voriconazole (1 %), an antifungal agent, is found beneficial in AKI followed by institution of oral as well as topical voriconazole drops. A novel combination treatment of chlorhexidine gluconate and natamycin (pimaricin) and debridement has been found successful for AK.

Voriconazole and chlorhexidine are also indicated for the treatment of Acanthamoeba infections (Cabello-Vílchez et al. 2014). Voriconazole oral monotherapy is also found successful in chronic stromal AK (Tu et al. 2010), whereas topical and intrastromal voriconazole is found successful in treating AK in cases of chlorhexidine- and hexamidine-resistant Acanthamoeba (Bang et al. 2010).

Moxifloxacin can be an adjuvant to consider as it is effectively prevents encystation of the amoeba which often complicates infection resolution. In addition, moxifloxacin is effective in preventing secondary bacterial infections (Martín-Navarro et al. 2013).

In addition, cycloplegic agents, which include atropine, cyclopentolate, homatropine, scopolamine, and tropicamide, are indicated for the pain relief in addition to nonsteroidal anti-inflammatory drugs. PHMB, also known as polyhexanide and polyaminopropyl biguanide, is commonly used as antiseptic in contact lens cleaning solutions and perioperative cleansers. The germicidal effect of PHMB (0.02 %) as eye drops prior to cataract surgery is well tolerated with minimal patient discomfort.

11.4.2 Chagas' Disease

Chagas' disease (CD), also known as American or African trypanosomiasis or sleeping sickness, is the infection caused by Trypanosoma cruzi and results from bite by a kissing bug. It is a major public health issue in many Central and South American countries (Santamaria et al. 2014). A palpebral and periorbital edema, known as Romana's sign, is a hallmark of acute CD.

Pharmacological agents in treatment: The antitrypanosomal agents include nifurtimox, eflornithine, melarsoprol, and benznidazole and are most successful (Dias et al. 2014). These agents are not commercially available for topical use. Thus, only oral or parenteral form which is used for CD is believed to be useful in the treatment of trypanosomiasis and its ocular manifestations (Barrett and Croft 2012).

Pharmacological basis of therapeutics and indications:

Nifurtimox is a 5-nitrofuran derivative available for oral and parenteral use in CD (Le Loup et al. 2011). Due to appearance of relapses (reported in about 50 % patients) with monotherapy, the combination of nifurtimox with melarsoprol is preferred owing to superior efficacy (Wolf et al. 2011). There is only report available showing the microfilaricidal effect of nifurtimox in the treatment of onchocerciasis, though failed to improve corneal lesions in the study (Fuglsang and Anderson 1978).

Eflornithine (α-difluoromethylornithine or DFMO) is termed as a "suicide inhibitor," irreversibly binding to the enzyme ornithine decarboxylase and preventing the natural substrate ornithine from accessing the active site (Heby et al. 2007). It is used with melarsoprol or nifurtimox (Burri and Brun 2003; Jennings 1988). Periocular injections of DFMO, which decreases polyamine levels, are believed to inhibit choroidal neovascularization (Lima e Silva et al. 2005). The side effects are transient and reversible. Seizures, hearing loss, and hematological abnormalities may occur.

Melarsoprol is a prodrug, which is metabolized to melarsen oxide (Mel Ox) as its active form which irreversibly binds with trypanothione and forms an adduct that inhibits trypanothione reductase and kills the parasitic cell. Due to high toxicity, oral melarsoprol is reserved only for the most dangerous of cases – stage 2 infections (Rodgers et al. 2011). It produces adverse effects similar to arsenic poisoning and may cause convulsions, fever, rashes, bloody stools, nausea, vomiting, and rarely encephalopathy.

Nifurtimox-eflornithine combination therapy which has superior efficacy is reserved for the treatment of second-stage CD or T. rhodesiense (Priotto et al. 2009).

Benznidazole acts by the production of free radicals and injurious to the sensitive T. cruzi as it possesses reduced detoxification capabilities (Medeiros 2009). In a clinical study, BENEFIT trial (BENznidazole Evaluation For Interrupting Trypanosomiasis) appears effective in chronic stages of CD (Coura and Borges-Pereira 2010). It is found successful in both adult and juvenile (Le Loup et al. 2011). The common side effects are ash and gastrointestinal disturbances and, rarely, peripheral neuropathy.

Posaconazole, a new drug, showed antitrypanosomal activity in patients with chronic CD in randomized clinical trials (Molina et al. 2014). Benznidazole is found to induce reduction, but not elimination, of circulating T. cruzi levels, whereas posaconazole led to a successful resolution of the infection, despite the maintenance of immunosuppressive therapy in CD (Pinazo et al. 2010).

11.4.3 Giardiasis

Giardiasis is caused by Giardia lamblia, transmitted from person-to-person through contaminated food and water (Lal et al. 2013). The ocular manifestations may include chorioretinitis, iridocyclitis, uveitis, and vitreal and retinal hemorrhage, described as "salt-and-pepper" changes (Turnbull et al. 2013; Corsi et al. 1998). No commercial formulations as eye drop/ointment are available for topical use in the eye.

Pharmacological agents in treatment: The recommended treatment includes metronidazole, albendazole, or paromomycin (Granados et al. 2012).

Pharmacological basis of therapeutics and indications:

Metronidazole is an antibiotic and an antiprotozoal drug used against amoebiasis, giardiasis, and trichomoniasis (Granados et al. 2012). It acts by inhibiting nucleic acid synthesis by disrupting the DNA of microbial cells. This function only occurs when metronidazole is partially reduced, and because this reduction usually happens only in anaerobic cells, it has relatively little effect upon human cells or aerobic bacteria. The common side effects of metronidazole are nausea, abdominal pain, headache, dizziness, and metallic taste (Pasupuleti et al. 2014).

Albendazole, a benzimidazole broad-spectrum anthelmintic drug, is used in the treatment of worm infestations such as roundworms, tapeworms, giardiasis, trichuriasis, filariasis, neurocysticercosis, hydatid disease, enterobiasis, and ascariasis (Granados et al. 2012). It causes degenerative changes and impairs the energetics of the worms. The common side effects are raised liver enzymes, abdominal pain, dizziness, headache, fever, nausea, and vomiting (Meltzer et al. 2014; Granados et al. 2012).

Paromomycin, also known as monomycin and aminosidine, is an aminoglycoside antibiotic. It inhibits protein synthesis by binding to 16S ribosomal RNA. It is an effective treatment for ulcerative cutaneous leishmaniasis apart from amoebiasis and leishmaniasis (Meltzer et al. 2014; Granados et al. 2012). It is found successful in the treatment of metronidazole-refractory giardiasis (Stover et al. 2012; Mørch et al. 2008). The common side effects are nephrotoxicity and ototoxicity with oral doses.

11.4.4 Leishmaniasis

Leishmaniasis is caused by obligate intracellular protozoans, hemoflagellates through the bite of a sandfly (Khadem and Uzonna 2014). It is a disease of the developing world, throughout Africa, Southern Europe, and Central Asia (Elmahallawy et al. 2014; Khyatti et al. 2014). Symptomatic ocular manifestations of visceral leishmaniasis are rare, but conjunctivitis, blepharitis, uveitis, keratitis, iritis, papillitis, and chorioretinitis occur with visceral leishmaniasis (Maude et al. 2014; Khalil et al. 2011; Yaghoobi et al. 2010; Sadeghian et al. 2005; Montero et al. 2003).

Pharmacological agents in treatment: Current strategies to control this disease are mainly based on chemotherapy. Due to high resistance and adverse effects, the antileishmanial drugs are used in combination treatment regimens (Sundar and Chakravarty 2015; Mahajan et al. 2015). Single dose of liposomal amphotericin B (LAmB), or multidrug therapy (L-AmB + miltefosine, L-AmB + paromomycin, or miltefosine + paromomycin), pentavalent antimonials, and paromomycin are usually used in the treatment of visceral leishmaniasis. The treatment is determined by where the disease is acquired, the species of Leishmania, severity of clinical lesions, type of infection, and its potential to develop into mucosal leishmaniasis (Khadem and Uzonna 2014). Bilateral, multifocal retinal hemorrhages get improved by specific antileishmanial therapy (Sundar and Chakravarty 2015; Montero et al. 2003).

11.4.4.1 Pharmacological Basis of Therapeutics and Indications

Amphotericin B is an effective antifungal and antiparasitic drug and is the first line of therapy for leishmaniasis (Sundar et al. 2011). Currently LAmB is the most effective anti-*Leishmania* drug and is administered by intravenous infusion (Sundar et al. 2010). However, LAmB limitations include efficacy, expensiveness, and nephrotoxicity. It is the first line of therapy for leishmaniasis and often used as a single dose with high success rate.

Like other polyene antifungals, it binds with the component of fungal cell membranes, forming a transmembrane channel, which causes leakage of monovalent ions and resultant fungal cell death. Combining intravitreal amphotericin B and voriconazole found a novel treatment strategy in the management of endophthalmitis caused by filamentous fungus. The ocular complications of interstitial keratitis were found successfully treated by amphotericin (Roizenblatt 1979).

The pentavalent antimonials are a group of compounds used for the treatment of leishmaniasis. The agents, sodium stibogluconate and meglumine antimoniate, are available either as slow intravenous or intramuscular injection, but due to resistance, amphotericin or miltefosine is now preferred. Combined stibogluconate and allopurinol may be an effective therapy in ocular leishmaniasis (Abrishami et al. 2002). Systemic sodium stibogluconate is found successful in cutaneous and ocular leishmaniasis (Sadeghian et al. 2005). The side effects are anemia, rash, headache, abdominal pain, myalgia, and raised liver enzymes.

Miltefosine is a phospholipid compound that kills Leishmania parasites and is the first (and still the only prescribed) oral drug in the treatment of leishmaniasis. Recently, it is approved by USFDA for any form of leishmaniasis including cutaneous or mucosal leishmaniasis. It acts as a protein kinase B (Akt) inhibitor in the microbial cell. It is also approved for topical treatment of leishmaniasis and appears promising for the topical treatment of Acanthamoeba infections (Walochnik et al. 2009).

Miltefosine was originally formulated as a topical treatment for cutaneous cancers (Sindermann and Engel 2006). The combination of LAmB and oral miltefosine is found successful in multiple relapses of visceral leishmaniasis in patient with HIV (Patole et al. 2014).

11.4.5 Malaria

Malaria is caused by the different species of Plasmodium (Plasmodium vivax, Plasmodium ovale, Plasmodium malariae, and Plasmodium falciparum) and transmitted by the bite of female anopheles mosquito. Ocular manifestations occur during infection with the following signs: retinal whitening, papilledema, and cotton wool spots.

Pharmacological agents: The antimalarials are used in the treatment of malaria, though the antimalarials chloroquine and hydroxychloroquine on long-term use may cause retinal toxicity in offspring of women exposed to antimalarials during pregnancy (Osadchy et al. 2011).

11.4.6 Microsporidiosis

Microsporidia are the intracellular pathogens that cause superficial punctate keratitis and stromal keratitis in both immunocompromised and immunocompetent individuals (Khandelwal et al. 2011). Ocular findings are generally limited to the conjunctiva and cornea and occur either by direct inoculation into eye structures or by dissemination systemically.

Pharmacological agents: The agents used in the treatment include albendazole, an anthelmintic agent; fumagillin, itraconazole, and voriconazole, antifungal agents; and metronidazole, an antiamoebic agent. Topically, propamidine isethionate is also used in the treatment. Oral medications, such as albendazole and itraconazole, have shown efficacy, but the risk of systemic adverse effects and drug-drug interactions exists (Loh et al. 2009). Combinations of medications, both topical and oral, have been attempted with varying success.

Pharmacological basis of therapeutics and indications:

Fumagillin is currently an orphan drug used within the European Union to treat microsporidiosis in immunocompromised or immunocompetent individuals (Kulakova et al. 2014; Chan et al. 2003). Treatment regimen includes topical fluoroquinolones (ciprofloxacin 0.3 %, moxifloxacin 0.5 %, gatifloxacin 0.5 %, levofloxacin 0.5 %, or norfloxacin 0.3 %) as monotherapy or in combination with topical fumagillin and/or systemic albendazole (Loh et al. 2009). The topical fumagillin and oral albendazole are found useful in microsporidial stromal keratitis following deep anterior lamellar keratoplasty (Ang et al. 2009). Fumagillin acts similar to angiogenesis inhibitors by blocking new blood vessel formation by binding to an enzyme methionine aminopeptidase.

Itraconazole is a broad-spectrum triazole antifungal agent that, like other azole antifungals, inhibits the fungal-mediated synthesis of ergosterol. It also inhibits both the hedgehog signaling pathway and angiogenesis. Oral itraconazole is found successful in the treatment of microsporidial keratoconjunctivitis (Sridhar and Sharma 2003). It also recommended in ocular, nasal, and paranasal sinus infection caused by Encephalitozoon cuniculi parasites when treatment with albendazole fails (Rossi et al. 1999).

Itraconazole administered topically, orally, and intravenously also has a high success rate in fungal keratitis and endophthalmitis (Jin et al. 2014; Mochizuki et al. 2013). Topical voriconazole (1 %) is found to be an effective treatment for keratitis due to microsporidia (Khandelwal et al. 2011) and in fungal corneal ulcers too (Parchand et al. 2012).

11.4.7 Toxoplasmosis

Toxoplasmosis is caused by an opportunistic parasite Toxoplasma gondii which infects about one third of the human population worldwide and appears as latent infection (Delair et al. 2011). Ocular toxoplasmosis frequently presents as a focal necrotizing retinitis or gray-white punctate lesions in the outer retina and retinal pigment epithelium (Park and Nam 2013; Antoniazzi et al. 2008).

Majority of cases of ocular toxoplasmosis are congenital (Noble 2007). Among the clinical manifestations of congenital ocular toxoplasmosis reported in infants are microphthalmia, enophthalmos, ptosis, nystagmus, choroidal colobomas, and strabismus (Pleyer et al. 2014; Maenz et al. 2014; Harrell and Carvounis 2014). Acute infection in newborns and patients infected with HIV may lead to an intense necrotizing chorioretinitis (Pleyer et al. 2014; Pfaff et al. 2014).

Pharmacological agents for treatment: Sulfonamides, pyrimethamine and/or sulfadiazine, folinic acid, trimethoprim/sulfamethoxazole (Opremcak et al. 1992), and macrolide antibiotics; azithromycin (Yazici et al. 2009); spiramycin (Cassaday et al. 1964); clindamycin (Tate and Martin 1977; Guldsten 1983); and antimalarial atovaquone, alone or in combination, are generally used in the treatment of toxoplasmosis and its ocular manifestations (de-la-Torre et al. 2011).

The first-line therapy of T. gondii-related chorioretinitis involves the use of pyrimethamine with sulfadiazine beyond the resolution of symptoms (Harrell and Carvounis 2014; Holland and Lewis 2002). The alternative regimens include the use of pyrimethamine with clindamycin, clarithromycin, or azithromycin.

The treatment regimens consisted of either pyrimethamine (100 mg for 1 day, then 25 mg bid), sulfadiazine (1 g qid), folinic acid (5 mg), and prednisone (60 mg then taper); clindamycin (300 mg qid), sulfadiazine (1 g qid), and prednisone (60 mg, then taper); or trimethoprim-sulfamethoxazole (160–800 mg bid for 2 weeks then 80–400 mg bid) (Harrell and Carvounis 2014). Randomized clinical trials showed that intravitreal clindamycin-dexamethasone is effective for *Toxoplasma* retinochoroiditis (Soheilian et al. 2011).

Trimethoprim-sulfamethoxazole is considered the best first-line treatment of *Toxoplasma* retinochoroiditis, with intravitreal clindamycin with dexamethasone an alternative for patients intolerant and unresponsive or with a contraindication (such as pregnancy) to trimethoprim-sulfamethoxazole. There is considerable evidence that administering trimethoprim-sulfamethoxazole combination can intermittently reduce the risk of recurrence. Corticosteroids are used as adjuvant, though a very recent Cochrane Review found no evidence from randomized controlled studies to support their use or indeed support concerns to anti-Toxoplasma treatment that may lead to worse outcomes (Vedula and Nguyen 2008).

A combination of pyrimethamine, sulfadiazine, and folinic acid is preferred as treatment for women in whom fetal infection has been confirmed or is highly suspected by a positive amniotic fluid polymerase chain reaction (Paquet 2013), whereas congenital toxoplasmosis appears suitably treated with combination of pyrimethamine, sulfadiazine, and leucovorin (Kaye 2011). As soon as the maternal infection is suspected, preventive treatment with spiramycin begins; the treatment is changed to a combination of pyrimethamine-sulfonamide if fetal infection is proven (Garcia-Méric et al. 2010).

Intravitreal clindamycin plus dexamethasone was found superior than conventional oral therapy including pyrimethamine, sulfadiazine, folinic acid, and prednisone in the treatment of active toxoplasmic retinochoroiditis (Baharivand et al. 2013). Adverse drug reaction appears as DRESS syndrome reported in pediatric patient following treatment with standard combination regimen includes oral sulfadiazine, pyrimethamine, folinic acid, and steroids for toxoplasma retinochoroiditis (Yusuf et al. 2013).

Pharmacological basis of therapeutics and indications:

Patients infected with HIV showing signs of previous infection receive primary prophylaxis with trimethoprim-sulfamethoxazole (Campos et al. 2014). In patients with AIDS showing toxoplasmic chorioretinitis, sulfadiazine, pyrimethamine, and folinic acid should be continued indefinitely following initial therapy. Folinic acid is added to prevent bone marrow toxicity, and spiramycin is considered relatively safe by USFDA for use in pregnancy. It is used popularly to prevent the toxoplasmosis and a popular choice in pregnancy (Asproudis et al. 2013; Garcia-Méric et al. 2010).

Pyrimethamine, an antimalarial drug, is used in the treatment of Toxoplasma gondii infections in immunocompromised patients such as HIV-positive individuals. It is typically given with a sulfadiazine and folinic acid (Butler et al. 2013). Sulfonamides inhibit dihydropteroate synthetase, an enzyme that participates in folic acid synthesis from para-aminobenzoic acid and works synergistically with pyrimethamine by blocking a different enzyme required for folic acid synthesis. Pyrimethamine may cause skin rash, gastrointestinal disturbances, headache, ataxia, and hematological side effects (Rajapakse et al. 2013).

Folinic acid is a folic acid derivative which is converted to tetrahydrofolate (the primary active form of folic acid) in vivo without relying on dihydrofolate reductase. Thus, folinic acid reduces side effects related to folate deficiency in the patient (Shea 2013).

Trimethoprim/sulfamethoxazole or co-trimoxazole, also known as SXT, TMP-SMX, TMP-SMZ, or TMP-sulfa, is a wide spectrum antimicrobial agent that consists of one part trimethoprim and five parts of sulfamethoxazole. It is used in the treatment of bacterial, fungal, and protozoal infections and shows greater effect when given together and behaves as bactericidal, though individually bacteriostatic (Manyando et al. 2013). The combination inhibits successive steps in the folate synthesis pathway. Trimethoprim causes a backlog of dihydrofolate (DHF), and this backlog works against the inhibitory effect the drug has on tetrahydrofolate biosynthesis; this is where the sulfamethoxazole comes in its role is in depleting the excess DHF by preventing it from being synthesized. It is antifolate in nature inhibiting both de novo folate biosynthesis and metabolism (Bentley 2009).

Atovaquone, a naphthoquinone compound, is an analog of ubiquinone with antipneumocystic activity. It is available in liquid form or oral suspension. Atovaquone (750 mg) orally given two to three times daily together with oral steroids is found effective in toxoplasmic retinochoroiditis (Winterhalter et al. 2010). Generally, co-trimoxazole is considered first-line agents, but atovaquone can be used in patients who cannot tolerate or are allergic to co-trimoxazole.

Macrolide antibiotics such as azithromycin and spiramycin and lincosamide antibiotic and clindamycin are also used to treat toxoplasmosis and various infections of the soft tissues (Hosseini et al. 2014; Yazici et al. 2009; Bonfioli and Orefice 2005). Azithromycin oral monotherapy is found effective and well tolerated for the treatment of active, non-vision-threatening toxoplasmic retinochoroiditis

(Balaskas et al. 2012). Azithromycin is an azalide, a subclass of macrolide antibiotic. The macrolides and lincosamides both act as a bacterial protein synthesis inhibitor by inhibiting ribosomal translocation through binding to the 50S rRNA of the large bacterial ribosome subunit. The common side effects of macrolides and lincosamides are nausea, vomiting, abdominal pain, nervousness, and dermatological reactions.

References

A controlled trial of oral acyclovir for iridocyclitis caused by herpes simplex virus. The Herpetic Eye Disease Study Group. Arch Ophthalmol. 1996;114(9):1065–72.

A controlled trial of oral acyclovir for the prevention of stromal keratitis or iritis in patients with herpes simplex virus epithelial keratitis. The Epithelial Keratitis Trial. The Herpetic Eye Disease Study Group. Arch Ophthalmol. 1997;115(6):703–12.

Acyclovir for the prevention of recurrent herpes simplex virus eye disease. Herpetic Eye Disease Study Group. N Engl J Med. 1998;339(5):300–6.

Altun A, Kurna SA, Sengor T, Altun G, Olcaysu OO, Aki SF, Simsek MH. Effectiveness of posaconazole in recalcitrant fungal keratitis resistant to conventional antifungal drugs. Case Rep Ophthalmol Med. 2014;2014:701653.

Barron BA, Gee L, Hauck WW, Kurinij N, et al. Herpetic Eye disease study. A controlled trial of oral acyclovir for herpes simplex stromal keratitis. Ophthalmology. 1994;101(12): 1871–82.

Biron KK, Elion GB. In vitro susceptibility of varicella-zoster virus to acyclovir. Antimicrob Agents Chemother. 1980;18(3):443–7.

Boston Interhospital Viral Study Group. Failure of high dose 5-iodo-2'-deoxyuridine in the therapy of herpes simplex virus encephalitis. Evidence of unacceptable toxicity. N Engl J Med. 1975;292(12):599–603.

Coster DJ, McKinnon JR, McGill JI, Jones BR, Fraunfelder FT. Clinical evaluation of adenine arabinoside and trifluorothymidine in the treatment of corneal ulcers caused by herpes simplex virus. J Infect Dis. 1976;133(Suppl):A173–7.

Davies ME, Bondi JV, Grabowski L, Schofield TL, Field AK. 2'-nor-2'deoxyguanosine is an effective therapeutic agent for treatment of experimental herpes keratitis. Antiviral Res. 1987;7(2): 119–25.

Dupuis A, Tournier N, Le Moal G, Venisse N. Preparation and stability of voriconazole eye drop solution. Antimicrob Agents Chemother. 2009;53(2):798–9.

Elion GB. Mechanism of action and selectivity of acyclovir. Am J Med. 1982;73(1A):7–13.

Foster CS, Stefanyszyn M. Intraocular penetration of miconazole in rabbits. Arch Ophthalmol. 1979;97(9):1703–6.

Gao H, Pennesi M, Shah K, Qiao X, Hariprasad SM, Mieler WF, et al. Safety of intravitreal voriconazole: electroretinographic and histopathologic studies. Trans Am Ophthalmol Soc. 2003; 101:183–9.

Goldblum D, Frueh BE, Sarra GM, Katsoulis K, Zimmerli S. Topical caspofungin for treatment of keratitis caused by Candida albicans in a rabbit model. Antimicrob Agents Chemother. 2005;49(4):1359–63.

Hurtado-Sarrió M, Duch-Samper A, Cisneros-Lanuza A, Díaz-Llopis M, Peman-Garcíia J, Vazquez-Polo A. Successful topical application of caspofungin in the treatment of fungal keratitis refractory to voriconazole. Arch Ophthalmol. 2010;128(7):941–2.

Kalavathy CM, Parmar P, Kaliamurthy J, Philip VR, Ramalingam MD, Jesudasan CA, Thomas PA. Comparison of topical itraconazole 1% with topical natamycin 5% for the treatment of filamentous fungal keratitis. Cornea. 2005;24(4):449–52.

Kaufman H, Martola E, Dohlman C. Use of 5-iodo-2'-deoxyuridine (IDU) in treatment of herpes simplex keratitis. Arch Ophthalmol. 1962a;68:235–9.
Kaufman HE, Heidelberger C. Therapeutic antiviral action of 5-trifluoromethyl-2'-deoxyuridine in herpes simplex keratitis. Science. 1964;145(3632):585–6.
Kaufman HE, Nesburn AB, Maloney ED. IDU therapy of herpes simplex. Arch Ophthalmol. 1962b;67:583–91.
Kaur IP, Rana C, Singh H. Development of effective ocular preparations of antifungal agents. J Ocul Pharmacol Ther. 2008;24(5):481–93. Review.
Khoo SH, Bond J, Denning DW. Administering amphotericin B—a practical approach. J Antimicrob Chemother. 1994;33(2):203–13.
Klotz SA, Zahid M, Bartholomew WR, Revera PM, Butrus S. Candida albicans keratitis treated successfully with itraconazole. Cornea. 1996;15(1):102–4.
Kobayashi D, Kondo K, Uehara N, Otokozawa S, Tsuji N, Yagihashi A, Watanabe N. Endogenous reactive oxygen species is an important mediator of miconazole antifungal effect. Antimicrob Agents Chemother. 2002;46(10):3113–7.
Lalitha P, Shapiro BL, Srinivasan M, Prajna NV, Acharya NR, Fothergill AW, et al. Antimicrobial susceptibility of Fusarium, Aspergillus, and other filamentous fungi isolated from keratitis. Arch Ophthalmol. 2007;125(6):789–93.
Larder BA, Darby G. Susceptibility to other antiherpes drugs of pathogenic variants of herpes simplex virus selected for resistance to acyclovir. Antimicrob Agents Chemother. 1986;29(5): 894–8.
Lee W, Benitez A, Goodman L, Baker BR. Potential Anticancer Agents. XL. Synthesis of the β-Anomer of 9-(D-Arabinofuranosyl)adenine. J Am Chem Soc. 1960;82:2648–9.
Li L, Wang Z, Li R, Luo S, Sun X. In vitro evaluation of combination antifungal activity against Fusarium species isolated from ocular tissues of keratomycosis patients. Am J Ophthalmol. 2008;146(5):724–8.
Lin HC, Chu PH, Kuo YH, Shen SC. Clinical experience in managing Fusarium solani keratitis. Int J Clin Pract. 2005;59(5):549–54.
Martinez R. Atualização no uso de agentes antifúngicos. J Bras Pneumol. 2006;32(5):449–60.
Morris MI, Villmann M. Echinocandins in the management of invasive fungal infections, part 1. Am J Health Syst Pharm. 2006;63(18):1693–703. Review.
Nicholson KG. Properties of antiviral agents. 1. Lancet. 1984;2(8401):503–6.
O'Day DM, Foulds G, Williams TE, Robinson RD, Allen RH, Head WS. Ocular uptake of fluconazole following oral administration. Arch Ophthalmol. 1990;108(7):1006–8.
O'Day DM, Ray WA, Head WS, Robinson RD. Influence of the corneal epithelium on the efficacy of topical antifungal agents. Invest Ophthalmol Vis Sci. 1984;25(7):855–9.
O'Day DM. Selection of appropriate antifungal therapy. Cornea. 1987;6(4):238–45. Review.
O'Day DM, Head WS, Robinson RD, Stern WH, Freeman JM. Intraocular penetration of systemically administered antifungal agents. Curr Eye Res. 1985;4(2):131–4.
Panda A, Sharma N, Angra SK. Topical fluconazole therapy of Candida keratitis. Cornea. 1996;15(4):373–5.
Prajna NV, Krishnan T, Mascarenhas J, Rajaraman R, Prajna L, Srinivasan M, Raghavan A, Oldenburg CE, Ray KJ, Zegans ME, McLeod SD, Porco TC, Acharya NR, Lietman TM, Mycotic Ulcer Treatment Trial Group. The mycotic ulcer treatment trial: a randomized trial comparing natamycin vs voriconazole. JAMA Ophthalmol. 2013;131(4):422–9.
Prajna NV, Mascarenhas J, Krishnan T, Reddy PR, Prajna L, Srinivasan M, et al. Comparison of natamycin and voriconazole for the treatment of fungal keratitis. Arch Ophthalmol. 2010; 128(6):672–8.
Prakash G, Sharma N, Goel M, Titiyal JS, Vajpayee RB. Evaluation of intrastromal injection of voriconazole as a therapeutic adjunctive for the management of deep recalcitrant fungal keratitis. Am J Ophthalmol. 2008;146(1):56–9.
Prusoff WH, Zucker M, Mancini WR, Otto MJ, Lin TS, Lee JJ. Basic biochemical and pharmacological aspects of antiviral agents. Antiviral Res. 1985;Suppl 1:1–10.

Rajaraman R, Bhat P, Vaidee V, Maskibail S, Raghavan A, Sivasubramaniam S, Rajasekaran J, Thomas PA, Kalavathy CM, Joseph PC, Abraham DJ. Itraconazole therapy for fungal keratitis. Indian J Ophthalmol. 1987;35(5–6):157–60.

Sacks SL, Scullard GH, Pollard RB, Gregory PB, Robinson WS, Merigan TC. Antiviral treatment of chronic hepatitis B virus infection: pharmacokinetics and side effects of interferon and adenine arabinoside alone and in combination. Antimicrob Agents Chemother. 1982;21(1):93–100.

Sharma N, Chacko J, Velpandian T, Titiyal JS, Sinha R, Satpathy G, Tandon R, Vajpayee RB. Comparative evaluation of topical versus intrastromal voriconazole as an adjunct to natamycin in recalcitrant fungal keratitis. Ophthalmology. 2013a;120(4):677–81.

Sharma S, Das S, Virdi A, Fernandes M, Sahu SK, Kumar Koday N, Ali MH, Garg P, Motukupally SR. Re-appraisal of topical 1% voriconazole and 5% natamycin in the treatment of fungal keratitis in a randomised trial. Br J Ophthalmol. 2015;99(9):1190–5.

Torres MA, Mohamed J, Cavazos-Adame H, Martinez LA. Topical ketoconazole for fungal keratitis. Am J Ophthalmol. 1985;100(2):293–8.

Travers JP, Patterson A. A controlled trial of adenine arabinoside and trifluorothymidine in herpetic keratitis. J Int Med Res. 1978;6(2):102–4.

Urbak SF, Degn T. Fluconazole in the management of fungal ocular infections. Ophthalmologica. 1994;208(3):147–56.

Van Bijsterveld OP, Post H. Trifluorothymidine versus adenine arabinoside in the treatment of herpes simplex keratitis. Br J Ophthalmol. 1980;64(1):33–6.

Vermes A, Guchelaar HJ, Dankert J. Flucytosine: a review of its pharmacology, clinical indications, pharmacokinetics, toxicity and drug interactions. J Antimicrob Chemother. 2000;46(2):171–9.

Wagstaff AJ, Faulds D, Goa KL. Aciclovir. A reappraisal of its antiviral activity, pharmacokinetic properties and therapeutic efficacy. Drugs. 1994;47(1):153–205.

Wilhelmus KR. The treatment of herpes simplex virus epithelial keratitis. Trans Am Ophthalmol Soc. 2000;98:505–32.

Wilson 2nd FM. Adverse external ocular effects of topical ophthalmic medications. Surv Ophthalmol. 1979;24(2):57–88.

Yoon KC, Jeong IY, Im SK, Chae HJ, Yang SY. Therapeutic effect of intracameral amphotericin B injection in the treatment of fungal keratitis. Cornea. 2007;26(7):814–8.

Agarwal AK, Ram J, Singh R. Sparfloxacin-associated corneal epithelial toxicity. BMJ Case Rep. 2014;19:2014.

Ahmed S, Kuruvilla O, Yee DC, et al. Intraocular penetration of systemic antibiotics in eyes with penetrating ocular injury. J Ocul Pharmacol Ther. 2014;30(10):823–30.

Akyol-Salman I, Azizi S, Mumcu UY, et al. Comparison of the efficacy of topical N-acetylcysteine and a topical steroid-antibiotic combination therapy in the treatment of meibomian gland dysfunction. J Ocul Pharmacol Ther. 2012;28(1):49–52.

Andreoli CM, Wiley HE, Durand ML, et al. Primary meningococcal conjunctivitis in an adult. Cornea. 2004;23(7):738–9.

Baneke A. Review: targeting trachoma: strategies to reduce the leading infectious cause of blindness. Travel Med Infect Dis. 2012;10(2):92–6.

Benson CE, Soliman MK, Knezevic A, et al. Bilateral papillitis and unilateral focal chorioretinitis as the presenting features of syphilis. J Ophthalmic Inflamm Infect. 2015;5:16.

Blanco AR, SudanoRoccaro A, Spoto CG, et al. Susceptibility of methicillin-resistant Staphylococci clinical isolates to netilmicin and other antibiotics commonly used in ophthalmic therapy. Curr Eye Res. 2013;38(8):811–6.

Cagini C, Piccinelli F, Lupidi M, et al. Ocular penetration of topical antibiotics: study on the penetration of chloramphenicol, tobramycin and netilmicin into the anterior chamber after topical administration. Clin Experiment Ophthalmol. 2013;41(7):644–7.

Chang VS, Dhaliwal DK, Raju L, Kowalski RP. Antibiotic resistance in the treatment of staphylococcus aureus keratitis: a 20-year review. Cornea. 2015;34(6):698–703.

Chen C, Chen Y, Wu P, et al. Update on new medicinal applications of gentamicin: evidence-based review. J Formos Med Assoc. 2014;113(2):72–82.

Chew FL, Soong TK, Shin HC, et al. Topical piperacillin/tazobactam for recalcitrant pseudomonas aeruginosa keratitis. J Ocul Pharmacol Ther. 2010;26(2):219–22.

Cosar CB, Cohen EJ, Rapuano CJ, et al. Clear corneal wound infection after phacoemulsification. Arch Ophthalmol. 2001;119(12):1755–9.

Darling EK, McDonald H. A meta-analysis of the efficacy of ocular prophylactic agents used for the prevention of gonococcal and chlamydial ophthalmianeonatorum. J Midwifery Womens Health. 2010;55(4):319–27.

Donnenfeld ED, O'Brien TP, Solomon R, et al. Infectious keratitis after photorefractive keratectomy. Ophthalmology. 2003;110(4):743–7.

Erdem E, Abdurrahmanoglu S, Kibar F, et al. Posttraumatic keratitis caused by Elizabeth kingiameningosepticum. Eye Contact Lens. 2013;39(5):361–3.

Foulks GN, Borchman D, Yappert M, et al. Topical azithromycin and oral doxycycline therapy of meibomian gland dysfunction: a comparative clinical and spectroscopic pilot study. Cornea. 2013;32(1):44–53.

Freitas D, Alvarenga L, Sampaio J, et al. An outbreak of Mycobacterium chelonae infection after LASIK. Ophthalmology. 2003;110(2):276–85.

Fukuda M, Ohashi H, Matsumoto C, et al. Methicillin-resistant Staphylococcus aureus and methicillin-resistant coagulase-negative Staphylococcus ocular surface infection efficacy of chloramphenicol eye drops. Cornea. 2002;21(7 Suppl):S86–9.

Garg P, Mathur U, Sony P, et al. Clinical and antibacterial efficacy and safety of besifloxacin ophthalmic suspension compared with moxifloxacin ophthalmic solution. Asia Pac J Ophthalmol (Phila). 2015;4(3):140–5.

Garnock-Jones KP. Azithromycin 1.5% ophthalmic solution: in purulent bacterial or trachomatous conjunctivitis. Drugs. 2012;72(3):361–73.

Gentile RC, Shukla S, Shah M, et al. Microbiological spectrum and antibiotic sensitivity in endophthalmitis: a 25-year review. Ophthalmology. 2014;121(8):1634–42.

Graffi S, Peretz A, Naftali M. Endogenous endophthalmitis with an unusual infective agent: Actinomyces neuii. Eur J Ophthalmol. 2012;22(5):834–5.

Heller W, Cruz M, Bhagat YR, et al. Gatifloxacin 0.5% administered twice daily for the treatment of acute bacterial conjunctivitis in patients one year of age or older. J Ocul Pharmacol Ther. 2014;30(10):815–22.

Hsiao CH, Chuang CC, Tan HY, Ma DH, Lin KK, Chang CJ, Huang YC. Methicillin-resistant Staphylococcus aureus ocular infection: a 10-year hospital-based study. Ophthalmology. 2012;119(3):522–7. doi: 10.1016/j.ophtha.2011.08.038. Epub 2011 Dec 15.

Jain R, Murthy SI, Motukupally SR, et al. Use of topical colistin in multiple drug-resistant Pseudomonas aeruginosa bacterial keratitis. Cornea. 2014;33(9):923–7.

Katibeh M, Ziaei H, Mirzaei M, et al. Perioperative prophylaxis for endophthalmitis after cataract surgery in iran. J Ophthalmic Vis Res. 2015;10(1):33–6.

Keenan JD, Moncada J, Gebre T, et al. Chlamydial infection during trachoma monitoring: are the most difficult-to-reach children more likely to be infected? Trop Med Int Health. 2012;17(3): 392–6.

Kessel L, Flesner P, Andresen J, et al. Antibiotic prevention of postcataract endophthalmitis: a systematic review and meta-analysis. Acta Ophthalmol. 2015;93(4):303–17.

Koh S, Maeda N, Soma T, Hori Y, Tsujikawa M, Watanabe H, Nishida K. Development of methicillin-resistant staphylococcus aureus keratitis in a dry eye patient with a therapeutic contact lens. Eye Contact Lens. 2012;38(3):200–2.

Leeming JP. Treatment of ocular infections with topical antibacterials. Clin Pharmacokinet. 1999;37(5):351–60.

Li B, Miño de Kaspar H, Haritoglou C, et al. Comparison of 1-day versus 1-hour application of topical neomycin/polymyxin-B before cataract surgery. J Cataract Refract Surg. 2015;41(4): 724–31.

Linertová R, Abreu-González R, García-Pérez L, et al. Intracameral cefuroxime and moxifloxacin used as endophthalmitis prophylaxis after cataract surgery: systematic review of effectiveness and cost-effectiveness. Clin Ophthalmol. 2014;8:1515–22.

Khalil MA, Sonbol FI. Investigation of biofilm formation on contact eye lenses caused by methicillin resistant Staphylococcus aureus. Niger J Clin Pract. 2014;17(6):776–84.
Mason BW, Howard AJ, Magee JT. Fusidic acid resistance in community isolates of methicillin-susceptible Staphylococcus aureus and fusidic acid prescribing. J Antimicrob Chemother. 2003;51(4):1033–6.
McDonald EM, Ram FS, Patel DV, et al. Topical antibiotics for the management of bacterial keratitis: an evidence-based review of high quality randomised controlled trials. Br J Ophthalmol. 2014;98(11):1470–7.
Mehta S, Armstrong BK, Kim SJ, et al. Long-term potency, sterility, and stability of vancomycin, ceftazidime, and moxifloxacin for treatment of bacterial endophthalmitis. Retina. 2011;31(7): 1316–22.
Munir WM, Rosenfeld SI, Udell I, et al. Clinical response of contact lens-associated fungal keratitis to topical fluoroquinolone therapy. Cornea. 2007;26(5):621–4.
Newman PE, Hider P, Waring 3rd GO, Hill EO, Wilson LA, Harbin TS. Corneal ulcer due to Achromobacter xylosoxidans. Br J Ophthalmol. 1984;68(7):472–4.
Nguyen AT, Hong AR, Baqai J, Lubniewski AJ, Huang AJ. Use of topical besifloxacin in the treatment of Mycobacterium chelonae Ocular Surface Infections. Cornea. 2015;34(8):967–71.
Mamalis N. Ocular methicillin-resistant Staphylococcus aureus. J Cataract Refract Surg. 2014;40(11):1757–8. doi: 10.1016/j.jcrs.2014.09.016. Epub 2014 Oct 23.
Ortega-Usobiaga J, Llovet-Osuna F, Djodeyre MR, et al. Incidence of corneal infections after laser in situ keratomileusis and surface ablation when moxifloxacin and tobramycin are used as postoperative treatment. J Cataract Refract Surg. 2015;18.
Papa V, Aragona P, Scuderi AC, et al. Treatment of acute bacterial conjunctivitis with topical netilmicin. Cornea. 2002;21(1):43–7.
Park YM, Kwon HJ, Lee JS. Microbiological study of therapeutic soft contact lenses used in the treatment of recurrent corneal erosion syndrome. Eye Contact Lens. 2015;41(2):84–6.
Penha FM, Rodrigues EB, Maia M, et al. Retinal and ocular toxicity in ocular application of drugs and chemicals – part II: retinal toxicity of current and new drugs. Ophthalmic Res. 2010;44(4): 205–24.
Rajapakse S, Chrishan SM, Samaranayake N, et al. Antibiotics for human toxoplasmosis: a systematic review of randomized trials. Pathog Glob Health. 2013;107(4):162–9.
Rautaraya B, Sharma S, Ali MH, et al. A 3½-year study of bacterial keratitis from Odisha, India. Asia Pac J Ophthalmol (Phila). 2014;3(3):146–50.
Ritterband DC, Shah M, Seedor J. Antibiotic prophylaxis in clear corneal cataract surgery. Arch Ophthalmol. 2003;121(2):296. author reply 296.
Robert PY, Adenis JP. Comparative review of topical ophthalmic antibacterial preparations. Drugs. 2001;61(2):175–85.
Ryan ET, Durand M. Ocular disease. In: Tropical infectious diseases: principles, pathogens and practice. Saunders Elsevier 2011. p. 991–1016.
Sharma R, Jhanji V, Satpathy G, et al. Coinfection with Acanthamoeba and Pseudomonas in contact lens-associated keratitis. Optom Vis Sci. 2013b;90(2):e53–5.
Sharma T, Kamath MM, Kamath MG, et al. Aqueous penetration of orally and topically administered moxifloxacin. Br J Ophthalmol. 2015;30.
Smith A, Pennefather PM, Kaye SB, Hart CA. Fluoroquinolones: place in ocular therapy. Drugs. 2001;61(6):747–61.
Snyder RW, Glasser DB. Antibiotic therapy for ocular infection. West J Med. 1994;161:579–84.
Sobolewska B, Doycheva D, Deuter C, et al. Treatment of ocular rosacea with once-daily low-dose doxycycline. Cornea. 2014;33(3):257–60.
Sridhar J, Kuriyan AE, Flynn Jr HW, et al. Endophthalmitis caused by Pseudomonas aeruginosa : clinical features, antibiotic susceptibilities, and treatment outcomes. Retina. 2015;35(6):1101–6.
Suemori S, Sawada A, Komori S, et al. Case of endogenous endophthalmitis caused by Streptococcus equisimilis. Clin Ophthalmol. 2010;4:917–8.
Tinley C, Van Zyl L, Grötte R. Poststreptococcal syndrome uveitis in South African children. Br J Ophthalmol. 2012;96(1):87–9.

Trichet E, Cohen-Bacrie S, Conrath J, et al. Nocardia transvalensis keratitis: an emerging pathology among travelers returning from Asia. BMC Infect Dis. 2011;11:296.

Vazirani J, Basu S. Role of topical, subconjunctival, intracameral, and irrigative antibiotics in cataract surgery. Curr Opin Ophthalmol. 2013;24(1):60–5.

Veldman P, Colby K. Current evidence for topical azithromycin 1% ophthalmic solution in the treatment of blepharitis and blepharitis-associated ocular dryness. Int Ophthalmol Clin. 2011;51(4):43–52.

Kos VN, Desjardins CA, Griggs A, Cerqueira G, Van Tonder A, et al. Comparative genomics of vancomycin-resistant staphylococcus aureus strains and their positions within the Clade Most Commonly Associated with Methicillin-Resistant S. aureus Hospital-Acquired Infection in the United States. mBio. 2012;3(3):e00112–12.

Wang L, Tsang H, Coroneo M. Treatment of recurrent corneal erosion syndrome using the combination of oral doxycycline and topical corticosteroid. Clin Experiment Ophthalmol. 2008;36(1): 8–12.

Williams L, Malhotra Y, Murante B, et al. A single-blinded randomized clinical trial comparing polymyxin B-trimethoprim and moxifloxacin for treatment of acute conjunctivitis in children. J Pediatr. 2013;162(4):857–61.

Abrishami M, Soheilian M, Farahi A, Dowlati Y. Successful treatment of ocular leishmaniasis. Eur J Dermatol. 2002;12(1):88–9.

Andersen SL, Oloo AJ, Gordon DM, Ragama OB, Aleman GM, Berman JD, Tang DB, Dunne MW, Shanks GD. Successful double-blinded, randomized, placebo-controlled field trial of azithromycin and doxycycline as prophylaxis for malaria in western Kenya. Clin Infect Dis. 1998;26(1): 146–50.

Ang M, Mehta JS, Mantoo S, Tan D. Deep anterior lamellar keratoplasty to treat microsporidial stromal keratitis. Cornea. 2009;28(7):832–5.

Antoniazzi E, Guagliano R, Meroni V, Pezzotta S, Bianchi PE. Ocular impairment of toxoplasmosis. Parassitologia. 2008;50(1–2):35–6.

Asproudis I, Koumpoulis I, Kalogeropoulos C, Sotiropoulos G, Papassava M, Aspiotis M. Case report of a neonate with ocular toxoplasmosis due to congenital infection: estimation of the percentage of ocular toxoplasmosis in Greece caused by congenital or acquired infection. Clin Ophthalmol. 2013;7:2249–52.

Baharivand N, Mahdavifard A, Fouladi RF. Intravitreal clindamycin plus dexamethasone versus classic oral therapy in toxoplasmic retinochoroiditis: a prospective randomized clinical trial. Int Ophthalmol. 2013;33(1):39–46.

Balaskas K, Vaudaux J, Boillat-Blanco N, Guex-Crosier Y. Azithromycin versus Sulfadiazine and Pyrimethamine for non-vision-threatening toxoplasmic retinochoroiditis: a pilot study. Med Sci Monit. 2012;18(5):CR296–302.

Bang S, Edell E, Eghrari AO, Gottsch JD. Treatment with voriconazole in 3 eyes with resistant Acanthamoeba keratitis. Am J Ophthalmol. 2010;149(1):66–9.

Barrett MP, Croft SL. Management of trypanosomiasis and leishmaniasis. Br Med Bull. 2012;104: 175–96.

Bentley R. Different roads to discovery; Prontosil (hence sulfa drugs) and penicillin (hence beta-lactams). J Ind Microbiol Biotechnol. 2009;36(6):775–86.

Bonfioli AA, Orefice F. Toxoplasmosis. Semin Ophthalmol. 2005;20(3):129–41.

Burri C, Brun R. Eflornithine for the treatment of human African trypanosomiasis. Parasitol Res. 2003;90(Supp 1):S49–52.

Butler NJ, Furtado JM, Winthrop KL, Smith JR. Ocular toxoplasmosis II: clinical features, pathology and management. Clin Experiment Ophthalmol. 2013;41(1):95–108.

Cabello-Vílchez AM, Martín-Navarro CM, López-Arencibia A, Reyes-Batlle M, Sifaoui I, Valladares B, Piñero JE, Lorenzo-Morales J. Voriconazole as a first-line treatment against potentially pathogenic Acanthamoeba strains from Peru. Parasitol Res. 2014;113:755–9.

Campos FA, Andrade GM, Lanna Ade P, Lage BF, Assumpção MV, Pinto JA. Incidence of congenital toxoplasmosis among infants born to HIV-coinfected mothers: case series and literature review. Braz J Infect Dis. 2014;18(6):609–17.

Cassaday JV, Bahler JW, Hinken MV. Spiramycin for toxoplasmosis. Am J Ophthalmol. 1964;57:227–35.

Chan CM, Theng JT, Li L, Tan DT. Microsporidial keratoconjunctivitis in healthy individuals: a case series. Ophthalmology. 2003;110(7):1420–5.

Corsi A, Nucci C, Knafelz D, Bulgarini D, Di Iorio L, Polito A, De Risi F, Ardenti Morini F, Paone FM. Ocular changes associated with Giardia lamblia infection in children. Br J Ophthalmol. 1998;82(1):59–62.

Coura JR, Borges-Pereira J. Chagas disease: 100 years after its discovery. A systemic review. Acta Trop. 2010;115(1–2):5–13.

Delair E, Latkany P, Noble AG, Rabiah P, McLeod R, Brézin A. Clinical manifestations of ocular toxoplasmosis. Ocul Immunol Inflamm. 2011;19(2):91–102.

de-la-Torre A, Stanford M, Curi A, Jaffe GJ, Gomez-Marin JE. Therapy for ocular toxoplasmosis. Ocul Immunol Inflamm. 2011;19(5):314–20.

Dias JCP, Coura JR, Yasuda MAS. The present situation, challenges, and perspectives regarding the production and utilization of effective drugs against human Chagas disease. Rev Soc Bras Med Trop. 2014;47(1):123–5.

Elmahallawy EK, Sampedro Martinez A, Rodriguez-Granger J, Hoyos-Mallecot Y, Agil A, Navarro Mari JM, Gutierrez FJ. Diagnosis of leishmaniasis. J Infect Dev Ctries. 2014;8(8):961–72.

Fuglsang H, Anderson J. A preliminary trial of nifurtimox in the treatment of onchocerciasis. Tropenmed Parasitol. 1978;29(3):335–8.

Garcia-Méric P, Franck J, Dumon H, Piarroux R. Management of congenital toxoplasmosis in France: current data. Presse Med. 2010;39(5):530–8.

Gaynor BD, Amza A, Kadri B, Nassirou B, Lawan O, Maman L, Stoller NE, Yu SN, Chin SA, West SK, Bailey RL, Rosenthal PJ, Keenan JD, Porco TC, Lietman TM. Impact of mass azithromycin distribution on malaria parasitemia during the low-transmission season in Niger: a cluster-randomized trial. Am J Trop Med Hyg. 2014;90(5):846–51.

Granados CE, Reveiz L, Uribe LG, Criollo CP. Drugs for treating giardiasis. Cochrane Database Syst Rev. 2012;12:CD007787. doi: 10.1002/14651858.CD007787.pub2.

Guldsten H. Clindamycin and sulphonamides in the treatment of ocular toxoplasmosis. Acta Ophthalmol (Copenh). 1983;61(1):51–7.

Harrell M, Carvounis PE. Current treatment of toxoplasma retinochoroiditis: an evidence-based review. J Ophthalmol. 2014;2014:273506.

Heby O, Persson L, Rentala M. Targeting the polyamine biosynthetic enzymes: a promising approach to therapy of African sleeping sickness, Chagas' disease, and leishmaniasis. Amino Acids. 2007;33(2):359–66.

Holland GN, Lewis KG. An update on current practices in the management of ocular toxoplasmosis. Am J Ophthalmol. 2002;134:102–14.

Hosseini SM, Abrishami M, Mehdi ZM. Intravitreal clindamycin in the treatment of unresponsive zone one toxoplasmic chorioretinitis: a case report. Iran Red Crescent Med J. 2014;16(11), e15428.

Jennings FW. Chemotherapy of trypanosomiasis: the potentiation of melarsoprol by concurrent difluoromethylornithine (DFMO) treatment. Trans R Soc Trop Med Hyg. 1988;82(4):572–3.

Jin KW, Jeon HS, Hyon JY, Wee WR, Suh W, Shin YJ. A case of fungal keratitis and onychomycosis simultaneously infected by Trichophyton species. BMC Ophthalmol. 2014;14:90.

Kaye A. Toxoplasmosis: diagnosis, treatment, and prevention in congenitally exposed infants. J Pediatr Health Care. 2011;25(6):355–64.

Khadem F, Uzonna JE. Immunity to visceral leishmaniasis: implications for immunotherapy. Future Microbiol. 2014;9(7):901–15.

Khalil EA, Musa AM, Younis BM, Elfaki ME, Zijlstra EE, Elhassan AM. Blindness following visceral leishmaniasis: a neglected post-kala-azar complication. Trop Doct. 2011;41(3):139–40.

Khandelwal SS, Woodward MA, Hall T, Grossniklaus HE, Stulting RD. Treatment of microsporidia keratitis with topical voriconazole monotherapy. Arch Ophthalmol. 2011;129(4):509–10.

Khyatti M, Trimbitas RD, Zouheir Y, Benani A, El Messaoudi MD, Hemminki K. Infectious diseases in North Africa and North African immigrants to Europe. Eur J Public Health. 2014;24 Suppl 1:47–56.

Kowalski RP, Abdel Aziz S, Romanowski EG, Shanks RM, Nau AC, Raju LV. Development of a practical complete-kill assay to evaluate anti-Acanthamoeba drugs. JAMA Ophthalmol. 2013;131(11):1459–62.

Kulakova L, Galkin A, Chen CZ, Southall N, Marugan JJ, Zheng W, Herzberg O. Discovery of novel antigiardiasis drug candidates. Antimicrob Agents Chemother. 2014;58(12):7303–11.

Lal A, Baker MG, Hales S, French NP. Potential effects of global environmental changes on cryptosporidiosis and giardiasis transmission. Trends Parasitol. 2013;29(2):83–90.

Le Loup G, Pialoux G, Lescure FX. Update in treatment of Chagas disease. Curr Opin Infect Dis. 2011;24(5):428–34.

Lima e Silva R, Saishin Y, Saishin Y, Akiyama H, Kachi S, Aslam S, Rogers B, Deering T, Gong YY, Hackett SF, Lai H, Frydman BJ, Valasinas A, Marton LJ, Campochiaro PA. Suppression and regression of choroidal neovascularization by polyamine analogues. Invest Ophthalmol Vis Sci. 2005;46(9):3323–30.

Lin HC, Hsiao CH, Ma DH, Yeh LK, Tan HY, Lin MY, Huang SC. Medical treatment for combined Fusarium and Acanthamoeba keratitis. Acta Ophthalmol. 2009;87(2):199–203.

Loh RS, Chan CM, Ti SE, Lim L, Chan KS, Tan DT. Emerging prevalence of microsporidial keratitis in Singapore: epidemiology, clinical features, and management. Ophthalmology. 2009; 116(12):2348–53.

Maenz M, Schlüter D, Liesenfeld O, Schares G, Gross U, Pleyer U. Ocular toxoplasmosis past, present and new aspects of an old disease. Prog Retin Eye Res. 2014;39:77–106.

Mahajan R, Das P, Isaakidis P, Sunyoto T, Sagili KD, Lima MA, Mitra G, Kumar D, Pandey K, Van Geertruyden JP, Boelaert M, Burza S. Combination Treatment for Visceral Leishmaniasis Patients Coinfected with Human Immunodeficiency Virus in India. Clin Infect Dis. 2015;61(8):1255–62. doi: 10.1093/cid/civ530. Epub 2015 Jun 30.

Manyando C, Njunju EM, D'Alessandro U, Van Geertruyden JP. Safety and efficacy of co-trimoxazole for treatment and prevention of Plasmodium falciparum malaria: a systematic review. PLoS One. 2013;8(2), e56916.

Martín-Navarro CM, López-Arencibia A, Arnalich-Montiel F, Valladares B, Piñero JE, Lorenzo-Morales J. Evaluation of the in vitro activity of commercially available moxifloxacin and voriconazole eye-drops against clinical strains of Acanthamoeba. Graefes Arch Clin Exp Ophthalmol. 2013;251(9):2111–7.

Maude RJ, Ahmed BU, Rahman AH, Rahman R, Majumder MI, Menezes DB, Abu Sayeed A, Hughes L, MacGillivray TJ, Borooah S, Dhillon B, Dondorp AM, Faiz MA. Retinal changes in visceral leishmaniasis by retinal photography. BMC Infect Dis. 2014;14:527.

Medeiros FPM. Current situation and new perspectives for the treatment of Chagas disease. Prospects for production and distribution of benznidazole. Rev Soc Bras Med Trop. 2009;42(Supl II):79.

Meltzer E, Lachish T, Schwartz E. Treatment of giardiasis after nonresponse to nitroimidazole. Emerg Infect Dis. 2014;20(10):1742–4.

Mochizuki K, Niwa Y, Ishida K, Kawakami H. Intraocular penetration of itraconazole in patient with fungal endophthalmitis. Int Ophthalmol. 2013;33(5):579–81.

Molina I, Gómez i Prat J, Salvador F, Treviño B, Sulleiro E, Serre N, Pou D, Roure S, Cabezos J, Valerio L, Blanco-Grau A, Sánchez-Montalvá A, Vidal X, Pahissa A. Randomized trial of posaconazole and benznidazole for chronic Chagas' disease. N Engl J Med. 2014;370(20): 1899–908.

Montero JA, Ruiz-Moreno JM, Sanchis E. Intraretinal hemorrhage associated with leishmaniasis. Ophthalmic Surg Lasers Imaging. 2003;34(3):212–4.

Mørch K, Hanevik K, Robertson LJ, Strand EA, Langeland N. Treatment-ladder and genetic characterisation of parasites in refractory giardiasis after an outbreak in Norway. J Infect. 2008;56(4):268–73.

Noble A. Cataracts in congenital toxoplasmosis. J AAPOS. 2007;11:551–4.
Opremcak EM, Scales DK, Sharpe MR. Trimethoprim-sulfamethoxazole therapy for ocular toxoplasmosis. Ophthalmology. 1992;99(6):920–5.
Osadchy A, Ratnapalan T, Koren G. Ocular toxicity in children exposed in utero to antimalarial drugs: review of the literature. J Rheumatol. 2011;38(12):2504–8.
Paquet C. Yudin MH; Toxoplasmosis in pregnancy: prevention, screening, and treatment. Society of Obstetricians and Gynaecologists of Canada. J Obstet Gynaecol Can. 2013;35(1):78–81.
Parchand S, Gupta A, Ram J, Gupta N, Chakrabarty A. Voriconazole for fungal corneal ulcers. Ophthalmology. 2012;119(5):1083.
Park YH, Nam HW. Clinical features and treatment of ocular toxoplasmosis. Korean J Parasitol. 2013;51(4):393–9.
Pasupuleti V, Escobedo AA, Deshpande A, Thota P, Roman Y, Hernandez AV. Efficacy of 5-nitroimidazoles for the treatment of giardiasis: a systematic review of randomized controlled trials. PLoS Negl Trop Dis. 2014;8(3), e2733.
Patole S, Burza S, Varghese GM. Multiple relapses of visceral leishmaniasis in a patient with HIV in India: a treatment challenge. Int J Infect Dis. 2014;25:204–6.
Pfaff AW, de-la-Torre A, Rochet E, Brunet J, Sabou M, Sauer A, Bourcier T, Gomez-Marin JE, Candolfi E. New clinical and experimental insights into Old World and neotropical ocular toxoplasmosis. Int J Parasitol. 2014;44(2):99–107.
Pinazo MJ, Espinosa G, Gállego M, et al. Successful treatment with posaconazole of a patient with chronic Chagas disease and systemic lupus erythematosus. Am J Trop Med Hyg. 2010;82: 583–7.
Pleyer U, Schlüter D, Mänz M. Ocular toxoplasmosis: recent aspects of pathophysiology and clinical implications. Ophthalmic Res. 2014;52(3):116–23.
Priotto G, Kasparian S, Mutombo W, Ngouama D, Ghorashian S, Arnold U, Ghabri S, Baudin E, Buard V, Kazadi-Kyanza S, Ilunga M, Mutangala W, Pohlig G, Schmid C, Karunakara U, Torreele E, Kande V. Nifurtimox-eflornithine combination therapy for second-stage African Trypanosoma brucei gambiense trypanosomiasis: a multicentre, randomised, phase III, non-inferiority trial. Lancet. 2009;374(9683):56–64.
Rodgers J, Jones A, Gibaud S, Bradley B, McCabe C, Barrett MP, Gettinby G, Kennedy PG. Melarsoprol cyclodextrin inclusion complexes as promising oral candidates for the treatment of human African trypanosomiasis. PLoS Negl Trop Dis. 2011;5(9), e1308.
Roizenblatt J. Interstitial keratitis caused by American (mucocutaneous) leishmaniasis. Am J Ophthalmol. 1979;87(2):175–9.
Rossi P, Urbani C, Donelli G, Pozio E. Resolution of microsporidial sinusitis and keratoconjunctivitis by itraconazole treatment. Am J Ophthalmol. 1999;127(2):210–2.
Sadeghian G, Nilfroushzadeh MA, Moradi SH, Hanjani SH. Ocular leishmaniasis: a case report. Dermatol Online J. 2005;11(2):19.
Santamaria C, Chatelain E, Jackson Y, Miao Q, Ward BJ, Chappuis F, Ndao M. Serum biomarkers predictive of cure in Chagas disease patients after nifurtimox treatment. BMC Infect Dis. 2014;14:302.
Shea B. Folic acid or folinic acid for reducing side effects of methotrexate for people with rheumatoid arthritis. J Evid Based Med. 2013;6(3):202–3.
Sindermann H, Engel J. Development of miltefosine as an oral treatment for leishmaniasis. Trans R Soc Trop Med Hyg. 2006;100 Suppl 1:S17–20.
Soheilian M, Ramezani A, Azimzadeh A, et al. Randomized trial of intravitreal clindamycin and dexamethasone versus pyrimethamine, sulfadiazine, and prednisolone in treatment of ocular toxoplasmosis. Ophthalmology. 2011;118(1):134–41.
Sridhar MS, Sharma S. Microsporidial keratoconjunctivitis in a HIV-seronegative patient treated with debridement and oral itraconazole. Am J Ophthalmol. 2003;136(4):745–6.
Stover KR, Riche DM, Gandy CL, Henderson H. What would we do without metronidazole? Am J Med Sci. 2012;343(4):316–9.

Sunada A, Kimura K, Nishi I, Toyokawa M, Ueda A, Sakata T, Suzuki T, Inoue Y, Ohashi Y, Asari S, Iwatani Y. In vitro evaluations of topical agents to treat Acanthamoeba keratitis. Ophthalmology. 2014;121(10):2059–65.

Sundar S, Chakravarty J, Agarwal D, Rai M, Murray HW. Single-dose liposomal amphotericin B for visceral leishmaniasis in India. N Engl J Med. 2010;362(6):504–12.

Sundar S, Chakravarty J. An update on pharmacotherapy for leishmaniasis. Expert Opin Pharmacother. 2015;16(2):237–52.

Sundar S, Sinha PK, Rai M, Verma DK, Nawin K, Alam S, Chakravarty J, Vaillant M, Verma N, Pandey K, Kumari P, Lal CS, Arora R, Sharma B, Ellis S, Strub-Wourgaft N, Balasegaram M, Olliaro P, Das P, Modabber F. Comparison of short-course multidrug treatment with standard therapy for visceral leishmaniasis in India: an open-label, non-inferiority, randomised controlled trial. Lancet. 2011;377(9764):477–86.

Tate Jr GW, Martin RG. Clindamycin in the treatment of human ocular toxoplasmosis. Can J Ophthalmol. 1977;12(3):188–95.

Taylor WR, Richie TL, Fryauff DJ, Picarima H, Ohrt C, Tang D, Braitman D, Murphy GS, Widjaja H, Tjitra E, Ganjar A, Jones TR, Basri H, Berman J. Malaria prophylaxis using azithromycin: a double-blind, placebo-controlled trial in Irian Jaya, Indonesia. Clin Infect Dis. 1999;28(1): 74–81.

Tu EY, Joslin CE, Shoff ME. Successful treatment of chronic stromal acanthamoeba keratitis with oral voriconazole monotherapy. Cornea. 2010;29(9):1066–8.

Turnbull AM, Lin Z, Matthews BN. Severe bilateral anterior uveitis secondary to giardiasis, initially misdiagnosed as a side effect of metronidazole. Eye (Lond). 2013;27(10):1225–6.

Vedula SS, Nguyen QD. Corticosteroids for ocular toxoplasmosis. Cochrane Database Syst Rev. 2008;4:CD007417.

Walochnik J, Obwaller A, Gruber F, Mildner M, Tschachler E, Suchomel M, Duchêne M, Auer H. Anti-acanthamoeba efficacy and toxicity of miltefosine in an organotypic skin equivalent. J Antimicrob Chemother. 2009;64(3):539–45.

Winterhalter S, Severing K, Stammen J, Maier AK, Godehardt E, Joussen AM. Does atovaquone prolong the disease-free interval of toxoplasmic retinochoroiditis? Graefes Arch Clin Exp Ophthalmol. 2010;248(8):1187–92.

Wolf A, Boulliat C, Coillot C, Rouault M, Gaillard K, Beranger C, Oliver M. Nifurtimox, a bright future for treatment of Chagas disease. Med Trop (Mars). 2011;71(2):131–3.

Yaghoobi R, Maraghi S, Bagherani N, Rafiei A. Cutaneous leishmaniasis of the lid: a report of nine cases. Korean J Ophthalmol. 2010;24(1):40–3.

Yazici A, Ozdal PC, Taskintuna I, Kavuncu S, Koklu G. Trimethoprim/Sulfamethoxazole and azithromycin combination therapy for ocular toxoplasmosis. Ocul Immunol Inflamm. 2009;17(4):289–91.

Yusuf IH, Sahare P, Hildebrand GD. DRESS syndrome in a child treated for toxoplasma retinochoroiditis. J AAPOS. 2013;17(5):521–3.

Chapter 12
Chemotherapy for Ocular Cancers

Bhavna Chawla, Rachna Seth, and Laxmi Moksha

Abstract Tumors occur in various locations of ocular structures. They may be benign or malignant. At times the tumors are managed non-surgically using pharmacological agents. Many times chemotherapy is used as an adjunct to surgical excision and enucleation. The prognosis of the ocular tumours solely depends on the early diagnosis, nature and the location of the tumor. This chapter extensively discusses about the clinical features, classification, diagnostic criteria for the ocular tumors and neoplasm, chemotherapeutic agents used in orbital and ocular tumors of childhood like retinoblastoma, drugs used for the treatment for the surface neoplasm and the underlying pharmacological modalities.

12.1 Orbital and Ocular Tumors of Childhood

Bhavna Chawla and Rachna Seth

Ocular and orbital tumors are neoplasms that develop in or around the eyes, respectively. They may be benign (noncancerous) or malignant (cancerous). Benign tumors are more common than malignant tumors. Among benign tumors, cystic lesions are the

B. Chawla, MS (Ophthalmol) (✉)
Ocular Oncology and Pediatric Ophthalmology Service,
Dr. Rajendra Prasad Center for Ophthalmic Sciences,
All India Institute of Medical Sciences, New Delhi, India
e-mail: bhavna2424@hotmail.com

R. Seth, MD
Division of Pediatric Oncology, Department of Pediatrics,
All India Institute of Medical Sciences, New Delhi, India

L. Moksha, MPharm
Ocular Pharmacology and Pharmacy,
Dr. Rajendra Prasad Center for Ophthalmic Sciences,
All India Institute of Medical Sciences, New Delhi, India

T. Velpandian (ed.), *Pharmacology of Ocular Therapeutics*,
DOI 10.1007/978-3-319-25498-2_12

commonest, followed by vascular lesions. Among malignant tumors, rhabdomyosarcoma is the most common. A brief classification system is shown in Table 12.1.

12.1.1 Clinical Approach

A thorough clinical assessment including ophthalmological, general physical and systemic examination should be undertaken. Investigations include a complete hemogram in which total and differential leukocytic counts, peripheral blood smear, imaging of the orbit and the eye with B-scan ultrasonography, and CT scan/MRI are being examined. In cases with suspected malignancy, a metastatic workup should include a chest X-ray and ultrasonography of abdomen, kidney and renal function tests. Fine-needle aspiration cytology or incisional biopsy may be required to establish the clinical diagnosis. Other investigations in selected cases include a bone marrow aspiration/biopsy, lumbar puncture, bone scan/positron emission tomography (PET)/CT scan, and fine-needle aspiration cytology (FNAC) or biopsy of regional lymph node, if enlarged.

12.1.2 Retinoblastoma

Retinoblastoma is the most common primary intraocular tumor of infancy and childhood. It is a tumor of the embryonic neural retina. It has an incidence of 1 in every 20,000 live births. About 90 % cases are diagnosed by the age of 3–4 years and 98 % by 5 years. Bilateral disease is diagnosed earlier then unilateral disease. The burden of the disease is more in developing nations especially Latin America, Africa, and Asia including India. It contributes to 4 % of all pediatric cancers. Retinoblastoma is highly sensitive to chemotherapy, and survival rates in developed countries are greater than 90 %. There is marked disparity in the mortality associated with retinoblastoma between developed and developing countries. In the developing world, 40–70 % of children with retinoblastoma die as opposed to only 3–5 % in the developed counties. This is predominantly due to delayed diagnosis leading to advanced disease (extraocular disease) at presentation (Hurwitz et al. 2011 and Dimaras et al. 2012).

12.1.2.1 Genetics and Inheritance

The retinoblastoma gene (RB1), encoded on chromosome 13q14, was the first described tumor suppressor gene. Constitutional loss of one RB1 allele causes cancer predisposition, and loss of the second allele in a developing retinal cell leads to retinoblastoma.

Retinoblastoma can be sporadic or inherited. Sporadic tumors are unilateral and unifocal and occur at an older age, while inherited tumors occur at an earlier age and are often bilateral and multifocal. One-third of all cases have bilateral tumors. All cases with bilateral disease have germline mutations of RB1 and are heritable

Table 12.1 Summary of orbital and ocular tumors of childhood (Shields JA and Shields CL, 2001)

Type of tumor	Characteristics
1. Cystic lesions A. Developmental cysts (a) Dermoid, epidermoid, and choristoma (b) Teratoma (c) Congenital cystic eye (d) Colobomatous cyst B. Acquired cysts (a) Parasitic cysts: hydatid, cysticercus (b) Epithelial cysts (appendage/implantation) (c) Lacrimal duct cysts (d) Aneurysmal bone cyst (e) Optic nerve sheath meningocele C. Developing from adjacent structures (a) Mucocele/mucopyocele (b) Dacryocele (c) Encephalocele/meningocele	Cystic lesions are the commonest orbital lesions seen in the pediatric age group Dermoid cysts are benign developmental choristomas sequestered in fetal suture lines at the time of closure Cysts containing squamous epithelium without dermal appendages are called epidermoid cysts Choristomatous tumors containing derivatives of all 3 germinal layers are teratomas Congenital cystic eyes and colobomatous cysts are rare developmental anomalies Acquired cysts are less common than developmental cysts Mucocele and mucopyocele originate from paranasal sinuses, while dacryocele originates from the lacrimal sac Encephalocele or meningocele result from congenital bony defects that permit herniation of intracranial tissues These are usually benign in nature
2. Vascular lesions (a) Hemangioma (capillary/cavernous) (b) Lymphangioma (c) Orbital varix (d) Arteriovenous malformation (e) Organized hematoma (hematic cyst/cholesterol granuloma) (f) Hemangiopericytoma (g) Sturge-Weber syndrome	Hemangiomas are hamartomatous growths composed of proliferating capillary endothelial cells, whereas malformations are developmental anomalies of capillary, venous, arterial, or lymphatic vessels Hemangiomas can progress or regress with age although vascular malformations remain relatively static, with growth of lesions correlating with growth of the child Hemangiopericytoma is a benign tumor of pericytes Sturge-Weber syndrome is a capillary malformation of leptomeninges with or without ocular or facial involvement Most vascular tumors are usually benign in nature, but some of them like hemangiopericytoma can have a malignant course
3. Inflammatory lesions (a) Preseptal and orbital cellulitis (b) Idiopathic orbital inflammatory syndrome (c) Other inflammatory diseases	Inflammatory lesions can be of infective or noninfective origin Preseptal and orbital cellulitis are infective diseases of preseptal and post-septal orbital tissues, respectively Idiopathic orbital inflammatory disease (orbital pseudotumor) is an inflammatory proptosis of childhood. It significantly differs from the adult form Bilaterality, episodic recurrence, and systemic manifestations like headache, nausea, vomiting, and lethargy are common features Thyroid eye disease, the commonest inflammatory lesion of adults, rarely occurs in children Inflammatory diseases are benign lesions

Table 12.1 (continued)

Type of tumor	Characteristics
4. Histiocytic and lymphoproliferative lesions (a) Langerhans cell histiocytosis (histiocytosis X, Hand-Schuller-Christian disease, and Letterer-Siwe disease) (b) Non-Langerhans cell histiocytosis (juvenile xanthogranuloma) (c) Leukemia and lymphoma (d) Sinus histiocytosis	Histiocytic disorders are caused by abnormal accumulation of cells of the mononuclear phagocytic system (dendritic cells and macrophages) which are derived from the bone marrow stem cells Leukemia (lymphocytic more than myelocytic) commonly involves the orbit in children Lymphoma in children very rarely involves the orbit Burkitt lymphoma is the most likely form to involve the orbit These tumors can have a benign or malignant course Lymphoma and leukemia are always malignant
5. Mesodermal tumors (a) Fibroma/myofibromatosis (b) Lipoma (c) Leiomyoma (d) Fibrous dysplasia (e) Giant cell granuloma (f) Sarcoma (osteosarcoma, leiomyosarcoma, fibrosarcoma, malignant fibrous histiocytoma, and alveolar soft part sarcoma) (g) Rhabdomyosarcoma	Mesodermal tumors are tumors of the soft tissues and fibro-osseous tissues of the orbit They can be benign or malignant Rhabdomyosarcoma is the most common malignant tumor of the orbit in children In general, mesenchymal tumors are classified into benign or malignant disease, depending upon histopathological features like number of mitotic figures, nuclear cytoplasmic ratio, invasion of adjacent structures, etc. Sarcomas always have a malignant course
6. Neurogenic tumors (a) Glioma (b) Meningioma (c) Neurofibroma (d) Schwannoma (e) Esthesioneuroblastoma (f) Paraganglioma (g) Melanotic neuroectodermal tumor of infancy	Glioma is the most important orbital tumor of neural origin in children. It is usually a low-grade astrocytoma Approximately 20 % of gliomas are associated with neurofibromatosis 1 Plexiform neurofibroma is nearly always associated with neurofibromatosis 1 Meningioma and schwannoma are rare in children Most of these tumors are benign, although paraganglioma can be benign or malignant Esthesioneuroblastoma is a malignant tumor
7. Lacrimal gland tumors (a) Pleomorphic adenoma (benign mixed tumor) (b) Adenoid cystic carcinoma (c) Adenocarcinoma (malignant mixed tumor)	Lacrimal gland tumors are less common in children as compared to adults A malignant tumor of the lacrimal gland is more common than a benign lesion in childhood Pleomorphic adenoma is a benign tumor, whereas adenoid cystic carcinoma and adenocarcinoma are malignant tumors
8. Metastatic tumors (a) Neuroblastoma (b) Ewing sarcoma (c) Wilms tumor (d) Rhabdomyosarcoma (rarely)	The orbit is the most common site of ocular metastasis in children Neuroblastoma is the most frequent source of orbital metastasis in childhood Other tumors that can metastasize to the orbit are Ewing sarcoma and Wilms tumor These are always malignant in nature
9. Intraocular tumors with orbital spread (a) Retinoblastoma (b) Medulloepithelioma	These are intraocular tumors that can progress to orbital tumors in the advanced stage Retinoblastoma is a malignant tumor Medulloepithelioma can be either benign or malignant

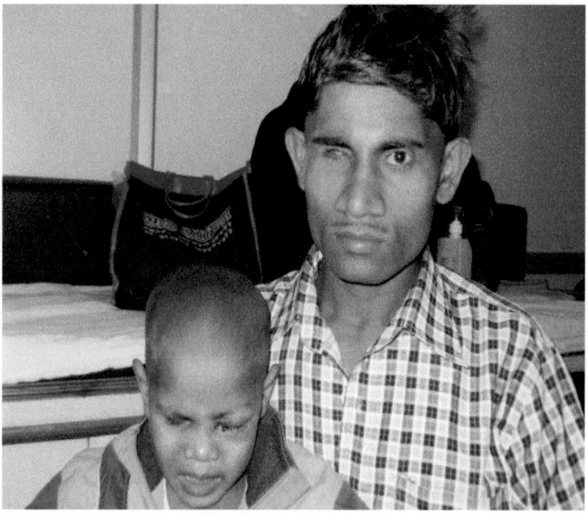

Fig. 12.1 Familial retinoblastoma

(Fig. 12.1). Only a small proportion of unilateral tumors are heritable. Alfred Knudson's "two-hit" model of oncogenesis proposes that two mutational events are required for development of retinoblastoma. In inherited retinoblastoma, the first hit is the mutation in the RB1 inherited in the germline, and the second is acquired in the somatic retinal cell. In sporadic retinoblastoma, both mutations occur in the somatic retinal cell. Most cases of hereditary retinoblastoma have spontaneous new germline mutation, while their parents have both wild-type RB1 alleles. The risk of an offspring inheriting an RB1 mutation from a parent with germline mutation of RB1 is 50 % and 97 % of these offsprings with the inherited mutation will go on to develop retinoblastoma. A constitutional (germline) mutation of RB1 also causes an increased risk of a second cancer of the lung, soft tissue, bladder, skin, bone, and brain, and this risk is even higher when these patients are treated with radiation therapy for their retinoblastoma. A small proportion (10–15 %) of unilateral tumors are also hereditary.

12.1.2.2 Clinical Presentation

Leukocoria (white pupillary reflex) is the most common presentation (Fig. 12.2). Retinoblastoma must be differentiated from Coat's disease, cataract, toxocariasis, and retinopathy of prematurity which may also present with leukocoria. Pain may be present secondary to glaucoma; other presenting features are strabismus, redness of the eye, and poor vision. Orbital inflammation and fungating orbital mass are signs of advanced disease (Fig. 12.3). In developing countries, retinoblastoma presents very late in its extraocular stage, either with an orbital mass (proptosis) or with distant metastasis in the bone, bone marrow, lymph nodes, and central nervous system (Fig. 12.4a, b) Chawla et al. (2015).

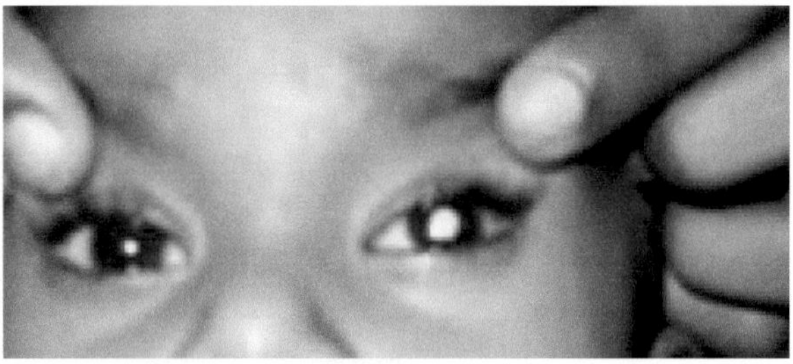

Fig. 12.2 Leukocoria

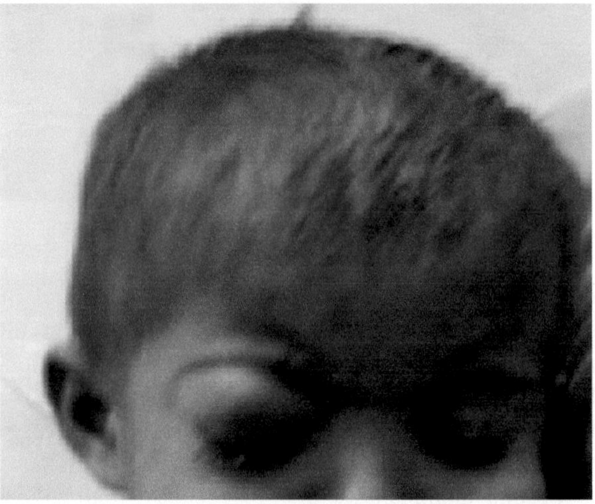

Fig. 12.3 Orbital cellulitis

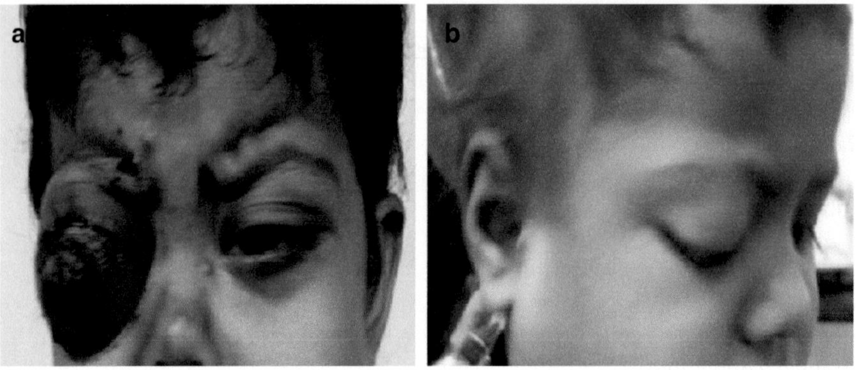

Fig. 12.4 (**a**) Extraocular metastatic retinoblastoma. (**b**) RB with lymph node metastasis

12.1.2.3 Diagnosis

Diagnosis is established by characteristic ophthalmologic findings, often requiring examination under anesthesia. Imaging studies such as ultrasound, CT scan or MRI (preferable) scans are used for assessment of orbital, optic nerve, and intracranial extension (Fig. 12.5).

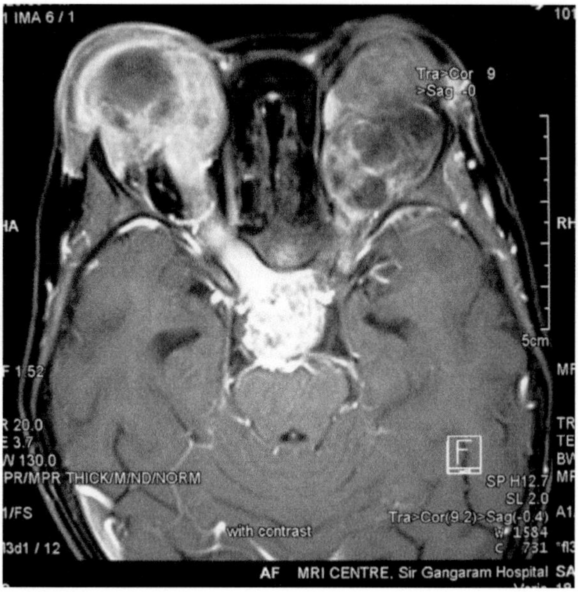

Fig. 12.5 Bilateral extraocular retinoblastoma with CNS metastasis

Rarely, children with hereditary retinoblastoma have pineal tumor (trilateral retinoblastoma) that may be found on imaging. CSF and bone marrow evaluation should only be done if indicated clinically, or by other imaging studies (i.e., in advanced disease).

Both eyes should be examined under general anesthesia.

Second malignant neoplasms are a major concern in retinoblastoma survival. Approximately 30 % of individuals cured of hereditary forms of RB will have a second malignancy within 30 years. Osteosarcoma is the commonest second malignancy; other second neoplasms include rhabdomyosarcoma and melanoma.

12.1.2.4 Classification and Staging

Intraocular

Intraocular retinoblastoma is localized to the eye and may be confined to the retina or may extend to involve other structures such as the choroid, ciliary body, anterior chamber, and the optic nerve head. Intraocular retinoblastoma does not extend beyond the eye into the tissues around the eye or to other parts of the body. For intraocular disease, enucleation is curative in more than 95 % of patients with advanced unilateral disease.

Extraocular

Extraocular retinoblastoma has extended beyond the eye. It may be confined to the tissues around the eye (orbital retinoblastoma), or it may have spread to the central nervous system, bone marrow, or lymph nodes (metastatic retinoblastoma).

Classification of Intraocular RB

Reese-Ellsworth Classification for Intraocular Tumors

Reese and Ellsworth developed a classification system for intraocular retinoblastoma that has been shown to have prognostic significance for maintenance of sight and control of local disease at a time when surgery and external beam radiation therapy (EBRT) were the primary treatment options:

Group I: very favorable for maintenance of sight

1. Solitary tumor, smaller than 4 disk diameters (DD), at or behind the equator
2. Multiple tumors, none larger than 4 DD, all at or behind the equator

Group II: favorable for maintenance of sight

1. Solitary tumor, 4–10 DD at or behind the equator
2. Multiple tumors, 4–10 DD, behind the equator

Group III: possible for maintenance of sight

1. Any lesion anterior to the equator
2. Solitary tumor, larger than 10 DD, behind the equator

Group IV: unfavorable for maintenance of sight

1. Multiple tumors, some larger than 10 DD
2. Any lesion extending anteriorly to the ora serrata

Group V: very unfavorable for maintenance of sight

1. Massive tumors involving more than one half of the retina
2. Vitreous seeding

International Classification of Intraocular Retinoblastoma

With the introduction of systemic chemotherapy as the primary modality for globe salvage in intra ocular disease, there is a new grouping system for retinoblastoma, which may offer greater precision in stratifying risk for newer therapies. The International Classification of Retinoblastoma that is used in the current Children's Oncology Group treatment studies and in some institutional studies has been shown to assist in predicting those eyes that are likely to be cured without the need for enucleation or external beam radiotherapy.

12.1.2.5 Staging

The patients of are usually diagnosed upon ophthalmic examination based on the International Classification System for Retinoblastoma (Table 12.2). The (International Retinoblastoma Staging System (IRSS) shown in Table 12.3a) is based on histopathology and imaging findings and takes into account that EORB with spread to regional lymphnode (LN) has a rate of overall survival comparable to non metastatic extraocular retinoblastoma (EORB).

Table 12.2 International Classification System for Retinoblastoma (Murphree 2005)

Group	Clinical features
A Very low risk	All tumors are 3 mm or smaller, confined to the retina, and located at least 3 mm from the foveola and 1.5 mm from the optic nerve.
B Low risk	Retinal tumors may be of any size or location not in Group A. No vitreous or subretinal seeding allowed. A small cuff of subretinal fluid extending no more than 5 mm from the base of the tumor is allowed.
C Moderate risk	Eyes with only focal vitreous or subretinal seeding and discrete retinal tumors of any size and location. Vitreous or subretinal seeding may extend no more than 3 mm from tumor. Up to 1 quadrant of subretinal fluid may be present.
D High risk	Eyes with diffuse vitreous or subretinal seeding and/or massive, nondiscrete endophytic or exophytic disease.
E Very high risk eyes	*Eyes with one or more of the following:* Neovascular glaucoma Massive intraocular hemorrhage Aseptic orbital cellulites Phthisis or pre-phthisis Tumor anterior to anterior vitreous face Tumor touching the lens Diffuse infiltrating retinoblastoma

Table 12.3a International Retinoblastoma Staging System (IRSS)

Stage	Description	
Stage 0	Eye has not been enucleated and no dissemination of disease	
	Conservative treatment	
Stage I	Eye enucleated, completely resected histologically	
Stage II	Eye enucleated, microscopic residual tumor in form of:	
	(i) Tumor invasion into extrascleral space	
	(ii) Tumor invasion into cut end of ON	
Stage III	Regional extension	(a) Overt orbital disease
		(b) Preauricular or cervical lymph node extension
Stage IV	Metastatic disease	(a) Hematogenous metastasis (without CNS involvement)
		1. Single lesion
		2. Multiple lesions
		(b) CNS extension (with or without any other site of regional or metastatic disease)
		1. Prechiasmatic lesion
		2. CNS mass
		3. Leptomeningeal and CSF disease

12.1.2.6 Treatment for Retinoblastoma

Principles

The first aim of treatment is survival of the child with preservation of the globe and vision being secondary goals (Table 12.3b). With improved survivorship, focus on

Table 12.3b Broad principles of chemotherapy

Modality	Schedule	Indication/classification
Chemoreduction for large I/O tumors	2–6 cycles before consolidative therapy up to 12 cycles	ICRB groups B–D Globe salvation
Chemoprophylaxis	6 cycles	Any high-risk histopathological features Invasion of the anterior chamber, iris, ciliary body Massive choroid invasion Invasion of sclera Post-laminar ON invasion
Adjuvant chemotherapy for microscopic residual disease	(12 cycles)	Extrascleral involvement Invasion of ON reaching cut end
Neoadjuvant chemotherapy (NACT)	2–3 cycles	Stage III EORB (orbital mass/ON involvement on MRI OR anterior fungating mass clinically)
High-dose chemotherapy with autologous SCT		Stage IV/metastatic RB

cosmesis with the use of prosthetic eye has also become important. Treatment depends on size and location of the tumor and whether it is unilateral or bilateral. Therapeutic plans usually require a multidisciplinary approach. Treatment should be highly individualized. Systemic chemotherapy has become the cornerstone of therapy for retinoblastoma and primarily includes vincristine, carboplatin, and etoposide. Chemotherapy may be administered through local routes also. Systemic chemotherapy may be used for primary chemoreduction, as an adjunct modality or for treatment of metastasis. The major concern is to avoid enucleation and/or external beam radiation, and trends are toward conservative treatment in intraocular disease.

In cases of unilateral disease with large tumors where no useful vision can be preserved, enucleation must be performed early; a delay leads to progressive disease. In children with bilateral disease, systemic chemotherapy is used to shrink the tumors, followed by local treatment with transpupillary thermotherapy or cryotherapy in order to preserve vision. Newer routes of drug administration including periocular, intravitreal, and selective intra-arterial chemotherapy have improved outcomes particularly in intraocular retinoblastoma (Shields et al. 1993; Banavali 2004).

Chemotherapeutic Agents

The main objectives of chemotherapy are eye salvage, vision preservation, avoidance of enucleation and EBRT. Systemic chemotherapy is usually combined with intensive local therapy. The various chemotherapeutic drugs used in treatment of retinoblastoma include Carboplatin, etoposide, vincristine, methotrexate,

Table 12.4a Standard chemotherapy protocol for RB

Drug	Dosage/route	Schedule	Side effects/remarks
Vincristine (VCR) Vinca alkaloid Facilitates apoptosis	1.5 mg/m^2/day/IV 0.05 mg/kg/day for children <3 years Max dose 2.0 mg	Day 1	Neurotoxicity Myelosuppression, intravenous Avoid extravasation
Carboplatin Platinum coordinator compound which cross-links DNA	560 mg/m^2/day 18.6 mg/kg/day for children <3 years	Day 1	Nephrotoxicity, ototoxicity, neurotoxicity, hypomagnesemia Intravenous Escalation of dose is done depending on stage of disease
Etoposide Inhibits DNA	150 mg/m^2/day 5 mg/kg/day for children <3 years	Day 1 & 2	Allergic reactions, hepatotoxicity, CNS toxicity, hypotension, AML, mucositis Intravenous Escalation of dose is done depending on stage of disease

Cycles every 3–4 weeks
Ensure ANC >1.0 and platelet count >1,00,000/cumm
LFT and RFT must be done before every cycle

Table 12.4b Classification of Chemotherapeutic agents used in orbital and ocular tumors

Class of agents	Drug	Effect on cell cycle
Platinum coordination complexes	Cisplatin, carboplatin, oxaliplatin	Cell cycle-nonspecific (CCNS) agents
Vinca alkaloids	Vincristine	Cell cycle-specific (CCS) agents
Epipodophyllotoxins	Etoposide	Cell cycle-specific (CCS) agents
Antitumor Antibiotics	Doxorubicin, idarubicin	Cell cycle-nonspecific (CCNS) agents
Camptothecins	Topotecan	Cell cycle-nonspecific (CCNS) agents
Nitrogen mustard	Melphalan, Thio-TEPA, cyclophosphamide	Cell cycle-nonspecific (CCNS) agents

cyclophosphamide, melphalan, doxorubicin, and triethylene melamine in various combinations. The most common and effective combination comprises vincristine, carboplatin, and etoposide (Tables 12.4a and b). This forms the standard of care for intraocular retinoblastoma. Combination chemotherapy is usually administered in monthly cycles varying usually from 2 to 12 cycles depending on extent of disease and histopathologic features. The indications for chemotherapy include (i) intraocular retinoblastoma, (ii) extraocular retinoblastoma, (iii) recurrent retinoblastoma, (iv) trilateral retinoblastoma, and (v) palliative care of retinoblastoma (Chawla et al. 2013).

Newer chemotherapeutic agents include 2-deoxy-D-glucose and anti-VEGF agent bevacizumab, and administration of chemotherapy (melphalan, carboplatin) via intra-arterial, subconjunctival, and intravitreal routes is likely to improve cure rates in retinoblastoma. External beam radiation therapy should only be considered in cases where chemotherapy and focal therapy fail. Radiation therapy leads to orbital deformity, sicca syndrome, cataracts, radiation retinopathy, neovascular glaucoma, and increased risk of second malignancy. Brachytherapy and episcleral plaque radiotherapy are other modes of radiation therapy which have less morbidity. Several reports have documented long-term survival of patients with metastatic disease treated with high-dose chemotherapy with autologous bone marrow transplantation. Routine eye examination should be done in these children till they are over 7 years of age. All first-degree relatives of children with known or suspected hereditary retinoblastoma should have eyes examined for retinomas or retinal scars. Patients with hereditary form of the disease are at a high risk of other cancers particularly osteosarcoma, soft tissue sarcomas, malignant melanoma, and carcinomas. In the developing countries, early enucleation of unilateral disease is critical for reducing mortality related to retinoblastoma (Chabner et al. 2011 and Chu and Sartorelli 2012).

12.1.3 Chemotherapeutics for Orbital and Ocular Tumors

Various chemotherapeutic agents classified in Table 12.4 are used in the treatment and management of orbital and ocular tumors.

Platinum Coordination Compounds The platinum coordination compounds are not alkylating agents in true sense as these compounds use platinum instead of alkyl groups to form dimers of DNA. Following are the few mentioned platinum compounds that are mainly used in the treatment of ocular surface cancers.

Carboplatin

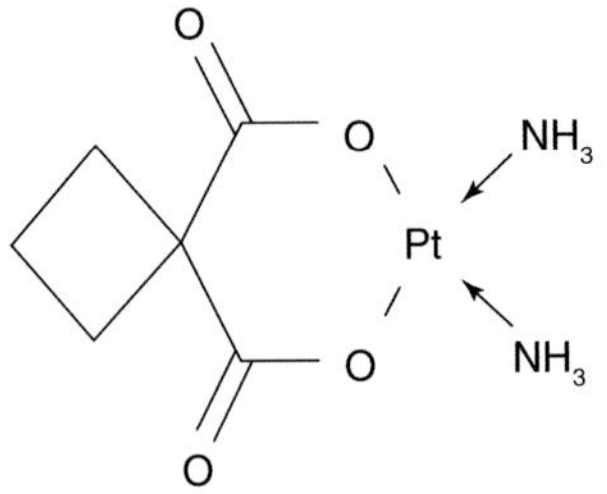

Oxaliplatin

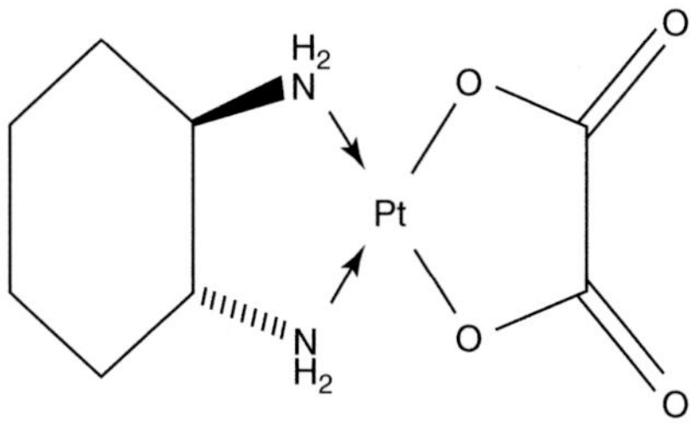

Cisplatin

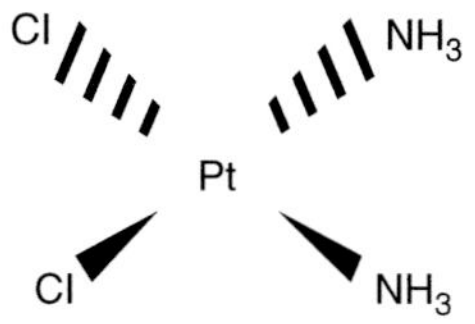

Cisplatin Cisplatin is a divalent inorganic water-soluble heavy metal coordination complex that must be activated by the process of aquation to form positively charged complex. The aquated species react with nucleophilic sites on DNA. Plasma protein binding of cisplatin is 90 %. It enters rapidly inside tissues, and is predominantly excreted via glomerular filtration, but slow rate of excretion has been observed (43 % in 5 days). Gastrointestinal distress, mild hematotoxicity, nephrotoxicity, and neurotoxicity may be induced by cisplatin (Chu and Sartorelli 2012; Rodriguez-Galindo 2010).

Carboplatin Carboplatin is similar to cisplatin in its mode of action, resistance, and clinical activity, but this second-generation platinum heavy metal coordination complex is better tolerated and is less toxic when compared to cisplatin. Carboplatin has less plasma protein binding that is why it is rapidly excreted from the kidneys (plasma $t_{1/2}$- 2h). In comparison to cisplatin, it is less likely to cause tinnitus but has greater myelosuppressant action.

Cisplatin and carboplatin are divalent, inorganic, water-soluble heavy metal, whereas oxaliplatin is a tetravalent complex which goes inside the cells by an active Cu^{2+} transporter, CTR1 and cross-link DNA in different ways (Kruh 2003). These complexes inside the cell get hydrolyzed producing highly reactive species which form both interstrand and intrastrand cross-link adducts which lead to the activation of many signal transduction pathways, viz., ATR, p53, p73, and MAPK pathways (Siddik 2003).

Cisplatin resistance is generally observed in patients on therapy. Cisplatin has cross resistance with carboplatin, but this is not a case with oxaliplatin. In vitro studies have revealed that oxaliplatin is found to be highly active in cisplatin-resistant cancer cells; further studies have to be conducted to prove this in vivo. Mutagenicty, teratogenicity, and carcinogenicity may be observed with platinum compounds (Chabner et al. 2011; Chu and Sartorelli 2012; Tripathi 2008; Rodriguez-Galindo 2010).

Vinca Alkaloids Vinka alkaloids are group of anti-mitotic and anti-microtubule agents that are naturally extracted from the Madagascar pink periwinkle plant, *Catharanthus roseus* or *Vinca rosea*. The agent which is being used in the treatment of retinoblastoma is vincristine. Resistance has been observed due to the efflux of drugs from the tumor cells via the membrane transporters.

Vincristine Vincristine is asymmetrical dimeric compound known to be a "spindle poison." Vincristine reversibly binds to β-tubulin and blocks its polymerization with α-tubulin into microtubules thereby causing metaphase arrest. It acts in the M phase of the cancer cell cycle. Vincristine is given parenterally and binds to plasma proteins (75 %), metabolized extensively by liver cytochromes, and its metabolites are mainly excreted in bile. Dose reduction is recommended in patients with hepatic dysfunction (bilirubin >3 mg/dl). Most prominent toxicity caused by vincristine is neurological viz., peripheral neuritis, areflexia, and paralytic ileus along with this severe constipation, colicky abdominal pain, obstruction, jaw pain, and vocal cord paralysis; weakness and loss of deep tendon reflex may also be observed. Other adverse effects are alopecia, optic atrophy, syndrome of inappropriate antidiuretic hormone secretion (SIADH), mild nausea, and vomiting (Chabner et al. 2011; Chu and Sartorelli 2012; Tripathi 2008; Rodriguez-Galindo 2010).

Vincristine

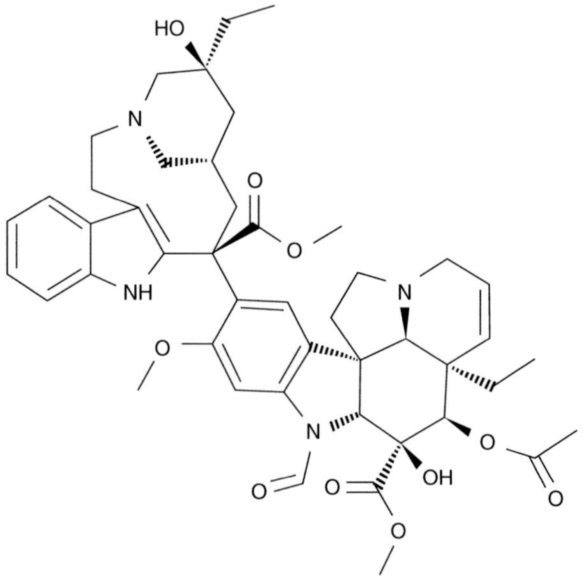

Epipodophyllotoxins These are naturally occurring substances extracted from the root of mandrake or Mayapple American plant (*Podophyllum peltatum*), and its derivatives are being mainly used as anticancer compounds.

Etoposide It is a semisynthetic derivative of podophyllotoxin, a plant glycoside. This drug is not mitotic inhibitor but blocks cell growth in late S and G2 phases of the cell cycle. It acts through DNA degradation process by forming a ternary complex with topoisomerase II and DNA and inhibits nucleoside transport and inhibition of mitochondrial electron transport. After intravenous injection, it binds to plasma protein and distributes to most of the tissues. Etoposide follows renal elimination, and dose modification is required for patient with renal impairment. Most common adverse effects due to etoposide are leukopenia, alopecia, gastrointestinal disturbances, and bone marrow suppression (Chabner et al. 2011; Chu and Sartorelli 2012; Rodriguez-Galindo 2010).

Etoposide

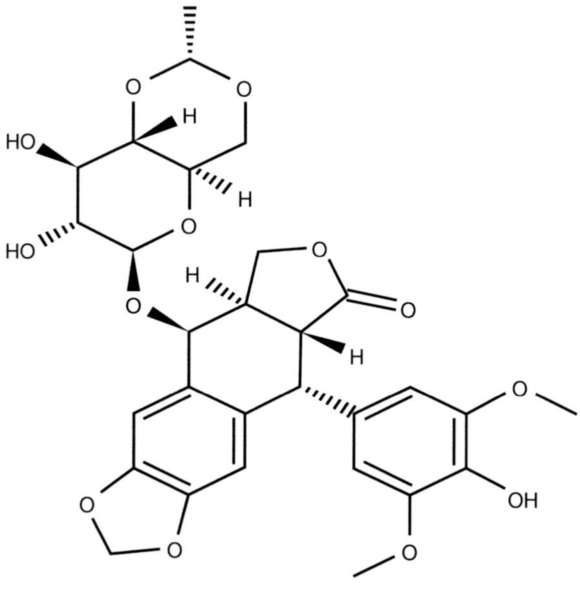

Antitumor Antibiotics (Anthracyclines) Anthracyclines are isolated from the fungus *Streptomyces peucetius* var. *caesius*. Analogs of naturally produced anthracycline; Idarubicin and doxorubicin, both are the antitumor agents used mainly for the treatment of retinoblastoma.

Doxorubicin and idarubicin These antitumor agents have a tetracycline ring attached to sugar moiety. Doxorubicin and idarubicin intercalate between base pairs and inhibit topoisomerase II leading to consequent blockade of DNA and RNA synthesis, also DNA strand scission. It also binds to membranes to alter fluidity and ion transport. Anthracyclines generate free radicals (semiqunone and oxygen free radicals) in solution as well as both in normal and malignant tissues. These form hydrogen peroxide and hydroxyl radicals to damage DNA and oxidize DNA bases. Multidrug resistance is found in tumor cells against anthracyclines. Anthracyclines must be administered by parenteral route, get metabolized in the liver, and be excreted in urine and bile. Bone marrow suppression, gastrointestinal distress, and severe alopecia are the most common adverse effects while cardiotoxicity as the most distinctive side effect (Chabner et al. 2011; Chu and Sartorelli 2012; Rodriguez-Galindo 2010).

Doxorubicin

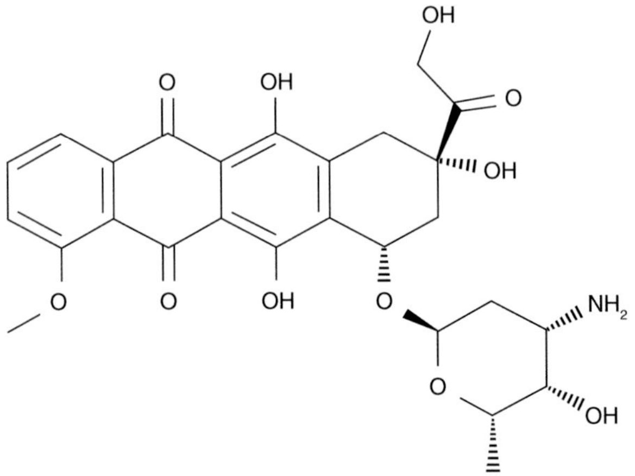

Idarubicin

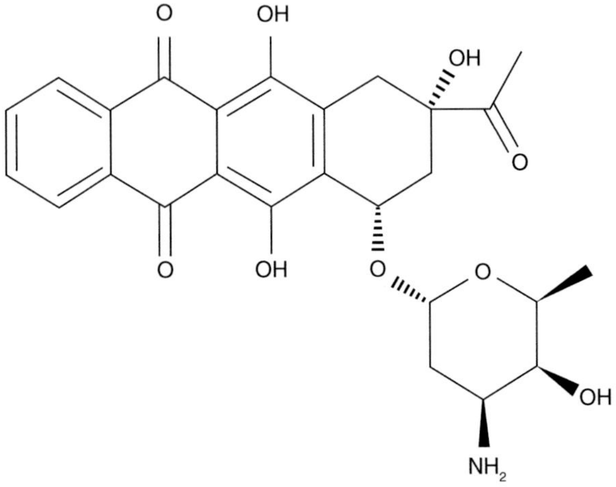

Camptothecins (Topotecan) Camptothecins group of cytotoxic quinoline alkaloid isolated from the bark and stem of Chinese tree *Camptotheca acuminate* have been found to be active against cancer. Topotecan is a semisynthetic analogue of camptothecin which binds to topoisomerase I-DNA complex and causes single-strand breaks in DNA further not allowing relegation of single-strand breaks. It acts mainly in S phase and arrests cell cycle at G2 phase. Topotecan is metabolized via pH-dependent hydrolysis of the lactone ring yielding hydroxyl acid (inactive) in plasma. Their metabolites are excreted in urine, so dose modification is required in patients with renal impairment. The most common adverse effect of topotecan is myelosuppression especially neutropenia along with diarrhea (Chabner et al. 2011; Chu and Sartorelli 2012; Tripathi 2008; Rodriguez-Galindo 2010).

Topotecan

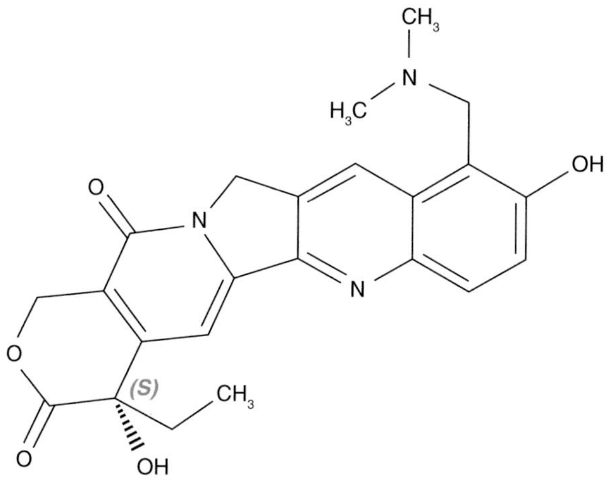

Nitrogen Mustard Nitrogen mustards are cell cycle-nonspecific alkylating agents (CCNS). These drugs involve the intramolecular cyclization to form an ethyleneimonium ion that may directly or through formation of carbonium ion transfer an alkylate nucleophilic group of DNA bases on N-7 position of gaunine leading to cross-linking of bases, abnormal base pairing, and DNA strand breakage (Chabner et al. 2011; Chu and Sartorelli 2012; Tripathi 2008; Rodriguez-Galindo 2010).

Melphalan Melphalan is a type of alkylating agent that attaches the alkyl group to the guanine base at N-7 of the imidazole ring thereby causing linkages between strands of DNA. Melphalan is given through intravenous infusion having plasma t1/2 45–90 min. The main route of elimination is through urine. Bone marrow depression is its most common toxicity along with other rare complications such as infection, diarrhea, and pancreatitis (Chabner et al. 2011; Chu and Sartorelli 2012; Tripathi 2008).

Thio-TEPA It is an organophosphorous compound having tetrahedral phosphorus and three ethyleneimine groups and does not require to form active intermediate. Thio-TEPA and triethylenephasphoraminde (TEPA), its primary metabolite, react with DNA phosphate groups to produce cross-linking of DNA strands. Thio-TEPA has shorter plasma t1/2 (2.5 h) as compared to that of TEPA (t1/2–17.5 h). Thio-TEPA and its metabolite follow urine as main route of elimination. Main toxicities caused due to Thio-TEPA and its active metabolite are myelosuppression and neurotoxicity; sometimes higher doses cause leukopenia, thrombocytopenia, anemia, coma, and seizures (Chabner et al. 2011; Chu and Sartorelli 2012; Rodriguez-Galindo 2010).

Cyclophosphamide Cyclophosphamide is an alkylating agent from oxazaphosphorine group. It's a produg, and hepatic biotransformation by cytochrome P450 enzyme forms different metabolites, viz., aldophosphamide, ketocyclophosphamide, phosphoramide mustard, and acrolein. Some of the metabolites of cyclophosphamide have wide range of antitumor activity. It is well absorbed orally. Immunosuppression is its most prominent effect. Gastrointestinal irritation, alopecia, and myelosuppression are other side effects (Chabner et al. 2011; Chu and Sartorelli 2012; Tripathi 2008; Rodriguez-Galindo 2010).

Melphalan

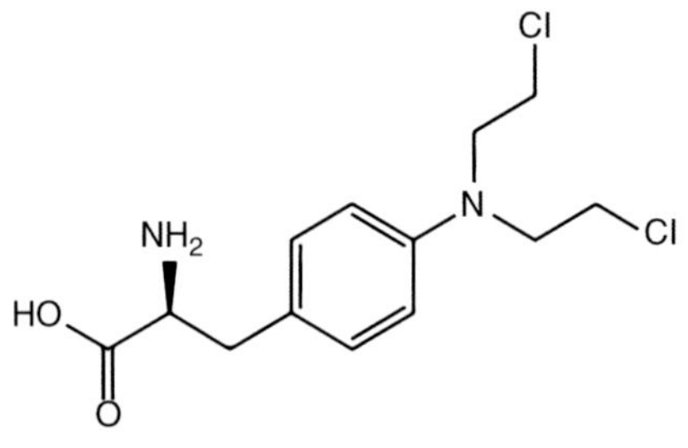

Thio-TEPA

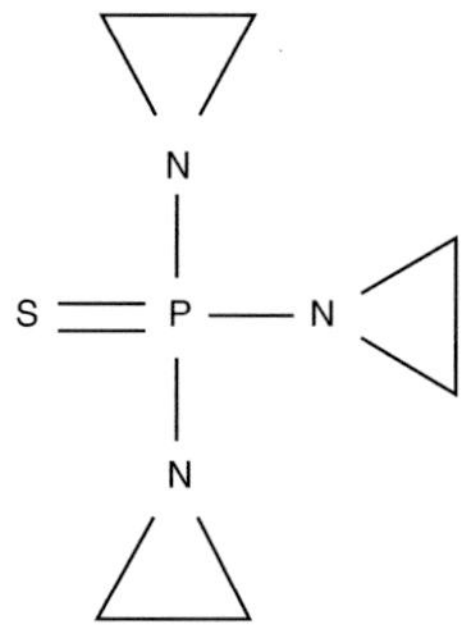

Cyclophosphamide

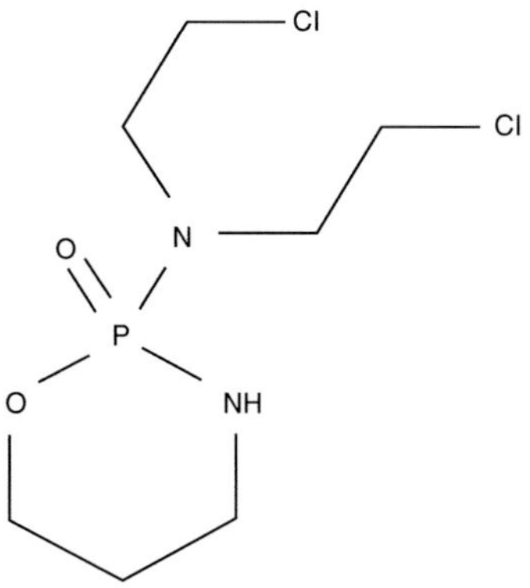

12.1.4 Prognosis

Most tumors that are confined to the eye are cured. Cures are infrequent when extensive orbital/optic nerve extension has occurred or the patient has distant metastasis. The reported mortality is 20–30 % with tumor invasion posterior to lamina cribrosa, and 78 % with involvement of the cut end of optic nerve. CNS metastasis carries a very high mortality. With the advent of hematopoietic stem cell transplantation (HSCT) and aggressive chemotherapy, the outcomes of extensive diseases are showing some improvement.

12.1.5 Management of Extraocular Disease

Patients with extraocular disease have a very poor prognosis with respect to survival. Recently, there has been encouraging data to suggest that patients with regional extraocular disease may benefit from a combination of conventional chemotherapy and external beam radiation (EBR) and those with distant metastatic disease may benefit from high-dose chemotherapy and EBR in conjunction with bone marrow stem cell transplantation. Regional extraocular disease includes patients with orbital and preauricular disease and patients with residual disease at the optic nerve surgical margin.

Chantada et al. (2009) reported a 5-year EFS rate of 84 % in 15 patients with orbital or preauricular disease treated with chemotherapy that included vincristine, doxorubicin, and cyclophosphamide or vincristine, idarubicin, cyclophosphamide, carboplatin, and etoposide. These patients also received EBR of 4500 cGy administered to the optic nerve chiasm for patients with orbital disease and to the involved nodes for those with preauricular lymphadenopathy.

Patients with metastatic extraocular disease have a poor prognosis when treated with regimens of conventional doses of chemotherapy. There are several reports now suggesting that high-dose chemotherapy with stem cell rescue combined with EBR for areas of bulky disease at diagnosis is beneficial, with some long-term survivors among patients with metastatic disease not involving the central nervous system (CNS). It is rare for a patient with metastatic CNS involvement to survive using the therapies described above.

12.1.5.1 Metastatic Tumors

There are a variety of metastatic tumors that involve the orbit/eye/surrounding structures (Fig. 12.6a–c). The patient's age at presentation helps differentiate among the possible tumor types. In children, the most common metastatic lesions include neuroblastoma, Ewing tumor, chloroma, and Langerhans cell histiocytosis. Neuroblastomas in pediatric patients are the most common metastatic tumor to spread to the orbit and have been reported in up to 40 % of patients. These tumors arise from the adrenal medulla or parasympathetic or sympathetic structures, often spreading to both orbits, where they frequently cause an abrupt onset of exophthalmos and bilateral eyelid edema and ecchymosis. Ewing tumor is a malignant bone lesion that classically involves the limbs, ribs, or pelvis. When this tumor metastasizes to the orbit, it usually presents as an abrupt hemorrhagic exophthalmos. Chloromas are the extramedullary form of acute myelogenetic leukemia. This lesion is also heralded by the onset of acute hemorrhagic exophthalmos. Langerhans cell

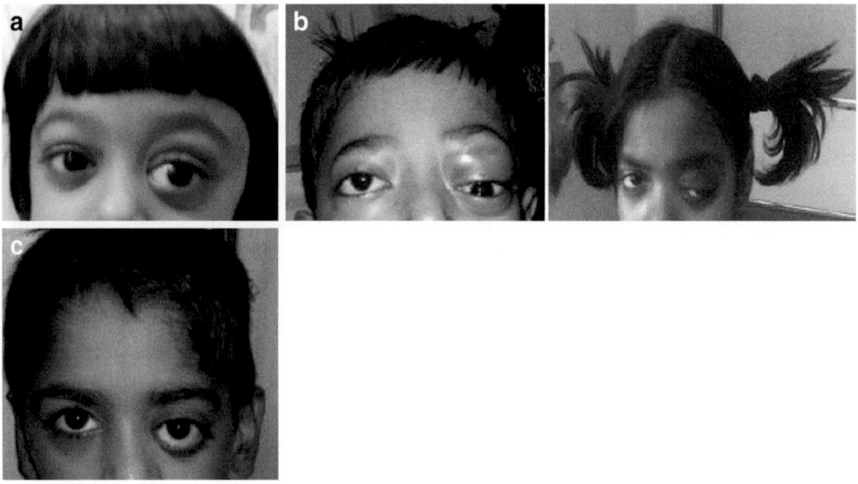

Fig. 12.6 (**a**) Proptosis and raccoon eye in a case of metastatic neuroblastoma. (**b**) Proptosis (chloroma) in children diagnosed with acute myeloid leukemia. (**c**) Proptosis in a child diagnosed with Langerhans cell histiocytosis (LCH)

histiocytosis is a term used to describe three similar but separate multisystem diseases: eosinophilic granulomatosis (or histiocytosis X), Hand-Schüller-Christian disease, and Letterer-Siwe disease. Only the first two subclasses cause orbital disease: eosinophilic granulomatosis with solitary granulomatous proliferation may occur in the orbit, causing painful eye swelling and exophthalmos, whereas Hand-Schüller-Christian disease has exophthalmos as part of its clinical triad, as well as diabetes insipidus and lesions of the bone.

12.2 Drugs Used in Ocular Surface Squamous Neoplasia

Moksha Laxmi

Ocular surface squamous neoplasia (OSSN) encompasses the wide spectrum of tumors termed for precancerous and cancerous epithelial lesions of the cornea, the limbus, and the conjunctiva (Lee and Hirst in 1995). It ranges from simple dysplasia, carcinoma in situ, conjunctival intraepithelial neoplastic lesions to invasive squamous cell carcinoma (Lee and Hirst 1995). It has been reported that before finalizing the terminology "ocular surface squamous neoplasia," several terminologies were in use viz., epithelioma, epithelial plaque, Bowenoid epithelioma, epidermalization/dyskeratosis, Epithelial hyperplasia with/without dyskeratosis, precancerous condition of the bulbular conjunctiva, precancerous epithelioma of the limbus, dyskeratotic epibulbar, limbal epithelioma, conjunctival intraepithelial neoplasia, corneal intraepithelial neoplasia, conjunctival and corneal invasive neoplasia, and ocular surface epithelial dysplasia (Lee and Hirst 1992, 1995; Pizzarello and Jakobiec 1978).

OSSN is the most common neoplasia of the ocular surface occurring worldwide, and peak incidence is found at latitude of 16° South. Age standardized rate worldwide is reported to be 0.18 and 0.08 cases/year/100 000 among males and females, respectively (Nagaiah et al. 2010; Grulich et al. 2007; Gichuhi et al. 2013).

The risk factors involved in the overgrowth of corneal, limbal and conjunctival epithelium are reported to be due to solar ultraviolet (UV) exposure, mutation of the p53 gene (tumor suppressor gene), immune-compromised conditions, heavy cigarette smoking and human papilloma virus infections (Gichuhi et al. 2013; Carreira et al. 2013; Gichuhi et al. 2014). The other potential risk factors leading to OSSN are vitamin A deficiency, exposure to petroleum products, chemicals such as trifluridine and arsenicals, ocular surface injury, etc. (Lee and Hirst 1995 and Basti and Mascai 2003; Boese et al. 2013 and Gichuhi et al. 2014).

Various diagnostic tools and methods opted for the diagnosis of OSSN are tissue histology after incisional or excisional biopsy (Papaioannou et al. 2008), impression cytology (Tananuvat et al. 2008), close careful examination with slit-lamp biomicroscopy, gonioscopy, fundus examination (Tananuvat and Lertprasertsuke 2012), anterior segment optical coherence tomography (OCT) (Kieval et al. 2012), and confocal microscopy (Xu et al. 2012). Traditional treatment modalities used for the OSSN are surgical excision, cryotherapy, radiotherapy, topical chemotherapy, and immunotherapy. The most common practice for OSSN is surgical excision, but there is relatively high recurrence rate after surgical excision. Therefore, along with surgery, adjunctive cryotherapy has been reported to reduce the recurrence rate of OSSN (Pe'er 2005; Lee and Hirst 1995; Basti and Mascai 2003; Kiire et al. 2010 and Rudkin et al. 2011). Apart from surgical interventions as primary treatment modality, post surgical topical chemotherapy has also been attempted.

Drugs such as mitocycin C, 5-fluorouracil and interferon α2b are used in topical chemotherapy (Midena et al. 1997; Midena et al. 2000; Panda et al. 2008; Yeatts et al. 2000; Kim and Abramson 2008).

12.2.1 Mitomycin C

Mitomycin (MMC) is a water-soluble antineoplastic antibiotic isolated from *Streptomyces caespitosus* having molecular weight of 334 daltons. After entering the cell, it looses methoxy group after the reduction of quinone and gets converted to bi- or trifunctional alkylating agent to inhibit DNA synthesis. It is available in the lyophilized form for injections and for other topical ocular formulations. It has been used for many ocular conditions such as conjunctival-corneal intraepithelial neoplasia, primary acquired melanomas with atypia, and as an adjunct in conditions such as pterygium and trabeculectomy. It has also been reported to be beneficial in modulating the postoperative healing process after excimer laser keratomileusis. For most of the procedures, MMC is used as topical eye drops (0.02–0.04 %) and used only for few days. Mitomycin showed a shorter half-life after reconstitution, and in the acidic condition, it is reported to undergo degradation by aziridine ring opening (Velpandian et al. 2005). Extemporaneously prepared MMC at pH between 7 and 8 and stored in the refrigerator can increase the duration of its stability. The topical use of mitomycin C was first described by Frucht-Pery et al. in 1994 and the drug have shown the reduction in the recurrence rate of OSSN in eyes but usually cause epithelial toxicity, conjunctivitis, and photophobia. Although Mitomycin C is usually well tolerated by patients but it causes dose dependent cellular toxicity (Sepulveda et al. 2010).

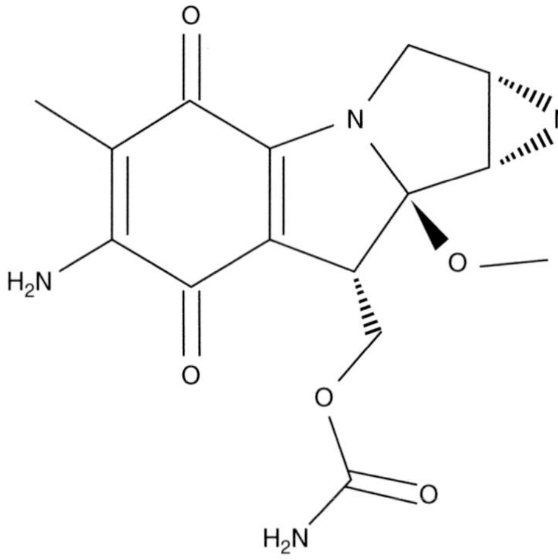

12.2.2 5-Fluorouracil

5-Fluorouracil a pyrimidine analogue is an antimetabolite used topically for the treatment of preinvasive ocular surface neoplasia. Keizer et al (1986) for the first time reported the use of 5-FU for the treatment of premalignant ocular surface lesion. 5-Fluorouracil is converted in cells to 5-fluoro-2'-deoxyuridine-5'-monophosphate which inhibit thymidylate synthase and leads to cell death thereby inhibiting RNA processing, and incorporation of FdUMP into DNA inhibits DNA synthesis. 5-FU is used in the clinical studies with dose of 1 % 4 times a day for 4 weeks continuously appears to be well tolerated in the majority of patients. Topical solution of 1 % 5-FU applied alone or as an adjunct to excision in cycles of 4 days "on" followed by 30 days "off" until lesion was resolved showed no long term side effects (Midena et al. 2000; Rudkin et al. 2011;Yeatts et al. 2000). Blumenkranz et al (1984) reported that 5-FU shows dose dependent inhibition of rabbit conjunctival fibroblast proliferation and requires the minimum concentration of 0.2 mg/ml to inhibit the cell growth. Topical administration of 1 % 5-FU to the patients four times/day for 4 weeks given alone or combined therapy have shown a long-term safe and effective treatment (Parrozzani et al. 2011). The common side effects associated with 5-FU reported by Yeatts et al. (2000) and Rudkin and Muecke (2011) are lid toxicity, eyelid skin erythema, superficial keratitis, epiphora, and corneal epithelial defects, conjunctival and corneal inflammation. 5-FU is easy to handle by patients and inexpensive as compared to the drugs used for the treatment of OSSN.

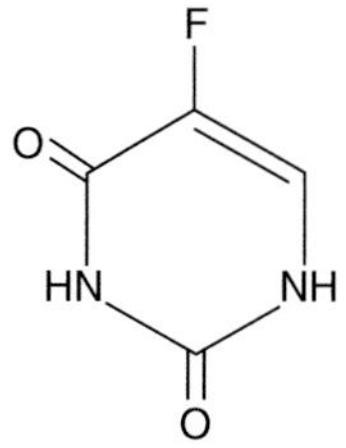

12.2.3 Interferon Alpha 2B

Interferon alpha 2b(IFNα2b), an endogenous glycoprotein (type 1 interferon) consists of 165 amino acid residues produced using recombinant DNA technology (Intron-A Schering Corp.). It is reported that Maskin in 1994 used IFNα2b first time for the treatment of OSSN. The IFNα2b eye drops are most well tolerated among all three antineoplastic agents with minimal side effects and inhibit the growth of various cancerous cells via JAK-STAT signal transduction pathway. It induces apoptosis to inhibit the proliferation of the cancerous cells via two pathways, viz., signal transduction through TNF-α as well as releasing cytochrome C by mitochondria. Both of these pathways lead to the activation of caspase signaling cascade, further resulting in cell death (Chiariello et al. 2000; Bazhanova 2005; Tagliaferri et al. 2005; Holcombe and Lee 2006; Bekisz et al. 2010). Interferon α2b topical drops instilled four times a day at the dose of 1Million IU/ml was compared with surgical excision. This study concluded that both topical interferon alfa-2b and aggressive surgical excision were found to be effective for the treatment of primary OSSN (Sturges et al. 2008). The study conducted by Shields et al (2013) in 80 patients reported that using IFNα2b eye drops and/or injection combined with surgical excision when necessary, provides complete control in all types of OSSN. Topical IFNα2b well tolerable drug with fewer ocular side effects when compared to other chemotherapeutic agents. The rare side effects are corneal epithelial microcysts, follicular conjunctivitis and keratitis, fever fatigue neuropathy and retinopathy etc. after topical or systemic administration (Poothullil and Colby 2006; Boehm and Huang 2004; Nemet et al. 2006; Aldave 2007; Vann and Karp 1999; Purvin 1995 and Guyer et al. 1993)

The above mentioned topical antineoplastic agents are well recognized in the management of non invasive OSSN having different levels of efficacy when compared to each other; MMC (88 %) > 5-FU (87 %) > IFNα-2b (80 %). These topical chemotherapeutic agents are not reported to be used as neoadjuvant or adjuvant therapy in cases with incomplete excised OSSN (Tananuvat and Lertprasertsuke 2012).

References

Aldave AJ, Nguyen A. Ocular surface toxicity associated with topical interferon α-2b. Br J Ophthalmol 2007;91:1087–8.

Banavali S. Evidence based management for retinoblastoma. Indian Journal of Medical and Pediatric Oncology 2004;25:35–45.

Basti S, Mascai MS. Ocular surface squamous neoplasia. Cornea 2003;22(7):687–704.

Bazhanova ED. Participation of interferon-alpha in regulation of apoptosis. J Evol Biochem Phys 2005;41(2):127–33.

Bekisz J, Baron S, Balinsky C, Morrow A, dan Zoon KC. Antiproliferative properties of type I and type II interferon. Pharmaceuticals (Basel) 2010;3(4):994–1015.

Blumenkranz MS, Claflin A, Hajek AS. Selection of therapeutic agents for intraocular proliferative disease. Cell culture evaluation. Arch Ophthalmol 1984;102(4):598–604.

Boehm MD, Huang AJ. Treatment of recurrent corneal and conjunctival intraepithelial neoplasia with topical interferon alfa 2b. Ophthalmology 2004;111:1755–61.

Boese E, Rogers GM, Kitzmann AS. A very unusual case of ocular surface squamous neoplasia. EyeRounds.org. 14 Feb 2013. Available from: http://EyeRounds.org/cases/163-OSSN.htm. Accessed 22 June 2015.

Carreira H, Coutinho F, Carrilho C, Lunet N. HIV and HPV infections and ocular surface squamous neoplasia: systematic review and meta-analysis. Br J Cancer 2013;109(7):1981–8.

Chabner BA, Bertino J, Cleary J, et al. Cytoxic agents. In: Brunton LL (ed). The pharmacological basis of therapeutics. The McGraw-Hill Companies, Inc. 12th ed, 2011:1665–755.

Chantada GL, Guitter MR, Fandino AC, Raslawski EC, de Davila MT, Vaiani E, et al. Treatment results in patients with RB and invasion to cut end of ON. Pediatr Blood cancer 2009;52:218–22.

Chawla B, Jain A, Azad R. Conservative treatment modalities in retinoblastoma. Indian J Ophthalmol 2013;61(9):479–85. doi: 10.4103/0301-4738.119424. Review. PMID: 24104705

Chawla B, Hasan F, Azad R, Seth R, Upadhyay AD, Pathy S, Pandey RM. Clinical presentation and survival of retinoblastoma in Indian children. Br J Ophthalmol 2015 Jun 10. pii: bjophthalmol-2015-306672. doi:10.1136/bjophthalmol-2015-306672. [Epub ahead of print] PMID: 26061162

Chiariello M, Gomez E, Gutkind JS. Regulation of cyclin-dependent kinase (Cdk) 2 Thr-160 phosphorylation and activity by mitogen-activated protein kinase in late G1 phase. Biochem J. 2000;349(3):869–76.

Chu E, Sartorelli AC Cancer Chemotherapy. In: Katzung BG, Masters SB, Trevor AJ (Eds). Basic and Clinical Pharmacology. New York, NY: McGraw-Hill Companies, Inc. 12th ed, 2012: 949–76.

Dimaras H, Kimani K, Dimba EAO, Gronsdah P, White A, Chan SL, Gallie BL. Retinoblastoma. Lancet 2012;379:1436–46.

Frucht-Pery J, Rozenman Y. Mitomycin C therapy for corneal intraepithelial neoplasia. Am J Ophthalmol 1994; 117:164–8.

Gichuhi S, Sagoo MS, Weiss HA, Burton MJ. Epidemiology of ocular surface squamous neoplasia in Africa. Trop Med Int Health 2013;18(12):1424–43.

Gichuhi S, Sagoo MS, Ohnuma S, Burton MJ. Pathophysiology of ocular surface squamous neoplasia. Exp Eye Res 2014;129:172–82.

Grulich AE, van Leeuwen MT, Falster MO, Vajdic CM. Incidence of cancers in people with HIV/AIDS compared with immunosuppressed transplant recipients: a meta-analysis. Lancet 2007;370:59–67.

Guyer DR, Tiedeman J, Yannuzzi LA, et al. Interferon-associated retinopathy. Arch Ophthalmol 1993;111:350–6.

Holcombe DJ, Lee GA. Topical interferon alfa-2b for the treatment of recalcitrant ocular surface squamous neoplasia. Am J Ophthalmol 2006;142(4):568–71.

Hurwitz RL, Shields CL, Shields JA, Cheves-Barrios P, Gombos D, Hurwitz MY, Chintagumpala MM. Retinoblastoma. In: Pizzo PA, Poplack DG, editors. Principles and practices of pediatric oncology. Philadelphia: Lippincott Williams & Wilkins; 2011. p. 809–37.

de Keizer RJ, de Wolff-Rouendaal D, van Delft JL. Topical application of 5-fluorouracil in premalignant lesions of cornea: conjunctiva and eyelid. Doc Ophthalmol 1986;64(1):31–42.

Kieval JZ, Karp CL, Abou Shousha M, Galor A, Hoffman RA, Dubovy SR, et al. Ultra-high resolution optical coherence tomography for differentiation of ocular surface squamous neoplasia and pterygia. Ophthalmology 2012;119(3):481–6.

Kiire CA, Srinivasan S, Karp CL. Ocular surface squamous neoplasia. Int Ophthal Mol Clin 2010;50(3):35–46.

Kim JW, Abramson DH. Topical treatment options for conjunctival neoplasms. Clin Ophthalmol 2008;2(3):503–15.

Kruh GD. Lustrous insights into cisplatin accumulation: copper transporters. Clin Cancer Res 2003;9:5807–9.

Lee GA, Hirst LW. Incidence of ocular surface epithelial dysplasia in metropolitan Brisbane. A 10-year survey. Arch Ophthalmol 1992;110:525–7.

Lee GA, Hirst LW. Ocular surface squamous neoplasia. Surv Ophthalmol 1995;39(6):429–50.

Linn Murphree A. Intraocular retinoblastoma: The case for a new group classification. Ophthalmol Clin North Am 2005;18:41–53.

Maskin SL. Regression of limbal epithelial dysplasia with topical interferon. Arch Ophthalmol 1994;112(9):1145–6

Midena E, Boccato P, Angeli CD. Conjunctival squamous cell carcinoma treated with topical 5- fluorouracil. Arch Ophthalmol 1997;115(12):1600–1.

Midena E, Angeli CD, Valenti M, et al. Treatment of conjunctival squamous cell carcinoma with topical 5-fluorouracil. Br J Ophthalmol 2000;84(3):268–72.

Nagaiah G, Stotler C, Orem J, Mwanda WO, Remicka SC. Ocular surface squamous neoplasia in patients with HIV infection in sub-Saharan Africa. Curr Opin Oncol 2010;22(5):437–42.

Nemet AY, Sharma V, and Benger R. Interferon alpha 2b treatment for residual ocular surface squamous neoplasia unresponsive to excision, cryotherapy and mitomycin-C. Clin Exp Ophthalmol 2006;34:375–7.

Panda A, Pe'er J, Aggarwal A, et al. Effect of topical mitomycin C on corneal endothelium. Am J Ophthalmol 2008;145(4):635–8.
Papaioannou IT, Melachrinou MP, Drimtzias EG, Gartaganis SP. Corneal-conjunctival squamous cell carcinoma. Cornea 2008;27(8):957–8.
Parrozzani R, Lazzarini D, Alemany-Rubio E, Urban F, Midena E. Topical 1% 5-fluorouracil in ocular surface squamous neoplasia: a long-term safety study. Br J Ophthalmol 2011;95(3):355–9. doi: 10.1136/bjo.2010.183244. Epub 2010 Aug 7.
Pe'er J. Ocular surface squamous neoplasia. Ophthalmol Clin North Am. 2005;18(1):1–13.
Pizzarello LD, Jakobiec FA. Bowen's disease of the conjunctiva: a misnomer. In: Jakobiec FA, editor. Ocularand adnexal tumors. Birmingham: Aesculapius; 1978. p. 553–71.
Poothullil AM, Colby KA. Topical medical therapies for ocular surface tumors. Semin Ophthalmol 2006;21:161–9.
Purvin VA. Anterior ischemic optic neuropathy secondary to interferon alfa. Arch Ophthalmol 1995;113:1041–4.
Rodriguez-Galindo C. Chemotherapy management in retinoblastoma. In: Rodriguez-Galindo C, Wilson MW (eds). Retinoblastoma. Springer, New York. 1st ed. 2010:67–73.
Rudkin AK, Dodd T, Muecke JS. The differential diagnosis of localized amelanotic limbal lesions: a review of 162 consecutive excisions. Br J Ophthalmol 2011;95:350–4.
Rudkin AK, Muecke JS. Adjuvant 5-fluorouracil in the treatment of localised ocular surface squamous neoplasia. Br J Ophthalmol 2011;95(7):947–50. doi:10.1136/bjo.2010.186171. Epub 2011 Jan 20.
Sepulveda R, Pe'er J, Midena E, Seregard S, Dua HS, Singh AD. Topical chemotherapy for ocular surface squamous neoplasia: current status. Br J Ophthalmol 2010;94(5):532–5. doi: 10.1136/bjo.2009.160820. Epub 2009 Sep 23. Review. PMID: 19776089
Shields CL, Shields JA, Baez KA, Cater JR, Potter P. Choroial invasion of RB: metastatic and clinical risk factors. Br J Ophthalmol 1993;77:544–8.
Shields JA, Shields CL. Pediatric ocular and periocular tumors. Pediatr Ann 2001;30:491–501.
Shields CL, Kaliki S, Kim HJ, Al-Dahmash S, Shah SU, Lally SE, Shields JA. Interferon for ocular surface squamous neoplasia in 81 cases: outcomes based on the American Joint Committee on Cancer classification. Cornea. 2013;32(3):248–56.
Siddik ZH. Cisplatin: mode of cytotoxic action and molecular basis of resistance. Oncogene 2003;22(47):7265–79.
Sturges A, Butt AL, Lai JE, Chodosh J. Topical interferon or surgical excision for the management of primary ocular surface squamous neoplasia. Ophthalmology 2008;115(8):1297–302, 1302.e1. doi: 10.1016/j.ophtha.2008.01.006. Epub 2008 Feb 21.
Tagliaferri P, Caraglia M, Budillon A, et al. New pharmacokinetic and pharmacodynamic tools for interferon-alpha (IFN-α) treatment of human cancer. Cancer Immunol Immunother 2005;54(1):1–10.
Tananuvat N, Lertprasertsuke N. Ocular Surface Squamous Neoplasia. In: Srivastava S, editor. Intraepithelial neoplasia. Publisher InTech. Published online 08 Feb 2012. Published in print edition February; 2012. www.intechopen.com. p. 35–62.
Tananuvat N, Lertprasertsuk N, Mahanupap P, Noppanakeepong P. Role of impression cytology in diagnosis of ocular surface neoplasia. Cornea 2008;27:269–74.
Tripathi KD. Chemotherapy of neoplastic diseases. In: Essentials of medical pharmacology. 6th ed. New Delhi: Jaypee Brothers Medical Publishers 2008; p. 819–34.
Vann RR, Karp CL. Perilesional and topical interferon alfa-2b for conjunctival and corneal neoplasia. Ophthalmology 1999;106:91–7.
Velpandian T, Saluja V, Ravi AK, Kumari SS, Mathur R, Biswas NR, Ghose S. Evaluation of the stability of extemporaneously prepared ophthalmic formulation of mitomycin C. J Ocul Pharmacol Ther. 2005;21(3):217–21.
Xu Y, Zhou Z, Xu Y, Wang M, Liu F, Qu H, et al. The clinical value of in vivo confocal microscopy for diagnosis of ocular surface squamous neoplasia. Eye (Lond) 2012;26(6):781–7.
Yeatts RP, Engelbrecht NE, Curry CD, et al. 5-Fluorouracil for the treatment of intraepithelial neoplasia of the conjunctiva and cornea. Ophthalmology 2000;107(12):2190–5.

Chapter 13
Ocular Diagnostic Agents

Manu Saini, Madhu Nath, and Murugesan Vanathi

Abstract Eye is the most accessible and easily visualized organ in the human body; due to this feature ophthalmic dyes have a significant role in ophthalmology to aid effective diagnosis of ocular condition. These dyes are extensively used for the differential diagnosis in various ocular pathological conditions such as corneal abrasions, congestion, micro aneurysm, blood vessel proliferations in retina and ischemia etc.

This chapter discusses about the handful of dyes such as trypan blue, rose bengal, indocynine green, brilliant blue, lissamine green and triamicolone actetonide etc., for their clinical utility, and their adverse effects.

Diagnostic agents are the pharmacological and non-pharmacological agents used in the detection of ocular deformities, ailments, and pathophysiological aspects. Dyes emerged recently as important and effective diagnostic adjuvants to enhance visualization of ocular tissues. Dye is an organic compound that contains chromophoric and auxochromic groups attached to a benzene ring, the color being attributable to the chromophores and the dying property to the salt-forming auxochromes (Norm 1969).

Dyes that provide color to living tissues or cells are called vital dyes. In cataract surgery, the blue dye trypan blue (TB) gained widespread use because of its staining ability to the anterior capsule and easier intraoperative removal of this fine, semi-transparent membrane. In vitreoretinal surgery, greening and bluish vital dyes such as indocyanine green (ICG) and brilliant blue (BriB) also facilitated visualization and removal of preretinal membranes as a result of their different affinities to intra-

M. Saini, MD • V. Murugesan, MD (✉)
Cornea Services, Dr. Rajendra Prasad Center for Ophthalmic Sciences, All India Institute of Medical Sciences, New Delhi, India
e-mail: vanathi_g@yahoo.com

M. Nath, RN (H), MSc (Clin Res)
Department of Ophthalmology, Dr. Rajendra Prasad Center for Ophthalmic Sciences, All India Institute of Medical Sciences, New Delhi, India

T. Velpandian (ed.), *Pharmacology of Ocular Therapeutics*,
DOI 10.1007/978-3-319-25498-2_13

ocular collagen and cellular elements. Vital dyes have also been used in corneal, glaucoma, orbit, strabismus, and conjunctival surgery.

In this chapter, we will discuss various dyes used in diagnosing ocular pathology, including their pharmacology, clinical utility, and their adverse effects mentioned below.

13.1 Sodium Fluorescein

This dye has been extensively used in the ocular diagnostics. Sodium fluorescein is a water-soluble salt of fluorescein, with empirical formula (C_{20} H_{10} Na_2 O_5) and of molecular weight 376 g/mol. This dye is also known as resorcinolphthalein sodium, or uranine, synthesized by Nobel prize winner in chemistry (1905) Adolf Von Bayer in 1871. Being a xanthenes group member which are primarily synthesized by the petroleum derivatives, fluorescein is a highly fluorescent compound (Wolfe 1986). This dye physically appears orange red in color in dry or concentrated solution form (Jacobs 1992). Dye concentration and pH can affect the intensity of fluorescence. Maximum fluorescence occurs at a pH of 7.4, but for angiographic use, pH is adjusted in a range of 8–9.8 for stability (Jacobs 1992). Sodium fluorescein shows peak excitation between 465 and 490 nm wavelength, corresponds to blue light, and emits florescence at the yellow green wavelength of 520–530 nm (Fig. 13.1).

The dye is visualized when illuminated in blue filter, appears florescent green, and is detectable in concentration between 0.1 and 0.0000001 % topically. For angiographic studies, sodium fluorescein is used extensively in clinical settings. The dose of 10–25 % fluorescein is injected through peripheral vein in a single bolus dose. Dye diffuses out rapidly from the capillaries except the retinal and central nervous system vasculature due to tight capillary junction in these location. On intravenous injection,

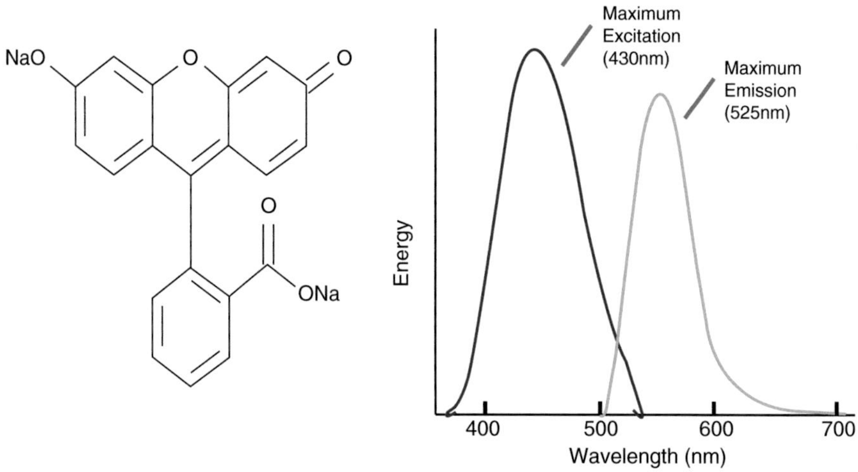

Fig. 13.1 Molecular structures of fluorescein sodium and wavelength spectra peak excitation and emission

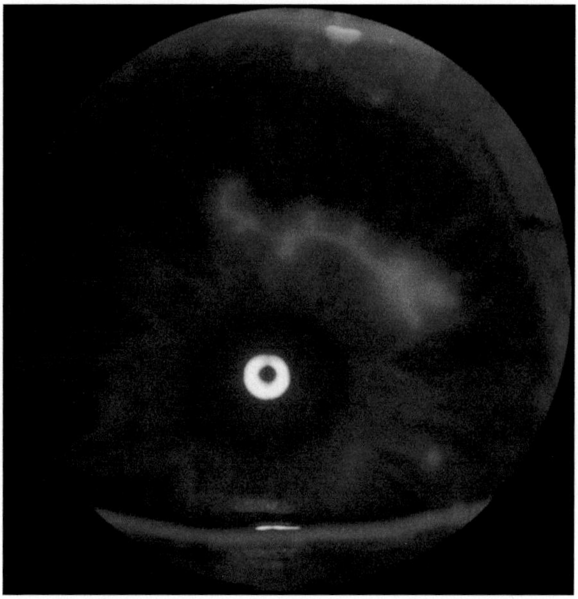

Image 13.1 Infectious epithelial keratitis stained with fluorescein

70–80 % of dye molecules bind to plasma proteins, and the remaining free or unbound molecules fluoresce on excitation by appropriate exciting wavelength (Morris 2002). It undergoes both hepatic and renal metabolism but is excreted principally through urine within 24–36 h of the administration. As it is small molecule, it can be excreted through milk also; therefore, its administration should be avoided in lactating mothers.

13.1.1 Ophthalmic Use

The primary purpose of fluorescein staining is to detect epithelial defects and to assist in the diagnosis of erosions, corneal abrasion, and keratitis. It has been a useful dye in assessing the rate of healing of corneal epithelial lesions. Fluorescein staining is also used to evaluate the status of the precorneal tear film with respect to tear breakup time (BUT) (Norm 1969) and contact lens fitting (Wolfe 1986) to evaluate tear volume and clearance, to measure corneal epithelial and endothelial permeability (Lass et al. 1985 and Kim 2000), and to detect aqueous humor flow and leakage, (Seidel test).

Fluorescein dye is also used to evaluate the tear secretion and tear turnover on the ocular surface in the fluorescein clearance test (Mishima et al. 1966). After a standardized amount of fluorescein is placed in the conjunctival sac, its concentration in the tear fluid is collected on Schirmer test strips placed in the inferior conjuctival fornix at 10-min intervals and visually compared to photographic standards. A reduced tear turnover rate is diagnosed by persistent fluorescein staining of the Schirmer test strips (Benedetto et al. 1984). Staining is enhanced with cell degeneration or death, which increases membrane permeability and manifests whenever there is a disruption of cell–cell junctions. Its staining is not blocked by tear compo-

Table 13.1 Clinical uses of sodium fluorescein in ocular conditions

1.	Lacrimal system	(a) Tear breakup time (dry eyes) (b) Jones test, dye disappearance test (blockage of lacrimal system)
2.	Cornea	(a) Detect epithelial defect (corneal abrasion, superficial punctate keratopathy) (b) Seidel's test (wound leak) (c) Contact lens fitting
3.	Anterior chamber	(a) Applanation Tonometry (b) Detect iris neovascularisation (c) TBUT (d) Clearance test
4.	Retina	(a) Fluorescein angiography

nents such as albumin and mucin or tear substitutes such as carboxycellulose (Feenstra and Tseng 1992). In addition, fluorescein sodium is routinely used for applanation tonometry, to check the patency of lacrimal passageways. Sodium fluorescein is extensively used in the retinal angiography to rule out ischemic, neovascularized, or obstructive pathology of the retina and choroid of the eye. (Table 13.1).

13.1.2 Adverse Effects

Sodium fluorescein is well tolerated by most patients, but angiography is an invasive procedure with an associated risk of complication or adverse reaction. Transient nausea and occasional vomiting are the most common reactions and require no treatment (Montavale 2006). These mild reactions typically occur 30–60 s after injection and last for about 1–2 min. More basic pH of this dye leads to painful experience at the site of injection, simultaneously extravasations of fluorescein dye can cause severe complications in the some patients although it is rare.

13.2 Trypan Blue

Trypan blue (TB) is a vital dye, first synthesized in 1904 by German scientist Paul Ehrlich. Trypan blue is an azo-based, hydrophilic, tetrasulfonated blue acid dye. Trypan blue is derived from toluidine which is a derivitized product of toluene, which has molecular formula of $C_{34}H_{28}N_6O_{14}S_4$ with the molecular weight of 872.88 g mol^{-1}. Trypan blue derived its name from trypanosomes, a parasite which causes sleeping sickness. An analog of trypan blue, suramin, is used for the treatment of trypanosomiasis (Morgan et al. 2011). This dye is also known as diamine blue and Niagara blue (Fig. 13.2).

Trypan blue is used as cell membrane-staining dye and extensively used to determine the viability of cells. Trypan blue will stain dead cells with permeable membrane blue, while the dye is excluded by most living cells and their intact membranes thereby allowing visual determination of living versus dead cells.

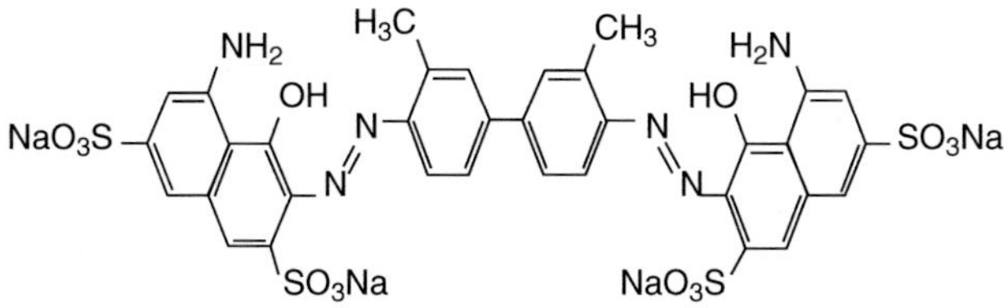

Fig. 13.2 Molecular structure of trypan blue dye

13.2.1 Ophthalmic Utilization

TB is used in both penetrating and deep lamellar keratoplasties. For penetrating keratoplasty, 0.02 % TB solution may be injected into the anterior chamber via a paracentesis to stain the descemmets membrane (DM) of the donor as well as the recipient corneal tissue. Dye exposure may promote close alignment of edges of host and donor DM, thus improving graft stability and minimizing surgically induced astigmatism (Roos and Kerr Muir 2005).

The vital dyes Indocynine Green (ICG) and TB aid in visualization of conjunctival cyst capsules (Kobayashi et al. 2002). Intraoperative injection of TB provides various advantages in cataract surgery. Surgical TB injection may promote higher rates of success of capsulorhexis in phacoemulsification for cases with inadequate red reflexes (Kothari et al. 2001 and Nodarjan et al. 2001). The blue vital stain allows staining of anterior and posterior capsules in children younger than 5, thereby enhancing effectiveness for completing the Continous Curvilinear Capsulorhexis (CCC) (Brown et al. 2004 and Saini et al. 2003). Wollensak and coauthors found TB staining led to an increase in elastic stiffness and a significant decrease in ultimate extensibility in the anterior capsule. This effect was probably due to the photosensitizing action of TB to physical cross-linking of collagen through yielding of free oxygen radicals, which causes a change in elastic behavior (Satofuka et al. 2004). Most clinical studies prefer 0.1 % TB to stain the anterior capsule, but effective staining has been also achieved with concentrations as low as 0.06 % (Chang et al. 2005). The minimum incubation time reported for successful capsule staining ranges from 5 seconds to 2 min (Saini et al. 2003). Trypan blue is also predominately used for assessing cell viability of cultured cells (Stevens 1993).

13.2.2 Adverse Effects

Side effects reported include discoloration of high water content hydrogen intraocular lenses; a relative contraindication for TB is the use of hydrophilic expandable acrylic intraocular lenses (IOLs), which have the highest water content (73.5 %) of currently manufactured implants and inadvertent staining of the posterior lens capsule and vitreous face followed use of trypan blue. Staining of the posterior lens capsule or staining of the vitreous face is generally self-limited, lasting up to one week.

13.3 Rose Bengal

Rose bengal (4,5,6,7-tetrachloro-2′,4′,5′,7′-tetraiodofluorescein) was originally prepared in 1884 by Gnehm. It is an iodine derivative of fluorescein which has vital staining properties; it is also called true histological stain. This is also a hydroxyanthene dye of a similar molecular structure to fluorescein. Additional halides give it its red color and also render it toxic. This toxicity is further enhanced by exposure to visible light. Rose bengal is classically well known to stain dead and devitalized cells, but now it is also reported to stain nuclear components of healthy cells (Fig. 13.3).

13.3.1 Ophthalmic Uses

It stains dead or degenerated epithelial cells, not normal cells, and is used to help in the diagnosis of corneal abrasion, keratitis, keratoconjunctivitis sicca, lagophthalmos, and meibomian gland dysfunction. In meibomian gland dysfunction, even though the tear volume appears to be normal, rose bengal staining may occur on the inferior or superior bulbar conjunctiva under the eyelids, which is outside the exposure zones (Uchiyama et al. 2007). With more severe inflammation, staining spreads and may affect the cornea in addition to the exposed conjunctiva. In nocturnal lagophthalmos, rose bengal staining is limited to the inferonasal corneal and conjunctival epithelium with a discrete line of demarcation between stained and unstained tissue. In contrast, rose bengal stains only the affected superior bulbar conjunctiva and the superior cornea in superior limbic keratoconjunctivitis.

Rose bengal is used to diagnose dendritic herpetic corneal ulcers (Uchiyama et al. 2007) and to delineate the extent of corneal and conjunctival neoplasms (Machado et al. 2009).

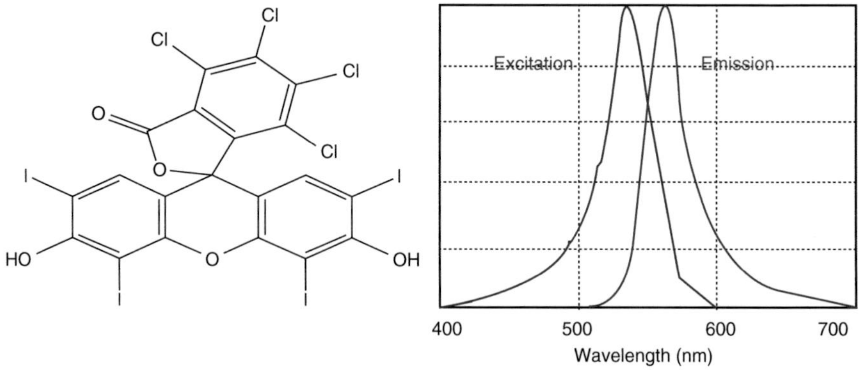

Fig. 13.3 Chemical structure of rose bengal (4,5,6,7-tetrachloro-2′,4′,5′,7′-tetraiodofluorescein) and fluorescence spectra (depicted)

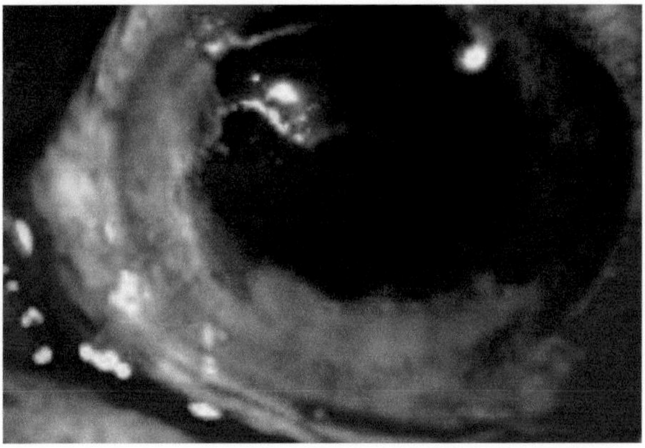

Image 13.2 Neurotrophic keratopathy stained with rose bengal

13.3.2 Adverse Effects/Toxicity

Rose bengal has also been known to have intrinsic cellular toxicity. Studies have shown that rose bengal has a dose-dependent, toxic effect on human corneal epithelial cells in vitro that is further enhanced by light exposure. Lastly, it's widely known to cause patient discomfort, particularly stinging sensation upon instillation, which can become severe, is often a deterrent from using rose bengal.

13.4 Indocyanine Green

Initially developed by Kodak Research Laboratories in 1955 for the near-infrared (NIR) photography, indocyanine green dye was approved for clinical use in 1956 (Engel et al. 2008; Bjoronsson et al. 1982). The chemical name for indocyanine green is 1 H benz[e]indolium, 2-[7-[1,3-dihydro-1,1-dimethyl-3-(4-sulfobutyl)-2H-benz[e]indol-2-ylidene]-1,3,5-heptatrienyl]-1,1-dimethyl-3-(4-sulfobutyl)-,hydroxide, inner salt, sodium salt. For retinal angiography, it has been used from early 1970s. ICG absorbs mainly between 600 nm and 900 nm and emits fluorescence between 750 and 950 nm. Near-infrared light is known to penetrate biological tissues such as skin and blood more efficiently than visible light therefore, they are best suited for tissue imaging (Fig. 13.4).

13.4.1 Ophthalmic Uses

ICG adheres well to the extracellular matrix components of the ILM, such as collagen type 4, laminin, and fibronectin (Wilson 1976). The first use of ICG in Macular Hole (MH) surgery was with a dye concentration of 0.5 %. After RPE changes and visual field defects appeared, a lower concentration was thought to be safer (T John

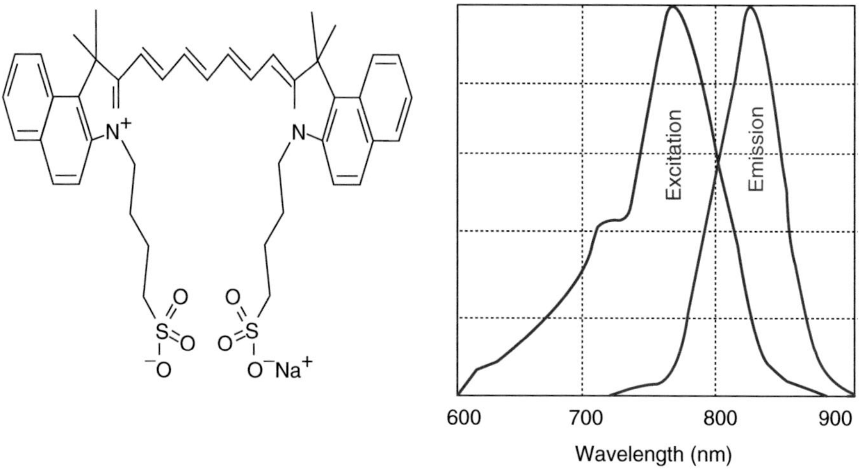

Fig. 13.4 Molecular structures of indocyanine green and its fluorescence spectra (depicted)

2003). ICG has been also used to facilitate Inner Limiting Membrane (ILM) peeling in other diseases: ICG-assisted ILM peeling in diabetic macular edema, proliferative diabetic vitreoretinopathy (PDVR), idiopathic Epiretinal Membrane (ERM) and proliferative vitreoretinopathy (PVR).

ICG is principally used for choroidal angiography. ICG is injected intravenously and circulate to reach the choroidal and retinal circulation. Due to its nature, ICG stays in the retinal and choroidal vessels; this allows the distinct outlines of the vessels of the choroid to be seen and identified. ICG is sometimes used to complement fluorescein angiography (FA). FA is often referred to retinal angiography, while ICG angiography is referred to choroidal angiography.

13.4.2 Adverse Effects/Toxicity

ICG is mainly metabolized by the liver and excreted through bile ducts; its toxicity is low as it is not absorbed through intestinal mucosa. Under UV exposure, ICG dissociates into a number of toxic substances which are still unknown substances (Toczylowska et al. 2014). The intravenous LD50 values measured in animals were 60 mg/kg in mice and 87 mg/kg in rats (Laperche et al. 1977). Its usage has been reported with analphylactic reactions, hypotension, tachycardia, dyspnea, and urticaria only in individual cases.

13.5 Lissamine Green

Lissamine green (LG) B is a synthetically produced organic acid dye with two aminophenyl groups having empirical formula of $C_{27}H_{25}N_2NaO_7S_2$ and molecular weight 576.62 g/mol. Synonyms include acid green S, wool green S or C, and fast light green. The staining profile of LG has been demonstrated to be comparable of rose bengal. However, LG is less irritating and is better tolerated by patients (Gandorfer et al. 2004). Lissamine green stains ocular surface epithelial cells that are unprotected by mucin or glycocalyx, as well as cells that have been damaged. LG is available in impregnated paper strips containing 1.5 mg of the dye. A drop of sterile saline is added to the strip and the dye is placed into the lower fornix of the eye by capillary action (Fig. 13.5).

13.5.1 Ophthalmic Use

Vital dyes such as lissamine green and rose bengal are used for detection of conjunctival xerosis associated with vitamin A deficiency (Rodrigues et al. 2005) and for ocular surface evaluation in keratoconjuctivitis sicca patients. The sensitivity of rose bengal has been described to be lower than that of lissamine green because of masking of the rose bengal stain by the pigmented and hyperemic conjunctiva (Hamrah et al. 2011).

13.5.2 Adverse Effects/Toxicity

The staining profile of LG has been demonstrated to be comparable to that of rose bengal. Rose bengal dye stains proliferating corneal epithelial cells and affects their viability; LG does not. This profiling makes better patient tolerance and nontoxic effect of LG.

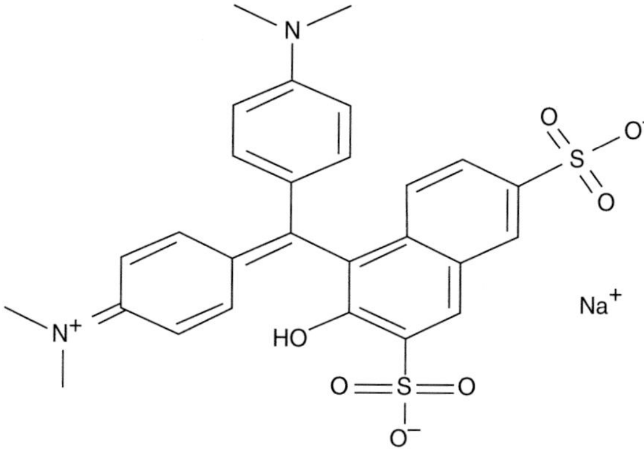

Fig. 13.5 Molecular structure of lissamine green

13.6 Triamcinolone Acetonide

Triamcinolone (TA) is a synthetic corticosteroid with empirical formula of $C_{24}H_{31}FO_6$ and molecular weight of 434.49 g/mol that is well known for its anti-inflammatory, anti-permeability, and antifibrotic properties, which justifies its use in inflammatory and vascular ophthalmic diseases (Sauter 1976). This water-insoluble steroid is used in ophthalmic surgery with the dose of 1–4 mg (25–100 μl) administered intravitreally (Emran and Sommer 1979).

13.6.1 Ophthalmic Use

TA upon intravitreal injection helps in visualization of vitreous and internal limiting membrane. The-insoluble crystals of TA integrate into loosely organized collagen fibers and hence get interwoven into the collagen bundles of vitreous (Peyman et al. 2000). When vitreous is removed surgically, the left over collagen fibers retained in the retina allow visualization of the internal limiting membrane, and epiretinal membrane thus helps in ophthalmic surgeries which are specifically called chromoviterectomy (Shah et al. 2004). Vitreo-retinal surgeons prefer the use of appropriate dyes for the vitrectomy surgery, and hence few dyes are popular in the ophthalmic surgery such as indocyanine green (ICG), trypan blue (TB), and recently TA (Couch and Bakri 2008).

13.6.2 Adverse Effects/Toxicity

Laboratory studies examined the effects of TA on various types of retinal cells, including ARPE19, human glial cells, neurosensory cells, ganglion cells, or choroidal fibroblasts. A few studies have indicated that TA may promote severe toxicity to choroidal fibroblasts and RPE cells (Narayanan et al. 2006). In addition, some investigators feel the preservative enhances the toxic effect (Chang et al. 2007). In contrast, a few researchers found a safe in vitro profile of TA to RPE cells. However, further invivo experimental studies in rabbits showed that up to 8mg intravitreal TA was found to be safe (Ye et al 2014).

13.7 Infracyanine Green

Infracyanine Green (IFCG) differs from ICG, in that it contains no iodine and can be dissolved directly into a 5 % glucose solution, generating an iso-osmotic solution of 294→314 mmol/kg, avoiding a hypo-osmotic preparation. It is therefore postulated that IFCG is less likely to produce cell damage than ICG. IFCG is less likely to produce retinal phototoxicity than ICG, as absorption has been found to be lower between 600 and 700 nm. It is therefore postulated that IFCG is less likely to produce phototoxic damage when used in conjunction with surgical endoillumination (Floman and Zor 1977) (Fig. 13.6).

13.7.1 Ophthalmic Use

IFCG also binds with high affinity to the acellular ILM. Ullern et al. demonstrated that IFCG stains ILM homogenously, but not epiretinal membranes (Wolfe. 1986), and thus assisting in ILM peeling in vitero-retinal surgeries.

13.7.2 Adverse Effects/Toxicity

Adverse effects/toxicity brief report by Haritoglou et al. 2004 has shown retinal damage in cadaveric eyes exposed to IFCG and light.

13.8 Gadolinium Sodium

Gadolinium (Gd) diethylenetriamine pentaacetic acid (DTPA) is a Food and Drug Administration-approved passive T1 magnetic resonance (MR) contrast agent clinically approved for assessing blood flow and vascular leakage in the eye, the brain, and the body (Fig. 13.7).

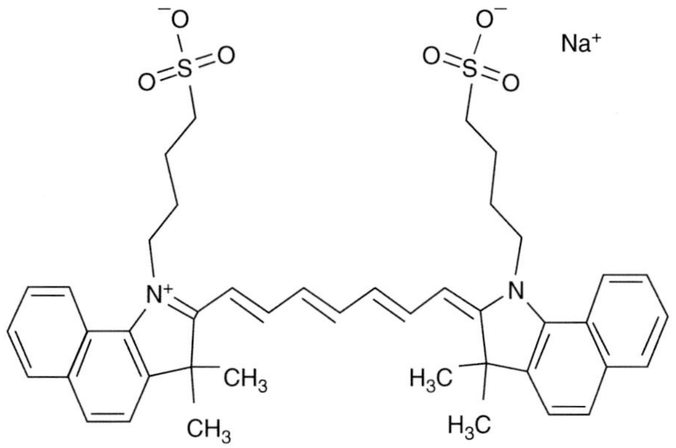

Fig. 13.6 Molecular structure of infracyanine green

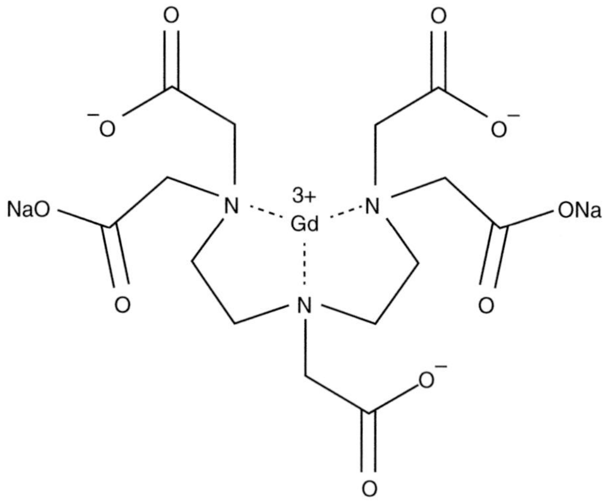

Fig. 13.7 Molecular structure of gadolinium sodium

13.8.1 Ophthalmic Use

Berkowitz et al. (1992) showed that Gd-DTPA is a promising method for investigating breakdown of the blood–retinal barrier (BRB). These authors only mentioned that the compound enters the vitreous space and it's directly correlated with the extent of blood–retinal barrier breakdown. Hence, this dye could be a useful marker in determining the breakage in the tight junction of ocular barriers as this molecule is not actively transported inside the eye. This agent has also been evaluated to assess the fate of topically administered eye drops. A study by Mao et al. (2010) assessed the corneal permeability of topical eye drop solutions added with various corneal penetrating accelerators and gadolinium-diethylene triamine pentaacetic acid (Gd-DTPA) by nuclear magnetic resonance imaging (MRI). This compound basically diffuses and follows aqueous humor kinetics, and as the systemically injected contrast gathers in anterior or posterior chamber of eye, it gives high contrast T1-weighted MRI images (Bert et al. 2006).

13.8.2 Future Aspects

Though it's in very prime stage of ocular imaging, this technique could be successfully used for the patients suspected for ocular barrier breakdown such as diabetic retinopathy. This agent would also be of immense help in studying the aqueous humor dynamics in the glaucoma-affected population.

13.8.3 Adverse Effects/Toxicity

A study from Yoshikawa et al. in 1998 showed that gadolinium created no local irritation in the eyes of rabbits and normal volunteers, although complication can arise from high dosage in renal functions.

13.9 Conclusion

Dyes have always been an integral part of diagnostic area specifically eye. The specific nature of dyes makes it unique in diagnosing various ocular pathologies.

References

Benedetto DA, Clinch TE, Laibson PR. In vivo observation of tear dynamics using fluorophotometry. Arch Ophthalmol. 1984;102:410–2.

Berkowitz BA, Tofts PS, Sen HA, Ando N, de Juan Jr E. Accurate and precise measurement of blood-retinal barrier breakdown using dynamic Gd-DTPA MRI. Invest Ophthalmol Vis Sci. 1992;33(13):3500–6.

Bert RJ, Caruthers SD, Jara H, et al. Demonstration of an anterior diffusional pathway for solutes in the normal human eye with high spatial resolution contrast-enhanced dynamic MR imaging. Invest Ophthalmol Vis Sci. 2006;47:5153–62.

Björnsson OG, Murphy R, Chadwick VS. Physicochemical studies of indocyanine green (ICG): absorbance/ concentration relationship, pH tolerance and assay precision in various solvents. Experientia. 1982;38(12):1441–2.

Brown SM, Graham WA, McCartney DL. Trypan blue in pediatric cataract surgery. J Cataract Refract Surg. 2004;30(10):2033.

Chang YS, Tseng SY, Tseng SH. Comparison of dyes for cataract surgery. Part 2: efficacy of capsule staining in a rabbit model. J Cataract Refract Surg. 2005;31(4):799–804.

Chang YS, Wu CL, Tseng SH, et al. Cytotoxicity of triamcinolone acetonide on human retinal pigment epithelial cells. Invest Ophthalmol Vis Sci. 2007;48(6):2792–8.

Couch SM, Bakri SJ. Use of triamcinolone during vitrectomy surgery to visualize membranes and vitreous. Clin Ophthalmol. 2008;2(4):891–6.

Emran N, Sommer A. Lissamine green staining in the clinical diagnosis of xerophthalmia. Arch Ophthalmol. 1979;97:2333–5.

Engel E, Schraml R, Maisch T, et al. Light-induced decomposition of indocyanine green. Invest Ophthalmol Vis Sci. 2008;49(5):1777–83.

Feenstra RPG, Tseng SCG. Comparison of fluorescein and rose Bengal staining. Ophthalmology. 1992;99:605–17.

Floman N, Zor U. Mechanism of steroid action in ocular inflammation: inhibition of prostaglandin production. Invest Ophthalmol Vis Sci. 1977;16(1):69–73.

Gandorfer A, Haritoglou C, Kampik A, Charteris D. Ultrastructure of the vitreoretinal interface following removal of the internal limiting membrane using indocyanine green. Curr Eye Res. 2004;29(4–5):319–20.

Hamrah P, Alipour F, Jiang S, Sohn J-H, Foulks GN. Optimizing evaluation of Lissamine Green parameters for ocular surface staining. Eye (Lond). 2011;25(11):1429–34.

Haritoglou C, Gandorfer A, Gass CA, Kampik A. Histology of the vitreoretinal interface after staining of the internal limiting membrane using glucose 5% diluted indocyanine green and infracyanine green. Am J Ophthalmol. 2004;137:345–8.

Jackson TL. http://www.opsweb.org/?page=FA.

Jackson TL, Vote B, Knight BC, El-Amir A, Stanford MR, Marshall J. Safety testing of infracyanine green using retinal pigment epithelium and glial cell cultures. Invest Ophthalmol Vis Sci. 2004;45(10):3697–703.

Jacobs J. Fluorescein sodium – what is it? J Ophthalmic Photography. 1992;14:62.

John T. Use of indocyanine green in deep lamellar endothelial keratoplasty. J Cataract Refract Surg. 2003;29(3):437–43.

Kim J. The use of vital dyes in corneal disease. Curr Opin Ophthalmol. 2000;11:241–7.

Kobayashi A, Saeki A, Nishimura A, et al. Visualization of conjunctival cyst by indocyanine green. Am J Ophthalmol. 2002;133(2):827–8.

Kothari K, Jain SS, Shah NJ. Anterior capsular staining with trypan blue for capsulorhexis in mature and hypermature cataracts. A preliminary study. Indian J Ophthalmol. 2001;49(3): 177–80.

Laperche Y, Oudea MC, Lostanlen D. Toxic effects of indocyanine green on rat liver mitochondria. Toxicol Appl Pharmacol. 1977;41(2):377–87.

Lass JH, Spurney RV, Rm D, et al. A morphologic and fluorophotometric analysis of the corneal endothelium in type I diabetes mellitus and cystic fibrosis. Am J Ophthalmol. 1985;100: 783–8.

Machado LM, Castro RS, Fontes BM. Staining patterns in dry eye syndrome: rose Bengal versus lissamine green. Cornea. 2009;28(7):732–4.

Mao X, Zhang S, Hen H, Du L, Li G, Li B, Zhang H. Corneal permeability assay of topical eye drop solutions in rabbits by MRI. J Huazhong Univ Sci Technolog Med Sci. 2010;30(6):804–8.

Marsh RJ, Fraunfelder FT, McGill JI. Herpetic corneal epithelial disease. Arch Ophthalmol. 1976;94:1899–902.

Mishima A, Gasset A, Klyce Jr SD, Baum JL. Determination of tear volume and tear flow. Invest Ophthalmol. 1966;5:264–76.

Montavale. Physicians' desk reference for ophthalmic medicines montvale. Thompson PDR; 207, 2006.

Morgan HP, McNae IW, Nowicki MW, Zhong W, Michels PA, Auld DS, Fothergill-Gilmore LA, Walkinshaw MD. The trypanocidal drug suramin and other trypan blue mimetics are inhibitors of pyruvate kinases and bind to the adenosine site. J Biol Chem. 2011;286(36):31232–40.

Morris PF. Fluorescein sodium and indocyanine green: uses and side effects. In: Saine PJ, Tyler ME, editors. Ophthalmic photography: retinal photography, angiography and electronic imaging. 2nd ed. Boston: Butterworth-Heinemann; 2002. p. 137–65.

Narayanan R, Mungcal JK, Kenney MC, et al. Toxicity of triamcinolone acetonide on retinal neurosensory and pigment epithelial cells. Invest Ophthalmol Vis Sci. 2006;47(2):722–8.

Nodarian M, Feys J, Sultan G, Salvanet-Bouccara A. Capsulorhexis staining by trypan blue in mature cataract surgery. J Fr Ophtalmol. 2001;24(3):274–6.

Norn MS. Desiccation of the precorneal tear film. I. Corneal wetting-time. Acta Ophthalmol. 1969;47:865–80.

Peyman GA, Cheema R, Conway MD, Fang T. Triamcinolone acetonide as an aid to visualization of the vitreous and the posterior hyaloid during pars plana vitrectomy. Retina. 2000;20(5):554–5.

Rodrigues EB, Meyer CH, Farah ME, Kroll P. Intravitreal staining of the internal limiting membrane using indocyanine green in the treatment of macular holes. Ophthalmologica. 2005;219(5):251–62.

Roos JC, Kerr Muir MG. Use of trypan blue for penetrating keratoplasty. J Cataract Refract Surg. 2005;31(10):1867–9.

Saini JS, Jain AK, Sukhija J, et al. Anterior and posterior capsulorhexis in pediatric cataract surgery with or without trypan blue dye: randomized prospective clinical study. J Cataract Refract Surg. 2003;29(9):1733–7.

Satofuka S, Nakamura K, Negishi K, et al. Time course of lens capsule staining using trypan blue and indocyanine green: in vitro study in porcine eyes. J Cataract Refract Surg. 2004;30(8): 1751–4.

Sauter JJM. Diagnosis of xerophthalmia by vital staining. Trop Doct. 1976;6:91–3.

Shah GK, Rosenblatt BJ, Smith M. Internal limiting membrane peeling using triamcinolone acetonide: histopathologic confirmation. Am J Ophthalmol. 2004;138(4):656–7.

Stevens A, Altman, Lisa Panders et al. Comparison of trypan blue dye exclusion and flurometric assay for mammalian cell viability. Biotechnol. Prog 1993,9(6 closed up):671–674.

Toczylowska B, Elzbieta Z, Grazyna G, Daniel M, Anna G, Adam L. Neurotoxic effects of indocyanine green -cerebellar granule cell culture viability study Biomed. Opt Express. 2014; 5(3):800–16.

Uchiyama E, Aronowicz JD, Butovich IA, Mc Culley JP. Pattern of vital staining and its correlation with aqueous tear deficiency and meibomian gland dropout. Eye Contact Lens. 2007;33(4): 177–9.

Wilson II FM. Rose bengal staining of epibulbar squamous neoplasms. Ophthalmic Surg. 1976; 7(2):21–3.

Wolfe DR. Fluorescein angiography basic science and engineering. Ophthalmology. 1986;93: 1617–20.

Ye YF, Gao YF, Xie HT, Wang HJ.Pharmacokinetics and retinal toxicity of various doses of intravitreal triamcinolone acetonide in rabbits. Mol Vis. 2014;20:629–36.

Yoshikawa T, Hirota S, Ohno Y, Matsumoto S, Ichikawa S, Tomita M, Fukuda T, Sako M, Yokogawa S. Basic study of MR-dacryocystography. Nippon Igaku Hoshasen Gakkai Zasshi. 1998;58(13):758–60.

Chapter 14
Systemic Toxicity of Drugs Applied to the Eye

Hanuman Prasad Sharma, Arumugam Ramamoorthy Vijayakumar, and Thirumurthy Velpandian

Abstract When a drug is administered to treat, diagnose or mitigate any ocular condition, it may produce certain undesirable effects besides the desirable or therapeutic one. When a drug is administered systemically, its absorption in the eye is restricted by various factors including the ocular barriers. Still, certain drugs are able to breach this barrier and thus can cause toxicity. Similarly, drugs given topically or by the invasive ocular route can cross the blood ocular barrier to cause systemic toxicity. This chapter discusses the systemic toxicity of drugs applied on eye including the anti-glaucoma agents, drugs acting on autonomic nervous system, anti-inflammatory agents, antimicrobial agents, drugs used for ocular neovascularization conditions and preservatives used in ophthalmic preparations. This chapter also briefly describes about the ocular toxicity caused by the systemically administered drugs.

Wide variety of agents are used for diagnostic and therapeutic purposes for various ocular conditions. Although, intraocular and periocular injections are preferred for surgical anesthesia and acute therapeutic conditions, topical route is the convenient mode which is extensively used and well accepted for ophthalmic purposes. As transcorneal penetration of topically instilled eye medications are restricted due to its unique anatomy and physiology, the applied drugs are often used at higher concentration to achieve desired pharmacological response. Nasolacrimal drainage of excessively applied topical drug solution or unabsorbed drug washed away from pre-corneal area by lacrimal fluid are absorbed into systemic circulation. Potent drugs having lower therapeutic index getting absorbed through this route bypass hepatic first pass metabolism, reach

H.P. Sharma, M. Pharm • T. Velpandian, BPharm, MS (Pharmacol), PhD (✉)
Ocular Pharmacology and Pharmacy, Dr. Rajendra Prasad Center for Ophthalmic Sciences, All India Institute of Medical Sciences, New Delhi, India
e-mail: tvelpandian@hotmail.com

A.R. Vijayakumar, PhD
Ophthalmic Pharmaceutical Division, Appasamy Associates, Arumbakkam, Chennai, India

T. Velpandian (ed.), *Pharmacology of Ocular Therapeutics*,
DOI 10.1007/978-3-319-25498-2_14

adequate levels in blood and cause undesirable systemic side effects. They can also cause potential drug interaction with concurrent usage of other drugs.

Regulatory guidelines for ophthalmic drug testing: Currently there are no well-established guidelines for toxicological testing of ophthalmic drug. As per US FDA, a novel entity to be used via ocular route has to go through complete preclinical systemic and ocular toxicity evaluation in two animal species (rodent and nonrodent). But most of the drugs used in current ophthalmological practice were earlier approved to be used for other routes (oral or injectable) and subsequently approved for their ocular use. For these drugs, preclinical toxicological analysis need to be done on only one animal species as their toxicity data has already been established (US-FDA 2008). Furthermore, regulatory authorities emphasize more on local rather than systemic toxicity of ophthalmic drugs. Currently, these regulatory guidelines are lacking proper design and evaluation of the product. The increasing burden of comorbidities warrants thorough evaluation of these drugs during clinical trial studies. Moroever, based on the systemic drug levels reached after topical administration also, their expected systemic manifestations can be extrapolated.

14.1 Systemic Side Effects of Ophthalmic Drugs (See Table 14.1)

14.1.1 Antiglaucoma Drugs

Glaucoma is an irreversible cause of blindness in the world with more than 70 million affected individuals (Quigley and Broman 2006). Treatment of glaucoma warrants rigorous intraocular hypertension control by pharmacological or surgical interventions. Sometimes these pharmacological agents can produce systemic side effects. Prostaglandin analogue drops generally produce headache, flu-like symptom and myalgias (Goldberg et al. 2008). Latanoprost is reported to produce chest tightness in patients with glaucoma. Systemic PGF2α is known to produce significant cardiac effects, but the same is not reported with its ocular use. Prostaglandin-induced visceral nociceptor sensitization was thought to produce the reported side effect (Rajan et al. 2003). Topical beta blockers are known to produce several cardiac side effects like congestive heart failure, bradyarrhythmias and sinus arrest. These effects may be life threatening in some cases. Beta blockers are also known to produce respiratory side effects, even deaths have been reported in some cases with topical timolol. Hence, beta blockers are contraindicated in patients with cardiac and respiratory disorders (Shiuey and Eisenberg 1996). Alpha-2 agonists are known to cause depression and profound hypotension (especially in children). In specific, brimonidine produces somnolence, shortness of breath, dizziness, headache and low mood as its systemic side effects. Frequency of these side effects may vary from 20 to 50 % with high occurrence rate in elderly cases. Reports of apneic spells and cyanosis, hypothermia and hypotony related to CNS depression warrant avoidance of brimonidine in newborns, young infants and children with juvenile glaucoma younger than 12 years (Bowman et al. 2004; Enyedi and Freedman 2001).

Table 14.1 Ophthalmic drugs known to cause systemic side effects

Drug	MOA	Systemic side effects	References
Cycloplegics: Atropine, hyoscine, homatropine (rarely) and cyclopentolate	Muscarinic receptor antagonists	Dryness and flushing of skin, thirst, tachycardia, convulsion, coma and dysarthria (especially in infants), delirium and confusion (especially in elderly) and speech difficulties	Kanski (1969), Reilly et al. (1996), Shiuey and Eisenberg (1996)
Mydriatics: Phenylephrine[a] and ephedrine	Adrenergic receptor agonists	Tachycardia, palpitation, hypertension and myocardial infarction[a]	Fraunfelder and Meyer (1987), Kanski (1969), Reilly et al. (1996), Shiuey and Eisenberg (1996)
Miotics: Pilocarpine	Muscarinic receptor agonist	Nausea, vomiting, abdominal spasm, salivation, lacrimation, sweating, pulmonary edema, bronchial spasm and cardiovascular decompensation	Everitt and Avorn (1990), Reilly et al. (1996), Shiuey and Eisenberg (1996), Zimmerman and Wheeler (1982)
Physostigmine and demecarium	Anticholinesterase	Respiratory depression, muscle twitching and convulsion	Bartlett and Jaanus (1989)
Carbachol	Cholinergic agonist	Bladder tightness, difficulty in breathing, rashes, swelling of the mouth, face, lips and tongue, eye irritation, stomach cramps, and irregular heartbeat	Reilly et al. (1996)
Echothiophate iodide	Anticholinesterase (Irreversible)	Diarrhea, nausea, vomiting, bradycardia, arrhythmias and hypotension	Bartlett and Jaanus (1989), Reilly et al. (1996), Shiuey and Eisenberg (1996)

(continued)

Table 14.1 (continued)

Drug	MOA	Systemic side effects	References
Beta blockers	Blockade of beta adrenergic receptors	Precipitation of bronchospasm, congestive heart failure, bradyarrhythmias, sinus arrest and dyslipidemias	Everitt and Avorn (1990), Fraunfelder and Meyer (1987), Goldberg et al. (2008), Lama (2002), Reilly et al. (1996), Shiuey and Eisenberg (1996)
Alpha-2 agonists	Agonists for adrenergic alpha 2 receptors	Depression and profound hypotension (especially in children)	Goldberg et al. (2008)
Prostaglandin analogues	Increase uveoscleral outflow	Headache, flu-like symptoms and myalgias	Goldberg et al. (2008)
Antibacterials: Chloramphenicol	Inhibit bacterial protein synthesis	Aplastic anemia	Fraunfelder and Meyer (1987), Laporte et al. (1998)
Sulfacetamide	Competitive inhibition of p-aminobenzoic acid (PABA) utilization in folate synthesis	Stevens-Johnson syndrome and systemic lupus erythematosus	Gottschalk and Stone (1976), Mackie and Mackie (1979)
Chlortetracyclin and tetracycline[a]	Inhibit protein synthesis by binding to 30S ribosomal units	Skin discoloration, redness, excessive light sensitivity and resistance at extraocular site[a]	Duvall and Kershner (2006), Gaynor et al. (2005)
Neomycin	Interference with microbial protein synthesis	Allergic contact dermatitis	Aoki (1997)
Antiviral agents: Idoxuridine, trifluridine, vidarabine, ganciclovir acyclovir and foscarnet	Interferes with viral DNA formation	Contact dermatitis	Amon et al. (1975), Cirkel and van Ketel (1981), Holdiness (2001), Millan-Parrilla and de la Cuadra (1990)

(continued)

Table 14.1 (continued)

Drug	MOA	Systemic side effects	References
Preservatives: Benzalkonium chloride	Detergent	Bronchoconstriction	Beasley et al. (1987)
Anti-VEGF therapy	Binding to VEGF	Thrombosis, hemorrhage, hypertension, proteinuria, myocardial infarction, transient ischemic attacks, deep vein thrombosis, pulmonary embolism and thrombophlebitis	Semeraro et al. (2011)
NSAIDs	Inhibition of COX enzyme	Exacerbation of bronchial asthma	Gaynes and Fiscella (2002)
Steroids	Act on nuclear receptors to regulate expression of corticosteroid-responsive genes	Interference with glycemic control and cushingoid habitus	Bahar et al. (2011), Ozerdem et al. (2000)
Antiallergics: Olopatadine	Antihistaminics	Headache, hyperemia, hypersensitivity, nausea, pharyngitis, pruritus, rhinitis, sinusitis and taste perversion	Aoki (1997)
Ketotifen		Allergic contact dermatitis	
Local anesthetics	Blockade of sodium ion channels	Allergic reactions, arrhythmias, myocardial depression, cardiac arrest, irritation, lethargy, seizures and CNS depression leading to respiratory arrest	Eggleston and Lush (1996), Rubin (1995)

[a]Specific

14.1.2 Miotics, Mydriatics and Cycloplegics

In ophthalmology, mydriatics and cycloplegics are generally used for posterior segment evaluation like fundus photography, fluorescein angiography and OCT. Miotics are generally used for the management of angle-closure glaucoma. Due to their activity on the autonomic nervous system, these drugs may produce systemic side effects. Phenylephrine's activity on alpha receptors can produce cardiovascular complications (Kanski 1969; Reilly et al. 1996; Shiuey and Eisenberg 1996). In the same manner cycloplegics have various side effects related to CNS and cardiovascular systems. Few of the reported side effects are more common in children and elderly. Shorter duration of action and tendency to produce less systemic side effects make tropicamide a drug of choice among others (Kanski 1969; Reilly et al. 1996; Shiuey and Eisenberg 1996).

14.1.3 Drugs for Pathological Neovascularization

These drugs are used to treat neovascular ocular disorders such as age-related macular degeneration, diabetic retinopathy etc. For the localized benefit, usually anti-VEGF compounds are injected intravitreally for ocular neovascular conditions. The systemic absorption of these compounds from vitreous humor has been attributed to their systemic adverse effects may or may not be related to their action through VEGF pathway. Intravitreal pegaptanib is considered to be a safer drug as compared to ranibizumab or bevacizumab. A retrospective study including 1173 patients receiving bevacizumab reported acute blood pressure elevations (0.59 %), cerebrovascular accidents (0.5 %), myocardial infarctions (0.4 %) and iliac artery aneurysms (0.17 %) as systemic side effects (Wu et al. 2008). Contrary to this, study done by Hwang et al. in 2012 did not find any significant difference in the safety profile of bevacizumab compared to ranibizumab (Hwang et al. 2012). Similarly a recent meta-analysis also concluded treatment from the both drugs as safe (Wang and Zhang 2014). Systemic side effects occur during treatment with these drugs should be thoroughly monitored irrespective of their safety reports.

14.1.4 Anti-inflammatory Drugs

Topical nonsteroidal anti-inflammatory drugs (NSAIDs) are used to treat many inflammatory conditions of the eye. These drugs are considered to be safe and produce very less systemic side effects, though may exacerbate bronchial asthma in predisposed cases (Gaynes and Fiscella 2002). Interestingly one such case was reported with the use of diclofenac eye drops in a patient with a history of mild bronchial asthma. Patient reported attack of bronchial asthma after each instillation of diclofenac eye drops. Nasolacrimal duct occlusion helped the patient to control the attack (Sharir 1997). NSAID induced bronchial asthma is caused by the diversion of arachidonic acid to lipoxygenase pathway due to inhibition of cyclooxygenase-1 (COX-1) and increased release of cysteinyl leukotrienes (Cys-LTs) (Picado, 2006).

14.1.5 Antimicrobial Agents

Topical antimicrobial agents are routinely used for ocular surface infections. These agents are applied on eye as drop or semisolid formulations. Intraocular microbial infections are usually treated with intraocular and/or systemic antimicrobials. Ocular infections are treated rigorously, as they are sight threatening. Multiple ocular instillations pose a risk of systemic adverse effects to these drugs. Aplastic anemia, a controversial systemic side effect of topical chloramphenicol, is still in debate (Wiholm et al. 1998). Contradictory findings regarding the association of topical chloramphenicol with aplastic anemia warrant judicious use by ophthalmologists. Several ocular antimicrobial agents are associated with allergic reaction like contact dermatitis. Sulfacetamide can even produce systemic lupus erythematosus (Mackie and Mackie 1979). Idoxuridine is found to have a positive relationship with the pyrimidine structural group and allergic propensity (Amon et al. 1975). Cross-reactivity of idoxuridine with brominated and chlorinated congeners suggests detailed medical history for the known allergies must be taken before initiating the therapy. Ocular tetracycline-induced resistance at extraocular site (Gaynor et al. 2005) proposes rational use of these antimicrobials.

14.1.6 Ophthalmic Preservatives

To minimize accidental microbial contaminations, preservatives are added in the eye drops. Several classes of preservatives are used, viz., detergents (benzalkonium chloride, chlorobutanol), oxidants (sodium perborate), chelating agents (methylparaben) and metabolic inhibitors. They are reported to affect corneal cellular makeup (Epstein et al. 2009), however, the information about their contribution to systemic toxicity is inadequate due to the lack of evidences. Parabens are found to cause contact dermatitis when absorbed by damaged or broken skin (Soni et al. 2002), but similar reports from its ophthalmic use are lacking. Organomercurial preservative thimerosal is rarely used nowadays because of its cellular toxicity (Epstein et al. 2009). Benzalkonium chloride-induced bronchoconstriction was reported in asthmatic patients using ipratropium bromide solution through nebulizer. Though benzalkonium chloride is known to release histamine from mast cells (Beasley et al. 1987), ocular uses are not reported to cause such adverse effect. Anaphylactic reaction following nasal drop containing benzalkonium chloride as preservative is reported (Mezger et al. 2012); hence warrants thorough checks for such type of reaction with ophthalmic drops as well.

To conclude, ophthalmic drops are having potential to produce systemic side effects which may become severe and life threatening in some cases. Proper instillation techniques like "pouch technique" where drug is instilled in cul-de-sac (pouch) and eye is gently closed and excess drug is wiped away can reduce systemic absorption to larger extent and thus these systemic side effects can be avoided.

14.2 Ocular Toxicity of Systemically Administered Drugs

Once the drug enters the body, it is free to move and enter anywhere unless restricted owing to the tissue specificity or the drug molecule itself. In this regard the drugs taken systemically can enter the eye, though the eye has its own safety measures like blood-retinal barrier at the posterior portion and blood-aqueous barrier at the anterior portion. The quantity of drug reaching ocular tissues may not be similar to other tissues due to the presence of preferential uptake and efflux mechanisms of the eye via barriers, but constant medication at a steady state may be reaching adequate levels causing alteration in the functions of eye or the levels reaching the brain causing change in vision perception. As per classical WHO definition, side effects are unintended effect occurring at normal dose related to the pharmacological properties where adverse events are defined as a response to a drug which is noxious and unintended and which occurs at doses normally used in man for the prophylaxis, diagnosis, or therapy of disease or for the modifications of physiological function. As far as ocular side effect/adverse effects of drugs are concerned, seeing them in isolation may not comprehend the mechanisms involved; therefore, they are grouped according to the system through which it is altering the function to bring the reason for such side effects. Although all the effects cannot be explained with the current state of knowledge, their action as a exaggerated pharmacological response through known mechanism can be rationalized. The knowledge available in this area is very vast and covering them all together is beyond the scope of this chapter; therefore, further information in this area can be obtained from the extensive reviews of Gokulgandhi et al. (2012), Vijayakumar et al. (2011) etc.

References

Amon RB, Lis AW, Hanifin JM. Allergic contact dermatitis caused by idoxuridine. Patterns of cross reactivity with other pyrimidine analogues. Arch Dermatol. 1975;111(12):1581–4.

Aoki J. [Allergic contact dermatitis due to eye drops. Their clinical features and the patch test results]. Nihon Ika Daigaku Zasshi. 1997;64(3):232–7.

Bahar I, Vinker S, Kaisrman I. The effect of topical steroids on blood glucose profile in diabetic patients. J Clin Experiment Ophthalmol. 2011;2(2):1–3.

Bartlett JD, Jaanus SD. Drug affecting the autonomic nervous system. Clinical ocular pharmacology. 2nd ed. Butterworth-Heinemann, Reed Publishing, USA; 1989.

Beasley CR, Rafferty P, Holgate ST. Bronchoconstrictor properties of preservatives in ipratropium bromide (Atrovent) nebuliser solution. Br Med J. 1987;294(6581):1197–8.

Bowman RJ, Cope J, Nischal KK. Ocular and systemic side effects of brimonidine 0.2% eye drops (Alphagan) in children. Eye. 2004;18(1):24–6.

Cirkel PK, van Ketel WG. Allergic contact dermatitis to trifluorothymidine eyedrops. Contact Dermatitis. 1981;7(1):49–50.

Duvall B, Kershner R. Ocular side effects of systemically administered medications. Ophthalmic medications and pharmacology. 2nd ed. SLACK incorporated, USA; 2006

Eggleston ST, Lush LW. Understanding allergic reactions to local anesthetics. Ann Pharmacother. 1996;30(7–8):851–7.

Enyedi LB, Freedman SF. Safety and efficacy of brimonidine in children with glaucoma. J AAPOS. 2001;5(5):281–4.

Epstein SP, Ahdoot M, Marcus E, Asbell PA. Comparative toxicity of preservatives on immortalized corneal and conjunctival epithelial cells. J Ocul Pharmacol Ther. 2009;25(2):113–9.

Everitt DE, Avorn J. Systemic effects of medications used to treat glaucoma. Ann Intern Med. 1990;112(2):120–5.

Fraunfelder FT, Meyer SM. Systemic reactions to ophthalmic drug preparations. Med Toxicol Adverse Drug Exp. 1987;2(4):287–93.
Gaynes BI, Fiscella R. Topical nonsteroidal anti-inflammatory drugs for ophthalmic use: a safety review. Drug Saf. 2002;25(4):233–50.
Gaynor BD, Chidambaram JD, Cevallos V, Miao Y, Miller K, Jha HC, et al. Topical ocular antibiotics induce bacterial resistance at extraocular sites. Br J Ophthalmol. 2005;89(9):1097–9.
Gokulgandhi MR, Vadlapudi AD, Mitra AK. Ocular toxicity from systemically administered xenobiotics. Expert Opin Drug Metab Toxicol. 2012;8(10):1277–91.
Goldberg I, Moloney G, McCluskey P. Topical ophthalmic medications: what potential for systemic side effects and interactions with other medications? Med J Aust. 2008;189(7):356–7.
Gottschalk HR, Stone OJ. Stevens-Johnson syndrome from ophthalmic sulfonamide. Arch Dermatol. 1976;112(4):513–4.
Holdiness MR. Contact dermatitis from topical antiviral drugs. Contact Dermatitis. 2001; 44(5):265–9.
Hwang DJ, Kim YW, Woo SJ, Park KH. Comparison of systemic adverse events associated with intravitreal anti-VEGF injection: ranibizumab versus bevacizumab. J Korean Med Sci. 2012;27(12):1580–5.
Kanski JJ. Mydriatics. Br J Ophthalmol. 1969;53(6):428–9.
Lama PJ. Systemic adverse effects of beta-adrenergic blockers: an evidence-based assessment. Am J Ophthalmol. 2002;134(5):749–60.
Laporte JR, Vidal X, Ballarin E, Ibanez L. Possible association between ocular chloramphenicol and aplastic anaemia – the absolute risk is very low. Br J Clin Pharmacol. 1998;46(2):181–4.
Mackie BS, Mackie LE. Systemic lupus erythematosus – dermatomyositis induced by sulphacetamide eye drops. Australas J Dermatol. 1979;20(1):49–50.
Mezger E, Wendler O, Mayr S, Bozzato A. Anaphylactic reaction following administration of nose drops containing benzalkonium chloride. Head Face Med. 2012;8:29.
Millan-Parrilla F, de la Cuadra J. Allergic contact dermatitis from trifluridine in eyedrops. Contact Dermatitis. 1990;22(5):289.
Ozerdem U, Levi L, Cheng L, Song MK, Scher C, Freeman WR. Systemic toxicity of topical and periocular corticosteroid therapy in an 11-year-old male with posterior uveitis. Am J Ophthalmol. 2000;130(2):240–1.
Picado C. Mechanisms of aspirin sensitivity. Current allergy and asthma reports. 2006;6(3):198–202.
Quigley HA, Broman AT. The number of people with glaucoma worldwide in 2010 and 2020. Br J Ophthalmol. 2006;90(3):262–7.
Rajan MS, Syam P, Liu C. Systemic side effects of topical latanoprost. Eye. 2003;17(3):442–4.
Reilly KM, Chan L, Mehta NJ, Salluzzo RF. Systemic toxicity from ocular homatropine. Acad Emer Med. 1996;3(9):868–71.
Rubin AP. Complications of local anaesthesia for ophthalmic surgery. Br J Anaesth. 1995;75(1): 93–6.
Semeraro F, Morescalchi F, Parmeggiani F, Arcidiacono B, Costagliola C. Systemic adverse drug reactions secondary to anti-VEGF intravitreal injection in patients with neovascular age-related macular degeneration. Curr Vasc Pharmacol. 2011;9(5):629–46.
Sharir M. Exacerbation of asthma by topical diclofenac. Arch Ophthalmol. 1997;115(2):294–5.
Shiuey Y, Eisenberg MJ. Cardiovascular effects of commonly used ophthalmic medications. Clin Cardiol. 1996;19(1):5–8.
Soni MG, Taylor SL, Greenberg NA, Burdock GA. Evaluation of the health aspects of methyl paraben: a review of the published literature. Food Chem Toxicol. 2002;40(10):1335–73.
US-FDA. Nonclinical safety evaluation of reformulated drug products and products intended for administration by an alternate route. In: FDA, editor. Rockville: Center for Drug Evaluation and Research, Food and Drug Administration; 2008. p. 1–8.
Vijayakumar AR, Velpandian T, Saxena R. Ocular adverse effects of systemically administered drugs. In: Agarwal R, Agarwal P, (ed.). Essentials of ocular pharmacology. Malaysia: University Publication Centre (UPENA); 2011;1:343–64.

Wang W, Zhang X. Systemic adverse events after intravitreal bevacizumab versus ranibizumab for age-related macular degeneration: a meta-analysis. PLoS One. 2014;9(10):e109744.

Wiholm BE, Kelly JP, Kaufman D, Issaragrisil S, Levy M anderson T, et al. Relation of aplastic anaemia to use of chloramphenicol eye drops in two international case–control studies. BMJ. 1998;316(7132):666.

Wu L, Martinez-Castellanos MA, Quiroz-Mercado H, Arevalo JF, Berrocal MH, Farah ME, et al. Twelve-month safety of intravitreal injections of bevacizumab (Avastin): results of the Pan-American Collaborative Retina Study Group (PACORES). Graefe's archive for clinical and experimental ophthalmology. Albrecht Von Graefes Arch Klin Exp Ophthalmol. 2008;246(1):81–7.

Zimmerman TJ, Wheeler TM. Miotics: side effects and ways to avoid them. Ophthalmology. 1982;89(1):76–80.

Chapter 15
Extemporaneously Used Drug Formulations for Ocular Emergencies

Thirumurthy Velpandian and Ujjalkumar S. Das

Abstract Extemporaneously compounded formulations are often used in regular ophthalmic practice. Dispensing drug for ophthalmic purposes require adequate skills and experience to customize formulations for individuals. Compounding ophthalmic formulations is a precise task requiring strict control over pH, osmolarity, sterility and knowledge about their stability. This chapter covers benefits of extemporaneously compounded formulations, regulatory requirements of compounding pharmacy, components of ophthalmic formulations, requirements for active/auxiliary ingredients, sterilization procedures, packaging, cost effectiveness, related risk factors and stability of compounded formulations etc.

15.1 Introduction

Extemporaneously dispensed drug formulations are in use for a long time in ophthalmic practice and pharmacists/apothecaries have been involved in compounding of these agents. Unlike other areas of therapeutics, requirements for ophthalmologists are much different, and many of them are not available commercially. There is a lack of sizable market for these agents due to which, pharmaceutical companies do not pay much of attention toward these formulations and their innovations. As most of the extemporaneously dispensed formulations are meant for external application, lack of knowledge regarding their pharmaceutical stability in aqueous solutions for the extended period of time is a major hurdle. Commonly dispensed drugs in hospital pharmacy are meant for immediate usage; therefore, usually they are not

T. Velpandian, BPharm, MS(Pharmacol), PhD (✉) • U.S. Das, MPharm
Ocular Pharmacology and Pharmacy, Dr. Rajendra Prasad Centre for Ophthalmic Sciences, All India Institute of Medical Sciences, New Delhi, India
e-mail: tvelpandian@hotmail.com

T. Velpandian (ed.), *Pharmacology of Ocular Therapeutics*,
DOI 10.1007/978-3-319-25498-2_15

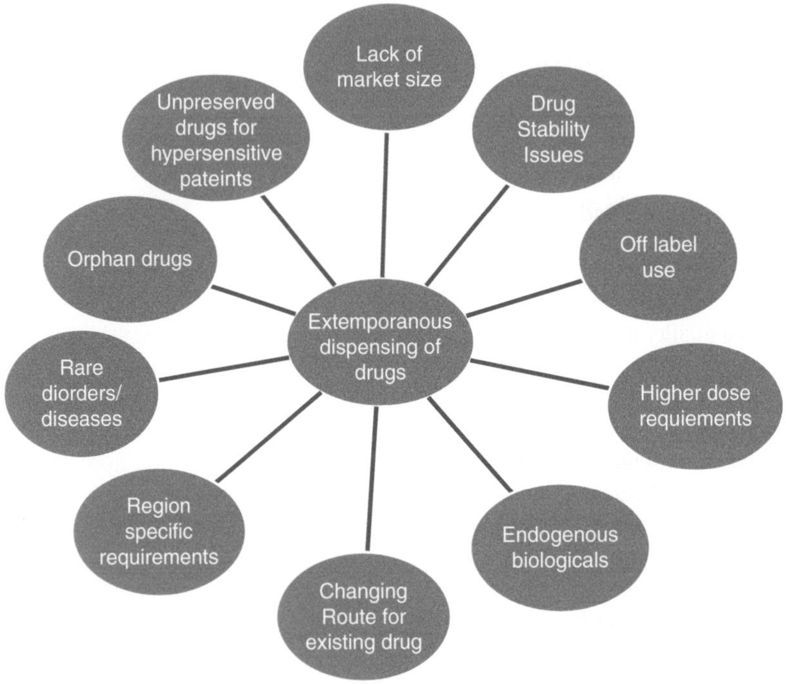

Fig. 15.1 Necessities of extemporaneously dispensed drug formulations for ocular therapeutics

preserved. A hospital attached with a good pharmacy dispensing facility with trained pharmacists in ophthalmic preparations is essential for such attempts while considering the dispensing practice. The possible reasons compelling for extemporaneously prepared ocular formulations are shown in the Fig. 15.1.

Considering the eye as an unique organ, understanding of its structure is very essential to develop ophthalmic dosage forms. Medications for ocular diseases have been developed as a special category of drug formulations, namely, ophthalmic products. It requires specific considerations during formulation optimization regarding sterility, stability, compatibility, tonicity, and other physicochemical characteristics relevant to sympathetic understanding of structure of the eye. In spite of commercially available branded ophthalmic drug products, the standard manner of compounding the drug products is another choice through the services of compounding pharmacists (Yuen et al. 2002).

Some examples of compounded substances used in ophthalmology are bevacizumab prepared for intravitreal injection, mitomycin C for surface neoplasms, fortified antibiotic drops used to treat corneal ulcers, and autologous serum or serum tears for the treatment of dry eye (Daniels 2010).

Although pharmaceutical industry has been involved in enhancing the armamentarium of ophthalmic preparations, extemporaneous compounding is often necessary for the successful treatment of specific ocular emergency cases (Giam et al. 2012).

In recent years the uses of extemporaneously compounded ophthalmic drug formulations have remarkably increased. It represents the growing knowledge of extemporaneously compounded ophthalmic drug formulations and attempts to standardize these products by suggesting strengths, routes of administration, appropriate vehicles, and methods for their preparation (Buurma et al. 2003). It is still now solely based on the experience and proficiency of compounding pharmacists on how to make them available in a ready-to-use form for patients. Ophthalmic preparations compounded in the way purely based on experience present a risk factor regarding effective assessment of quality and efficacy of the finally compounded product. It is an utmost important duty of pharmacists to ensure the compounded product will be of desired quality and stable for its indicated shelf life (Spark 2014).

According to the leading professional organizations for ophthalmology professionals (Tortora and Grabowski 2002), it is also imperative to have certain ophthalmic drugs handy in the ambulatory setting. Of course, ophthalmologists are not the only clinicians who use medications from compounding pharmacies. For years, many other medical practices, such as ambulatory surgery, orthopedic surgeries, pain management, pediatrics, etc., have relied on compounding pharmacies to supply frequently needed sterile drugs. Whenever the drug has been prescribed according to the best knowledge of physicians, it seems to be an evidence-based practice. When a drug formulation is prescribed to a patient, it is therapy, whereas, when a new drug or in a novel manner of administration, a particular drug formulation at specific strength/dosage is prescribed by clinicians, it is research. Extemporaneous preparations are generally being compounded to meet specific purposes in clinical trials.

In certain ocular emergencies, waiting or delay in treatment while waiting for extemporaneously prepared formulations might get into adverse consequence as shown in the Table 15.1.

One size cannot fill the requirement of particular medication for all patients; this is true in medicine as well (Spark 2014). Pharmaceutical industry produces medicines having a limited range of doses and dosage forms which meet the needs of most of the people, but there are some people who require drug/dosage forms that are not manufactured. When licensed manufactured pharmaceutical products do not meet a person's medicine requirements, then products prepared specifically for them in a pharmacy (extemporaneous preparations) can only fill the inevitability (IACP 2014; Williams et al. 2013).

The intention of this chapter is to explore the implications of extemporaneously prepared ophthalmic drug formulations in the treatment of several ocular diseases. It intends to provide a detail insight into the basic principle involved in extemporaneous ophthalmic preparations, its need, typical issues encountered in the compounding, and benefits in current therapeutics relevant to specific ocular emergency cases. This chapter focuses on different aspects, and physicochemical factors associated with its compounding, evaluation of its quality, safety, efficacy, and other critical parameters and stringent conditions required for its manufacturing in hospitals have been discussed. Future prospects of extemporaneous drug formulations have been discussed for better advancement of pharmacy practice toward the patient care.

Table 15.1 Outcomes of delayed treatment in ophthalmology practice

Drug	Recommended indications	Result of delayed treatment
Intravitreal antibiotics	Endophthalmitis	Permanent loss of vision and even loss of the eye itself
Fortified topical antibiotics	Bacterial corneal ulcers	Corneal perforation, corneal scarring, or partial or complete blindness within a short period
Intravitreal vascular endothelial growth factor (VEGF) inhibitors (e.g., bevacizumab)	Neovascularization, neovascular glaucoma (immediate and aggressive treatment is imperative)	Complete loss of vision
Mitomycin C	Treatment of failing glaucoma filtration procedures and intraoperative treatment at the time of glaucoma filtration surgery	Fibrosis, scarring, and blindness
Combination dilating drops	Diagnostic use in pediatric patients	Difficulty in receiving multiple eye drops and their related toxicity (especially pediatric patients)

15.2 Extemporaneous Ophthalmic Drug Formulations

The word "extemporaneous" is derived from the Latin *extempore* which is referring to *in accordance with the needs of the moment*. Extemporaneous dispensing is the science of medicinal preparations as a result of there being no commercially available medicinal product or required form of a medicinal product for the treatment of a patient. In other words, compounding can be referred as patient-specific production of medicinal substances rather than commercially manufactured drug products (Houck 2005).

"Extemporaneous compounding is defined as the preparation, mixing, assembling, packaging, and labeling of a medicinal product based on a prescription order from a licensed practitioner for the individual patient." The lack of commercially available formulations for patients with specific needs poses a challenge to gain access to the medicinal product in distinct form. This qualifies as off-license use of a medicine, whereby a licensed medicine is reformulated into a preparation that is made acceptable for the needs of the patient (Shargel 1997; Aquilina 2013; USP convention 2011).

"Good Manufacturing Practices" are the guidelines that pharmacists and manufacturers must follow to guarantee that a product is extemporaneously compounded appropriately (NABP 1993). Getting an approval for drugs for ocular specific personalized indication is a very difficult task, due to this extemporaneous preparations help in providing available medications as per need of individual by doing preparation of sterile formulations in aseptic conditions.

15.3 Benefits and Its Utility in Ophthalmology

Many of the medications commonly used in ophthalmology practice are either not available commercially as required by prescribers or do not have FDA approval for particular indication to be used in ocular case which explains why a required ophthalmic drug might not be manufactured as given below (Stokowski 2013; McElhiney 2013):

1. The product might not be stable enough or have a long enough shelf life to make it feasible to produce on a commercial scale. Some compounded antibiotic ophthalmic preparations (topicals and intraocular injections) are prepared from commercially available injections, but the stability of the drug in the solution or vehicle may only be 14 days or less when refrigerated.
2. Patients don't always tolerate the commercial products, usually due to the preservatives in case of pediatric ophthalmology and may need a compounded preparation, for example, benzalkonium chloride.
3. Some dyes are not commercially available, such as brilliant blue G, and compounders who specialize in high-risk compounded sterile preparations are needed to meet these needs of the ophthalmologists.
4. Concentration matters in case of ophthalmic products as per physician. A few commercially available antibiotic ophthalmic products are not concentrated or strong enough to treat a severe infection, so the pharmacist may have to prepare a fortified antibiotic ophthalmic solution that has a higher dose of drug and can be effective against a severe infection. For example, sodium ascorbate 10 % w/v is needed to treat corneal alkali burn.
5. Economics (for the drug manufacturer) may be a factor. It simply may not be profitable for a manufacturer to produce the ophthalmic on a commercial scale or for every class of patients.

15.3.1 Categories of Ophthalmic Products That Must Be Compounded (Stokowski 2013)

1. Formulations or combinations of drugs that are not commercially available. Examples are combination antimicrobial drops and combination anesthetic and dilating agents.
2. Patient-specific formulations that must be compounded individually. Examples are autologous serum eye drops that are compounded using the patient's own serum. Moreover formulations might also require the removal of ingredients that are not tolerated by the patient such as preservatives and antioxidants/bisulfites.
3. Discontinued yet still needed drugs. Drug makers might have discontinued the production of a drug because the market for the product is too small and it is no longer economically feasible to produce.

4. Repackaging of doses of available drugs. When the available dosage form is not appropriate for routine clinical need, drugs are fractionated and relabeled for use by clinicians (e.g., bevacizumab).
5. Manufacturing shortages. When critical drugs are in short supply at the point of manufacture, drugs can be compounded from bulk ingredients.
6. Ophthalmology practitioners have turned to compounded agents for economic reason. In the case of a drug frequently compounded for ophthalmic use – bevacizumab – cost entered into the equation.

15.3.2 Common Examples of Extemporaneously Dispensed Drugs

Various categories of drugs for ocular use are being dispensed in the hospital pharmacies which include several topical and intravitreal formulations given in Table 15.2.

15.3.3 Cost-Effective Dispensing of Bevacizumab (Anti-VEGF Antibody)

Anti-vascular endothelial growth factors (anti-VEGF) have revolutionized the treatment of many retinal diseases. The VEGF inhibitor bevacizumab (AVASTIN, Genentech, Inc.) was approved by the FDA for the treatment of colorectal cancer in 2004. Bevacizumab is a full-length, humanized monoclonal antibody directed against all the biologically active isoforms of vascular endothelial growth factor (VEGFA). Its potential for the treatment of ocular pathologies, such as choroidal neovascularization, age-related macular degeneration (AMD), diabetic retinopathy (DR), and retinal vein occlusion, has been well recognized by the ophthalmologists (Salvatore and Focke 2007).

Although found to be safe and effective in clinical ophthalmology practice, the ophthalmic use of bevacizumab comes under the off-label use, and therefore not manufactured in doses required for intravitreal injection (Wong and Kyle 2006). Subsequent to bevazicumab, ranibizumab (another anti VEGF antibody) was approved for ocular use by FDA (Biswas et al. 2011). Both of the agents were subsequently found to be equally clinically effective in treating AMD, but a huge difference between them is the cost. The per-dose cost of Avastin is \$30–\$50, but for Lucentis, it is \$2000. The reason for the discrepancy is that a 4-mL single-dose vial of Avastin can be divided by a compounding pharmacy into as many as 10–18 aliquots (depending on the techniques used) for individual injection, whereas Lucentis is supplied in the volume needed for a single injection for ophthalmic use (Schmucker et al. 2012; Velpandian et al. 2007).

The price difference was largely responsible for the decision by many ophthalmology practices to obtain their supplies of bevacizumab for intravitreal injection

Table 15.2 Common intravitreal medications (Biju 2007)

S. No.	Drug	Dosage strength	Indications
1.	Bevacizumab	1.25 mg/0.05 mL	Wet Age-related macular degeneration
2.	Ganciclovir	2.0 mg/0.1 mL	CMV retinitis in HIV patients, varicella-zoster retinitis, acute retinal necrosis
3.	Foscarnet	2.4 mg/0.1 mL	
4.	Vancomycin	1 mg/0.1 mL	Gram-positive bacterial endophthalmitis
5.	Ceftazidime	2.25 mg/0.1 mL	Gram-negative bacterial endophthalmitis
6.	Amikacin	0.4 mg/0.1 mL	
7.	Amphotericin B	0.1 mL of 5–10 μg/mL	Fungal Endophthalmitis
8.	Dexamethasone	0.4 mg/0.1 mL	Bacterial endophthalmitis
9.	Triamcinolone acetonide	0.1 mL of 4 mg/mL	Diabetic Macular edema, central retinal and branch retinal vein occlusions, wet age-related macular degeneration

from national compounding pharmacies, rather than using single-dose vials of ranibizumab. A recent study provided support for this decision, finding that given their similarities in efficacy, bevacizumab is more cost-effective than ranibizumab (Rogers et al. 2013; Velpandian et al. 2007). Compounding pharmacies prepare batches of bevacizumab in single-dose syringes/ampoules, in accordance with the prescription and make the aliquot available to ophthalmology specialists directly. This allows ophthalmologists to have the sterile, dispensed drug in hand when patients need unscheduled intravitreal injections and is essential for the provision of prompt, efficient, and effective patient care.

15.4 Comparison of FDA-Approved Branded/Generics and Compounded Drug Products

As such extemporaneously compounded drug products are not under any regulatory bodies like FDA, but at the same time, its quality is solely governed by the skill of compounding pharmacists, principles of pharmacy practice, and facilities available. State Board of Pharmacy is the only regulatory body oversees pharmacy practice including drug compounding. In the countries where there is no specific regulatory requirements regarding sterile compounding requirements, they must voluntarily adopt the requirements set by other regulatory agencies like USFDA for maintaining their standards and patient's safety. By necessity, compounded drugs are made under standards that are less stringent than those applied to FDA-approved products but, without any compromise on sterility and without adding any other active pharmaceutical ingredient (API). The branded products are FDA approved for particular

Table 15.3 Key differences between US FDA-approved and compounded drugs (Sellers and Utian 2012)

	FDA-approved drug	Compounded drug
Made "extemporaneously" after receipt of prescription	No	Yes
Reviewed by FDA for quality, safety, and efficacy prior to marketing/prescribing	Yes	No
Manufactured under federal GMP regulations	Yes	No
Labeling for safe prescribing and use required and regulated	Yes	No
Sterile products adhere to federal GMP sterility requirements	Yes	No
Benefit-risk assessment	Conducted by FDA at population level	Conducted by prescriber at patient level

Adapted from Sellers and Utian (2012) with permission
GMP good manufacturing practice

indication as well as they are under strict regulations for any adverse events reported. With the development of industrial manufacturing, the pharmacies transitioned into dispensaries which are under oversight and regulation. Therefore, extemporaneously prepared ophthalmic product must be prepared in a highly recommended facility and guidelines documented by FDA/USP for sterile compounding (Glass and Haywood 2006). Generally, extemporaneous formulations lack studies to document stability, bioavailability, pharmacokinetics, pharmacodynamics, and safety (Nahata and Allen 2008) unlike branded as well as generic drug products are systematically evaluated. Extemporaneously prepared drug formulations of already marketed drug products are exempted from reporting any adverse event to the FDA which is mandatory for FDA-approved products.

Following are the brief details given (Table 15.3) of key differences between FDA-approved (branded and generics) and compounded drug products.

15.4.1 Regulations in the USA and Other Countries

Government regulations must be implemented on all compounding pharmacies for their better functions and control standardization. Compounding pharmacies and pharmacists should be regulated by their individual State Board of Pharmacy, FDA, and the Drug Enforcement Agency (DEA) (Ann 2013; IACP 2012). The United States Pharmacopeia (USP <797>) sets the national standards for the process, testing, and verification of any medication prepared for administration to patients. Pharmacies with the Pharmacy Compounding Accreditation Board (PCAB) accreditation status have demonstrated that they meet the highest possible standards and are recognized as having another level of quality assurance for both sterile and non-sterile compounded preparations (Cabaleiro 2007, 2008; Murry 2008). Although, the guidelines are very clear in USFDA, other drug regulatory agencies in various countries are having their own regulatory methods and distribution of powers among various enforcement authorities on compounding pharmacies.

15.5 Ophthalmic Compounding/Dispensing

Extemporaneous compounding of ophthalmic drugs needs to be done with strict compliance of USFDA (USP <797> guidelines 2012). The ophthalmic preparations are sterile preparations according to the USP <797> standards and must be prepared in the sound sterile environment risks to patient health and safety are higher if sterile agents are improperly compounded. Drugs meant for ophthalmic treatment must ensure its sterility, otherwise contaminated ophthalmic medication with bacteria, fungi or particulate matters can further worsen the patient's ocular condition.

In ophthalmic compounding and dispensing, the formula (components) for the compounded medication is very important. Components that might be safe for oral or parenteral use could be toxic or irritating to the eye. To make the administration of the ophthalmic preparation comfortable for the patient, the pH and tonicity must be adjusted. Ophthalmic products should be prepared by taking into account the perfect balance between formulation characteristics (pH, osmolarity, preservation) and environmental factors (clean room, aseptic handling, and trained pharmacy professionals). The following factors given in Fig. 15.2 must be taken into account prior to make/dispense ophthalmic formulations extemporaneously.

Fig. 15.2 Illustrate common requirements of ophthalmic preparations

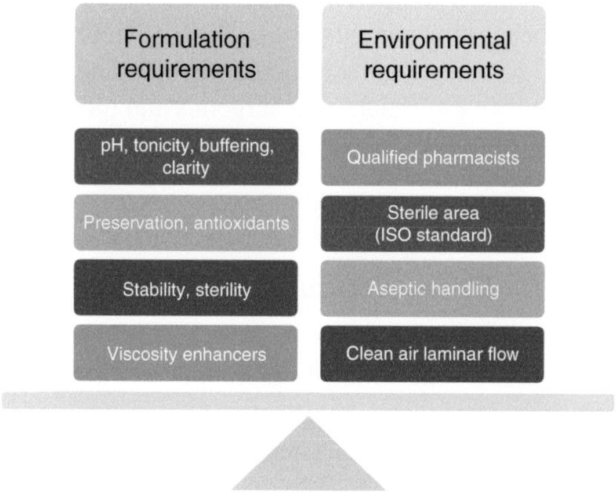

15.5.1 Dispensing Laboratory (Pharmacy): Minimum Requirements of the Hospital Pharmacy for Adopting Extemporaneous Dispensing

A suitable dispensing facility in the pharmacy would be having sterile room fitted with a centralized HEPA/ULPA filters or suitable filters to get clean air. These clean rooms maintain particulate-free air by using aforesaid filters employing laminar or turbulent airflow principles. The construction of these rooms must be done according to the laid down conditions of the state drug regulatory bodies like USFDA or EU. As ocular drugs are recognized as solutions meant for ocular use are sterile in nature, this unit must accompany a moist heat, dry heat, ethylene oxide (ETO) sterilizing instruments. The water used for the formulations used in pharmacy must meet the standards of water for injection according to the pharmacopeia. Generally, freshly distilled water is used for the formulations in dispensing pharmacy, and the use of deionized high purity water prepared by reverse osmosis systems is still a matter of debate for its substitution in the place of distilled water unless it reaches required quality in terms of chemical, microbiological, and pyrogen test of water for Injection according to the pharmacopeia (USFDA 2015 & CHSP 1996).

15.5.2 Components of Ophthalmic Formulations

Ophthalmic solutions are sterile solutions that are compounded and packed for installation into the eyes. It provides more uniform dosage forms. In addition to their sterility, their preparation requires the careful consideration of pharmaceutical factors as the need for antimicrobial agents, isotonicity, buffering, viscosity, and proper packaging. Safe, sterile compounded medications have long been essential tools available to ophthalmologists for urgent treatment of eye diseases and conditions, benefitting patients (Parke 2013). These products are compounded in the most sterile and safest manner possible in ensuring the safe availability of these medications for eye physicians and surgeons and the patients they serve (Nahata and Allen 2008).

15.5.3 Desired Qualities of Ophthalmic Solutions

The properties of an ideal ophthalmic solution are described below. These are not just desired properties but absolute requirements for ophthalmic solutions. Achieving all of these objectives simultaneously is sometimes impossible, and therefore appropriate compromises can be made, or another therapeutic option may be necessary (Dale et al. 2013; Sandle 2014):

A. *Sterility and clarity*: The preparation and packaging should be done in a sterile environment such as a laminar flow hood or a barrier isolator. A sterile, particle-free solution can be achieved by one of the following methods:

    1. The solution should be prepared in a manner similar to a parenteral preparation, using aseptic technique with sterile parenteral drug products as the solution ingredients and packaging the solution in a clean, particle-free, sterile container.
    2. It should be prepared by using non-sterile but high-quality ingredients and filtered using a 0.22- or 0.45-micron bacterial filter/0.1-micron mycoplasma-free filter into a dispensing container that is clean, particle-free, and sterile.
    3. If an autoclave is available, terminal steam sterilization can be used. In this case, the solution may be prepared using non-sterile but high-quality ingredients and packaged in an appropriate clean, particle-free container that is stable to the elevated temperature and pressure needed for steam sterilization. The preparation is then autoclaved in the dispensing container. Quality control procedures for steam sterilization must be used, for example, validation of the autoclave cycle through the use of biological and other indicators, as well as the use of monitoring devices that track and record time, temperature, and pressure. Since steam sterilization uses elevated temperature and pressure, consideration of drug stability is important before using this method.

       All ophthalmic solutions should be clear and free from any particulate matter. Foreign particles in an ophthalmic solution can cause damage to the eye by causing abrasions to the cornea and the membranes of the eyelids or other possible diseases such as endophthalmitis in case of intravitreal injections. Filtering the solutions with a 0.22-micron filter should remove all harmful particulate matter. The use of HPMC can improve the clarity of ophthalmic solutions. Adding Polysorbate 20 and Polysorbate 80, in a maximum concentration of 1 %, can also improve the clarity of ophthalmic solutions. Polysorbates, also known as polyoxyethylene sorbitan fatty acid esters, are solubilizing agents that help dissolve poorly soluble ingredients.

B. *Preservation*: When the solution is dispensed in a multidose container that is to be used over a period of time longer than 24 h or more, a preservative must be added to ensure microbiologic safety over the period of use. It is necessary to add preservative in the ophthalmic solutions to prevent microbiological contamination during use in ocular diseases. Usually preservative-free dispensed ophthalmic solutions should be used at earliest.
C. *pH*: Although solutions with the same pH as lacrimal fluid (7.4) are ideal, the outer surfaces of the eye tolerate a larger range, 3.5–8.5. The normal useful range to prevent corneal damage is 6.5–8.5. The final pH of the solution is often a compromise, because many ophthalmic drugs have limited solubility and stability at the desired pH of 7.4. Buffers or pH-adjusting agents or vehicles can be added to adjust and stabilize the pH at a desired level. Ophthalmic solutions are

ordinarily buffered at the pH of maximum stability of the drug(s) they contain. The buffers are included to minimize any change in pH during the storage life of the drug; this can result from absorbed carbon dioxide from the air or from hydroxyl ions from a glass container. Changes in pH can affect the solubility and stability of drugs; consequently, it is important to minimize fluctuations in pH. The buffer system should be designed sufficient to maintain the pH throughout the expected shelf life of the product, but with a low buffer capacity so that when the ophthalmic solution is instilled into the eye, the buffer system of the tears will rapidly bring the pH of the solution back to that of the tears. Low concentrations of buffer salts are used to prepare buffers of low buffer capacity.

D. *Isotonicity*: Solutions that are isotonic with tears are preferred. An amount equivalent to 0.9 % NaCl is ideal for comfort and should be used when possible. The eye can tolerate tonicities within the equivalent range of 0.6–2 % NaCl without discomfort. There are times when hypertonic ophthalmic solutions are necessary therapeutically or when the addition of an auxiliary agent required for reasons of stability supersedes the need for isotonicity. A hypotonic ophthalmic solution will require the addition of a substance (tonicity adjusting agent) to attain the proper tonicity range.

E. *Stability*: The stability of the ophthalmic formulation determines the therapeutic efficacy of drug product. As with all pharmaceutical solutions, ophthalmics must be chemically, physically, and microbiologically stable. It is the most intensive parameter toward the quality of ophthalmics. After every preparation, pharmacists should incorporate the beyond-use date on the compounded product.

F. *Therapeutic efficacy*: This is the only criteria which depends on the overall stability of active ingredient(s) in the product. The active ingredient(s) should be present in the most therapeutically effective form. This goal must often be compromised for reasons of solubility or stability of the active ingredient or patient comfort. For example, while many drugs are most active in their undissociated form, they are least soluble in this form. They may also be less stable at pH values that favor the undissociated form.

G. *Compatibility with the eye*: Most of the ingredients in ophthalmic solutions should be incorporated with prior knowledge of toxicity to the eye. The products should be free of chemicals or agents that cause allergy or toxicity to the sensitive membranes and tissues of the eye. Auxiliary agents, such as preservatives and antioxidants, should be added with care because many patients are sensitive to these substances. Before adding any auxiliary agent, it is recommended to check the history of patient about allergies and sensitivities.

Sourcing Bulk Drugs and Quality Control In the art of compounding, the most important aspect is the process to ensure the quality of the ingredients for compounding pharmacy. Unlike mass commercial production, in dispensing pharmacies, the bulk drug container needs to be opened multiple times for making small batches. Therefore, it is advised that the bulk drug must be immediately packed into multiple small airtight containers. Moreover, it is wise to check the bulk drug powders; it must be tested for infrared spectroscopy for its appropriateness at least once or twice in a year as per the standard operating procedure. The source of such drugs must be ensured that they comply with pharmacopoeial requirement and its material data sheet along with analysis.

15.5.4 Active Ingredients

The active ingredients used in ophthalmic liquids are available as pure powder, as sterile powder manufactured for parenteral administration, or as a sterile, parenteral solution of the desired ingredient. It is worth mentioning here that most of the ocular drugs are available as their corresponding salts. Therefore, one must remember to calculate their equivalent weight to the active drug component before making the formulation under extemporaneous prepared solutions. For example, homatropine HBr with the MW 356.25 g/mol must be calculated for its equivalence to homatropine having MW 275.34 g/mol unless otherwise specified.

15.5.5 Auxiliary Agents

Auxiliary agents added to ophthalmic solutions include buffers, tonicity adjustors, preservatives, antioxidants, and viscosity-inducing agents (Table 15.4).

15.5.6 Sterilization Procedures in Compounding Pharmacy

All ocular formulations are considered as sterile and have been treated like the way it has been treated for parenterals. Terminal sterilization is an ultimate parameter which makes most of the large volume and small volume parenterals to be sterile. However, for the drugs terminal sterilization can not be given for antibodies like bevacizumab maintaining aseptic zone right from the beginning of the initiation of process for dispensing.

Most of the cases, when vials are taken into compounding room, the main culprit for contamination comes from the carton boxes used for transportation. In order to maintain storing temperature, they are usually dispensed along with ice packs. Therefore, as soon as they are opened, they need to be surface cleaned with disinfectors like spirit or other suitable evaporable surface-sterilizing agents. Once the seal is broken, rubber seal needs to be surface sterilized with disinfectants. It is essential to leave for enough time to give right exposure time for the agents to sterilize the surface. In agents like umbilical cord serum or autologous serum or any other compounds having biological nature, it is wise to handle them aseptically and to use 0.22-micron sterile in-line filters before placing them in dispensing vials.

Table 15.4 List of various additives used in ophthalmic formulations (Hecht 2000)

Category	Examples
Buffers	Sorenson's phosphate buffer
	Citrate buffer
	Acetate buffer
	Boric acid buffer
Tonicity adjustors	Sodium chloride, sodium nitrate, sodium sulfate, dextrose, glycerol, propylene glycol, mannitol
Preservatives	Benzalkonium chloride (0.004–0.02 %)
	Benzethonium chloride (0.002–0.01 %)
	Chlorobutanol (0.5 %)
	Phenylmercuric acetate (0.001–0.01 %)
	Phenylmercuric nitrate (0.001–0.01 %)
	Thimerosal (0.005–0.02 %)
	Parahydroxybenzoates: Methyl paraben (0.1–0.2 %) Propyl paraben (0.02–0.04 %)
Antioxidants	Sodium bisulfite (0.01–0.5 %)
	Sodium metabisulfite (0.01–0.5 %)
	Thiourea (0.002–0.3 %)
	Disodium edetate (0.005–0.1 %)
Viscosity modifiers	Polyvinyl alcohol (0.1–4 %)
	Polyvinylpyrrolidone (0.1–2 %)
	Methylcellulose (0.2–2.5 %)
	Hydroxypropyl methylcellulose (0.2–2.5 %)
	Hydroxyethyl cellulose (0.2–2.5 %)
	Hydroxypropyl cellulose (0.2–2.5 %)
	Dextran 70 (0.1–3 %)
	Polyethylene glycol 400 (0.2–1 %)

15.5.7 *Packaging and Labeling of Ophthalmic Products*

Dropping vials meant for topical eye drops must have been made up of nontoxic high low-density polyethylene resin or polypropylene resin container having dropping nozzles and screwable cap with piercing tip. All the parts of the vials are usually packed appropriately and sterilized by either ^{60}Co gamma irradiation or by ethylene oxide gas sterilization using required protocols. These sterilizations must be accompanied by the use of indicator tapes to ensure the achievement of complete sterilization process. For its appropriate usage in laminar flow benches, they must be packed in small quantities and sealed in transparent polyethylene bags so that they can be used appropriately whenever there is a requirement of small quantity.

The pharmacist should dispense sterile ophthalmic products into multidose sterile container for packaging and labeling. If the patient is sensitive to the

Table 15.5 Sources of guidelines for aseptic processing

S. no.	Guidelines	References
1.	FDA Guidance for Industry 2004 on Drug Products Produced by Aseptic Processing	USFDA (2004)
2.	USP <1116> Microbiological Control and Monitoring of Aseptic Processing Environments	USP 35-NF30 <1116> (2012)
3.	ISO 13408 Aseptic Processing of Healthcare Products	ISO 13408–1 (1997)
4.	ISO 14698–1. Cleanrooms and Associated Controlled Environments–Biocontamination Control: Part 1: General Principles and Methods	ISO 14698–1 (2003)
5.	ISPE Baseline Guide to Sterile Manufacturing Facilities	ISPE (1999)

Adapted from Sandle et al. (2014) Sterile ophthalmic preparations and contamination control

preservative, it is possible to exempt by using preservative-free solution. FDA regulations for sterile ophthalmic products allow the use of unpreserved multi-dose packaging if it is packaged and well labeled to provide adequate efficacy and minimize the microbial contamination (21CFR 200.50).

15.5.8 Environmental Quality Monitoring

The final quality embedded in sterile ophthalmic formulations is the result of several attempts starting from quality status of the components incorporated, the process utilized, personnel performance, to the environmental conditions under which the dispensing is performed. The principal goal of environmental control is to achieve and maintain sterility and overall freedom from contamination (USP <797> 2012). Aseptic dispensing is an art for which well-qualified personnel (pharmacists) are required serving as an essential component in the pharmaceutical industry, hospital facility, and at clinical settings.

There are a number of guidelines available (Table 15.5) in relation to aseptic dispensing, the usual method of preparation of ophthalmic dosage forms. Aseptic processing is highly regulated, and there is considerable guidance in the US Code of Federal Regulations (CFR 21, such as CFR 21 Subpart C (211.42)), FDA documents, and in the EU GMP "Rules and Guidance for Pharmaceutical Manufacturers and Distributors" (Euradlex 2014).

15.6 Facility Design, Clean Rooms, and Aseptic Handling

Sterile pharmaceutical dispensing for ophthalmic formulations must be attempted in the facility specifically fabricated to have controlled atmosphere which is free from particulate matter microbial contamination (Sandle 2014). This clean room is

Table 15.6 Classification of Cleanrooms (USP <797> 2004) (International Organization of Standardization (ISO) Classification of Particulate Matter in Clean Room Air (limits are in particles 0.5 μm and larger per cubic meter (current ISO) and cubic feet (former Federal Standard No. 209E, FS209E)))

Class name		Particle Number (maximum limit)	
ISO class	U.S. FS 209E class	ISO, m^3	FS 209E, ft.^{3}
3	Class 1	35.2	1
4	Class 10	352	10
5	Class 100	3520	100
6	Class 1000	35,200	1000
7	Class 10,000	352,000	10,000
8	Class 100,000	3,520,000	100,000

expected to have separate zones where particulate matter and microbial load are controlled to specific limits according to the classification of clean roams in ISO standards (Table 15.6).

In these facilities, air filtration and temperature control are achieved by dedicated systems. For filtering air, high-efficiency particulate air filters (HEPA) are used to control air dynamics. HEPA filters are known to have the efficiency to remove particulate matter which is having more than 0.3 μm in size thereby having the efficiency to remove 99.97 % and has the probability of having particles having the size lesser than 0.3 μm contributing to 0.03 %. An ISO Class 5 environment (approximately equivalent to EU and WHO GMP Grade A or Class 100) is required for aseptic filling/dispensing of ophthalmic products (Table 15.6). To reach these requirements, temperature-controlled HEPA-filtered airflow is designed to dilute and remove airborne particles. Airflow adjustments according to floor design can lead to an improvement with better particle counts (Sundstrom et al. 2009).

As per the USP guidelines, sterile product preparation facilities utilize laminar airflow workbenches to provide an adequate critical site environment. This is either an enclosed barrier unidirectional airflow device or within an isolator. All sterile compounding in a community pharmacy/hospital pharmacy should be performed in clean room inside the laminar airflow hood. These hoods are designed to reduce the risk of airborne contamination during the preparation of sterile products. Laminar airflow hoods have two basic functions, namely, (1) to filter bacteria and exogenous materials from the air and (2) to maintain constant airflow out of the hood to prevent contaminated room air from entering the hood. Airflow velocity determines the filtering capacity of the hood. If airflow is reduced, the filter is presumed to be clogged with contaminants and must be cleaned. The airflow velocity of 0.3 m/s and 0.45 m/s for vertical and horizontal laminar hood, respectively, is recommended (USP <797> 2004). The clean room and laminar flow hood must be tested on regular basis for bacteria and endotoxin.

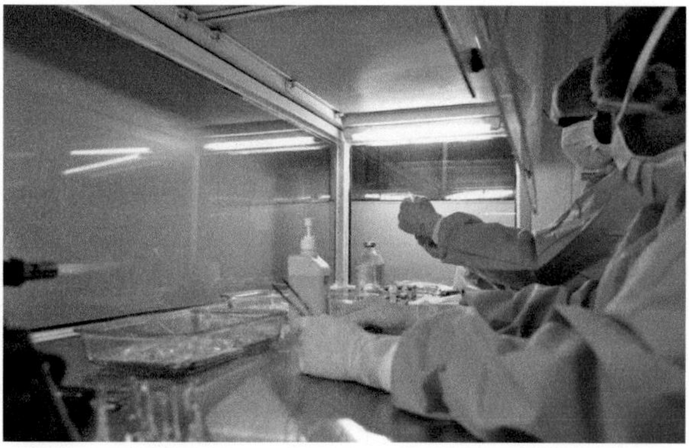

Fig. 15.3 Compounding pharmacy setup (Photograph Courtesy, Dr. RPCPharmacy, AIIMS, New Delhi (India))

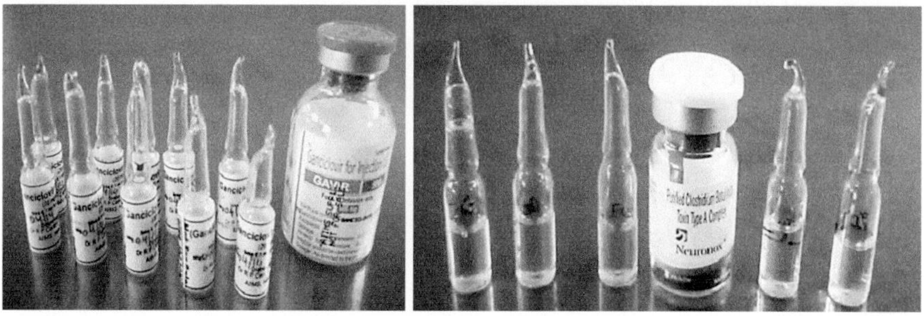

Fig. 15.4 Ganciclovir and botulinum toxin (Botox) aseptically dispensed in ampoules in smaller aliquots to enable intravitreal and intramuscular injections (Photograph Courtesy, Dr. RPC Pharmacy, AIIMS, New Delhi (India))

Engineering controls reduce the potential for airborne contamination in workspaces by limiting the amount and size of contaminants in the processing environment. Primary engineering controls are used and generally include horizontal flow clean benches, vertical flow clean benches, biological safety cabinets, and barrier isolators. Primary environmental control must provide at least ISO Class 5 quality of air to which sterile ingredients and components are directly exposed.

In aseptic dispensing, the process of preparation of ophthalmic products involves the careful handling of sterile materials in a controlled environment to control microbial and particulate contamination to acceptable levels. Careful considerations should be given to aseptic operations. These include the class of clean rooms, areas where the product is transferred into the aseptic processing area and where and how the product is to be dispensed. Regular monitoring of clean room, sterility, and contamination control is necessary to achieve the quality products through aseptic processing (Figs. 15.3 and 15.4).

15.7 Potential Risks Associated with Extemporaneous Compounding

Extemporaneous compounding of medicines poses significant risk, as the risks of using unlicensed medicines are combined with inherent risks associated with the pharmaceutical compounding process. Ophthalmic products compounded by trained pharmacy professionals have been associated with quality defects, infectious disease outbreaks, and other adverse events. In order to demonstrate the risks associated with compounding ophthalmic products, it is essential to understand the major factors that would affect the final quality of compounded products and at the same time create trouble to the patients. The major factors include compounding error (personnel), adverse reaction to any of the inactive ingredient, use of substandard drug quality, contamination during use, sterility issue, and use of contaminated products that ultimately leads to ocular complications especially during postoperative period. Other possibilities for the risks are non-validated stability of the product and packaging error.

15.7.1 Extemporaneous Ophthalmic Formulations and Its Related Risks

Pharmaceutical compounding is explored as being a very essential part of emergency care in ophthalmology practices. It has been utilized for preparing customized medications to meet the specific needs of physicians and patients both. Examples of commonly used ophthalmic medications that must be prepared by a compounding pharmacy are fortified antibiotics, preservative-free formulations, discontinued medications, and specialty items such as bevacizumab (Avastin) for intravitreal injection. It provides the better therapeutic option in cost-effective manner such as an improved therapeutic outcome resulted from compounded ophthalmic treatment (e.g., bevacizumab dispensed in multiple aliquots containing single dose).

Pharmaceutical compounding is also having higher potential of risks to patient's safety despite of its advantages. Poor pharmacy practices can result in contamination or in products that do not possess the required sterility and quality. Compounding pharmacies are not subject to the same regulations as large-scale drug manufacturers (Stevens and Matheson,1992).

15.7.2 Recent Outbreaks of Extemporaneously Compounded Products

Noncompliance with recognized standards, poor aseptic techniques, and contamination during dispensing are the most likely cause of the outbreaks (Table 15.7). The key to preventing these major catastrophic events depends on the

Table 15.7 List of recent outcomes of contaminated pharmacy-dispensed medications

Year	Compounded product	Ocular emergency	Source of dispensing	References
2013	Intravitreal injections of bevacizumab; repackaged into single-use syringes	5 patients developed severe endophthalmitis	Compounding pharmacy, Georgia	Lowes (2013)
2012	Vitrectomy with epiretinal peeling using brilliant blue G or had received intravitreal injections of triamcinolone	33 cases of fungal endophthalmitis; fungal species, including *Fusarium incarnatum-equiseti* species complex, *Rhodotorula*, *Bullera*, *Pseudomonas*, and *Enterobacter* were found in unopened vials	Compounding pharmacy, Florida	CDC (MMWR) (2012b)
2012	Epidural injections of 3 lots of preservative-free methylprednisolone acetate	461 people diagnosed with fungal meningitis and other infections and 32 individuals had died	New England Compounding Center (NECC), a compounding pharmacy in Framingham	CDC (MMWR) (2012a)
2011	Repackaged intravitreal injections of Avastin	12 patients developed streptococcal endophthalmitis; some had lost their vision	Compounding pharmacy, Miami	Goldberg et al. (2012), USFDA (2011)
2011	Injectable drug products	33 eye surgery patients in seven states suffered a rare fungal eye infection; partial to sever vision loss	Compounding pharmacy, Ocala, Fla	USFDA (2012)
2005	Trypan blue ophthalmic solution	Bacterial contamination of product leads to endophthalmitis	Veterans affairs hospital, Washington, D.C.	Wynkoop (2012)

implementation of and strict adherence to USP <797>guidelines for sterile product compounding (Staes et al. 2013).

15.7.3 *Increased Risks Associated with the Use of Ophthalmic Drugs in Connection with Surgery*

The risk of contamination and infection associated with the use of ophthalmic products during postoperative settings has been reported recently. The risk of infection is high when using same eye drop multidose bottle for both eyes. Based on the evidences, CDERs put forward the concept of the use of separate bottle for each eye recently that will help to minimize the risk of infection in post-surgical settings (CDER 2012).

15.7.4 Microbiological Contamination of Ophthalmic Products during Use

The ophthalmic products are highly associated with contamination by potentially harmful microorganisms during use. They should maintain sterility after opening since it would impact more on the stability of the product (21CFR 200.50. USFDA 2014).

In account to render the product to be remained sterile after opening the container, preservatives are included in the final formulation to hinder the microbial growth. However, such products may become contaminated in all approved configuration of multidose ophthalmic products. The reported rates of microbial contamination of ophthalmic products range from 0.07 to 35.8 % (Nentwich et al. 2007). Major types of bacteria which profoundly isolated from contaminated bottles include typical conjunctival flora (coagulase negative staphylococcus and diphtheroids) and other potential pathogens such as *Staphylococcus aureus* and *Pseudomonas* (Jokl et al. 2007; Rahman et al. 2006; Geyer et al. 1995; Livingstone et al. 1998).

The potential sites of contamination are the nozzle tip, cap, inside head space, and drop expelled from the bottle (Schein et al. 1992). The expelled volume from bottle during use through the way of nozzle would create it to be moist which serves as a reservoir for microbial contamination. The contaminating microorganisms may be introduced when this moist nozzle comes in contact with patients during use who inadvertently touch their eyes or skin with the dropper or tip of the bottle, which could contaminate the container. These microbes may subsequently then transmigrate to other portion of the bottle and bottle contents (Nentwich et al. 2007). There are other possibilities of introducing contaminating microorganisms when the bottle comes into contact with the fingers, lids, conjunctiva, or cornea. Microbial contamination has been reported in various products including artificial tears, lubricants, intraocular pressure (IOP) lowering medications, and anti-inflammatory products for postoperative use. Microbial contamination has been found in ophthalmic solutions that contain preservatives and those that do not (Seal 2007).

15.7.5 Infection Risk Associated with Eye Surgery

Eye surgery is often the most sterile operation conducted which made efforts to minimize the risk of postoperative infections or contamination (Taban et al. 2005).

Since the most natural protective barrier of the eye (most cases cornea) has been breached during surgical procedure, ocular tissues are at higher risk of infection after post-surgical conditions. Different types of eye surgeries have been taken into account for various purposes which are listed in Table 15.8. Endophthalmitis is one of the major postoperative infections to be caused after cataract surgery (Wycoff et al. 2010).

The patients are at higher risk of infection after surgery together with the use of contaminated eye drops that have been linked to severe adverse events which can result into blindness as well. There are some reported cases of infections which are due to the contaminated eye drops used in eye at post-surgical settings, for example, bacterial keratitis after the use of prednisolone acetate, timolol, and natamycin eye drops (Templeton 1982; Krishnan and Sengupta 2009; Schein et al. 1988). These issues have led the FDA to issue warning letters against the use of compounded products, and many have raised questions about the advantage of compounded products after ocular surgery (Schein et al. 1992).

15.7.6 Compounding Quality Act 2013 (USFDA 2015)

Recently, FDA has initiated new regulations to regulate compounding pharmacy in the states under new act, namely, Compounding Act 2013 title 1 "Drugs Quality and Security Act" legislation that contains important provisions relating to the oversight of compounding of human drugs. It has been noted by FDA that number of unwanted events (Table 15.8) due to contaminated compounded products have been enhanced tremendously. These events are due to poor control and regulations in the practice of pharmacy of the state board pharmacies (Drug Quality and Security Act 2013).

Table 15.8 Various types and rates of post-operative infections associated with ocular surgeries

Type of surgery	Reported rates and types of infection	Reference
Cataract surgery	Endophthalmitis	Taban et al. (2005)
	0.327 % (1970)	
	0.158 % (1980)	
	0.087 % (1990)	
	0.265 % (2005)	
	0.028 % (2009)	Wycoff et al. (2010)
Corneal surgery	0.02–0.2 % infectious keratitis	
1. Photorefractive keratectomy	0.02 %, bacterial keratitis	Wroblewski et al. (2006)
2. LASIK	0.04 %, infectious keratitis	Llovet (2010)
3. Laser surface ablation	0.2 %, infectious keratitis	De Rojas (2011)
4. Oculoplastic surgery	0.04 %, infectious keratitis	Lee et al. (2009)

This new law creates a new section 503B in the Federal Food, Drug, and Cosmetic Act (FDCA). Under section 503B, a compounder can become an *outsourcing facility*. An outsourcing facility will be able to qualify for exemptions from the FDA approval requirements and the requirement to label products with adequate directions for use, but not the exemption from CGMP requirements. Outsourcing facilities:

1. Must comply with CGMP requirements
2. Will be inspected by FDA according to a risk-based schedule
3. Must meet certain other conditions, such as reporting adverse events and providing FDA with certain information about the products they compound

FDA anticipates that state boards of pharmacy will continue their oversight and regulation of the practice of pharmacy, including traditional pharmacy compounding. It also intends to cooperate with state authorities to address pharmacy compounding activities to prevent them from any violation of the FDCA act.

15.8 Stability of Extemporaneous Drug Formulations

Stability is defined as the extent to which a preparation retains, within specified limits and throughout its period of storage and use, the same properties and characteristics that it possessed at the time of compounding (ICH 2003). The drug product dispensed should contain expiration date according to USFDA to assure its appropriateness (Expiration dating, 21 CFR 211.137) (USFDA 2015). The beyond-use date/expiration date is the date after which a compounded preparation is not to be used and is determined from the date the preparation is compounded. Because compounded preparations are intended for administration immediately or following short-term storage, their beyond-use dates may be assigned based on criteria different from those applied to assigning expiration dates to manufactured drug products.

It is an essential criterion for the pharmaceutical formulation to remain stable for the entire shelf life. The stability of extemporaneously formulated ophthalmic preparations is being closely correlated to their therapeutic efficacy. Extemporaneous ophthalmic formulations are required to be consumed within stipulated time duration since the stability of the therapeutic agent is variable. But it is necessary to define the optimal storage conditions and therefore need to have stability data available. There are no such regulations for the conduct of stability evaluation of extemporaneous preparations. In turn, recently the stability of extemporaneous drug formulations has given much more importance as supported by published literatures.

The prime concern about stability of ophthalmic formulations can be assessed in context of its physical stability (in order to detect potential precipitates, crystals, troubles, or coloration changes), chemical stability (pH, drug content, osmolality measurements), and sterility evaluation; otherwise they impact the stability at a major height.

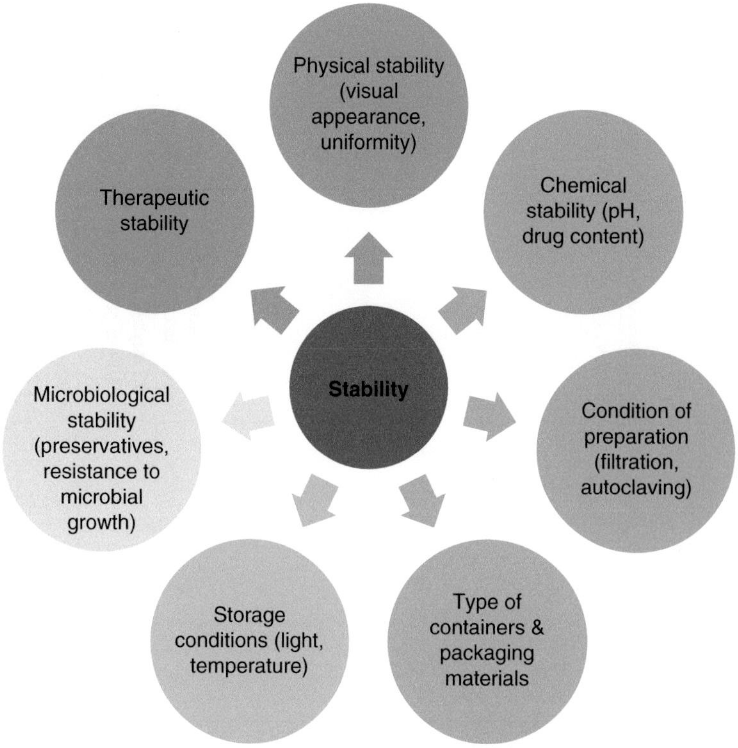

Fig. 15.5 Representing various factors affecting stability of ophthalmic formulations

The stability of ophthalmic formulations can be assessed by estimating the degradation products which are forming over the time at particular storage temperature. This can be evaluated by measurement of pH and osmolarity. The ophthalmic formulations are required to be sterile until opened (21CFR 200.50. USFDA 2014). It would appear that repeated opening of multidose container also adversely affects the chemical stability of active agents (Sautou 2010). This is the result of microbiological insult for the solution which indicated that multidose solution must be preserved. But most of the extemporaneous formulations are dispensed without preservative which in turn required to be used within couple of days. The stability of such formulations must be accounted and documented for their better efficacy.

The cardinal parameters that must be taken into account are enumerated in the figure (Fig. 15.5):

The examples that are given in Table 15.9 demonstrate the influence of different parameters, such as the type of formulation and storage conditions, together with the concentration, in the stability of an ophthalmic formulation.

Table 15.9 Listing stability of extemporaneous ophthalmic drug formulations

Ophthalmic drug formulations	Strength	Formulation contents	Stability				References
			Temperature			Duration	
			Frozen (−10 to −20 °C)	Refrig-erator (2–8 °C)	RT (23–25 °C)	Days/weeks/months	
Acetylcysteine eye drops	10 %w/v	0.025 % disodium edetate, 0.5 % chlorobutanol	–	*	–	60 days	Anaizi et al. (1997)
	20 %w/v						
5-Fluorouracil eye drops	1 mg/0.1 mL (1 %w/v)	Sterile saline 0.9 % NaCl	*	*	*	7 days	Fuhrman et al. (2000)
Caspofungin eye drops	0.5 %w/v	Water for injection	–	*	–	28 days	Neoh et al. (2012)
Cefazolin sodium eye drops (fortified)	50 mg/mL	Artificial tear; 0.3 % HPMC, 0.001 % Polyquad II (polyquaternium −1), 0.028 % sodium perborate as preservative, protected from light		*		28 days	Rojanarata et al. (2010), Charlton et al. (1998)
	1 %w/v	Citrate buffer pH 6.11–6.27, PVA, 0.001 % phenylmercuric borate, 0.4 % beta- phenylethyl alcohol	–	*	–	30 days stored with light protection	Kodym et al. (2012), Bowe et al. (1991)
	5 %w/v		–	–	*	9–15 days stored with light protection	
	33.5 mg/mL	Artificial tear, sterile saline	–	–	*	<7 days	Arici et al. (1999)
			–	*	–	>7 days	
Cefepime eye drops	1 %w/v	Sterile buffered solution	–	–	*	21–27 days	Kodym et al. (2011c)
	5 %w/v		–	–	*	18–21 days	

Chlorhexidine eye drops	0.02 %w/v	Sodium acetate buffer, pH 5.9; stored in light-resistant HDPE eyedroppers	–	*	*	6 months after being sealed	Shu-Chiao Lin et al. (2014)
						1 month after being opened	
Vancomycin eye drops	14 mg/mL	Sterile saline 0.9 %NaCl, 0.005 % BKC	–	–	*	60 days	Christine McLellan et al. (2008)
			*	–	–	6 months	
	31 mg/mL	Artificial tear	–	–	*	10 days	Khangtragool et al. (2011)
			–	*	–	28 days	
	31 mg/ml	Artificial tear, 0.3 % HPMC, 0.1 % dextran 70, 0.01 % BKC, 0.05 %disodium edetate	*	–	–	45 days	Fuhrman and Stroman (1998), Arici et al. (1999)
			–	*	–	10 days	
			–	–	*	7 days	
Voriconazole eye drops	2 %w/v (20 mg/mL)	Sterile water for injection, 0.01 % BKC	–	*	*	16 weeks	Al-Badriyeh et al. (2009), Senthilkumari et al. (2010)
	1 %w/v (10 mg/mL)		–	*	–	14 weeks (8 weeks at 40 °C)	
	1 %w/v	Sterile water for injection	*	–	–	90 days	AmorósReboredo et al. (2015)
			–	*	–	14 days	
Mitomycin C eye drops	0.015 %, 0.03 %, 0.06 %	Sterile phosphate buffer pH 8	* (–80)	*	–	28 days	Velpandian et al. (2005), Francoeur et al. (1999)
Infliximab eye drops	10 mg/mL	Artificial tear	*	*	–	45 days	Robert et al. (2014)
Melphalan solution for intravitreal injection	300 ug/mL (0.03 %)	Sterile saline 0.9 %NaCl	*	–	–	6 months	Buitrago et al. (2014)
			–	*	–	3 h	
			–	–	*	2 h	
Recombinant human interferon alpha-2b eye drops		Sterile water for injection, 0.01 % BKC	–	*	–	15 days	Ruiz et al. (2007)
			–	–	*	7 days	

(continued)

Table 15.9 (continued)

Ophthalmic drug formulations	Strength	Formulation contents	Stability				References
			Temperature			Duration	
			Frozen (−10 to −20 °C)	Refrigerator (2–8 °C)	RT (23–25 °C)	Days/weeks/months	
Phenylephrine	2 %w/v	Phosphate buffer in sterile water for injection, 0.9 %NaCl	–	–	*	60 days	Dreno et al. (2015)
	0.5 %w/v						
Cefuroxime	1 %w/v	Citrate buffer of pH 6.05–6.28; PVA; 0.001 % phenylmercuric borate; 0.4 % beta-phenylethyl alcohol	–	*	–	15 days	Kodym et al. (2011d)
	5 %w/v						
	10 mg/mL	0.9 % NaCl/ 0.2 % hyaluronate gel	–	*	–	21 days	Uhart et al. (2010)
			–	–	*	2 days	
Metronidazole	0.5 %w/v	0.9 % solution of NaCl, 5 % glucose, phosphate buffers pH 6.97–6.81, thiomersal, and phenylmercuric borate	–	–	*	24 months	Kodym et al. (2011b)
Ceftazidime	1 %w/v	Citrate buffer of pH 6.10–6.24, PVA, phenylmercuric borate	–	*	–	27–18 days (1 %)	Kodym et al. (2011a)
	5 %w/v					21–12 days (5 %)	
			–	–	*	3 days	
		2-Phenylethanol					
Cyclosporine	1 %w/v	Artificial tears (polyvinyl alcohol 1.4 % and povidone 0.6 %)	*	*	–	28 days	Fiscella et al. (1996)
	2 %w/v		–	–	*	7 days	
		Sterile castor oil	–	–	*	12 months	Chast et al. (2004)

Ticarcillin	5 mg/mL	Sterile saline 0.9 % NaCl	–	*	–	7 days	Blondeel et al. (2005)
			–	–	*	3 days	
			*	–	–	9 weeks	
Gentamicin	13.6 mg/mL (fortified)	Sterile saline	–	*	–	3 months	McBride et al. (1991)
			–	–	*	<7 days	Arici et al. (1999)
			–	*	–	>7 days	
Tobramycin	13.6 mg/mL	Sterile saline	–	*	–	3 months	McBride et al. (1991)
			–	–	*	<7 days	Arici et al. (1999)
			–	*	–	>7 days	
	15 mg/mL	Artificial tear	–	–	*	28 days	Charlton et al. (1998)
			–	*	*	1 month	Bowe et al. (1991)
Tropicamide	0.5 %w/v	Benzalkonium chloride (0.01%w/v), Disodium edetate, Sodium chloride, and Purified water	–	*	*	2 months	Pohloudek-Fabini et al. (1982), Benavides et al. (1997)
	1 %w/v						
Ganciclovir intravitreal injection	20 mg/0.1 mL	Normal saline	*	*	*	1 month	Morlet et al. (1995)
Pilocarpine	0.13 %w/v, 1 %w/v, 2 %w/v	Normal saline	–	–	*	1 month	Fagerstrom (2011), Pilatti et al. (1999)
						1 year (dark)	
Timolol	0.25 %w/v	Phosphate buffer, BKC (0.01 %)	–	–	*	2 month	Moorfields Pharmacist Handbook (2006)
	0.5 %w/v						
Avastin	2.5 mg/0.1 ml	Arginine acetate buffer, pH 4.5–5.5. polysorbate 20–0.04 %	–	*	–	6 months	Chen et al. (2009)
Homatropine	2 %w/v	Phosphate buffered saline	–	–	*	4 weeks	Moorfields Pharmacist Handbook (2006)

(continued)

Table 15.9 (continued)

Ophthalmic drug formulations	Strength	Formulation contents	Stability				References
			Temperature			Duration	
			Frozen (–10 to –20 °C)	Refrig-erator (2–8 °C)	RT (23–25 °C)	Days/weeks/months	
Autologous serum eye drops	Pure or diluted with saline	0.5 % chloramphenicol with boric acid 1.5 %, borax 0.3 % and purified water or saline	–	*	–	1 month	Fischer et al. (2012), Phasukkijwatana et al. (2011)
			*	–	–	6 months	
Amikacin intravitreal injection	0.1 mg/0.1 mL	Diluted with 0.9 % saline	–	*	–	1 month	Trissel (2009), Baum et al. (2012)
	0.4 mg/0.1 mL						
Cysteamine eye drops	0.5 %	0.9 % NaCl	*	–	–	180 days	Macdonald et al. (1990), Tsilou et al. (2003)
			–	*	–	14 days	
			–	–	*	7 days	
Disodium edetate solution	0.01 M	Sterile water for injection, sodium hydroxide (1 N) qs to pH 7	–	*	–	52 days	Moorfields Pharmacist Handbook (2006)
	0.05 M						
Sodium or potassium ascorbate	10 %w/v	Normal saline	–	*	–	52 days	Moorfields Pharmacist Handbook (2006), Davis et al. (1997)
Sodium citrate	10 %w/v	Normal saline	–	–	*	104 days	Moorfields Pharmacist Handbook (2006)
Retinoic acid	0.05 %w/v	Absolute alcohol, arachis oil	*	–	–	28 days	Reynolds and Closson (1993)
Botulinum toxin type A	20 IU	Normal saline (0.9 % NaCl)	*	*	–	2 weeks	Anderson (2004), Sloop et al. (1997)
Sodium hyaluronate	0.1 %w/v	Water for injection	–	*	–	7 days	Reynolds and Closson (1993)

Note: Preservative used for extemporaneously prepared drugs must be selected based on the pharmacy practice /in-house guidelines of the formulary
(*) & (–) represent presence and absence of respective storage condition, respectively; RT = Room temperature

15.9 Conclusion

Ophthalmic products require much more strict control over their specifications as compared to other dosage forms to ensure patient safety. In one hand, it requires specific considerations during formulation optimization regarding compatibility, tonicity, stability, and other physicochemical characteristics relevant to sympathetic understanding of structure of the eye. On the other hand, it should be dispensed or compounded by qualified pharmacist in clean room facility to maintain the desired quality and sterility in the final products.

References

Al-Badriyeh D, Li J, Stewart K, Kong DC, Leung L, Davies GE, Fullinfaw R. Stability of extemporaneously prepared voriconazole ophthalmic solution. Am J Health Syst Pharm. 2009;66(16): 1478–83. doi:10.2146/ajhp080110.

Aldricha DS, Bacha CM, Brown W, Chambers W, Fleitmana J, Hunt D, Marquesb MRC, Millee Y, Mitra AK, Platzer SM, Tice T, Tin GW. Ophthalmic preparations. 2013;39(5). (P)\\uspnetapp2\share\SHARE\USPNF\PRINTQ\pager\xmlIn\NEP_20130828110441_S200824.xml. Aug 28 2013 11:04:44.

All drug products intended for ophthalmic use must be sterile. 21 CFR 200.50. USFDA, 2014.

AmorosReboredo P, BastidaFernandez C, GuerreroMolina L, SoyMuner D, LopezCabezas C. Stability of frozen 1 % voriconazole ophthalmic solution. Am J Health Syst Pharm. 2015;72(6):479–82. doi:10.2146/ajhp140127.

Anaizi NH, Swenson CF, Dentinger PJ. Stability of acetylcysteine in an extemporaneously compounded ophthalmic solution. Am J Health Syst Pharm. 1997;54(5):549–53.

Anderson Jr ER. Proper dose, preparation, and storage of botulinum neurotoxin serotype A. Am J Health Syst Pharm. 2004;61(22 Suppl 6):S24–9.

Aquilina A. The extemporaneous compounding of paediatric medicines at Mater Dei Hospital. J Malta Coll Pharm Pract. 2013;19:28–30.

Arici MK, Sumer Z, Guler C, Elibol O, Saygi G, Cetinkaya S. In vitro potency and stability of fortified ophthalmic antibiotics. Aust N Z J Ophthalmol. 1999;27(6):426–30.

Aseptic Processing of Health Care Products. 1 – General requirements. Geneva: ISO 13408–1, International Standards Organization; 1997.

Baum JL. Chapter 26: Antibiotic use in ophthalmology. In: Duane's Ophthalmology. Ed: William Tasman. Vol 4, Lippincott Williams & Wilkins, Hagerstown, MD. 2006. Available at: http://www.oculist.net/downaton502/prof/ebook/duanes/pages/v4/v4c026.html

Benavides JO, Satchell ER, Frantz KA. Efficacy of a mydriatic spray in the pediatric population. Optom Vis Sci. 1997;74(3):160–3.

Biju J. Intravitreal injections. Kerala J Ophthalmol. 2007;XIX(1):46–57.

Biswas P, Sengupta S, Choudhary R, Home S, Paul A, Sinha S. Comparative role of intravitreal ranibizumab versus bevacizumab in choroidal neovascular membrane in age-related macular degeneration. Indian J Ophthalmol. 2011;5:191–6. [PMCID: PMC3120237] [PubMed: 21586838].

Blondeel S, Pelloquin A, Pointereau-Bellanger A, Thuillier A, Fernandez C. Effect of freezing on stability of a fortified 5 mg/mL ticarcillin ophthalmic solution. Can J Hosp Pharm. 2005;58(2):65–70.

Bowe BE, Snyder JW, Eiferman RA. An in vitro study of the potency and stability of fortified ophthalmic antibiotic preparations. Am J Ophthalmol. 1991;111(6):686–9.

Buitrago E, Lagomarsino E, Mato G, Schaiquevich P. Stability of melphalan solution for intravitreal injection for retinoblastoma. JAMA Ophthalmol. 2014;132(11):1372–3. doi:10.1001/jamaophthalmol.2014.2324.

Buurma H, de Smet PAGM, van den Hoff OP, Sysling H, Storimans M, Egberts ACG. Frequency, nature and determinants of pharmacy compounded medicines in Dutch community pharmacies. Pharm World Sci. 2003;25(6):280–7.
Cabaleiro J. Obtaining accreditation by the Pharmacy Compounding Accreditation Board, part 2: developing essential standard operating procedures. Int J Pharm Compd. 2007;11(5):397–9.
Cabaleiro J. Obtaining accreditation by the Pharmacy Compounding Accreditation Board, part 4: tips for "last minute" preparations. Int J Pharm Compd. 2008;12(5):432–3.
Centers for Disease Control and Prevention (CDC). Multistate outbreak of fungal infection associated with injection of methylprednisolone acetate solution from a single compounding pharmacy – United States, 2012. MMWR Morb Mortal Wkly Rep. 2012a;61:839–42.
Centers for Disease Control and Prevention (CDC). Notes from the field: multistate outbreak of post-procedural fungal endophthalmitis associated with a single compounding pharmacy-United States, March-April 2012. MMWR Morb Mortal Wkly Rep. 2012b;61:310–1.
Charlton JF, Dalla KP, Kniska A. Storage of extemporaneously prepared ophthalmic antimicrobial solutions. Am J Health Syst Pharm. 1998;55(5):463–6.
Chast F, Lemare F, Legeais JM, Batista R, Bardin C, Renard G. Cyclosporine 2 % eye drops preparation. J Fr Ophtalmol. 2004;27(6 Pt 1):567–76.
Chen YH, Wu PC, Shiea J, Lo LH, Wu YC, Kuo HK. Evaluation of the sterility, stability, and efficacy of bevacizumab stored in multiple-dose vials for 6 months. J Ocul Pharmacol Ther. 2009;25(1):65–9. doi:10.1089/jop.2008.0043.
Compounding quality act (Drug Quality and Security Act of 2013). USFDA 2015. Available at: http://www.fda.gov/Drugs/GuidanceComplianceRegulatoryInformation/PharmacyCompounding/ucm2007064.htm. Accessed on 28 Feb 2015.
CSHP. Guidelines for preparation of sterile products in pharmacies. 1996.
Daniels R. Compounding of ophthalmic drugs in the pharmacy. Special care must be taken. Pharm Unserer Zeit. 2010;39(4):306–11. doi:10.1002/pauz.201000377.
Davis AR, Ali QH, Aclimandos WA, Hunter PA. Topical steroid use in the treatment of ocular alkali burns. Br J Ophthalmol. 1997;81:732–4. doi:10.1136/bjo.81.9.732.
De Rojas V. Infectious keratitis in 18,651 laser surface ablation procedures. J Cataract Refract Surg. 2011;37(10):1822–31.
Division of Transplant and Ophthalmology Products Office of Antimicrobial Products of New Drugs. Center for Drug Evaluation and Research FDA; Dermatologic and Ophthalmic Drugs Advisory Committe. Silver Spring, MD. February 27, 2012. Accessed 21 Apr 2015.
Dreno C, Gicquel T, Harry M, Tribut O, Aubin F, Brandhonneur N, Dollo G. Formulation and stability study of a pediatric 2 % phenylephrine hydrochloride eye drop solution. Ann Pharm Fr. 2015;73(1):31–6. doi:10.1016/j.pharma.2014.06.006. Jul 14.
Euradlex. The Rules Governing Medicinal Products in the European Community, Annex 1, published by the European Commission: Brussels, 2014.
Fagerstrom R. A note on the stability of ophthalmic solutions containing pilocarpine hydrochloride alone and with eserine. J Pharm Pharmacol. 2011;15(1):479–82.
FDA warning regarding Pseudomonas endophthalmitis and keratitis from compounded contaminated indomethacin eye drops used after cataract surgery. New York Times (cited in Schein 1992 on December 9, 1990).
FDA Consumer Health Information / U.S. Food and Drug Administration: The special risks of pharmacy compounding. (Dec 2012) Available at: http://www.fda.gov/downloads/ForConsumers/ConsumerUpdates/UCM107839.pdf.
Fiscella RG, Le H, Lam TT, Labib S. Stability of cyclosporine 1 % in artificial tears. J Ocul Pharmacol Ther. 1996;12(1):1–4.
Fischer KR, Opitz A, Böeck M, Geerling G. Stability of serum eye drops after storage of 6 months. Cornea. 2012;31(11):1313–8. doi:10.1097/ICO.0b013e3182542085.
Food and Drug Administration. Guideline on Sterile Drug Products Produced by Aseptic Processing FDA, Rockville, 2004.
Francoeur AM, Assalian A, Lesk MR, Morin I, Tetreault F, Calleja K, Guttman A, Rauth M, Pan SS. A comparative study of the chemical stability of various mitomycin C solutions used in glaucoma filtering surgery. J Glaucoma. 1999;8:242–6.

Fuhrman Jr LC, Stroman RT. Stability of vancomycin in an extemporaneously compounded ophthalmic solution. Am J Health Syst Pharm. 1998;55(13):1386–8.

Fuhrman Jr LC, Godwin DA, Davis RA. Stability of 5fluorouracil in an extemporaneously compounded ophthalmic solution. Int J Pharm Compd. 2000;4(4):320–3.

Geyer O, et al. Microbial contamination of medications used to treat glaucoma. Br J Ophthalmol. 1995;79:376–9.

Giam JA, McLachlan AJ, Krass I. Characterizing specialized compounding in community pharmacies. Res Social Adm Pharm. 2012;8:240–52.

Glass BD, Haywood A. Stability considerations in liquid dosage forms extemporaneously prepared from commercially available products. J Pharm Pharm Sci. 2006;9(3):398–426.

Goldberg RA, Flynn Jr HW, Isom RF, Miller D, Gonzalez S. An outbreak of streptococcus endophthalmitis after intravitreal injection of bevacizumab. Am J Ophthalmol. 2012;153: 204–8.

Good compounding practices applicable to state-licensed pharmacies. In: Model State Pharmacy Act and Model Rules of the National Association of Boards of Pharmacy. Park Ridge, Ill: National Association of Boards of Pharmacy; 1993:C.1–5. 3.

Government Printing Office. Drug Quality and Security Act. 2013. http://www.gpo.gov/fdsys/pkg/BILLS-113hr3204enr/pdf/BILLS-113hr3204enr.pdf. Accessed on 28 Feb 2015.

Hecht G. Ophthalmic preparation. In: Gennaro AR, editor. Remington: the science and practice of pharmacy. 20th ed. Easton: Mack Publishing Co; 2000. p. 821–35.

Houck LK. Compounding: a well-established practice in 1938. Int J Pharm Compd. 2005;9(5):364–7.

IACP. Member Alert. 2012. Available at http://www.iacprx.org/displaycommon.cfm?an=1&subarticlenbr=277. Accessed 10 Apr 2015.

ICH. Stability testing of new drug substances and products Q1A (R2), 2003. http://private.ich.org/LOB/media/MEDIA419.pdf. Accessed 15 Feb 2015.

International Academy of Compounding Pharmacists. One size doesn't fit all; 2014, available from: http://www.iacprx.org/displaycommon.cfm?an=1&subarticlenbr=128. Cited 25 Apr 2014.

ISO 14698–1. Cleanrooms and associated controlled environments–Biocontamination Control: part 1: general principles and methods. Geneva: International Organisation for Standardization; 2003.

ISPE Baseline® Pharmaceutical Engineering Guide, Volume 3 - Sterile Manufacturing Facilities, International Society for Pharmaceutical Engineering (ISPE), First Edition, January 1999. Available at www.ispe.org

Jokl DHK, et al. Bacterial contamination of ophthalmic solutions used in an extended care facility. Br J Ophthalmol. 2007;91:1308–10.

Khangtragool A, Santidherakul S, Leesawat P. Stability of vancomycin 31 mg/mL in extemporaneous eye drops determined with capillary electrophoresis. Chiang Mai J Sci. 2011;38(4): 533–40.

Kodym A, Hapka-Zmich D, Gołab M, Gwizdala M. Stability of ceftazidime in 1 % and 5 % buffered eye drops determined with HPLC method. Acta Pol Pharm. 2011a;68(1):99–107.

Kodym A, Kaczyńska-Dyba E, Kubiak B, Kukuła H. Technology of eye drops containing metronidazole. Acta Pol Pharm. 2011b;68(1):109–14.

Kodym A, Pawłowska M, Rumiński JK, Bartosińska A, Kieliba A. Stability of cefepime in aqueous eye drops. Pharmazie. 2011c;66(1):17–23.

Kodym A, Wiśniewski A, Knioła D, Olejniczak M. Stability of cefuroxime in 1 % and 5 % buffered eye drops determined with HPLC method. Acta Pol Pharm. 2011d;68(4):555–64.

Kodym A, Bilski P, Domańska A, Hełminiak Ł, Jabłońska M, Jachymska A. Physical and chemical properties and stability of sodium cefazolin in buffered eye drops determined with HPLC method. Acta Pol Pharm. 2012;69(1):95–105.

Krishnan T, Sengupta S. Secondary pseudomonas infection of fungal keratitis following use of contaminated natamycin eye drops: a case series. Eye. 2009;23:477–9.

Lee EW, Holtebeck AC, Harrison AR. Infection rates in outpatient eyelid surgery. Ophthal Plast Reconstr Surg. 2009;25(2):109–10.

Lin S-C, et al. Formulation and stability of an extemporaneous 0.02 % chlorhexidine digluconate ophthalmic solution. J Formos Med Assoc. 2014;xx:1–8. http://dx.doi.org/10.1016/j.jfma.2014.08.003.

Ling MR. Extemporaneous compounding. The end of the road? Dermatol Ther. 1998;16(2):321–7.

Livingstone DJ, et al. Evaluation of an extended period of use for preserved eye drops in hospital practice. Br J Ophthalmol. 1998;82:473–5.

Llovet F. Infectious keratitis in 204, 586 LASIK procedures. Ophthalmology. 2010;117(2):232–8.

Lowes R. Compounding pharmacy crackdown continues with Avastin recall. Medscape Medical News. March 19, 2013. /viewarticle/781039. Accessed 2 May 2015.

Macdonald IM, Noel LP, Mintsioulis G, Clarke WN. The effect of topical cysteamine drops on reducing crystal formation within the cornea of patients affected by nephropathic cystinosis. J Pediatr Ophthalmol Strabismus. 1990;27(5):272–5.

McBride HA, Martinez DR, Trang JM, Lander RD, Helms HA. Stability of gentamicin sulfate and tobramycin sulfate in extemporaneously prepared ophthalmic solutions at 8 degrees C. Am J Hosp Pharm. 1991;48(3):507–9.

McElhiney LF. Compounding Guide for Ophthalmic Preparations. 1st Edition. American Pharmacists Association, Washington DC. 2013.

McLellan C, Pasedis S, Dohlman CH. Testing long term stability of vancomycin ophthalmic solution. Int J Pharm Compd. 2008;12(5):456–9.

Morlet N, Young S, Naidoo D, Fong T, Coroneo MT. High dose intravitreal ganciclovir for CMV retinitis: a shelf life and cost comparison study. Br J Ophthalmol. 1995;79:753–5.

Moorfields Eye Hospital NHS Foundation trust. Pharmacists Handbook. Moorfields Pharmaceuticals, 2006. Available at: http://mehhome/_uploads/documents/policy-documents/clinical-guidelines/moorfields-pharmacists-handbook-(2006).pdf.

Murry T. Accreditation by the pharmacy compounding accreditation board: raising the bar for patient care. Int J Pharm Compd. 2008;12(2):174–5.

Nahata MC, Allen LV. Extemporaneous drug formulations. Clin Ther. 2008;30(11):2112–9.

Nentwich MM, Kollmann KHM, Meshack J, Ilako DR, Schaller UC. Microbial contamination of multi-use ophthalmic solutions in Kenya. Br J Ophthalmol. 2007;91(10):1265–8.

Neoh CF, Jacob J, Leung L, Li J, Stathopoulos A, Stewart K, Kong DC. Stability of extemporaneously prepared 0.5-percent caspofungin eye drops: a potential cost-savings exercise. Antimicrob Agents Chemother. 2012;56(6):3435–7.

Parke DW. American Academy of Ophthalmology Issues Statement on Provisions to Pharmaceutical Compounding Quality and Accountability Act. 2013. Available at http://www.prnewswire.com/news-releases/american-academy-of-ophthalmology-issues-statement-on-provisions-to-pharmaceutical-compounding-quality-and-accountability-act-209358771.html. Assessed on 3 Apr 2015.

Pharmaceutical Compounding Expert Committee. Pharmaceutical compounding. In: United States Pharmacopeia 34/National Formulary 29. Rockville: United States Pharmacopeial Convention; 2011.

Phasukkijwatana N, Lertrit P, Liammongkolkul S, Prabhasawat P. Stability of epitheliotrophic factors in autologous serum eye drops from chronic Stevens-Johnson syndrome dry eye compared to non-autoimmune dry eye. Curr Eye Res. 2011;36(9):775–81. doi:10.3109/02713683.2011.587935.

Pilatti C, del CM, Chiale TC, Spinetto M. Stability of pilocarpine ophthalmic solutions. Drug Dev Ind Pharm. 1999;25(6):801–5.

Pohloudek-Fabini R, Martin E, Gallasch V. Contribution to the stability of tropicamide solutions. Pharmazie. 1982;37(3):184–7.

Rahman MQ, et al. Microbial contaminations of preservative free multiple application containers. Br J Ophthalmol. 2006;90:139–41.

Reynolds L, Closson R, editors. Extemporaneous ophthalmic preparations. Vancouver: Applied Therapeutics Inc; 1993. p. 288–90.

Robert MC, Spurr-Michaud S, Frenette M, Young D, Gipson IK, Dohlman CH. Stability and in vitro toxicity of an infliximab eye drop formulation. Int J Pharm Compd. 2014;18(5): 418–26.

Rogers C, Dakin HA, Wordsworth S. Cost-effectiveness of ranibizumab for neovascular age-related macular degeneration: 1 year IVAN results. Program and abstracts of the Association for Research in Vision Ophthalmology (ARVO) 2013 Annual Meeting; May 5–9, 2013; Seattle, Washington. Abstract 373.

Rojanarata T, Tankul J, Woranaipinich C, Potawanich P, Plianwong S, Sakulma S, Saehuan C. Stability of fortified cefazolin ophthalmic solutions prepared in artificial tears containing surfactant-based versus oxidant-based preservatives. J Ocul Pharmacol Ther. 2010;26(5): 485–90.

Ruiz L, Rodriguez I, Baez R, Aldana R. Stability of an extemporaneously prepared recombinant human interferon alfa-2b eye drop formulation. Am J Health Syst Pharm. 2007;64(16): 1716–9.

Salvatore G, Focke Z. Bevacizumab: off label use in ophthalmology. Indian J Ophthalmol. 2007;55(6):417–20.

Sandle T. Sterile Ophthalmic Preparations and Contamination Control. 2014. Available at http://www.ivtnetwork.com/article/sterile-ophthalmic-preparations-and-contamination-control.

Sautou V. Stability of ophthalmic preparation. 2010. Available at http://www.gerpac.eu/spip.php?article69. Accessed on 2 Mar 2015.

Schein OD, Wasson PJ. Microbial keratitis associated with contaminated ocular medications. Am J Ophthalmol. 1988;105(4):361–5.

Schein OD, et al. Microbial contamination of in-use ocular medications. Arch Ophthalmol. 1992;110:82–5.

Schmucker C, Ehlken C, Agostini HT, Antes G, Ruecker G, Lelgemann M, Loke YK. A safety review and meta-analyses of Bevacizumab and Ranibizumab: off-label versus gold standard. PLoS One. 2012;7(8), e42701. doi:10.1371/journal.pone.0042701.

Seal DV. Endophthalmitis prophylaxis – implications of the European society of cataract and refractive surgery endophthalmitis study. Eur Ophthalmol Rev. 2007;1:30–2. doi:10.17925/EOR.2007.00.01.30.

Sellers S, Utian WH. Pharmacy compounding primer for physicians. Curr Opin Drug. 2012;72(16):2043–50.

Senthilkumari S, Lalitha P, Prajna NV, Haripriya A, Nirmal J, Gupta P, Velpandian T. Single and multidose ocular kinetics and stability analysis of extemporaneous formulation of topical voriconazole in humans. Curr Eye Res. 2010;35(11):953–60.

Shargel L. Comprehensive pharmacy review. 3rd ed. Philadelphia: Lippincott Williams and Wilkins; 1997.

Sloop RR, Cole BA, Escutin RO. Reconstituted botulinum toxin type A does not lose potency in humans if it is refrozen or refrigerated for 2 weeks before use. Neurology. 1997;48(1):249–53.

Spark MJ. Compounding of medicines by pharmacies: An update. Maturitas. 2014. Available at http://dx.doi.org/10.1016/j.maturitas.2014.05.00.

Staes C, Jacobs J, Mayer J, Allen J. Description of outbreaks of health-care-associated infections related to compounding pharmacies, 2000–12. Am J Health Syst Pharm. 2013;70(15):1301–12.

Stevens JD, Matheson MM. Survey of the contamination of eye drops of hospital inpatients and recommendations for the changing of current practice in eyedrop dispensing. Br J Ophthalmol. 1992;76:36–8.

Sterile Drug Products Produced by Aseptic Processing — Current Good Manufacturing Practice. USFDA, Sep 2004. Available at: http://www.fda.gov/downloads/Drugs/.../Guidances/ucm070342.pdf.

Stokowski LA. The Compounding Controversy. Medscape. Jul 03, 2013.

Sundstrom S, Ljungqvist B, Reinmuller B. Some observations on airborne particles in the critical areas of a blow-fill-seal machine. PDA J Pharm Sci Technol. 2009;63(1):71–80.

Taban M, et al. Acute endophthalmitis following cataract surgery a systematic review of the literature. Arch Ophthalmol. 2005;123:613–20.

Templeton WC. Serratia keratitis transmitted by contaminated eyedroppers. Am J Ophthalmol. 1982;93(6):723–6.
The Ann. Deadly Meds. 2013. Available at http://www.theannmagazine.com/2013/01/04/deadly-meds/. Accessed 02 Mar 2015.
Tortora GJ, Grabowski SR, editors. Principles of anatomy and physiology. 10th ed. New York: Wiley; 2002. p. 866–73.
Trissel LA. Trissel's stability of compounded formulations. 4th ed. Washington, DC: American Pharmacists Association; 2009. p. 26–7.
Tsilou ET, Thompson D, Linblad AS, et al. A multicentre randomized double masked clinical trial of a new formulation of topical cysteamine for the treatment of corneal cystine crystals in cystinosis. Br J Ophthalmol. 2003;87(1):8–31.
Uhart M, Pirot F, Boillon A, Senaux E, Tall L, Diouf E, Burillon C, Padois K, Falson F, Leboucher G, Pivot C. Assessment of sodium hyaluronate gel as vehicle for intracameral delivery of cefuroxime in endophthalmitis prophylaxis. Int J Pharm. 2010;398(1–2):14–20. Available at doi:10.1016/j.ijpharm.2010.07.009. Epub 2010 Jul 15.
United states pharmacopoeia. General Chapter <1231> Water for pharmaceutical purposes, USP 29–NF24. Rockville, MD: United States Pharmacopeia Convention; 2006.
United States Pharmacopeia. General chapter <1116> microbiological control and monitoring of aseptic processing environments, USP 35–NF 30. Bethesda: United States Pharmacopeia; 2012.
US Department of Health and Human Services. US FDA. FDA alerts health care professionals of infection risk from repackaged avastin intravitreal injections. 2011. Available from URL: http://www.fda.gov/Drugs/DrugSafety/ucm270296.htm.
USP <797> The United States Pharmacopoeia 27 National Formulary 22 (USP-NF). Chapter 797: Pharmaceutical Compounding. 2004. USP Convention. 2008:1–61.
USP <797> United States Pharmacopeia. General chapter <1116> microbiological control and monitoring of aseptic processing environments, USP 35–NF 30. Bethesda: United States Pharmacopeia; 2012.
Velpandian T, Saluja V, Ravi A, Kumari SS, Mathur R, Ranjan N, Ghose S. Evaluation of the stability of extemporaneously prepared ophthalmic formulation of mitomycin C. J Ocul Pharmacol Ther. 2005;21(3):217–22. doi:10.1089/jop.2005.21.217.
Velpandian T, Sharma C, Garg SP, Mandal S, Ghose S. Safety and cost-effectiveness of single dose dispensing of bevacizumab for various retinal pathologies in developing countries. Indian J Ophthalmol. 2007;55:488–90. (PMCID: PMC2635973) (PubMed: 17951922).
Williams RD, Thompson J, Epley DK, Liebermann JM, Tan D. Letter on compounding pharmacies. American Association for Pediatric Ophthalmology and Strabismus. 2013. Available at http://www.aapos.org/news/show/109. Accessed 28 May 2013.
Wong D, Kyle G. Some ethical considerations for the "off-label" use of drugs such as Avastin. Avastin: ethical considerations. Commentaries. Br J Ophthalmol. 2006;90:1218–9.
Wroblewski KJ, Pasternak JF, Bower KS. Infectious keratitis after photorefractive keratectomy in the United States army and navy. Ophthalmology. 2006;113(4):520–5.
Wycoff CC, et al. Nosocomial acute-onset postoperative endophthalmitis at a University Teaching Hospital (2002–2009). Am J Ophthalmol. 2010;150:392–8.
Wynkoop K. Compounded products: use, regulation, and risk. OMIC digest. Fall 2012.
Yuen JR, Fiscella RG, Gaynes BI. Ophthalmic agents and managed care. J Manag Care Pharm. 2002;8(3):217–23.

Chapter 16
Preservatives for Topical Ocular Drug Formulations

Thirumurthy Velpandian

Abstract Although, the use of eye medications are known for their prolonged presence in the history, the concept of using preservatives in ocular drug formulations came to practice only after second World War. Usage of preservatives restricts the microbial growth in the opened ophthalmic drug formulations which are meant for multiple dosing. Preservatives used for ophthalmic formulations are not free from hurdles. This chapter explains the physical, chemical and biological preservation methods employed in ophthalmic dosage forms and the adverse effect of preservatives on eye.

16.1 Introduction

After the Second World War, quality control on sterility for ophthalmic product is a mandatory requirement. CFR 21/4 (2014) claims that the containers of ophthalmic preparations shall be sterile at the time of filling and closing and the container or individual carton shall be so sealed that the contents cannot be used without destroying the seal. It also cautions that all ophthalmic products must be manufactured to be sterile until they are opened. Ophthalmic solutions are dispensed in multidose containers which enable the patient to apply them frequently according to the dosing regimen. During that period, they need to be opened, used and closed, thus giving a window for microbial contamination. Moreover, the dropping nozzle, cap, inside head space and the drug coming out of the vial are the potential areas for contamination during usage (Coad et al. 1984; Schein et al. 1992).

T. Velpandian, BPharm, MS(Pharmacol), PhD
Ocular Pharmacology and Pharmacy, Dr. Rajendra Prasad Centre for Ophthalmic Sciences, All India Institute of Medical Sciences, New Delhi, India
e-mail: tvelpandian@hotmail.com

T. Velpandian (ed.), *Pharmacology of Ocular Therapeutics*,
DOI 10.1007/978-3-319-25498-2_16

Therefore, the sterile formulations are added with one or more suitable preservative substances to inhibit the growth of microorganisms. Usually, eye drop containers carry a caution label about the period of usage once if the container is opened to ensure the adequate protection against contamination. In general, ophthalmic formulations are made after giving due consideration about the requirements to preserve them against physical, chemical and biological changes while on storage and their usage (Brown and Norton 1965).

While manufacturing or compounding, eye drops are sterile and most of them undergo terminal sterilization ending up with moist heat sterilization. This process is applicable only for thermostable components in the formulation. Thermolabile compounds have classically been made in a place which is having strictly particulate matter and microbe-controlled environment followed by filter sterilization using 0.1–0.22 μm sterile filters. The steps involved in the drug formulation are usually optimized for preserving its physical, chemical and biological properties of all of their components.

16.2 Biological Preservation

The real task of preservation against microbe starts mainly after opening the multidosage vial. Usually, eye drops come with the warning that they should not be used beyond 1 month after opening the vial. Therefore, these formulations are protected against microbial contamination using preservatives. Classically detergents like benzalkonium chloride are extensively used in most of the formulations due to its excellent microbial protection properties but not free of potential problems. Comparative analysis of the advantage and concerns of preservatives are shown in Table 16.1.

16.3 Detergents

16.3.1 Benzalkonium Chloride

Gerhard Domagk, a German chemist who bagged a Nobel Prize for his discovery of sulphonamides (the first antimicrobials), observed that increasing nitrogen containing carbon chain length from 8 to 18 showed excellent antimicrobial activity. In 1935 he synthesized and studied the effect of benzalkonium chloride on microbes (DoMagk 1935). It was reported to have good inhibitory action of wide range of bacteria and yeast (Sevag and Ross 1944; Baker et al. 1941) After the Second World War, it was considered as nontoxic and extensively used as a cleansing agent for surgeons in the name of Zephiran and Germinal. Benzalkonium chloride (BKC) is a quaternary ammonium compound (cationic detergent) most widely used for the preservation in topical ophthalmic products. Its high water solubility and colourless and orderless nature having high thermal and chemical stability in aqueous formulations favoured

Table 16.1 Preservatives used in topical ophthalmic formulations along with their advantage and concern

Preservatives (type)	Example	Mechanism/property	Concern/Advantage
Detergents	*Benzalkonium chloride* (0.001–0.02%)	Disrupts microbial cell membrane due to its charge-related binding. Excellent disinfectant activity and wide spectrum	Disrupts corneal and conjunctival cell and induces apoptosis
	Polyquaternium-1 (0.001 %)	Similar to BKC	Less toxic than BKC
	Cetrimonium salt (0.005)	Similar to BKC	Corneal and conjunctival toxicity
Organomercuric compounds	*Thimerosal* (0.001–0.02 %)	Effective against bacteria, fungus and protozoa	Conjunctival and corneal epithelial cell toxicity reported
	Phenylmercuric nitrate (0.002–0.004 %)	Similar to thimerosal	Chemical incompatibility with salts of halides
Oxidizing agents	*Oxychloro complex* also called as purite (mixture of chlorine dioxide, chlorite and chlorate)	Inhibit microbial protein synthesis and by oxidizing glutathione	Lesser toxic than BKC
	Sodium perborate	Oxidizing microbial cell membranes and enzymes due to hydrogen peroxide generation	Lesser toxic than BKC
Ionic-buffered preservatives	*SofZia*	Combining antimicrobial strength of zinc, boron	Comparatively be safe for cornea but limited prevention for S. aureus
Substituted alcohols and phenols	*Chlorobutanol* (0.5 %)	Wider spectrum of activity on bacteria and fungus	Thermal instability, irritation on ocular surface and can cause corneal epithelial toxicity
	Phenylethyl alcohol		
Benzoic acid esters	Methylparaben, propylparaben	Poor antimicrobial activity	Poor water solubility, lesser toxicity as compared to BKC
Miscellaneous	*Sorbates* (0.1 %)	Broad-spectrum antimicrobial in lower pH	Stinging sensation and corneal irritation
	EDTA (0.01–0.1 %)	Chelates divalent cations in the microbe and potentiates the effect of other preservatives	Not used alone and also chelates precorneal cations less toxic as compared to BKC
	Hydroxymethylglycinate, silver chloride complex	Further studies required	Further studies required

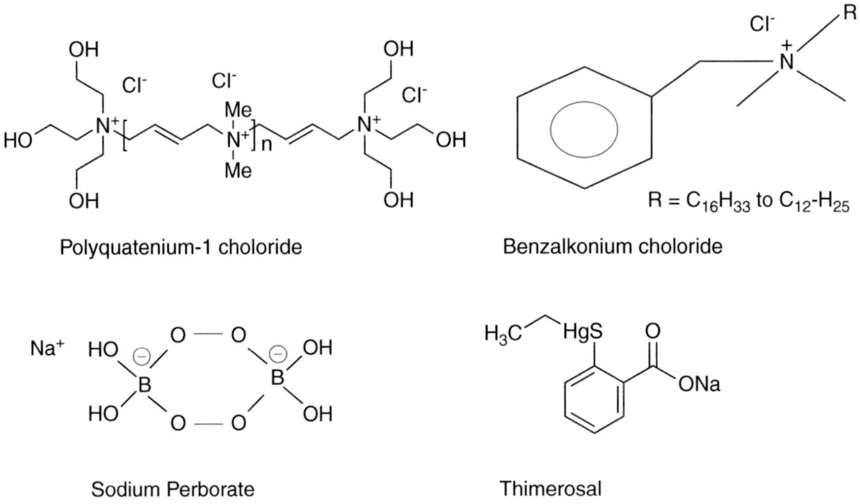

Fig. 16.1 Showing the chemical structures of benzalkonium chloride, polyquaternium (Polyquad), sodium perborate, thimerosal

its use for topical disinfectant and preservation. It is reported to be incompatible with anionic compounds such as salicylates and nitrates. It is a mixture of alkyl benzyldimethyammonium chlorides having different alkyl lengths. The highest antimicrobial activity was found to be between the alkyl group R having $C_{16}H_{33}$ to C_{12}–H_{25} (Fig. 16.1). BKC has been used in the concentrations varying from 0.001 to 0.02 %. Quaternary ammonium compounds are detergents as they have a cationic polar group and non-polar carbon chain. They are reported to cause tear film instability, loss of goblet cells, conjunctival squamous metaplasia and apoptosis, disruption of the corneal epithelium barrier, and damage to deeper ocular tissues (Baudouin et al. 2010). The tear film instability could be explained by their ability to disrupt the arrangement of monolipid layer. BKC increases corneal permeability of drugs by disrupting tight junctions of corneal epithelium (Chen et al. 2012). Ocular kinetics of radiolabelled BKC has been reported to achieve higher levels in anterior ocular tissues and retained over the period of 120 h. Moreover, it has also been reported to disappear rapidly from precorneal area (Green and Chapman 1986). Most of the studies on the intraocular penetration and topical disposition studies on benzalkonium were conducted when more sensitive analytical methods like mass spectroscopy were not available; therefore, comprehensive information is not available. However, transcorneal uptake of cationic compounds through organic cation transporters (OCT) has been reported by Nirmal et al. (2013) and partially explains the fate of quaternary ammonium compounds in the precorneal area.

Preservatives such as BKC, benzododecinium bromide, cetrimide, phenylmercuric nitrate, thimerosal (thi), methyl parahydroxybenzoate, chlorobutanol, and EDTA were compared for their cytotoxicity in human conjunctival cell line by exposing them for 15 min followed by 24 h recovery by Debbasch et al. (2001) and reported that quaternary amines are the most cytotoxic preservatives. They were found to induce apoptosis at lower concentration followed by necrosis at higher concentrations. Moreover, they have also implicated that superoxide anions may be responsible for the tissue damage caused on ocular surface.

16.3.2 Polyquaternium-1

It is a quaternary ammonium compound derivative brought by Alcon Labs as an effective preservative in multipurpose contact lens solutions. for chronic administration of travoprost in glaucoma. Studies that compared the preservatives such as Polyquad and BKC used in prostaglandin analogues on corneal surface changes reported that Polyquad showed higher degree of safety over BKC (Lee et al. 2014; Sezgin Akçay et al. 2014). Patient compliance to adhere to chronic drug regimen is high where ocular drugs related side effects are low. Although BAC is having its place as a preservative in ophthalmic products, Polyquad can be considered for chronic drug administration to have less problems with ocular surface disorder (Rolando et al. 2011; Labbé et al. 2006). Considering this safety, Polyquad has been used extensively in contact lens solutions. In this group of quaternary ammonium compounds, other members such as benzethonium chloride and cetylpyridinium chloride are also found occasionally in the drug formulations.

16.4 Organomercuric Compounds

Organomercuric compound do not share the toxicity of free mercury. Thimerosal, also called as merthiolate, is reported to have bacteriostatic, antifungal and antiprotozoal activity. It is used as a preservative in the concentration varying from 0.005 to 0.02 %. It is relatively slow acting but a stable compound used in contact lens solutions (later replaced with Polyquad and biguanides) As compared to all other preservatives, thimerosal 0.004 % when combined in solution with EDTA was effective against Acanthamoeba castellanii and Acanthamoeba polyphaga trophozoites and cysts (Silvany et al. 1991). Phenylmercuric nitrate or acetate is used in the concentration varying from 0.002 to 0.004 % in ophthalmic solutions. It is reported to have considerable antifungal activity, and its in vitro effect is significantly superior to those of benzalkonium chloride, natamycin and ketoconazole against ocular pathogenic filamentous fungi (Xu et al. 2013). Phenylmercuric nitrate has been reported to have incompatibility with halide salts of other compounds in the formulation.

16.5 Benzoic Acid Esters

Methyl- and propylparabens are rarely used as a preservative in ophthalmic solutions. Methylparaben is used in the concentration varying from 0.1 to 0.2 %. They show poor antimicrobial activity. Ocular irritation and stinging have been reported.

16.6 Phenols and Substituted Alcohols

16.6.1 Chlorobutanol

It is reported to have wider spectrum over Gram-positive and Gram-negative bacteria, P aeruginosa and fungi. It is used at the concentration of 0.5 % in the topical solutions. It is reported to undergo decomposition while on standing and at higher temperatures causing release hydrochloric acid which in turn reduces the pH of the aqueous solution. Therefore, the solution is buffered at 5–5.5 to improve its shelf life.

16.7 Oxidative Preservatives

16.7.1 Stabilized Oxychloro Complex

Stabilized oxychloro complex (SOC) is a preservative used at a low concentration such as 0.005 % in ophthalmic solutions. It is reported to have a broad spectrum of activity. This oxychloro complex is a mixture containing chlorine dioxide, chlorate and chlorite. It is reported to inhibit microbial protein synthesis and by oxidizing glutathione. Light causes SOC dissociation into chloride, oxygen, chlorine and sodium species. Chloride free radicals are involved in the oxidation process causing microbial kill (Noss and Olivieri 1985). Oral administration of 5 mg/L (0.0005 %) solution of SOC for 12 weeks was tested in human volunteers and was found to be safe (Lubbers et al. 1982).

16.7.2 Sodium Perborate

It was introduced in 1950 as a disinfectant for oral rinse and dental bleach (Saenz 1950). It is a odourless water-soluble sodium salt having a chemical formula $Na_2H_4B_2O_8$ (Fig. 16.1). It is prepared by mixing sodium borate with hydrogen peroxide in alkaline condition and available as hydrate in crystalline form. In aqueous solution, it releases hydrogen peroxide and borate, but it has been found to have an equilibrium with peroxoborate anion (McKillop and Sanderson 1995). It is considered as less toxic as compared to BKC in experimental studies.

16.7.3 sofZia Proprietary Ionic Buffer

SofZia is a preservation system developed by Alcon Laboratories as a proprietary ionic buffer system (Fort Worth, Texas) for antiglaucoma medication travoprost. This preservation system having composition containing borate, sorbitol, propylene glycol and zinc (Noecker 2007) has been reported to meet the requirement of US Pharmacopoeia standards for ophthalmic preservatives. This composition containing ingredients were all found to be safe for ocular use; therefore, it has been promoted for chronic drug therapy for glaucoma and dry eye (Rosenthal et al. 2006). Many studies found that preservation with SofZia composition equals effect with low toxicity on the ocular surface (Anwar et al. 2013). Use of boric acid in eye wash has been known for a long time, and antimicrobial action on pathogenic organisms of the eye was reported in the concentrations from 0.5 to 2 % solutions by Novak and Taylor in 1951. Similarly, antimicrobial activity of zinc salts has also been well known (Choi et al. 2010). Together with all at a given pH, SofZia has been reported to be effective as per US Pharmacopeia standards for ocular drug preservation. When travoprost with sofZia and BKC was compared, it has been found that SofZia did not meet European Pharmacopoeia criteria due to its limited effectiveness against Staphylococcus aureus. However, both products satisfied US and Japanese Pharmacopoeia criteria (Ryan et al. 2011).

16.7.4 Studies Comparing of Preservatives in Terms of Efficacy and Toxicity

Many studies are available comparing the toxicity of various preservatives; however, lack of uniformity in the dose, variation in the methods adopted for testing and diverse experimental conditions are the factors making it difficult to have head-to-head comparison among them. A study assessed the effect of drug preservatives such as benzalkonium chloride, Polyquad, purite and sofZia-like mixture on trabecular meshwork cells. This study reported that BKC and Polyquad caused significant DNA damage, cell viability and increased DNA fragmentation. BKC, Polyquad and purite all caused altered gene expression. However, all of these effects were found to be less by sofZia (Izzotti et al. 2015). Long-term use of topical drugs in conditions like glaucoma is reported to induce toxic immunopathological changes in the ocular surface. One-month topical administration of preservatives cetrimonium chloride (0.01 %), benzalkonium chloride (0.01 %), benzododecinium bromide (0.01 %), thiomersal (0.004 %) and methyl parahydroxybenzoate (0.05 %) were all reported to cause similar changes in rat cornea (Becquet et al. 1998). When sodium chlorite was compared with BKC, based on the depletion of intracellular glutathione in conjunctiva and corneal epithelial cells, Ingram et al. (2004) reported that best balance of high antibacterial toxicity with low ocular toxicity was achieved with sodium chlorite. Another study compared the toxicity of preservatives on cell viability in immortalized human conjunctival and corneal epithelial cells; this study concluded that the toxicity was found from higher to low in the order of thimerosal 0.0025 % > BKC (0.025 %) > chlorobutanol (0.25 %) > methylparaben (0.01 %) > sodium perborate (0.0 025 %) and EDTA (0.01 %). For long-term administration, BKC showed unfavourable outcome in most of the studies, but substitution of BAK with Polyquad or sofZia has resulted in significant improvement in conjunctival and corneal cells (Ammar et al. 2010).

Interestingly, a comparative study evaluating five brands of over-the-counter artificial tears having different preservatives such as benzalkonium chloride/EDTA, parabens, chlorobutanol, silver chloride complex and purite-stabilized oxychloro complex was inoculated with test microorganisms like Pseudomonas aeruginosa, Staphylococcus aureus and Candida albicans (Charnock 2006). This study revealed that only the artificial tear containing benzalkonium chloride/EDTA is suitable per European Pharmacopoeia (Charnock 2006). Therefore, microbial preservation in the countries where environmental microbial load is high with resistant microorganisms, caution must be exercised while using these preservatives.

16.7.5 Miscellaneous

16.7.5.1 Sodium Hydroxyl Methyl Glycinate

Recently, a new preservative solution containing sodium hydroxymethylglycinate (SHMG) and edetate disodium was studied for its usefulness in multiuse ophthalmic solutions by Ghelardi et al. (2013). The MIC values for SHMG for bacteria and fungi were found to be 0.0025 % to 0.0125 % and 0.125 % to 0.50 %, respectively. However, its safety about corneal toxicity has not been proven.

16.8 Sorbates

It is a chemical, 2,4-hexadienoic acid, first isolated from the unripe berries of a tree (Sorbus aucuparia). As a salt of sodium, potassium and calcium, it is used as antimicrobial agent for food preservation. They are used at the concentration varying from 0.1 to 0.2 % in eye drop formulations. In a randomized, double-masked, parallel-group comparison study, a slightly higher incidence of burning and stinging on instillation has been recorded in patients when timolol with sorbate was compared with timolol with BKC (Mundorf et al. 2004).

16.8.1 Ethylenediaminetetraacetic Acid

It is a well-known compound mostly used for chelating calcium. Interestingly, when it is used in combination with other agents, synergism increases the activity. Metal cations are the integral parts of the cell wall of Gram-negative bacteria (Gray and Wilkinson 1965). Therefore, EDTA has been successfully used along with other agents to increase the antimicrobial spectrum. Using along with BKC has been reported to inactivate resistant Pseudomonas aeruginosa (Richards 1971). Along with thimerosal (0.004 %), EDTA (0.1 %) has been reported to kill Acanthamoeba castellanii and Acanthamoeba polyphaga trophozoites and cysts (Silvany et al. 1991).

16.8.2 Polyhexamethylene Biguanide

Polyhexamethylene biguanide (PHMB) is mostly used as a preservative in multipurpose contact lens cleaning solutions. Contact lens usage led to microbial keratitis due to Acanthamoeba species causing severe ocular inflammation and visual loss. Therefore, PHMB has been used as a preservative in contact lens disinfecting solutions (Illingworth and Cook 1998). Either it is used alone or in combination with other agents, it is used for the treatment of Acanthamoeba keratitis at the concentration of 0.02 %.

16.9 Physical and Chemical Preservation

When a drug formulation is subjected for wet heat sterilization, there is a possibility of them getting degraded by the process of hydrolysis, oxidation, reacting with other components resulting in change of colour, loss of activity, degradation of active chemical component, change in pH, etc. In the formulation development, topical formulations are usually subjected for accelerated stability studies at different conditions. During the drug formulation process, decomposition of phenylmercuric nitrate up to 30 % in sulphacetamine solution during heat sterilization has been reported (Parkin 1993). In the aqueous solution, prevention of oxidation is a pharmaceutical hurdle. In the topical solution of epinephrine, antioxidants such as *N*-acetylcysteine and sodium metabisulphite are reported to increase the shelf life (Springer et al. 1981). Even packing lipid derivatives such as latanoprost in an inert atmosphere and storing at gas-tight containers are expected to increase the stability (Velpandian et al. 2015). This formulation factors also include pH in the chemical stability of eye drop formulations. Extemporaneously prepared mitomycin C at the pH between 7 and 8 and stored at low temperature has been reported to increase the duration of its stability (Velpandian et al. 2005).

16.10 Preservative-Free Ophthalmic Solutions

Preservatives are generally added in multidose solutions to reduce the risk of microbial contamination. However, repeated use of drug formulations containing preservatives for chronic treatment for dry eye and glaucoma can use adverse effect on the ocular surface. Therefore, preservative-free ophthalmic solutions came to market for those who cannot tolerate preservatives. Preservative-free solutions always carry the risk of getting environmental contamination quickly. However, it is compulsory that they need to be kept in refrigerator and maintain the low temperature 3–5 °C (non-freezing) to avoid microbial growth. A study conducted in the United Kingdom, to find out the incidence of microbial contamination of preservative-free drops dispensed from multiusage containers, showed that 8.5 % of preservative-free vials were found to be contaminated with microbes like Staphylococcus aureus, coagulase-negative staphylococcus, Bacillus spp., Serratia spp., Klebsiella oxytoca, Enterobacter cloacae, and alpha streptococcus after patient usage (Rahman et al. 2006). Usage of perborate type of preservatives is known to generate hydrogen peroxide and cause oxidation in microbes. Although oxidation is known to affect the stability of drug, their relevance to drug stability is not known.

16.11 Conclusion

Although much emphasis has been made on preservation techniques in ophthalmic products, still contamination in ocular drug formulations during patient usage is unavoidable. Ocular toxicity of preservatives is one of the important concerns as they can cause mild symptoms like irritation, discomfort, foreign body sensation, itching or burning to severe side effects due to chronic inflammation in long-term topical treatments. A delicate balance is embedded between corneal toxicity of preservatives and microbial contamination in eye drops in preservative-free solutions. Even after using preservatives, microbial contaminations are reported. A recent study showed that pathogenic strains such as Pseudomonas aeruginosa, Serratia marcescens, Acinetobacter lwoffii, Stenotrophomonas maltophilia, and Staphylococcus aureus were found as a microbial contamination in 1.5 % bottles of antiglaucoma eye drops used in the hospital (Teuchner et al. 2015). This study also showed the high incidence contamination in outpatients of glaucoma as compared to antibiotic and anaesthetic eye drops. For eye drops applied by the patients, the tip was more frequently contaminated than the drops and the residual internal fluid indicating that educating the patients on drop administration technique is essential. Therefore, adequate emphasis must be given for patient education about the hygiene, storage methods and appropriate drug application method that are very important in reducing the microbial contamination and improving their suitability for ocular use. Moreover, while prescribing for long-term use, the ophthalmologist must take the preservative into account to improve quality of life and compliance in order to improve the outcome of the therapy.

References

Ammar DA, Noecker RJ, Kahook MY. Effects of benzalkonium chloride-preserved, polyquad-preserved, and sofZia-preserved topical glaucoma medications on human ocular epithelial cells. Adv Ther. 2010;27(11):837–45. doi:10.1007/s12325-010-0070-1.

Anwar Z, Wellik SR, Galor A. Glaucoma therapy and ocular surface disease: current literature and recommendations. Curr Opin Ophthalmol. 2013;24(2):136–43. doi:10.1097/ICU.0b013e32835c8aba.

Baker Z, Harrison RW, Miller BF. Action of synthetic detergents on the metabolism of bacteria. J Exp Med. 1941;73(2):249–71.

Baudouin C, Labbé A, Liang H, Pauly A, Brignole-Baudouin F. Preservatives in eyedrops: the good, the bad and the ugly. Prog Retin Eye Res. 2010;29(4):312–34.

Becquet F, Goldschild M, Moldovan MS, Ettaiche M, Gastaud P, Baudouin C. Histopathological effects of topical ophthalmic preservatives on rat corneoconjunctival surface. Curr Eye Res. 1998;17(4):419–25.

Brown MRW, Norton DA. The preservation of ophthalmic preparation. J Soc Cosmet Chem. 1965;16:369–93.

Charnock C. Are multidose over-the-counter artificial tears adequately preserved? Cornea. 2006;25(4):432–7.

Chen W, Hu J, Zhang Z, Chen L, Xie H, Dong N, Chen Y, Liu Z. Localization and expression of zonula occludins-1 in the rabbit corneal epithelium following exposure to benzalkonium chloride. PLoS One. 2012;7(7):e40893. doi:10.1371/journal.pone.0040893. Epub 2012 Jul 18.

Choi EK, Lee HH, Kang MS, Kim BG, Lim HS, Kim SM, Kang IC. Potentiation of bacterial killing activity of zinc chloride by pyrrolidine dithiocarbamate. J Microbiol. 2010;48(1):40–3. doi:10.1007/s12275-009-0049-2. Epub 2010 Mar 11.

Coad CT, Osato MS, Wilhelmus KR. Bacterial contamination of eyedrop dispensers. Am J Ophthalmol. 1984;98(5):548–51.

Code of Federal Regulations Ophthalmic preparations and dispensers 21CFR200.50. http://www.accessdata.fda.gov/scripts/cdrh/cfdocs/cfcfr/CFRSearch.cfm?fr=200.50

Debbasch C, Brignole F, Pisella PJ, Warnet JM, Rat P, Baudouin C. Quaternary ammoniums and other preservatives' contribution in oxidative stress and apoptosis on Chang conjunctival cells. Invest Ophthalmol Vis Sci. 2001;42(3):642–52.

DoMAGK G. Eine neue Klasse von Desinfektionsmitteln. Deut med Woch- schr. 1935;61:829–32.

Epstein SP, Ahdoot M, Marcus E, Asbell PA. Comparative Toxicity of Preservatives on Immortalized Corneal and Conjunctival Epithelial Cells. Journal of Ocular Pharmacology and Therapeutics. 2009;25(2):113–19.

Ghelardi E, Celandroni F, Gueye SA, Salvetti S, Campa M, Senesi S. Antimicrobial activity of a new preservative for multiuse ophthalmic solutions. J Ocul Pharmacol Ther. 2013;29(6):586–90.

Gray GW, Wilkinson SG. The effect of ethylenediaminetetra-acetic acid on the cell walls of some gram-negative bacteria. J Gen Microbiol. 1965;39(3):385–99.

Green K, Chapman J. Benzalkonium chloride kinetics in young and adult albino and pigmented rabbit eyes. Cutan Ocul Toxicol. 1986;5(2):133–42.

Hugo WB, Foster JHS. Bactericid al effect on Pseudomanas aeruginosa of chemical agents for use in ophthalmic solutions. J. Pharm. Pharmacol. 1964; Suppl, 16:124–26.

Illingworth CD, Cook SD. Acanthamoeba keratitis. Surv Ophthalmol. 1998;42(6):493–508.

Ingram PR, Pitt AR, Wilson CG, Olejnik O, Spickett CM. A comparison of the effects of ocular preservatives on mammalian and microbial ATP and glutathione levels. Free Radic Res. 2004;38(7):739–50.

Izzotti A, La Maestra S, Micale RT, Longobardi MG, Saccà SC. Genomic and post-genomic effects of anti-glaucoma drug preservatives in trabecular meshwork. Mutat Res. 2015;772:1–9.

Labbé A, Pauly A, Liang H, Brignole-Baudouin F, Martin C, Warnet JM, Baudouin C. Comparison of toxicological profiles of benzalkonium chloride and polyquaternium-1: an experimental study. J Ocul Pharmacol Ther. 2006;22(4):267–78.

Lee HJ, Jun RM, Cho MS, Choi KR. Comparison of the ocular surface changes following the use of two different prostaglandin F2α analogues containing benzalkonium chloride or polyquad in rabbit eyes. Cutan Ocul Toxicol. 2014;34(3):195–202.

Lubbers JR, Chauan S, Bianchine JR. Controlled clinical evaluations of chlorine dioxide, chlorite and chlorate in man. Environ Health Perspect. 1982;46:57–62.

McKillop A, Sanderson WR. Sodium perborate and sodium percarbonate: cheap, safe and versatile oxidising agents for organic synthesis. Tetrahedron. 1995;51:6145–66.

Mundorf TK, Ogawa T, Naka H, Novack GD, Crockett RS, US Istalol Study Group. A 12-month, multicenter, randomized, double-masked, parallel-group comparison of timolol-LA once daily and timolol maleate ophthalmic solution twice daily in the treatment of adults with glaucoma or ocular hypertension. Clin Ther. 2004;26(4):541–51.

Nirmal J, Singh SB, Biswas NR, Thavaraj V, Azad RV, Velpandian T. Potential pharmacokinetic role of organic cation transporters in modulating the transcorneal penetration of its substrates administered topically. Eye (Lond). 2013;27(10):1196–203. doi:10.1038/eye.2013.146. Epub 2013 Jul 12.

Noecker RJ. SofZia preservative system meets United States Pharmacopoeia standards. 2007. http://www.eyeworld.org/article.php?sid=3734. Accessed 21 June 2015.

Noss CI, Olivieri VP. Disinfecting capabilities of oxychlorine compounds. Appl Environ Microbiol. 1985;50(5):1162–4.

Novak M, Taylor WI. Antibacterial action of boric acid in lacrima (tears). J Am Pharm Assoc Am Pharm Assoc. 1951;40(9):430–2.

Parkin JE. The decomposition of phenylmercuric nitrate in sulphacetamide drops during heat sterilization. J Pharm Pharmacol. 1993;45(12):1024–7.

Rahman MQ, Tejwani D, Wilson JA, Butcher I, Ramaesh K. Microbial contamination of preservative free eye drops in multiple application containers. Br J Ophthalmol. 2006;90(2):139–41.

Richards RM. Inactivation of resistant by antibacterial combinations. J Pharm Pharmacol. 1971;23:136S–40.

Rolando M, Crider JY, Kahook MY. Ophthalmic preservatives: focus on polyquaternium-1. Expert Opin Drug Deliv. 2011;8(11):1425–38.

Rosenthal RA, Buck SL, Henry CL, Schlech BA. Evaluation of the preserving efficacy of lubricant eye drops with a novel preservative system. J Ocul Pharmacol Ther. 2006;22(6):440–8.

Ryan Jr G, Fain JM, Lovelace C, Gelotte KM. Effectiveness of ophthalmic solution preservatives: a comparison of latanoprost with 0.02% benzalkonium chloride and travoprost with the sofZia preservative system. BMC Ophthalmol. 2011;11:8.

Saenz M. Nascent oxygen from sodium perborate in oral disinfection and hygiene. Odontoiatr Rev Iberoam Med Boca. 1950;7(83):617–50.

Schein OD, Hibberd PL, Starck T, Baker AS, Kenyon KR. Microbial contamination of in-use ocular medications. Arch Ophthalmol. 1992;110(1):82–5.

Sevag MG, Ross OA. Studies on the mechanism of the inhibitory action of zephiran on yeast cells. J Bacteriol. 1944;48(6):677–82.

Sezgin Akçay Bİ, Güney E, Bozkurt TK, Topal CS, Akkan JC, Ünlü C. Effects of polyquaternium- and benzalkonium-chloride-preserved travoprost on ocular surfaces: an impression cytology study. J Ocul Pharmacol Ther. 2014;30(7):548–53. doi:10.1089/jop.2013.0248. Epub 2014 Jun 5.

Silvany RE, Dougherty JM, McCulley JP. Effect of contact lens preservatives on Acanthamoeba. Ophthalmology. 1991;98(6):854–7.

Springer V, Struhár M, Chalabala M. Preparation of eye drops with zinc sulphate and adrenaline. Pharmazie. 1981;36(10):706–8.

Teuchner B, Wagner J, Bechrakis NE, Orth-Höller D, Nagl M. Microbial contamination of glaucoma eyedrops used by patients compared with ocular medications used in the hospital. Medicine (Baltimore). 2015;94(8):e583.

Velpandian T, Saluja V, Ravi AK, Kumari SS, Mathur R, Ranjan N, Ghose S. Evaluation of the stability of extemporaneously prepared ophthalmic formulation of mitomycin C. J Ocul Pharmacol Ther. 2005;21(3):217–22.

Velpandian T, Kotnala A, Halder N, Ravi AK, Archunan V, Sihota R. Stability of latanoprost in generic formulations using controlled degradation and patient usage simulation studies. Curr Eye Res. 2015;40(6):561–71.

Xu Y, He Y, Li X, Gao C, Zhou L, Sun S, Pang G. Antifungal effect of ophthalmic preservatives phenylmercuric nitrate and benzalkonium chloride on ocular pathogenic filamentous fungi. Diagn Microbiol Infect Dis. 2013;75(1):64–7.

Chapter 17
Miscellaneous Drugs and Agents for Ocular Use

Thirumurthy Velpandian, Santosh Patnaik, Ujjalkumar S. Das, Kanuj Mishra, Ramalingam Kalainesan Rajeshkumar, Hanuman Prasad Sharma, Monica Chaudhry, and Sharmilee Vetrivel

Abstract In the practice of ophthalmology and optometry, several agents are important for therapeutic, cosmetic and diagnostic purposes and cannot be grouped into a single category. They are governed by pharmacopeia or abide by regulatory requirements which are commercially available except few of the customized formulations compounded by hospital pharmacies. This chapter includes most of the formulations extensively used in routine ophthalmic practices like corneal preservative media used to store cornea for transplantation, tattooing solutions for cosmetic use in corneal opacity, agents used in acid or alkali burn, vitreous substitutes, vitreolytic agents, viscoelastic substances, topical immunosuppressants, local anesthetics, botulinum toxin, protease inhibitors, chelators, contact lens solutions and irritation solutions.

T. Velpandian, BPharm, MS(Pharmacol), PhD (✉) • S. Patnaik, M. Pharm • U.S. Das, MPharm • R.K. Rajeshkumar, MS BioTech, MPhil, PhD • H.P. Sharma, M. Pharm
Ocular Pharmacology and Pharmacy, Dr. Rajendra Prasad Center for Ophthalmic Sciences, All India Institute of Medical Sciences, New Delhi, India
e-mail: tvelpandian@hotmail.com

K. Mishra, MBiotech • S. Vetrivel, MBiotech
Department of Biotechnology, All India Institute of Medical Sciences, New Delhi, India

M. Chaudhary, M. Optom
Department of Optometry and Vision Science, Amity University, Haryana, India

T. Velpandian (ed.), *Pharmacology of Ocular Therapeutics*,
DOI 10.1007/978-3-319-25498-2_17

17.1 Introduction

There are several ophthalmic preparations which have not been classified under separate chapters but their importance and utility in routine ophthalmological practice warrant their mention. Hence this chapter has included culture medium for the preservation of corneas for transplant, tattooing dye for cosmetic use in corneal opacity, agents used in acid or alkali burn, vitreolytic agents, viscoelastic substances, topical immunosuppressants, local anesthetics, contact lens solutions and drug preservatives for ophthalmic use (Table 17.1).

Table 17.1 Shows the list of content being covered

1.	Corneal preservation media
2.	Tattooing solution
3.	Acid and alkali burn
4.	Vitreolytic agents and replacement agent
5.	Ocular use of immunosuppressants
6.	Local anesthetics
7.	Contact lens solution
8.	Drug preservatives used in ophthalmic solution
9.	Irrigating solutions

17.2 Corneal Preservation Media

Santosh Patnaik

Corneal blindness is the second most common preventable blindness in the world after cataract. In developing countries like India, out of 1% total corneal blind cases, half can be corrected by corneal transplant. Vitamin A deficiency, infections, trauma, improper use of contact lenses and inappropriate use of home remedies are the common causes of preventable blindness (Acharya et al. 2012). Worldwide approximately 45 million people are suffering from bilateral blindness and 135 million have severe bilateral vision impairment (Whitcher et al. 2001). As stated above, corneal transplant is a potential mean to correct treatable blindness. For the successful achievement of the transplant, a good cornea is of paramount importance. Previously corneas were stored in the moist chamber maintained at 4 °C. This technique was having a drawback of the endothelial insult due to the presence of the metabolic waste and other materials in aqueous humor. Corneal preservation witnessed a major breakthrough in 1965 when Capella, Kaufman and Robbins developed the technique of corneal tissue cryopreservation. This technique could able to maintain corneas for more than 1 year in transplantable state. Still the technique was suffering from few shortcomings like requirement of special equipment, trained technician and donor tissue removal in less than 6 h postmortem. In 1968, stocker developed a method to store the corneas in the homologous serum. This technique led him to transplant corneas stored for more than 4 days. This technique had a specific requirement of the serum of acceptor of the cornea (McCarey and Kaufman 1974). In 1968, Mizukawa and Manabe developed a preservation solution in which whole excised eyeball could be submerged. The medium was formulated using chondroitin sulfate, inosine, adenine, adenosine, penicillin and streptomycin. Almost 600 successful keratoplasties were done using this technique (Mizukawa and Manabe 1968). This revolutionary work became the basis for the development of future chondroitin sulfate-containing media. In March 1974, two scientists, Bernard E. McCarey and Herbert E. Kaufman, developed a storage medium which affected the storage of corneas in a greater way. The most important factor involved with this media was the non-requirement of the specialized techniques stated earlier. This modified tissue culture medium was given the name MK medium by them. MK medium is a mixture of medium 199 (containing cell nutrients, commercially made by Sigma Aldrich, US) and dextran with antibiotics. It is a buffered medium which has an osmolarity between 290 and 320 and a pH 7.4. After the development of medium, it was tested on the rabbit corneas where it is found to maintain them for 14 days (McCarey and Kaufman 1974). In 1984, intermediate storage medium was introduced by Kaufman and associates. Medium named K-sol contains 2.5 % chondroitin sulfate, modified medium 199 with HEPES. The medium contains gentamicin for the maintenance of the sterility. It was proposed to store and maintain them for 14 days, but acceptable storage days are from 4 to 7 days (Lindstrom 1990). After K-sol intermediate storage media Dexsol was introduced in 1988 by Chiron Ophthalmics Inc. In addition to 1% dextran, Dexsol contains 1.35 % of chondroitin sulfate (Kaufman et al. 1991). In order to study the corneal deturgescence ability of chondroitin sulfate, a study was done by Lindstrom and associates. They found that 1.5 % chondroitin sulfate was needed to maintain the normal human corneal thickness at 4 °C and 34 °C (Lindstrom 1990). In order to preserve corneas for longer time, Optisol was introduced by Chiron Ophthalmics Inc. which has 2.5 % of chondroitin sulfate along with 1 % dextran. A comparative study done between Dexsol and Optisol with human corneas found that corneas stored in Optisol were significantly less thick than with Dexsol (Kaufman et al. 1991). In the European countries, eye banks usually use organ culture medium. Organ culture method provides several advantages like long storage time, acceptance of corneas of longer postmortem time and detection of microbial contamination prior to transplant (Pels 1997; Frueh and Bohnke 2000). Components of organ culture are Eagle's minimum essential medium (MEM) supplemented with 2 % fetal bovine serum (FBS). Few eye banks in Europe were found to use up to 8 % FBS (Armitage 2011). Several studies have shown superiority of the organ culture over hypothermic media (Armitage et al. 2014; Bohnke 1991). These days, adjoining of the two storage techniques, i.e., hypothermic and organ culture, is a current research area in the field of corneal storage (Haug et al. 2013) (Fig. 17.1).

To summarize, corneal storage media have done a long journey starting from short-term compromised storage to long-term improved storage. Still a lot is expected to happen to increase the lifespan of corneas to decrease the burden of preventable vision loss worldwide.

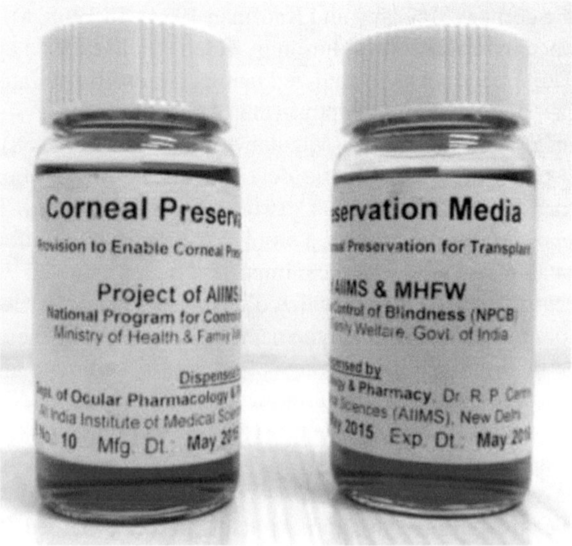

Fig. 17.1 Corneal preservation (McCareyKufman Media) media (Courtesy Dr. RPC (Pharmacy), AIIMS, N. Delhi, India)

17.3 Tattooing Solution

Santosh Patnaik

Tattooing solutions are used to mask the disfigured cornea. Tattooing solutions are used by ophthalmologist for cosmetically repairing the corneal opacities. There are different solutions used to tattoo the cornea. Tattooing with copper sulfate was introduced by Galen. In 1870 DeWecker used Indian ink for staining the cornea by mechanical means. In 1925 Professor Knapp introduced a method for coloring the discolored cornea by using gold chloride solution into the corneal stroma. The corneal tattooing should be done in such a way that it gives a good cosmetic effect along with permanent staining of the entire corneal opacity (Ziegler 1922; Pitz et al. 2002).

Gold or platinum chloride solutions are used for tattooing the discolored cornea. It is a simple, safe and effective method for coloring the cornea brown or black as compared to previously used Indian ink. For tattooing 2 % gold chloride or 2 % platinum chloride solution is used. The affected cornea is anesthetized by topical anesthesia and the corneal epithelium is removed from the area to be stained. Then with the help of a cotton-tipped applicator, 2 % gold chloride solution is applied to the affected area followed by 2 % hydrazine hydrate solution, till the affected area turns brown or black as desired. The tattooing technique with platinum chloride is similar to gold chloride tattooing (Duggan and Nanavati 1936; Pradhan et al. 2015) (Fig. 17.2).

Tattooing of the corneal opacities is a useful technique for the patients who are intolerant to cosmetic contact lenses. Tattooing of the cornea has got several advantages over wearing contact lenses. The patient is free from the maintenance of wearing a contact lens. In patient with peripheral corneal opacities with vision,

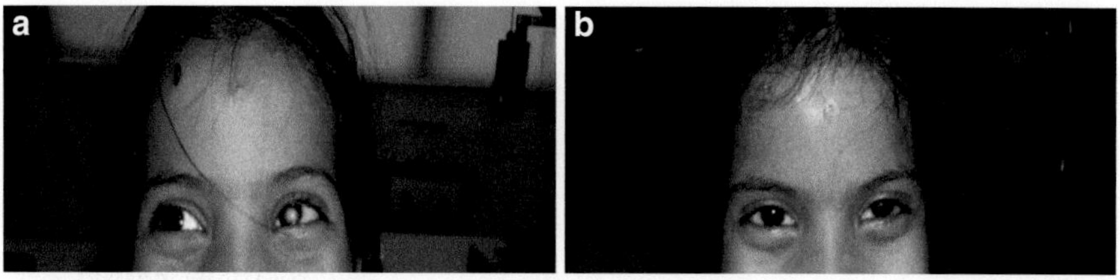

Fig. 17.2 (**a**) Preoperative left eye. (**b**) Post-tattooing left eye (Photograph courtesy Tarun Arora MD, Dr. RP Centre for Ophthalmic Sciences, AIIMS, N. Delhi)

corneal tattooing is an alternative to correct the cosmetic complaint without hampering the vision, whereas a colored contact lens may do so. It also gives social acceptance to the people (Pitz et al. 2002; Mannis et al. 1999).

17.4 Acid and Alkali Neutralizers

Ujjalkumar S. Das

Chemical ocular burns constitute true ophthalmic urgencies affecting extensively the cornea, surface epithelium, conjunctiva, anterior segment and limbal stem cell system leading devastating consequences, viz., chronic pain, disfigurement and vision impairment (Spector and Fernandez 2008). It is necessary to be diagnosed and treated at the earliest to prevent from potentially blinding ocular injuries and morbidity. It needs intensive evaluation of the burn, and prompt interventions should be given immediately to restore the integrity of ocular surface and tissues. Typically its occurrence is due to accidental ingress of corrosive substances into the surface of the eye or periocular tissues. Understanding the pathogenesis of these traumatic situation leads to the development of novel agents for the treatment. The major goal of the therapy is to rejuvenate the ocular surface and corneal clarity at optimal level needed for good sight.

17.4.1 Classification of Ocular Surface Burns

Several classification systems of ocular burns do exist. Most often it is categorized either by the causative agent (physicochemical or radiation or thermal) or by assessing the extent of damage to ocular tissues particularly the corneal, limbal and conjunctival tissues at the time of injury.

Ocular burns are broadly classified into the following types:

1. *Thermal burns*
   Thermal injuries to the eye are due to exposure to direct flame, firework explosions, steam, boiling water, or molten metal (commonly aluminum). This constitutes a rare event, but most of the parts of the eye affected in this insult are

eyelids, eyebrows and eyelashes due to the rapidity of lid reflex which protects the eye itself and visual acuity.

2. *Chemical burns*
   It is due to accidental exposure of the eye to chemical agents such as acid, alkali and other agents. Mostly the eye is affected by chemical burn and it accounts approximately 11.5–22.1 % of ocular injuries (Clare G et al. 2012). This type of insult to the eye can be accounted by the extent of damage to the cornea, conjunctiva and limbal tissue.
3. *Ocular injuries after radiation exposure*
   Direct exposure of light rays of variable wavelength is known to affect the eye due to its potential devastating effect. Several ocular tissues such as the corneal surface, retina and conjunctiva are recognized to absorb UV radiation (wavelengths 290–400 nm), infrared rays (wavelength >700 nm) and visible solar light (wavelengths 400–700 nm) which affect their functions after prolonged exposure time. UV damage to the corneal epithelium results in an inflammatory keratitis known as superficial punctuate keratitis (Brozen and Fromm 2006; Taylor 1989). Prolonged exposure to infrared radiation damages the anterior lens and may lead to cataract formation (e.g., glassblower's cataracts). Prolonged exposure to visible solar light may rarely result in retinal injury and subsequent visual loss (Roberts 2001).
4. *Ocular injuries after biological exposure*
   Biological exposure refers to contact of the eye to human blood or body fluids (saliva, semen, urine) which can serve as a potential source of infection. Blood-borne pathogens include hepatitis B virus (HBV), hepatitis C virus (HCV) and HIV lead to infection if it makes direct contact with the mucous membrane of the eye. The probability of infection is related to the amount (volume) and concentration (viral load) of the biological exposure (Zaleznik 2007; CDC 2003).

17.4.2 Roper-Hall System of Classification of Ocular Chemical Injuries

The classification system to categorize the chemical ocular injuries is first proposed by Ballen (1964) which was later modified based on the severity of damage to the cornea, limbal (limbal ischemia) and conjunctival tissues which divides the ocular chemical injuries into 4 grades (Roper-Hall 1965). Till now there are several

Table 17.2 Classification of ocular surface burns by Roper-Hall

	Clinical finding		
Grade	Cornea	Conjunctiva/limbus	Prognosis
I	Corneal epithelial damage	No limbal ischemia	Good
II	Corneal haze, iris details visible	<1/3 limbal ischemia	Good
III	Total epithelial loss, stromal haze, iris details obscured	1/3–1/2 limbal ischemia	Guarded
IV	Cornea opaque, iris and pupil obscured	>limbal ischemia	Poor

Table 17.3 Newer classification of ocular surface burns

Grade	Prognosis	Clinical findings	Conjunctival involvement	Analog scale
I	Very good	0 clock hours of limbal involvement	0 %	0/0 %
II	Good	≤3 clock hours of limbal involvement	≤30 %	0.1–3/1–29.9 %
III	Good	>3–6 clock hours of limbal involvement	>30–50 %	3.1–6/31–50 %
IV	Good to guarded	>6–9 clock hours of limbal involvement	>50–75 %	6.1–9/51–75 %
V	Guarded to poor	>9 to < clock hours of limbal involvement	>75 to <100 %	9.1–11.9/75.1–99.9 %
VI	Very poor	Total limbus (12 clock hours) involved	Total conjunctiva (100 %) involved	12/100 %

classification systems available, but Roper-Hall classification is widely used by clinicians for prompt recognition of the severity of disease (Table 17.2).

17.4.3 Dual System of Classification (Newer Classification of Ocular Chemical Injuries)

Dua et al. (2001) proposed a new classification for ocular chemical injuries which is a modification to Roper-Hall classification. This modification has taken into account the extent of limbal involvement in clock hours and the percentage of conjunctival involvement. This system classifies chemical surface burns into six grade (Table 17.3).

17.4.4 Pathophysiology

Understanding pathogenesis of these severe ocular traumatic conditions leads to the better prognosis rate of the disease and provides treatment options. Severity and recovery both depend on the type of causative agent, volume, concentration, duration of exposure and extent of penetration into ocular tissues (Pfister and Pfister 2005a, b). The mechanism followed by acid and alkali burn is quite different and explained as below.

17.4.4.1 Acid Burns

Acids dissociate into hydrogen ions and anion in the cornea. This usually occurs when a strong acid has a pH of less than 4. The hydrogen molecule damages the ocular surface by altering the pH, while the anion causes protein denaturation, precipitation and coagulation. Protein coagulation creates a barrier and thus generally prevents deeper penetration of acids and is responsible for the ground glass appearance of the corneal stroma following acid injury. Hydrofluoric acid is an exception; it behaves like an alkaline substance because the fluoride ion has better penetrance through the stroma, leading to the same spectrum and more extensive anterior segment disruption (Pfister and Pfister 2005a).

After entering into anterior chamber, it reacts with collagen resulting in shortening of collagen fibers which cause a rapid increase in intraocular pressure (IOP). After severe acid burns with ciliary body damage, decrease in levels of aqueous ascorbate has been demonstrated.

17.4.4.2 Alkali Burns

Alkaline substances are lipophilic and can penetrate cell membranes. They dissociate into a hydroxyl ion and a cation in the ocular surface. The hydroxyl ion saponifies cell membrane fatty acids, while the cation interacts with stromal collagen and glycosaminoglycans. This interaction facilitates deeper penetration into and through the cornea and into the anterior segment. Subsequent hydration of glycosaminoglycans results in stromal haze. Collagen hydration causes fibril distortion and shortening, leading to trabecular meshwork alterations that can result in increased intraocular pressure (IOP). Additionally, the inflammatory mediators released during this process stimulate the release of prostaglandins, which can further increase IOP (Pfister and Pfister 2005b). The damage to the corneal and conjunctival epithelium leads to the damage of the limbal stem cell causing limbal stem cell deficiency (LSCD). This in turn resulted in opacification and neovascularization in the cornea (Table 17.4).

Table 17.4 Examples of causative agents in acid and alkali burns (Spector and Fernandez 2008)

	Products	Chemical
Acid burns	Toilet cleaner	Sulfuric acid (80 %)
	Battery fluid	Sulfuric acid (30 %)
	Pool cleaners	Sodium or calcium hypochlorite (70 %)
	Bleaches	Sodium hypochlorite (3 %)
	Vinegar	Acetic acid
	Glass polishers, rust removal agents, silicon production agents	Hydrofluoric acid
	Food- and leather-processing compounds	Hydrochloric acid
Alkali burns	Lime	Calcium or magnesium carbonate
	Plaster and mortar	Calcium hydroxide
	Oven and drain cleaner	Sodium or potassium hydroxide
	Fireworks and sparklers	Magnesium hydroxide
	Ammonia (chemical agents and fertilizers)	Ammonium hydroxide
	Dishwater detergent	Sodium tripolyphosphate

17.4.5 *Therapeutic Interventions for Management*

Immediate initiation of management for ocular chemical injuries influences the final outcome favorably, namely, restoration of the normal ocular surface anatomy and lid position, control of glaucoma and restoration of corneal clarity. Management of chemical burns is based on the basic mechanism of the initial incident and the subsequent inflammatory response. It can be subdivided into the following types based on the timing of the treatment.

17.4.5.1 Emergency Therapy

After an acute chemical burn, copious irrigation is necessary to wash out the offending chemicals. Irrigation is performed with isotonic saline or lactate ringer solution or Morgan Lens to change pH to physiological levels and provide medication to the cornea and conjunctiva. This is followed by removal of any remaining particles from the ocular surface with a moist cotton tip or fine-tipped forceps (Eslani et al. 2014). Thus, emergency therapy represents the first line of management of ocular injuries and whose efficacy significantly affects further prognosis of the injury.

17.4.5.2 Acute Phase Treatment

Acute phase treatment proceeds emergency treatment and is based on the ophthalmic evaluation of the injuries done at emergency stage. It basically employs broad-spectrum topical antibiotic, cycloplegic and antiglaucoma therapy to promote reepithelialization, support repair and control inflammation. The different modalities (Table 17.5) employed in the acute phase treatment aim at reestablishment and maintenance of an intact and healthy corneal epithelium, control of the balance between collagen synthesis and collagenolysis and minimizing the adverse sequelae that often follow a chemical injury (Singh et al. 2013).

Table 17.5 Different treatment modalities for acute phase of chemical injuries

Treatment	Drugs
Promoting reepithelialization	Tear substitutes, bandage soft contact lens, Boston scleral lens, autologous serum, retinoic acid, epidermal growth factor and fibronectin, systemic ascorbic acid
Repair and minimizing ulceration	Ascorbate, collagenase inhibitors including cysteine, acetylcysteine, sodium ethylenediamine tetra acetic acid (EDTA), calcium EDTA, penicillamine and citrate
Anti-inflammatory therapy	Corticosteroids like topical prednisolone 0.5 % in conjunction with topical ascorbate 10 %

17.4.5.3 Early Reparative Phase Treatment

If an intact epithelium is not achieved by the 14th day after injury, then corticosteroids dosage is tapered and discontinued and aggressive therapy is followed through the use of lubricants, punctual plugs, punctal occlusion with cautery, bandage contact lens and tarsorrhaphy. In addition antibiotic, ascorbate, citrate and antiglaucoma therapy are continued and examination for the formation of symblepharon and corneal thinning are done (Singh et al. 2013). A symblepharon ring can be placed in the fornices to effectively prevent symblepharon formation. Proteinase inhibitors such as aprotinin and collagenase inhibitors such as cysteine, acetylcysteine and chelators such as sodium ethylenediamine tetra acetic acid (EDTA), calcium EDTA, penicillamine, citrate and especially tetracyclines have been found to prevent corneal thinning in chemically burned corneas (Wagoner 1997).

17.4.5.4 Surgical Management

Surgical management falls in the late reparative phase of treatment when an intact epithelium has not developed by the 21st day after injury leading to a significant risk of permanent vision loss (Eslani et al. 2014). The primary goal of early surgical management is to maintain the globe and promote reepithelialization. Early surgical management starts with initial debridement of the necrotic material, amniotic membrane transplantation and tectonic grafting if necessary. Late surgical interventions including limbal stem cell transplantation and keratoplasty are aimed at restoring the normal ocular surface anatomy and visual function (Singh et al. 2013).

17.5 Vitreous Substitutes

Kanuj Mishra

The vitreous body is a natural polymeric hydrogel composed primarily of type 2 collagen and hyaluronic acid and performs the essential physiological functions of intraocular pressure maintenance and ocular nourishment. Disruptions in this delicate architecture lead to the separation of its components (syneresis), creating the conditions for vitreoretinal disease (Foster 2008). Vitreous substitutes have been in use for almost a century to repair numerous complex vitreoretinal conditions successfully, such as most retinal detachments, giant retinal tears, macular holes and complex detachments. The ideal vitreous substitute should mimic the native vitreous in both form and function and be transparent, nontoxic, elastic and biocompatible for the long term. For practical reasons, it should also be easily manipulable during surgery, easily available, stable during storage, injectable through a small syringe and available at a reasonable cost. Advances in vitreoretinal surgical techniques, instrumentation and material technology have led to an array of agents from which vitreoretinal surgeons can choose (Torsten and Caroline 2007). The vitreous substitutes can be classified based on their availability, composition and physical properties into the following types:

17.5.1 Conventional Vitreous Substitutes

17.5.1.1 Air

This was the earliest vitreous substitutes developed by Ohm in 1911 when he treated retinal detachment with injection of sterile air into the vitreous cavity. Now the gases are mainly used intraoperatively in pneumatic retinopexy, at the end of vitrectomy surgery to facilitate retinal reattachment. Air facilitates and maintains retinal reattachment through the high surface tension of the gas bubble (Foster 2008).

17.5.1.2 Expansile Gas-Based Substitutes

Expansile gases have been used since the early 1970s and are the most effective short-term vitreous substitutes for retinal detachment repair since the early 1990s. These gases are colorless, odorless, heavier than air and nontoxic to the human eye. Sulfur hexafluoride (SF6) and perfluoropropane (C3F8) are the common class of gas-based substitutes available and are used in non-expansile concentrations to fill the vitreous cavity in pneumatic retinopexy. Gas-based substitutes have the highest surface tension of all vitreous fluid replacements (70 dyn/cm) which aids them to be expansile and to maintain a tamponade effect (Torsten and Caroline 2007). They are replaced with aqueous humor, avoiding a second surgery to remove them (Kleinberg et al. 2011).

17.5.1.3 Liquids

Perfluorocarbon

Perfluorocarbon liquid (PFCL) are fluorinated, carbon-containing hydrophobic compounds that are clear, colorless and odorless. These liquids were developed as blood substitutes due to their inert nature and ability to carry oxygen. The intraoperative uses of perfluorocarbon liquids depend on their high specific gravity (1.7–2.03) by the property of which a unique gravitational force is applied on the dependent portion of retina (Azad 2012). Commonly used PFCLs are perfluoro-n-octane (C8F18), perfluorodecalin (C10F18), perfluoroperhydrophenanthrene (C14F24) and perfluorohexyloctane (C6F13C8H18). Perfluorocarbon liquids have been successfully used in the management of proliferative vitreoretinopathy (PVR), repair of detachments secondary to ocular trauma and removal of dislocated crystalline lenses. Perfluorocarbon liquids are being primarily as a short-term intraoperative vitreous substitute and long-term complications are rare (Foster 2008).

Silicone Oil (SO)

The use of silicone oil as a long-acting vitreous substitute was pioneered by Cibis in 1962 for complex retinal detachments (Yang et al. 2014). Silicone oil refers to the polymers of polydimethylsiloxane and is the only substance currently accepted for long-term vitreous replacement. The most commonly available silicone oils have viscosities of 1000 centistokes (cS) and 5000 cS and contain trimethylsiloxyl-terminated polydimethylsiloxane, but standards have yet to be established and batch variation may exist. Silicone oil is slightly lighter than water with a specific gravity of 0.97 and during substitution, a silicone globule floats on a residual aqueous base inside the eye. Silicone oil represents a more versatile replacement than air or gas and is widely used for giant retinal breaks, hypotony due to chronic uveitis, infectious retinitis and finally retinal detachments where postoperative positioning is not possible. Postsurgical and late complications of intraocular silicone oil fills are common and may require removal of the oil earlier than the desired duration (Foster 2008).

The available replacements each have their specific advantages and drawbacks (Table 17.6). Hence the recent thrust is on the development of substitutes that not only serve as retinal tamponades but also satisfy biomechanical aspect of vitreous. These recently developed substitutes can be classified into two types – newer vitreous substitutes and experimental vitreous substitutes based on their stage of development.

Table 17.6 Advantages and disadvantages of different class of vitreous replacements

Class	Advantage	Disadvantage
Air	Inexpensive Readily available	Less intravitreal residence time (2–3 days) Cataract corneal endothelial damage, raised IOP
Expansile gas-based substitutes	Good success rate, exceeding 90 % for retinopexy	Limited to treating the upper retina gas-induced cataract formation corneal endothelial changes raised IOP central retinal artery occlusion
Perfluorocarbon	The low viscosity of PFCLs allows for tissue manipulation, injection and removal	During prolonged usage decrease in vitreous clarity, compromise of the trabecular meshwork with subsequent IOP rises and subretinal migration of droplets through residual breaks
Silicone oil	Suppression of future neovascularization bactericidal properties has 70 % success rate in preserving anatomical integrity	Emulsification, corneal decompensation, band keratopathy, cataract and secondary glaucoma. SO removal has been accompanied by visual acuity loss, hypotony and corneal abnormalities

17.5.2 Newer Vitreous Substitutes

17.5.2.1 Semifluorinated Alkanes

Semifluorinated alkanes (SFAs), also known as partially fluorinated alkanes (PFAs) or fluorinated alkanes, were investigated for their vitreous replacement properties in the early 2000s. SFAs were initially used as a solvent for SO and then as a temporary vitreous substitute for special cases of retinal detachment when silicone oil failed to function properly. Their low specific gravity (compared to PFCLs) and high interface tension (compared to silicone oil) are thought to produce less retinal damage and bridge larger retinal breaks (Azad 2012). Clinical trials have shown SFAs to be tolerated for extended periods of 2–3 months and they are being pioneered the first internal tamponade agents to be used beyond the intraoperative setting (Kleinberg et al. 2011).

17.5.2.2 Silicone Oil/Semifluorinated Alkanes Combinations

This combination takes advantage of the high viscosity of SO and high specific gravity of the SFAs to produce a vitreous substitute with a good tamponade effect and lesser chance of emulsification. Depending on the ratio of the two liquids, either a homogenous clear solutions (heavy silicone oils) or separated solutions (double fills) are developed (Azad 2012). Double fill (DF) was developed with the goal of having the light SO support the superior retina, while the heavier SFA supports the inferior retina. DF has been reported to have the best results in complicated surgeries with large inferior retinal breaks. Heavy silicone oil (HSO) is heavier than water and is created by combining SO and a PFA in such a way as to create a homogenous solution. HSO is being promoted as a long-term replacement agent for complex retinal detachments involving inferior proliferative vitreoretinopathy (Kleinberg et al. 2011).

17.5.3 Experimental Vitreous Substitutes

17.5.3.1 Hydrogels

Hydrogels are three-dimensional hydrophilic polymers that swell in aqueous solutions without dissolving and form a gel network through cross-linkage. They are clear viscoelastic gel that strongly resembles the natural vitreous humor (Azad 2012). Hydrogels were the first biomaterials synthesized for human use, but in vivo research on hydrogels as vitreous replacements is still in the animal model stage. Because of the early experimental nature of the materials, complications and efficacy associated with hydrogels are not well known.

17.5.3.2 Implants

Implantable devices may be able to support the retina without the need of a potentially immunoreactive intravitreally injected solution. Foldable capsular vitreous bodies (FCVB) injected with saline showed good biocompatibility and retinal support in rabbit eyes over a 180-day implantation time. However, the feasibility of a synthetic implant in the human eye is untested and longer-term animal data are first needed to assess the potential use of this approach (Kleinberg et al. 2011).

The intraocular vitreous body is a highly complex macromolecular structure and despite significant progress over the past few decades, ideal, universal vitreous substitute does not exist. Recently, in situ-forming zwitterionic hydrogels have been developed as a promising vitreous substitute (Chang et al. 2015). Thus, advancements in material sciences coupled with extensive molecular understanding of vitreous components could aid in a plethora of compound that could facilitate longer and more efficient vitreous replacement.

17.5.4 Chemical Agents for Vitreolysis

The earliest definition of vitreolytic agents was given by Sebag et al. 1998 as "agents that alter the molecular organization of vitreous in an effort to reduce or eliminate its role in disease."

The vitreous is involved in multiple diseases when an incomplete posterior vitreous detachment (PVD) occurs. Incomplete PVD is considered pathological when associated with focal adhesions, causing vitreomacular traction (VMT) syndrome, vitreopapillary adhesion, tractional diabetic macular edema (DME), peripheral retinal breaks and rhegmatogenous retinal detachment or when associated with vitreoschisis (hyaloid delamination), predisposing to epiretinal membrane, macular hole and diabetic retinopathy neovessel proliferation and recurrence (Gandorfer 2012).

Vitreous liquefaction and posterior vitreous separation have to be done through pharmacological vitreolysis to obtain a safe and complete PVD. There are several vitreolytic agents that have been studied to date. They can be categorized as "enzymatic" or "nonenzymatic," according to their mechanism of action and as "liquefactants (induce a vitreous liquefaction) or interfactants" (induce dehiscence at the vitreoretinal interface on the basis of their biological effect) (Table 17.7). Some of the most studied vitreolytic agents are discussed below:

17.5.4.1 Enzymatic Vitreolytic Agents

Dispase

Dispase is a protease which cleaves fibronectin, collagen IV and collagen I (to a lesser extent). Studies in animal and human models document the efficacy of dispase to cleave the attachment between the posterior hyaloid and the internal limiting membrane (ILM), with minimal morphological changes to the inner retina (Tezel

Table 17.7 Classification of vitreolytic agents on the basis of their mechanism of action and biological effects

	Interfactants	Liquefactants	Combination
Enzymatic	Dispase	Hyaluronidase	Plasmin
		Collagenase	Microplasmin
			tPA/plasminogen
			Nattokinase
			Chondroitinase
Nonenzymatic	RGD peptides		Vitreosolve

et al. 1998; Oliveira et al. 2002). Despite its usefulness as an adjunct in facilitating surgical creation of PVD harmful effects including proliferative vitreoretinopathy, retinal hemorrhages, cataract, lens subluxation and retinal toxicity have been reported (Jorge et al. 2003; Wang et al. 2004; Zhu et al. 2006; Frenzel et al. 1998; Kralinger et al. 2006; Ivastinovic et al. 2012).

Hyaluronidase

Hyaluronidase is the only agent for enzymatic vitreolysis which has been evaluated in phase III clinical trials (Kuppermann et al. 2005). Hyaluronidase cleaves the glycosidic bonds of hyaluronan as well as other mucopolysaccharides resulting in dissolution of the hyaluronan and collagen complex and subsequent vitreous liquefaction. Hyaluronidase has been considered as liquefactant because of its property of dissolving the glycosaminoglycan network of the vitreous gel. But several other studies have concluded hyaluronidase alone to be ineffective in inducing PVD suggesting a combination of vitreolytic agents with hyaluronidase (Zhi-Liang et al. 2009; Wang et al. 2005; Narayanan and Kuppermann 2009).

Collagenase

Collagenase is a liquefactant obtained from *Clostridium histolyticum* which selectively cleaves the type II collagen that constitutes the fibrillar network of the vitreous gel. Cleaved type II collagen forms soluble proteolyzed fragments allowing for spontaneous denaturation and further degradation by nonspecific proteases. Its liquefactant action has been successfully established in animal models, and found to be associated with inner limiting membrane damage and disruption of retinal architecture (O'Neill and Shea 1973) or histological and electrophysiological toxicity (Moorhead et al. 1980, 1983).

Plasmin and Ocriplasmin

Plasmin is a nonspecific serine protease with a critical role in fibrinolysis and the most studied vitreolytic agent. It directly degrades fibrin and other extracellular matrix components including laminin and fibronectin (Liotta et al. 1981; Uemura et al. 2005; Li et al. 2002) and may also indirectly generate increased levels of other nonspecific proteases such as matrix metalloproteinases and elastase (Bandello et al. 2013). These downstream activities enhance the primary action of plasmin in weakening the vitreoretinal insertion. Thus, it is capable of degrading the vitreous gel and of cleaving further ECM structures, serving as a liquefactant as well as an interfactant. Various preclinical studies have concluded plasmin to be an excellent vitreolytic agent through ERG examinations and histological analysis at doses up to 4 U and with exposure times ranging from 30 min to 1 week in which no pathological tissue damage and functional changes were noted (Bandello et al. 2013). However, the process for isolating autologous plasmin is cumbersome and the enzymatic activity is dependent on multiple variables including the level of plasminogen in the blood. As a result, the amount of enzymatic activity obtained is variable and difficult to quantify.

Ocriplasmin, formerly known as microplasmin, is a recombinant product of plasmin which alleviated most of the problems associated with autologous plasmin (Chen et al. 2008; Sebag et al. 2007). It is a truncated form of plasmin that lacks the five kringle domains of plasmin but contains the protease domain making it a smaller molecule than plasmin (27 kD compared to 80 kD) but with similar enzymatic activity. Advantage of being recombinant is that microplasmin can be produced in large quantity supplementing the need of use in different dose-ranging studies. Animal and ex vivo studies demonstrate that microplasmin creates both posterior vitreous detachment and vitreous liquefaction without evidence of retinal toxicity.

Nattokinase and Chondroitinase

Nattokinase is serine protease produced by *Bacillus subtilis* and is derived from fermented soybean, whereas chondroitinase is a protease able to degrade chondroitin sulfate, a glycosaminoglycan. They both act as liquefactant and interfactant. Both have been studied in animal models, but conclusive data on safety and efficacy are lacking (Takano et al. 2006; Hermel and Schrage 2007; Staubach et al. 2004).

17.5.4.2 Nonenzymatic Vitreolytic Agents

RGD Peptides

Integrins are proteins of the plasma membrane that mediate the adhesion of cells to each other and to the extracellular matrix and carry signals in both directions across the membrane. The extracellular ligands that interact with integrins include laminin, collagen, fibrinogen, fibronectin and many other proteins that have the sequence recognized by integrins: Arg-GIy-Asp (RGD). Synthetic RGD peptides are known to compete for integrin-binding sites, which results in disruption of integrin-ECM interaction and subsequent loosening of attachments. They are considered as interfactants because of their possible role in disrupting vitreoretinal adhesion of the membrane.

Despite fewer studies on rabbit model (Oliveira et al. 2002) where RGD peptides made PVD easier during vitrectomy procedure, no further studies have been published.

17.6 Ocular Use of Immunosuppressants

Ramalingam Kalainesan Rajeshkumar

Transplantation and immunosuppressants are two sides of the coin. The earliest description of human organ transplantation is from the fourth century BC ancient Chinese text in which the eminent Chinese surgeon Tsin Yue-Jin reported to have exchanged the hearts of two soldiers, while the original concept of corneal transplantation can be attributed to the Greek physician Galen (130–200 AD) who proposed superficial keratectomy as a means of restoring corneal transparency (Moffatt et al. 2005). Corneas represent the most commonly transplanted tissue worldwide and all surgical procedures of corneal transplantation demands optimized immunosuppression to maximize transplantation success (Tan et al. 2012).

Table 17.8 represents different classes of immunosuppressants used for ocular transplantation along with their doses.

17.7 Thrombolytics

Ramalingam Kalainesan Rajeshkumar

Thrombus is a pathological condition due to intravascular blood clotting. Thrombolytics are group of drugs used to dissolve thrombi and fibrin deposits, e.g., tissue plasminogen activator (tPA), urokinase, streptokinase, etc.

17.7.1 Occlusion in Vessels of Eye

The central retinal artery occlusion (CRAO) and central retinal vein occlusion (CRVO) are the major problem associated with the eye which needs to be treated with thrombolytic agents. Embolism is the most common cause of CRAO, the major source of this being atherosclerotic plaques in carotid artery disease (Varma et al. 2013).

17.7.2 Treatment with Thrombolytics

CRAO is treated by intra-arterial thrombolysis using tPA or urokinase (50 mg tPA over 60 min) infused at the origin of the ophthalmic artery and also by intravenous thrombolysis with tPA (Valerie 2008).

Table 17.8 Immunosuppressants for ocular transplantation

	Drugs	Mechanism of action	Route of administration	Transplantation type	Dose (Alone or in combinations)	References
1.	Corticosteroids	Anti-inflammatory and immunosupressive actions are due to glucocorticoid agonism by altering the transcription of genes involved in the process.	Systemic	Keratoplasties	Methylprednisolone – 1 g/day IV for first 3 days followed by 1 mg/kg oral, Dexamethasone – 8 mg/day OD	Gregory and Kanna (2011), Krensky et al. (2011), Suh et al. (2006)
2.	Cyclosporine	Cyclosporine binds to cytosolic immunophilins (cyclophillins) of T lymphocytes forming a complex which inhibits the calcineurin. Normally,Calcineurin catalyzed dephosphorylation allows the movement of the nuclear factor of activated T cells (NFAT) required for transcription of interleukin-2 and other cytokines (lymphokines). Therefore, this Cyclosporine-cyclophillin complex inhibits calcineurin preventing signal transductions which ultimately leads to the reduced functioning of effector T-Cells.	Systemic or Topical 2 %	Keratoplasties, limbal transplantation	Pre-operative 5–7 mg/kg, 1–2 mg/kg post-operative Topical 2 %	Gerber et al. (1998), Sahu (2011), Sinha et al (2010)
3.	Mycophenolate mofetil	Inhibits inosine monophosphate dehydrogenase which is key enzyme for guanine nucleotide synthesis and T-lmphocyte proliferation.	Systemic	Keratoplasties	1000 mg/day BD	Chan and Holland (2013), Natsumeda and Carr (1993)

4.	Tacrolimus	FK-506 or fujimycin, is a macrolide calcineurin inhibitor binds to immunophillin FKBP-12 (FK506 binding protein) FK-506-FKBP-12 complex which inhibits calcineurin, which further inhibits the both T-lymphocyte signal transduction and IL-2 transcription. It ultimately leads to reduced function of effector T-cells.	Systemic	Keratoplasties	4000 mg/day BD	Chan and Holland (2013), Krensky et al. (2011)
5.	Cyclophosphamide	Alkylation of DNA by phosphoramide mustard, a toxic metabolite of cyclophosphamide causing suppressionof cellular and humoral immunity.	Systemic	Limbal transplantation	750 mg/m^2 IV for first 3 days followed by 1–2 mg/kg oral	Burkhart et al. (2011), Suh et al. (2006)
6.	Basiliximab/gene therapy	Basiliximab,a glycoprotein is a chimeric anti-intcrleukin-2 receptor monoclonal antibody which binds to alpha chain subunit of the IL2 receptor (CD25 antigen), on the surface of activated T-lymphocytes halting T cells replication and B cells activation thereby preventing these cells to stimulate an immune response against the organ transplant.	Under investigation			Birnbaum et al. (2008)

17.8 Botulinum Toxin

Ramalingam Kalainesan Rajeshkumar

17.8.1 Introduction

It is the most potent poison known and is lethal at doses as low as 0.05 μg. It is produced by the bacterium *Clostridium botulinum* which produces seven antigen-specific toxin type A, B, C, D, E, F and G (Gonnering 1993). Among these, type A is mostly used and rarely type B is used in the ocular treatments (Table 17.9). Type A is more potent in low doses and in nonresponsive case, type B is used. But type B suffers from the adverse reaction of diffusing to adjacent tissues.

17.8.2 Mechanism of Action

Botulinum toxin blocks neuromuscular transmission by antagonizing the serotonin-mediated calcium ion release in the peripheral cholinergic nerve endings and thus prevents acetylcholine being released from the presynaptic terminals (Dutton 1996). Botulinum toxin interferes with transmission not only at the neuromuscular junction but also in the cholinergic autonomic parasympathetic and postganglionic sympathetic nervous system. As such it is increasingly found useful in the treatment of various disorders of the autonomic nervous system (Naumann et al. 1999).

Table 17.9 Ocular Use of Botulinum Toxin A

	Type/region	Disease condition
1	Eyelid	Facial dystonia – blepharospasm
		Hemifacial spasm
		Reduce lid retraction, e.g., thyroid eye disease
		Apraxia of lid opening
		Induce ptosis in exposure keratopathy
		Lower lid spastic entropion
2	Strabismus	Infantile esotropia/acquired esotropia
		Intermittent exotropia
		Nerve palsies
		Thyroid eye disease-related strabismus
		Congenital nystagmus
3	Cosmetic	Glabellar lines
		Crow's feet
		Bunny lines

17.8.3 Side Effects

Fever, increased muscle tone, injection site problems such as bleeding, bruising, irritation, pain, tenderness, swelling, erythema, inflammation, hypersensitivity, infections, muscle weakness, pain in the extremities and unexplained or unexpected bruising, difficulty with swallowing, infection, neck pain, uncontrolled twisting movements of the neck.

17.9 Chelators

Chelation therapy is the removal of excess of heavy metals from the body using chelators. Therapy involves topical administration of chelating agents; these agents will bind to heavy metals/minerals in the eye and help in the removal process.

17.9.1 Disodium EDTA

Disodium EDTA is a sodium salt of ethylenediamine tetraacetic acid which is mainly used for ophthalmic chelation therapy. It is mainly used in the treatment of calcific band keratopathy (CBK) which is a condition characterized by the deposition of calcium in the superficial layers of the cornea, most frequently in the interpalpebral zone (Najjar et al., 2004). These opaque calcium deposits are separated from the limbus by a clear region. Disodium EDTA is also used to treat chemical exposure of eye to Calcium hydroxide burns and Zinc chloride injury. It has been used as emergency treatment to decontaminate the eye after injury by zinc chloride and for emergency management.

17.9.1.1 Treatment and dosage

EDTA formulation for ophthalmic use is not commercially available. It can be freshly prepared 0.35 to 1.85% in standard isotonic ophthalmic irrigation solutions which does not contain calcium such as isotonic saline. This solution can be used by irrigation for 15 to 20 minutes to remove calcium deposits. Disodium EDTA is lipid-insoluble and does not penetrate the corneal epithelium. In case of calcium deposits in the deep stroma, the epithelium must be debrided before irrigation or direct application using sterile cotton. In this method applicator is soaked in the diluted EDTA solution and applied against the calcium until its dissolution. This requires from 5 to 45 minutes of EDTA application, depending on the density of the calcium (Ellis, 1981).

17.9.1.2 Side effects

Sodium EDTA is toxic to the corneal stroma causing corneal edema, chemosis and severe inflammation etc. To minimize these adverse effect it should be applied for the shortest possible duration (Ellis, 1981).

17.9.2 Protease Inhibitors and Ocular Diseases

Ramalingam Kalainesan Rajeshkumar

The presence of proteases is well known in the living organisms. It catalyzes hydrolysis of target proteins and it regulates the fate, localization and activity of many substrates; creates new bioactive molecules; contributes to process cellular information and transducer; amplifies molecular signals; modulate protein-protein interactions; etc. Expression of these proteases or increase in the cellular level leads to consequences like corneal and retinal degenerative disorders, neurodegenerative disorders, inflammation, cardiovascular diseases, etc. (Pescosolido et al. 2014). Protease activity is being controlled by protease-inhibitor system. The balance between proteases and protease-inhibitor system plays a key role in maintaining cellular and tissue homeostasis (Lopez et al. 2008).

17.9.3 Aprotinin

Aprotinin is a broad-spectrum serine protease inhibitor. It is a competitive serine protease inhibitor which complexes with and blocks the active sites of enzymes (Skondra et al., 2009). The binding is reversible and dissociation depends on the pH. It is showing better results to treat ocular inflammation in experimental uveitis. Aprotinin is also used to inhibit fibrinolysis of the human fibrin glue which is used in corneal surgery and keratoplasty etc (Por et al., 2009; Sharma et al., 2003).

17.10 Local Anesthetics

Hanuman Prasad Sharma

History Cocaine was the first agent used by Carl Koller and Sigmund Freud as local anesthetic (LA) in 1884 to enucleate dog's eye without pain (Freud 1884). Later in 1885, Leonard Corning injected 2 % cocaine solution in the spine of a dog which resulted in the loss of sensation within 5 min (Corning 1885). The high toxic-

Table 17.10 **Use of LAs in ophthalmology**

Topical	Injectable
Contact lens fitting, tonometry, ophthalmic surgeries, gonioscopy, electroretinography, minor ophthalmic procedures – corneal scrapping and lacrimal duct dilation	Retrobulbar injection, eyelid infiltration, facial nerve block, subtenon injection, subconjunctival and intracameral injections

ity of the cocaine led to the development of the procaine by Alfred Einhorn in 1904. He found that the benzoyl group of the cocaine called as "anesthesiophoric" group by Paul Ehrlich was responsible of its anesthetic property (Einhorn 1899).

In general, local anesthetics (LAs) are the chemical agents used in the arrest of the neuronal sensation at local site of application. LAs are useful in several application sites like topical, spinal and local. Though topical anesthetic agents are sufficient for most of the procedures (Table 17.10), injectables are also required in certain cases (Bartletta and Reddy 1995).

Mechanism of action of local anesthetics LAs act by blocking the sodium channels in the neurons. Sodium channel consists of four domains (DI–DIV) containing six helices each (S1–S6). Sodium channel represents three states of functioning – (1) closed state at potential below −70 mV, (2) open state at potential above −40 which comes after depolarization of transmembrane potential to the level of threshold and (3) state of inactivation which comes after peak sodium current (Scholz 2002). LAs bind to their receptors situated within sodium channels and increase the threshold of the opening of the channels (Tripathi 2008). Besides sodium channels, LAs also bind to voltage-dependent and voltage-independent potassium channels. This binding occurs at very high concentration of the LAs. LAs also bind to calcium channels because of the structural resemblance to sodium channels. The sensitivity of the L type calcium channel is more than that of the other types (Scholz 2002).

Structural properties Based on the structure LAs are classified as amides and esters.

Generally a LA agent has a lipophilic center made up of carbocyclic or heterocyclic ring system and a hydrophilic center made up of secondary or tertiary amines. Hydrophilic center is attached to the ester or amide which forms a bridge between both the centers (Fig. 17.3). Lipophilic center of the LAs governs lipid solubility and penetration to the cells and hydrophilic center governs the water solubility which facilitates the movement into the cell. For a drug to be a good LA, it should have a balance of both of the centers.

Use in Ophthalmology Lignocaine is generally used subconjunctivally before intravitreal injection. A study was also carried out in patients for topical or subconjunctival anesthesia using lignocaine. It was concluded at last that more than 80 % of the patients preferred subconjunctival injection over topical anesthesia

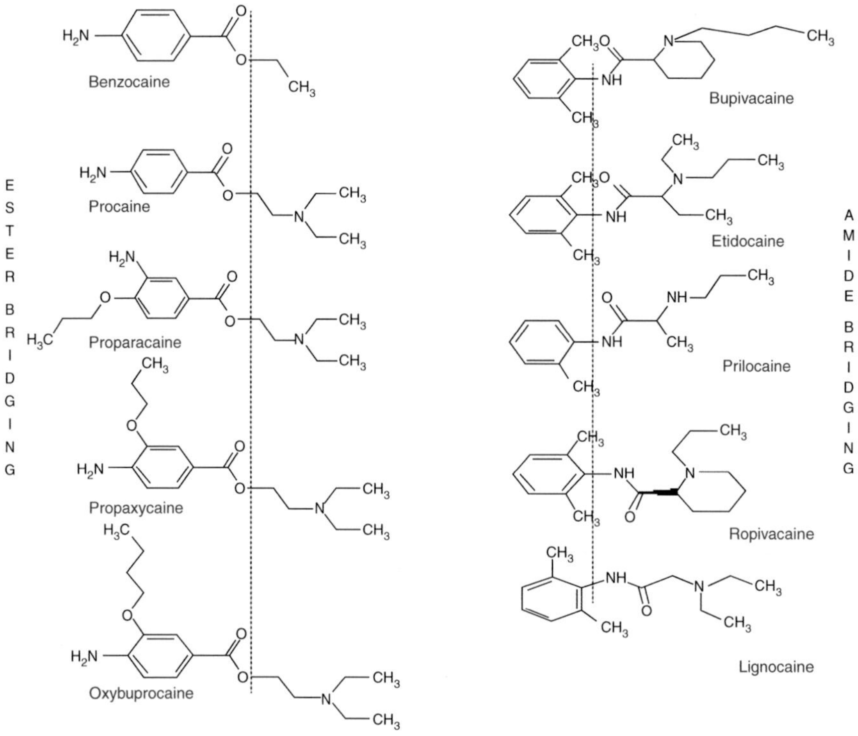

Fig 17.3 Structures of commonly used local anesthetics having ester and amide bridge (indicated by vertical line)

for intravitreal injection (Cohen et al. 2014). In an important study, a detailed review was done for the pain relief from topical medications after photorefractive keratectomy (PRK). It was found that tetracaine should not be the choice of the LA because of its effect on delaying corneal reepithelialization (Faktorovich and Melwani 2014). Lignocaine, which is used in a routine basis for the local anesthesia, is found to have pupil dilatation effect as well; hence, it was used intracamerally for the cataract surgery. Lignocaine administered by subtenon route was also found to prevent intraoperative floppy iris syndrome (IFIS) in patients taking oral alpha receptor antagonists (Klysik and Korzycka 2014). Table 17.11 represents some commonly used LAs with their pharmaceutical form and drug content.

Adverse reactions to LAs Though topical anesthetic agents are well tolerated, they may be a part of drug abuse if used at home repeatedly. Topical ocular anesthetic abuse can lead to superficial punctate keratitis, persistent epithelial defects, stromal/ring infiltrates, corneal edema, endothelial damage and ocular inflammation and can be misdiagnosed often as *Acanthamoeba* keratitis (Patel and Fraunfelder 2013). All

Table 17.11 Commonly used LAs with pharmaceutical form and strength

Name	Pharmaceutical formulation	%
Benzocaine	Ophthalmic solution	5 %
	Cream	6 %
	Gel	15 and 20 %
	Ointment	5 and 20 %
	Lotion	0.8 %
	Liquid	20 %
	Spray	20 %
Bupivacaine	Parenteral	0.25, 0.5 and 0.75 %
Lignocaine	Parenteral	0.5, 1, 1.5, 2 and 4 %
	Topical	2.5 %
	Ointment	5 %
	Cream	0.5 and 4 %
	Gel	0.5 and 2.5 %
	Solution	2, 2.5, and 4 %
	Patch	23 and 46 mg/2 cm^2
Procaine	Parenteral	1, 2 and 10 %
Proparacaine	Topical	0.5 %
Prilocaine	Parenteral	4 %
Ropivacaine	Parenteral	0.2, 0.5, 0.75, and 1 %
Tetracaine	Topical	0.5 and 1 %
	Cream	7 %
	Ointment	7 %
	Gel	4 %

LAs of ester chemical class are known to cause allergic reactions. This selective class behavior is due to the development of para-aminobenzoic acid (PABA) metabolite which doesn't happen with amide class of LAs. Though parabens (methylparaben) also produce same PABA metabolite and LAs containing methyl- or propylparaben as preservative can also produce same allergic reaction. Proparacaine is an exception of ester class which is not metabolized to PABA and can be used with caution in patients sensitive to PABA metabolites (Eggleston and Lush 1996; Ramos-Esteban and Cruz 2011). LAs can produce systemic toxicities including cardiac toxicities such as arrhythmias, myocardial depression and cardiac arrest and CNS toxicities like irritation, lethargy, seizures and CNS depression leading to respiratory arrest. Bupivacaine is known to produce more cardiotoxicity than any other LAs. The reason behind is the blockage of the significant fraction of sodium channels of the heart as bupivacaine dissociates slowly during diastole. Few of the adverse effects related to the techniques used (regional block, subconjunctival and subtenon injection) are conjunctival chemosis, subconjunctival hemorrhage, retrobulbar hemorrhage, globe perforation, amaurosis, myotoxicity and facial nerve block (Ramos-Esteban and Cruz 2011; Rubin 1995).

17.11 Contact Lens Solution in Ocular Therapeutics

Monica Choudhry

The solution used for care of contact lenses is important to keep lenses free from microbial contamination, free of deposits and hydrated in the eye. Deposits are culprits which lead to spoilage, chemical changes in the lens material and further binding of microorganisms. The common sources are dirty fingers, tear and ocular secretions, cosmetics and environment. Contact lens users are more prone to microbial keratitis and significantly higher risk in patients who sleep with lenses (Alfonso et al. 1986).

Common microorganisms isolated from contact lenses are *Pseudomonas.* Coagulase-negative staphylococci and *Propionibacterium* spp. were also the common isolates from all ocular sites examined and constituted the normal ocular microbiota. Other bacteria, including members of the families *Enterobacteriaceae* and *Pseudomonadaceae*, were isolated infrequently from all sites but most frequently from contact lens cases (Willcox et al. 1997).

The contact lens care system should follow the following criteria. It has to be sterile and maintain the sterility when in use. The chemicals in it should be nontoxic to the ocular tissue. At the same time, it should not degenerate or alter the desired contact lens material or parameters. The compatibility of contact lens care system has to be good for most of the other eye care solutions or drops.

The contact lens care system sterility test: Stand-alone and regimen testing are two tests used to certify the sterility of the care solution . Three strains of bacteria from ATCC *Pseudomonas aeruginosa*, *Serratia marcescens* and *Staphylococcus aureus* and two fungal strains, *Candida albicans* and *Fusarium solani*, are used for testing.3 log reduction (99.9 %) for bacteria and 1 log reduction (90 %) for fungi are the minimum to pass the stand-alone test. The biocidal efficacy of all the care solutions against *Acanthamoeba* is still a challenge.

Care systems can also be contaminated and at the same time patient may be asymptomatic. Pathogens like *Acanthamoeba* and *Pseudomonas* have also been isolated from the care system bottles (Donzis et al. 1987). Contact lens cases show a significant higher incidence of contamination (Wilson et al. 1990). The microbial flora isolated from the contact lens containers had no correlation with microbial flora of the conjunctiva (Fleiszig and Efron 1992). Thus, the care system of contact lens consists of three main steps: cleaning, rinsing and soaking.

Cleaning agents This step is a must for all reusable lenses and it is done to remove all debris and contamination buildup during the wear. It is best done at night or after lens removal. The cleaning agent mainly consists of a surfactant which has a hydrophobic and hydrophilic component. It solubilizes the debris and emulsifies the lipids. The surfactant forms the surface layer with the hydrophobic region and loosens the debris or deposits. These surfactants are mostly effective against the lipid and the protein deposits but are less effective against the bound or denatured deposits. The formation of denatured proteins and its binding to the lens forms the basis of recommendation of disposable lenses. The surfactants are mostly nonionic and anionic as they generally will be inert and not react to polymers of the soft lens materials. Cationic, ionic surfactants are used only in disinfecting systems and not as cleaners. Poloxamine and polaxamers are two common surfactants.

Rinsing 0.9 % saline forms the basis of all rinsing solutions. The purpose of rinsing is to remove the loosened debris and the microorganisms after the cleaning step. Saline is also used in thermal disinfection and scleral lenses as a filling solution. Saline is of two types: (a) preserved and (b) unpreserved. Preserved saline has preservatives lie thiomersal (0.001 %) sorbic acid, sorbate, etc., buffering agent and EDTA (0.1 %). This can be used for a period of approximately 1 month after opening. Unpreserved saline for rinsing is the unit dose formulations which have to be discarded after one-time use.

Disinfection Everyday after use, the microorganism from the normal flora of the eye adhere to the contact lens and lens has to be disinfected for the next-day use. This step is must for reusable lenses. One-day disposables are discarded after every use and do not undergo this step. Microorganisms like pseudomonas and staphylococcus are not the usual flora and likely to cause microbial keratitis. The eye has a protective mechanism and tear components like immunoglobulins, lysozymes and lactoferrin play this role. The epithelium of the eye acts as a barrier and prevents the harmful pathogens from entering the cornea. Any abrasion or break in the epithelium can lead to manifestation of infection in the eye.

Other ingredients of contact lens solution are osmolarity agents, chelating agents, buffers, cushioning agents, cleaning agents and disinfecting agents.

Osmolarity Agents NaCl balances the osmolarity of the contact lens solutions. the osmolarity is maintained between 290–310 mOsm.

Chelating agents They bind with proteins and metals which may prevent lens deposits. It also enhances the antimicrobial property. EDTA is a commonly used chelating agent.

Buffers Buffering agents are added to maintain optimum pH which will impact the comfort on insertion. It also indirectly enhances the antimicrobial property of the solution. Phosphate, citrate and borate are some examples of buffers. The pH of contact lens solution ranges from 7.3 to 7.70.

Comfort and Conditioning agents Surfactants and copolymers are often used to increase initial comfort upon lens insertion. Poloxamer and tyloxapol enhance the wettability and improve the comfort by cushioning effect.

Antimicrobial agents The care bottles have both preservatives and disinfectants in them. Preservatives are chemicals which prevent microbial growth in the bottle once it is opened. Disinfectants are those which reduce the level of microorganisms such that they are no longer harmful to the eye. The concentration of these preservatives and disinfectants is important as it is imperative that they should not cause any harmful ocular effect and at the same time be harsh enough to kill microorganisms.

Some of the patients may be toxic to these chemicals and may manifest symptoms of toxicity like dryness, irritation and reduced wearing time.

Some of the disinfectants are:

1. *Hydrogen peroxide*: H_2O_2 is a fast effective disinfectant against most of the bacteria, fungi, viruses and protozoa. It has a unique property of disintegrating into water and oxygen and thus least toxic to the ocular tissue. Most systems recommend 4–6 h of disinfection with 3 % or hours for 0.6 %. It is advocated to be effective against *Acanthamoeba* cysts also. After disinfection the H_2O_2 must be neutralized before insertion of contact lens in the eye. Compounds like platinum disc, catalase, sodium pyruvate and sodium thiosulfate are examples of neutralizing agents.
2. *Thiomersal*: It is an old-generation organomercury compound with thiosalicylic component. It is very effective antiseptic and antifungal agent but not in use thesedays due to toxicity reports.
3. Quaternary ammonium compounds: These are less effective for Gram-negative bacteria and fungi so are used as combination with other disinfectants. Benzalkonium chloride was the first-generation disinfectant in this category. It was used with PMMA (hard lenses). With the invention of soft material (HEMA) use of BKC reduced because BKC binds to the material of soft contact lenses and produce toxic effects to the eye.

Newer-generation compounds were then developed like polyquaternium 1 (Polyquad) and are found to be less toxic than BKC.

Wetting agents These are important as they form a smooth surface over the lens, creating a smooth tear film over it . This enhances the comfort and improves the quality of vision. Wetting agents are viscosity building compounds. Some of the examples of wetting agents are polyvinyl alcohol and polyvinylpyrrolidone, methyl cellulose and hypromellose. Hyaluronan (HA)-glycosaminoglycan is a natural lubricating ingredient found in tears, conjunctiva, corneal epithelium and even vitreous. It plays an important role of hydration of corneal epithelium and stabilization of precorneal tear film. It holds water and has been added as an ingredient on soft lenses to hold moisture for almost the whole day. It is thus an effective wetting agent too.

Protein removers Deposits start forming immediately over the lens on insertion. They are important as they help in adaptation and brain accepting the lens as part of the eye. Denatured protein deposits over contact lenses can lead to many complications such as giant papillary conjunctivitis and dry eye symptoms. Frequent replacement is the answer or using protein removal enzyme treatment is suggested. Proteolytic enzymes like papain are non-ocular toxic and used as protein-removing tablets for reusable lenses.

Multipurpose solution To improve compliance and reduce infection risks, care solutions are formulated in multipurpose form as a single bottle which cleans, rinses and disinfects.

17.11.1 Dyes in Evaluation of Contact Lenses

Fluorescein: in sterile paper strips at 20 % concentration are used for the assessment of rigid contact lens fitting and corneal integrity. It is a water-soluble, yellow-colored compound which does not penetrate the cornea unless epithelial damage. This property makes fluorescein an important dye used in contact lens clinics. It is used for evaluating the fitting assessment and assessing the corneal integrity. Fluorescein should not be used with hydrogel lenses (soft lenses) as it is absorbed by the material and can spoil the lens permanently. High-molecular-weight fluorescein (376) can only be used with soft lenses for assessment of fitting.

Rose Bengal dye: it is a red fat-soluble dye which is available in 1 % concentration sterile single-dose strips. Its action is different from fluorescein as it stains the dead cells or tissues only. Thus, it is used in conditions to locate the degenerative tissue in the sclera, conjunctiva and cornea prior to the fitting and post-fitting follow-ups of contact lens users. It stains the mucus in the tear film also. In dry eyes, the positive stain area of Rose Bengal dye helps locate the degenerative areas and helps in predicting the lens tolerance . This dye is irritating; therefore, should be used in small quantities. It can also leave a stain on the lids and the facial tissue hence should be used carefully.

17.11.2 Local Anesthetics Used in Contact Lens Practice

Anesthetics are used to make diagnostic rigid lens fit easy and tolerable for the first-time wearer. It is also used in obtaining an impression of the eye for the sclera lens fitting. The choice of local anesthetics is usually proparacaine because of its rapid onset and short duration of action. They are also nontoxic and do not interfere with rigid lenses. Use with soft lenses is not recommended.

17.11.3 Antibiotics in Contact Lens Practice

Corneal ulcers (Galentine et al. 1984) or microbial keratitis is a rare but serious complication in contact lens users. Soft lens users are at higher risk mostly due to noncompliance. *Pseudomonas* keratitis is the predominant causative agent. Fungal, viral and *Acanthamoeba* keratitis are rare. The offending bacteria are usually sensitive to antibiotics and the treatment outcome is usually good (Sharma et al. 2003).

Silicone hydrogel-based soft lenses release less drug than hydrogel-based soft lenses. The uptake and release of different drugs and drug interaction may vary with different types of soft lens materials (Karlgarda et al. 2003).

Soft contact lenses are used as therapeutic lenses and the penetration of drug through the contact lens is better than the subconjunctival route. Soft lenses can be used for sustained release drug delivery.

17.11.4 Other Drugs Used in Contact Lenses

Decongestants may be used temporarily to relieve congestion in the earlier stages of lens adaptation. Regular use is not recommended. Many of them interact with the soft lenses and can spoil lenses.

Antiallergic drugs Mast cell inhibitors are commonly prescribed to patients who develop seasonal allergies and also use contact lenses. Here again since the absorption and release of these drugs with soft lenses is not well studied, they should be avoided to be used with soft lenses.

Anti-inflammatory drugs Steroids are risky to be used with contact lenses. Treatment should be done without them simply because contact lens users become further at risk of infections.

17.12 Irrigating Solution

Sharmillee Vetrivel

An irrigating solution refers to the formulation containing sodium, potassium, magnesium, calcium, chloride and bicarbonate ions as well as dextrose and glutathione in proportions to maintain the anatomical and physiological integrity of tissues. Ocular irrigating solution represents an indispensable requirement in case of current surgical techniques such as cataract removal, pars plana lensectomy, vitrectomy and anterior chamber reconstruction (clinical ophthalmic). Irrigating solution has been reported to have deleterious effects on ocular tissues (McDermott et al. 1988). Reports have observed that prolonged irrigation causes transient postoperative corneal decompensation during cataract removal procedures (Christiansen et al. 1976). Thus, the development of a clinically effective ocular irrigating solution requires a clear understanding of the metabolic requirements of the anterior segment, particularly the corneal endothelium.

Corneal endothelial safety is the guideline for developing intraocular irrigating solutions (Joussen et al. 2000). Corneal endothelial cells are especially sensitive to surgical damage because of their exposed position as the innermost corneal

Table 17.12 Components of ocular irrigating solution with their respective functions

Component	Function
Sodium ion	Maintains extracellular cation and isotonicity
Magnesium ions	Cofactor for adenosine triphosphatase, responsible for fluid transport across cell membranes
Calcium ions	To maintain the endothelial junction
Potassium ions	Contribute to replenish intracellular cation to maintain the Na+/K+ ratio for endothelial ionic pumps
Bicarbonate	Mimicking the bicarbonate buffer system of aqueous humor
Dextrose	Substrate for various metabolic pathways
Glutathione	To aid the metabolic pump mechanism

layer encircling the anterior chamber and their limited ability to regenerate. In addition the failure of the endothelium to perform its fluid transport function for short periods of time will result in corneal thickening and decreased vision. Thus, taking into account the vulnerability of corneal endothelium, an ophthalmic irrigating solution to protect the endothelium should as closely as possible resemble its natural bathing fluid – aqueous humor (Garabedian and Roehrs 1984). Research has indicated the composition of the irrigating solution to be more important to endothelial survival than irrigation volume and time (Matsuda et al. 1984). In that concert, various formulations including fortified balanced salt solution (BSS Plus) and Ringer's lactate have been developed to aid successful irrigation. But the essential components of the modified irrigating solutions are listed in Table 17.12 along with its function. Another point of concern is the corneal temperature which is lower than the body temperature. The central corneal temperature is 30.7–35.0 °C. Cooling the irrigation solution has been shown to maintain intraoperative mydriasis but also prevent postoperative corneal swelling (McDermott et al. 1988).

The available irrigating solutions are comparable in their role in intraocular irrigation during surgical procedures and extraocular irrigation during foreign body removal. But there is still a need for improved ophthalmic irrigating solutions to continue, particularly in view of new surgical techniques which may probe deeper into the eye and require several hours of operating time. These sterile solutions are suitably adjusted to maintain physiological tonicity and pH.

References

Acharya P, et al. Evidence for autoregulation and cell signaling pathway regulation from genome-wide binding of the Drosophila retinoblastoma protein. G3 (Bethesda). 2012;2(11):1459–72.

Alfonso E, Mandelbaum S, Fox MJ, Forster RK. Ulcerative keratitis associated with contact lens wear. Am J Ophthalmol. 1986;101(4):429–33.

Armitage WJ. Preservation of human cornea. Transfus Med Hemother. 2011;38(2):143–7.

Armitage WJ, et al. The suitability of corneas stored by organ culture for penetrating keratoplasty and influence of donor and recipient factors on 5-year graft survival. Invest Ophthalmol Vis Sci. 2014;55(2):784–91.

Azad SV. Vitreous substitutes. Delhi J Ophthalmol. 2012;23(1):9–13. http://doi.org/10.7869/djo.2012.34.
Ballen PH. Treatment of chemical burns of the eye. Eye Ear Nose Throat Mon. 1964;43:57–61.
Bandello F, La Spina C, Iuliano L, Fogliato G, Parodi MB. Review and perspectives on pharmacological vitreolysis. Ophthalmologica. 2013;230(4):179–85. http://doi.org/10.1159/000354547.
Bartletta MA, Reddy IK. Clinical pharmacology of the anterior segment of the eye. In: Reddy IK, editor. Ocular therapeutics and drug delivery. Pennsylvania: Technomic Publishing Company; 1995. p. 218–21.
Biousse V. Thrombolysis for acute central retinal artery occlusion: is it time? American journal of ophthalmology. 2008;146(5):631–4.
Birnbaum F, Jehle T, Schwartzkopff J, Sokolovska Y, Böhringer D, Reis A, Reinhard T. Basiliximab following penetrating risk-keratoplasty-a prospective randomized pilot study. Klin Monbl Augenheilkd. 2008;225(1):62–5.
Bohnke M. Donor tissue for keratoplasty. Report of experiences by the Hamburg cornea bank. Klin Monbl Augenheilkd. 1991;198(6):562–71.
Brozen R, Fromm C. Ultraviolet keratitis. Emedicine. 2006. Available at: http://www.emedicine.com/EMERG/topic759.htm. Accessed on 2 May 2015.
Burkhart C, Morrell D, Goldsmith L. Dermatological Pharmacology. In: Brunton LL, Chabner BA, Knollmann BC, editors. Goodman & Gilman's the pharmacological basis of therapeutics. 12th ed. USA: The McGraw-Hill; 2011. p. 1803.
CDC. Exposure to blood: what healthcare personnel need to know. 2003. Available at: http://www.cdc.gov/ncidod/dhqp/pdf/bbp/Exp_to_Blood.pdf. Accessed 3 May 2015.
Chan CC, Holland EJ. Immunosuppression in ocular surface stem cell transplantation. In: Holland EJ, Mannis MJ, Lee WB, editors. Ocular surface disease: cornea, conjunctiva and tear film. London: Elsevier Saunders; 2013. p. 385–90.
Chang J, Tao Y, Wang B, Guo B, Xu H, Jiang Y, Huang Y. An in situ-forming zwitterionic hydrogel as vitreous substitute. J Mater Chem B. 2015;3(6):1097–105. http://doi.org/10.1039/C4TB01775G.
Chen W, Huang X, Ma X-W, Mo W, Wang W-J, Song H-Y. Enzymatic vitreolysis with recombinant microplasminogen and tissue plasminogen activator. Eye (Lond). 2008;22(2):300–7. http://doi.org/10.1038/sj.eye.6702931.
Christiansen JM, Kollarits CR, Fukui H, Fishman ML, Michels RG, Mikuni I. Intraocular irrigating solutions and lens clarity. Am J Ophthalmol. 1976;82(4):594–7.
Clare G. Amniotic membrane transplantation for acute ocular burns. Cochrane Database Syst Rev. 2012;(9):CD009379.
Cohen SM, Billiris-Findlay K, Eichenbaum DA, Pautler SE. Topical lidocaine gel with and without subconjunctival lidocaine injection for intravitreal injection: a within-patient study. Ophthal Surg Lasers Imaging Retina. 2014;45(4):306–10.
Corning JL. Spinal anaesthesia and local medication of the cord. N Y Med J. 1885;42:183–5.
Donzis PB, Mondino BJ, Weissman BA, Bruckner DA. Microbial contamination of contact lens care systems. Am J Ophthalmol. 1987;104(4):325–33.
Dua HS, King AJ, Joseph A. A new classification of ocular surface burns. Br J Ophthalmol. 2001;85(11):1379–83.
Duggan JN, Nanavati BP. Tattooing of corneal opacity with gold and platinum chloride. Br J Ophthalmol. 1936;20(7):419–25.
Dutton JJ. Botulinum-A toxin in the treatment of craniocervical muscle spasms: short- and long-term, local and systemic effects. Survey of ophthalmology. 1996;41(1):51–65.
Eggleston ST, Lush LW. Understanding allergic reactions to local anesthetics. Ann Pharmacother. 1996;30(7–8):851–7.
Einhorn A. On the chemistry of local anesthetics. Munch Med Wochenschr. 1899;46:1218–20.
Ellis PP. Therapeutic agents. Ocular therapeutics and pharmacology. 6 ed. London: The C. V. mosby company; 1981. p. 265–6.
Eslani M, Baradaran-Rafii A, Movahedan A, Djalilian AR. The ocular surface chemical burns. J Ophthalmol. 2014:1–9. Article ID 196827. Available at http://dx.doi.org/10.1155/2014/196827.

Faktorovich EG, Melwani K. Efficacy and safety of pain relief medications after photorefractive keratectomy: review of prospective randomized trials. J Cataract Refract Surg. 2014;40(10): 1716–30.

Fleiszig SM, Efron N. Microbial flora in eyes of current and former contact lens wearers. J Clin Microbiol. 1992;30(5):1156–61.

Foster WJ. Vitreous substitutes. Exp Rev Ophthalmol. 2008;3(2):211–8. http://doi.org/10.1586/17469899.3.2.211.

Frenzel EM, Neely KA, Walsh AW, Cameron JD, Gregerson DS. A new model of proliferative vitreoretinopathy. Invest Ophthalmol Vis Sci. 1998;39(11):2157–64. Retrieved from http://www.ncbi.nlm.nih.gov/pubmed/9761295.

Freud S. Uber Coca. Zentralbl Ges Ther. 1884;2:289–314.

Frueh BE, Bohnke M. Prospective, randomized clinical evaluation of Optisol vs organ culture corneal storage media. Arch Ophthalmol. 2000;118(6):757–60.

Galentine PG, Cohen EJ, Laibson PR, Adams CP, Michaud R, Arentsen JJ. Corneal ulcers associated with contact lens wear. Arch Ophthalmol. 1984;102(6):891–4.

Gandorfer A. Pharmacologic vitreolysis: rationale, potential indications, and promising agents. Retina. 2012;32 Suppl 2:S221–4. http://doi.org/10.1097/IAE.0b013e31825bc4df.

Garabedian ME, Roehrs RE. US 4550022 A. Filing date Feb. Tissue irrigating solution. 22 Feb 1984.

Gerber DA, Bonham CA, Thomson AW. Immunosuppressive agents: recent developments in molecular action and clinical application. Transplant Proc. 1998;30(4):1573–9.

Gonnering RS. Pharmacology of botulinum toxin. International ophthalmology clinics. 1993;33(4):203–26.

Gregory ME, Kanna R. Transplantation of limbal stem cells. In: Boyd S, Gutierrez AM, McCulley JP, editors. Atlas and text of corneal pathology and surgery. New Delhi: Jaypee-Highlights USA: Medical Publishers; 2011. p. 523–48.

Haug K, et al. Donor cornea transfer from Optisol GS to organ culture storage: a two-step procedure to increase donor tissue lifespan. Acta Ophthalmol. 2013;91(3):219–25.

Hermel M, Schrage NF. Efficacy of plasmin enzymes and chondroitinase ABC in creating posterior vitreous separation in the pig: a masked, placebo-controlled in vivo study. Graefes Arch Clin Exp Ophthalmol. 2007;245:399–406.

Ivastinovic D, Langmann G, Aigelsreiter A, Georgi T, Wedrich A, Velikay-Parel M. Dispase-assisted vitrectomy for epiretinal prostheses implantation. Acta Ophthalmol. 2012;90(2):e163–5. http://doi.org/10.1111/j.1755-3768.2010.02084.x.

Jorge R, Oyamaguchi EK, Cardillo JA, Gobbi A, Laicine EM, Haddad A. Intravitreal injection of dispase causes retinal hemorrhages in rabbit and human eyes. Curr Eye Res. 2003;26(2): 107–12. Retrieved from http://www.ncbi.nlm.nih.gov/pubmed/12815529.

Joussen AM, Barth U, Cubuk H, Koch H. Effect of irrigating solution and irrigation temperature on the cornea and pupil during phacoemulsification. J Cataract Refract Surg. 2000;26(3): 392–7.

Karlgarda CCS, Wonga NS, Jonesc LW, Moresolia C. In vitro uptake and release studies of ocular pharmaceutical agents by silicon-containing and p-HEMA hydrogel contact lens materials. Int J Pharm. 2003;257(1–2):141–51.

Kaufman HE, et al. Optisol corneal storage medium. Arch Ophthalmol. 1991;109(6):864–8.

Kleinberg TT, Tzekov RT, Stein L, Ravi N, Kaushal S. Vitreous substitutes: a comprehensive review. Surv Ophthalmol. 2011;56(4):300–23. http://doi.org/10.1016/j.survophthal.2010.09.001.

Klysik A, Korzycka D. Sub-Tenon injection of 2% lidocaine prevents intra-operative floppy iris syndrome (IFIS) in male patients taking oral alpha-adrenergic antagonists. Acta Ophthalmol. 2014;92(6):535–40.

Kralinger MT, Kieselbach GF, Voigt M, Hayden B, Hernandez E, Fernandez V, Parel J-M. Experimental model for proliferative vitreoretinopathy by intravitreal dispase: limited by zonulolysis and cataract. Ophthalmologica. 2006;220(4):211–6. http://doi.org/10.1159/000093073.

Krensky AM, Bennett WM, Vincenti F. Immunosuppressants, tolerogens and immunostimulants. In: Brunton LL, Chabner BA, Knollmann BC, editors. Goodman and Gilman's the pharmacological basis of therapeutics. 12th ed. USA: The McGraw-Hill; 2011. p. 1005–29.

Kuppermann BD, Thomas EL, de Smet MD, Grillone LR. Safety results of two phase III trials of an intravitreous injection of highly purified ovine hyaluronidase (Vitrase) for the management of vitreous hemorrhage. Am J Ophthalmol. 2005;140(4):585–97. http://doi.org/10.1016/j.ajo.2005.06.022.

Li X, Shi X, Fan J. Posterior vitreous detachment with plasmin in the isolated human eye. Graefe's Arch Clin Exp Ophthalmol. 2002;240(1):56–62. Retrieved from http://www.ncbi.nlm.nih.gov/pubmed/11954782.

Lindstrom RL. Advances in corneal preservation. Trans Am Ophthalmol Soc. 1990;88:555–648.

Liotta LA, Goldfarb RH, Brundage R, Siegal GP, Terranova V, Garbisa S. Effect of plasminogen activator (urokinase), plasmin, and thrombin on glycoprotein and collagenous components of basement membrane. Cancer Res. 1981;41(11 Pt 1):4629–36. Retrieved from http://www.ncbi.nlm.nih.gov/pubmed/6458354.

Lopez-Otin C, Bond JS. Proteases: multifunctional enzymes in life and disease. The Journal of biological chemistry. 2008;283(45):30433–7.

Mannis MJ, Eghbali K, Schwab IR. Keratopigmentation: a review of corneal tattooing. Cornea. 1999;18(6):633–7.

Matsuda M, Tano Y, Edelhauser HF. Comparison of intraocular irrigating solutions used for pars plana vitrectomy and prevention of endothelial cell loss. Jpn J Ophthalmol. 1984;28(3): 230–8.

McCarey BE, Kaufman HE. Improved corneal storage. Invest Ophthalmol. 1974;13(3):165–73.

McDermott ML, Edelhauser HF, Hack HM, Langston RH. Ophthalmic irrigants: a current review and update. Ophthalmic Surg. 1988;19(10):724–33.

Mizukawa T, Manabe R. Recent advances in keratoplasty, with special reference to the advantages of liquid preservation. Nihon Ganka Kiyo. 1968;19(12):1310–8.

Moffatt SL, Cartwright VA, Stumpf TH. Centennial review of corneal transplantation. Clinical & experimental ophthalmology. 2005;33(6):642–57.

Moorhead LC, Redburn DA, Kirkpatrick DS, Kretzer F. Bacterial collagenase. Proposed adjunct to vitrectomy with membranectomy. Arch Ophthalmol. 1980;98(10):1829–39. Retrieved from http://www.ncbi.nlm.nih.gov/pubmed/6252879.

Moorhead LC, Chu HH, Garcia CA. Enzyme-assisted vitrectomy with bacterial collagenase. Time course and toxicity studies. Arch Ophthalmol. 1983;101(2):265–74. Retrieved from http://www.ncbi.nlm.nih.gov/pubmed/6297438.

Najjar DM, Cohen EJ, Rapuano CJ, Laibson PR. EDTA chelation for calcific band keratopathy: results and long-term follow-up. American journal of ophthalmology. 2004;137(6):1056–64.

Narayanan R, Kuppermann BD. Hyaluronidase for pharmacologic vitreolysis. Dev Ophthalmol. 2009;44:20–5. http://doi.org/10.1159/000223941.

Natsumeda Y, Carr SF. Human type I and II IMP dehydrogenases as drug targets. Ann N Y Acad Sci. 1993;696:88–93.

Naumann M, Jost WH, Toyka KV. Botulinum toxin in the treatment of neurological disorders of the autonomic nervous system. Archives of neurology. 1999;56(8):914–6.

O'Neill R, Shea M. The effects of bacterial collagenase in rabbit vitreous. Can J of Ophthalmol. 1973;8(2):366–70. Retrieved from http://www.ncbi.nlm.nih.gov/pubmed/4350501.

Oliveira LB, Meyer CH, Kumar J, Tatebayashi M, Toth CA, Wong F, Epstein DL, McCuen 2nd BW. RGD peptide-assisted vitrectomy to facilitate induction of a posterior vitreous detachment: a new principle in pharmacological vitreolysis. Curr Eye Res. 2002;25:333–40.

Patel M, Fraunfelder FW. Toxicity of topical ophthalmic anesthetics. Expert Opin Drug Metab Toxicol. 2013;9(8):983–8.

Pescosolido N, Barbato A, Pascarella A, Giannotti R, Genzano M, Nebbioso M. Role of Protease-Inhibitors in Ocular Diseases. Molecules. 2014;19(12):20557–69.

Pels L. Organ culture: the method of choice for preservation of human donor corneas. Br J Ophthalmol. 1997;81(7):523–5.

Pfister RR, Pfister DA. Alkali injuries of the eye. In: Fundamentals of cornea and external disease. Cornea. 2005a;2:1285–93.
Pfister DA, Pfister RR. Acid injuries of the eye. Fundamentals of cornea and external disease. Cornea. 2005b;2:1277–84.
Pitz S, et al. Corneal tattooing: an alternative treatment for disfiguring corneal scars. Br J Opthalmol. 2002;86(4):397–9.
Por YM, Tan YL, Mehta JS, Tan DT. Intracameral fibrin tissue sealant as an adjunct in tectonic lamellar keratoplasty for large corneal perforations. Cornea. 2009;28(4):451–5.
Pradhan S, Das M, Panigrahi AK, Prajna NV. Severe Conjunctival Reaction Following Attempted Corneal Tattooing. JAMA Ophthalmol. 2015; 133(7): 854–6.
Ramos-Esteban JC, Cruz MA. Complications associated with local ophthalmic anesthesia techniques. In: Boyd S, Wu L, editors. Management of complications in ophthalmic surgery. New Jaypee-Highlights Medical Publishers, Panama Republic of Panama; 2011. p. 1–6.
Roberts JE. Ocular phototoxicity. J Photochem Photobiol B. 2001;64(2–3):136–43.
Roper-Hall MJ. Thermal and chemical burns. Trans Ophthalmol Soc U K. 1965;85:631–53.
Rubin AP. Complications of local anaesthesia for ophthalmic surgery. Br J Anaesth. 1995;75(1):93–6.
Sahu CC. Comprehensive notes in ophthalmology. 1st ed. New Delhi: Jaypee Brothers Medical Publishers; 2011. p. 39–136.
Scholz A. Mechanisms of (local) anaesthetics on voltage-gated sodium and other ion channels. Br J Anaesth. 2002;89(1):52–61.
Sebag J, Ansari RR, Suh KI. Pharmacologic vitreolysis with microplasmin increases vitreous diffusion coefficients. Graefe's Arch Clin Exp. 2007;245(4):576–80. http://doi.org/10.1007/s00417-006-0394-3.
Sebag J. Pharmacologic vitreolysis. Retina. 1998;18(1):1–3.
Sharma S, Gopalakrishnan S, Aasuri MK, Garg P, Rao GN. Trends in contact lens–associated microbial keratitis in Southern India. Ophthalmology. 2003;110(1):138–43.
Sharma A, Kaur R, Kumar S, Gupta P, Pandav S, Patnaik B, et al. Fibrin glue versus N-butyl-2-cyanoacrylate in corneal perforations. Ophthalmology. 2003;110(2):291–8.
Singh P, Tyagi M, Kumar Y, Gupta KK, Sharma PD. Ocular chemical injuries and their management. Oman J Ophthalmol. 2013;6(2):83–6.
Sinha R, Jhanji V, Verma K, Sharma N, Biswas NR, Vajpayee RB. Efficacy of topical cyclosporine A 2% in prevention of graft rejection in high-risk keratoplasty: a randomized controlled trial. Graefes Arch Clin Exp Ophthalmol. 2010;248(8):1167–72.
Skondra D, Noda K, Yu H, Schering A, Gragoudas E, Hafezi-Moghadam A. Aprotinin Reduces Intraocular Inflammation in Endotoxin Induced Uveitis. IOVS. 2009;50(13):6046.
Spector J, Fernandez WG. Chemical, thermal, and biological ocular exposures. Emerg Med Clin North Am. 2008;26(1):125–36.
Staubach F, Nober V, Janknecht P. Enzyme assisted vitrectomy in enucleated pig eyes: a comparison of hyaluronidase, chondroitinase, and plasmin. Curr Eye Res. 2004;29:261–8.
Suh LH, Akpek EK, Stark WJ. Tectonic lamellar keratoplasty for Mooren's and Mooren's-like corneal ulcers. In: John T, editor. Step by step anterior and posterior lamellar keratoplasty. 5th ed. New Delhi: Jaypee Brothers Medical Publishers (P) Ltd; 2006. p. 259–76.
Takano A, Hirata A, Ogasawara K, Sagara N, Inomata Y, Kawaji T, Tanihara H. Posterior vitreous detachment induced by nattokinase (subtilis in NAT): a novel enzyme for pharmacologic vitreolysis. Invest Ophthalmol Vis Sci. 2006;47:2075–9.
Tan DT, Dart JK, Holland EJ, Kinoshita S. Corneal transplantation. Lancet. 2012;379(9827): 1749–61.
Taylor HR. The biological effects of UV-B on the eye. Photochem Photobiol. 1989;50(4): 489–92.
Tezel TH, Del Priore LV, Kaplan HJ. Posterior vitreous detachment with dispase. Retina. 1998;18(1):7–15. Retrieved from http://www.ncbi.nlm.nih.gov/pubmed/9502275.
Tripathi KD. Essentials of medical pharmacology. 6th ed. New Delhi: Jaypee Brothers Medical Publishers; 2008.

Uemura A, Nakamura M, Kachi S, Nishizawa Y, Asami T, Miyake Y, Terasaki H. Effect of plasmin on laminin and fibronectin during plasmin-assisted vitrectomy. Arch Ophthalmol. 2005;123(2):209–13. http://doi.org/10.1001/archopht.123.2.209.

Varma DD, Cugati S, Lee AW, Chen CS. A review of central retinal artery occlusion: clinical presentation and management. Eye. 2013;27(6):688–97.

Wagoner MD. Chemical injuries of the eye: current concepts in pathophysiology and therapy. Surv Ophthalmol. 1997;41(4):275–313.

Wang F, Wang Z, Sun X, Wang F, Xu X, Zhang X. Safety and efficacy of dispase and plasmin in pharmacologic vitreolysis. Invest Ophthalmol Vis Sci. 2004;45(9):3286–90. http://doi.org/10.1167/iovs.04-0026.

Wang Z-L, Zhang X, Xu X, Sun X-D, Wang F. PVD following plasmin but not hyaluronidase: implications for combination pharmacologic vitreolysis therapy. Retina. 2005;25(1):38–43. Retrieved from http://www.ncbi.nlm.nih.gov/pubmed/15655439.

Whitcher JP, Srinivasan M, Upadhyay MP. Corneal blindness: a global perspective. Bull World Health Organ. 2001;79(3):214–21.

Wiegand TW, Baumal CR. The status of vitreous substitutes. 2007. Retrieved 27 May 2015, from http://www.retinalphysician.com/articleviewer.aspx?articleID=100295.

Willcox M, Power KN. Potential sources of bacteria that are Isolated from contact lenses during wear. Optom Vis Sci. 1997;74(12):1030–8.

Wilson LA, Sawant AD, Simmons RB, Ahearn DG. Microbial contamination of contact lens storage cases and solutions. Am J Ophthalmol. 1990;110(2):193–8.

Yang W, Yuan Y, Zong Y, Huang Z, Mai S, Li Y, Qian X, Liu Y, Gao Q. Preliminary study on retinal vascular and oxygen-related changes after long-term silicone oil and foldable capsular vitreous body tamponade. Sci Rep. 2014;4:5272. http://doi.org/10.1038/srep05272.

Zaleznik D. Patient information: blood and body fluid exposure. 2007. Available at: http://patients.uptodate.com/topic.asp?file¼inf_immu/8025. Accessed 3 May 2015.

Zhi-Liang W, Wo-Dong S, Min L, Xiao-Ping B, Jin J. Pharmacologic vitreolysis with plasmin and hyaluronidase in diabetic rats. Retina. 2009;29(2):269–74. http://doi.org/10.1097/IAE.0b013e3181923ff0.

Zhu D, Chen H, Xu X. Effects of intravitreal dispase on vitreoretinal interface in rabbits. Curr Eye Res. 2006;31(11):935–46. http://doi.org/10.1080/02713680600932142.

Ziegler SL. Multicolor tattooing of the cornea. Trans Am Ophthalmol Soc. 1922;20:71–87.

Chapter 18
Cellular Therapy for Ocular Diseases

Sujata Mohanty

Abstract Over the past decade several investigations have been performed to study the regenerative capacity of different type of stem cells such as adult and embryonic stem cells for their application in Opthalmology. In particular, limbal epithelial stem cells have shown most promising results for ocular surface reconstruction. This book chapter discusses current approaches used in stem cell therapy and the challenges faced along with the future scope of advancements to use stem cell in other ocular degenerative conditions.

18.1 Introduction

The dramatic advances in the field of stem cell research have raised the possibility of using stem cells to treat a variety of eye diseases. These diseases are considered excellent candidates for stem cell therapy because the eye is an immune-privileged site, meaning transplanted cells are not as likely to be rejected as foreign cells compared with transplantations elsewhere.

S. Mohanty, PhD
Stem Cell Facility, DBT-Centre for Excellence of Stem Cell Research,
All India Institute of Medical Sciences, Ansari Nagar, New Delhi, 110029, India
e-mail: drmohantysujata@gmail.com

T. Velpandian (ed.), *Pharmacology of Ocular Therapeutics*,
DOI 10.1007/978-3-319-25498-2_18

The prominent ones are inherited retinal diseases, like age-related macular degeneration and retinitis pigmentosa, and diseases affecting the cornea, such as hypersensitivity reaction-mediated Stevens–Johnson syndrome, and chemical and thermal burns. These diseases cause significant visual loss, and currently, there are limited treatments for these conditions. Stem cell transplantation in these cases holds the potential to restore vision and provide treatment.

Broadly, stem cells are categorized into embryonic stem cells (ESCs) and adult stem cells (ASCs). ESCs are highly proliferative and show higher degree of plasticity and can be differentiated into various other tissue lineages as compared to ASCs. ESCs have been differentiated in vitro into eye neural cells and retinal pigmented epithelium cells (RPE) (Banin et al. 2006; Hirano et al. 2003). However, ASCs are preferred over ESCs because of ethical concerns due to the formation of teratoma by their uncontrolled proliferation. Stem/progenitor cells from various adult tissues have been used as a source of cell therapy in eye disorders, limbal stem cells being the major player.

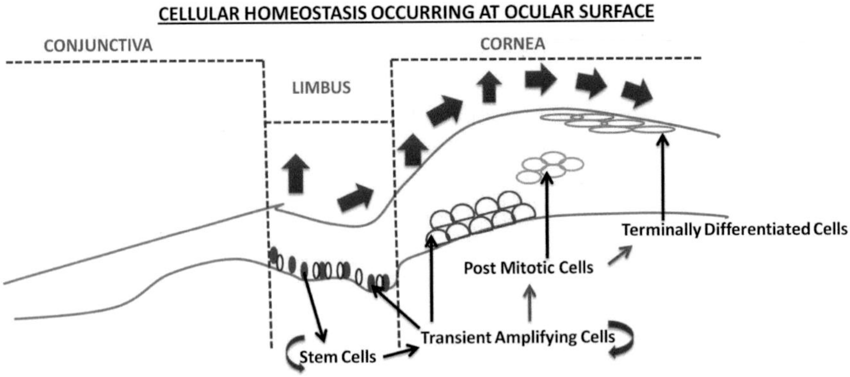

Stem Cells for corneal epithelium are located in the basal cell layer at the limbus, which divide to form transient amplifying cells. They latter undergo mitosis and differentiation while moving towards the central cornea and into more superficial strata.

18.1.1 Limbal Epithelium

Limbus region of the eye houses limbal epithelial stem cells (LESC). This niche is thought to be located in the palisades of Vogt (Hirano et al. 2003) which is an optimal microenvironment for stem cell growth (Goldberg et al. 1982; Lagali et al. 2013; Goldberg and Bron 1982). However, there is no specific marker for the LESC, and therefore, the expression of putative stem cell markers and lack of differentiation-related marker (K3/K12), morphology (Arpitha et al. 2005), clone formation assay

(Pellegrini et al. 1999), and DNA retention study (Schermer et al. 1986; Cotsarelis et al. 1989) are considered for the identification of LEST cells (Budak et al. 2005; De Paiva et al. 2005; Di Iorio et al. 2005).

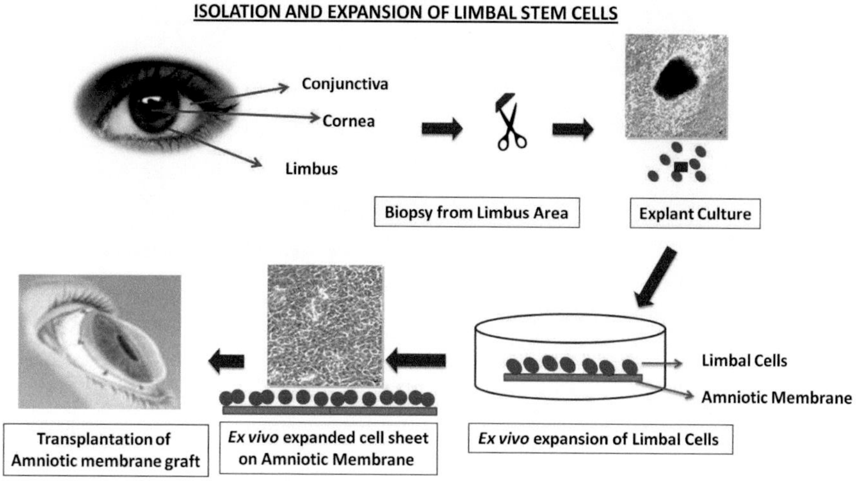

There has been a great deal of improvisation in the technique of isolation of LESC for clinical use.

1. *Conjunctival limbal autograft (CLAU)*: In its simplest form, conjunctival limbal autograft has been successfully used in the treatment of unilateral LSCD. However, there is a concern of inducing LSCD in the donor eye, therefore leading to its modification involving a smaller source tissue in conjunction with in vivo expansion. While these methods have been successful for patients with unilateral LSCD , similar approaches with conjunctival limbal allograft (due to bilateral LSCD) have been largely unsuccessful due to high frequency of immune rejection Since the first report in 1989 by Kenyon and Tseng, CLAU has become a widely accepted technique in the management of unilateral total LSCD (Kenyon and Tseng 1989)
2. *Corneal stem cell allograft transplantation*: Allograft transplantation for the patients suffering from bilateral total LSCD or whose fellow eye is not suitable as a graft source. Generally, allograft transplantation includes cadaveric keratolimbal allograft (KLAL) and living-related conjunctival limbal allograft (Lr-CLAL) (Shanmuganathan et al. 2007; Huang et al. 2011; Lam et al. 2000; Rao et al. 1999). Due to high risk of immune rejection, both methods offer poor long-term outcomes.
3. *Simple limbal epithelial transplantation (SLET)*: The use of amniotic membrane for in vivo expansion of smaller graft tissue improved the success rate of limbal epithelial transplant (Meallet et al. 2003; Mittal et al. 2006). Amniotic membrane

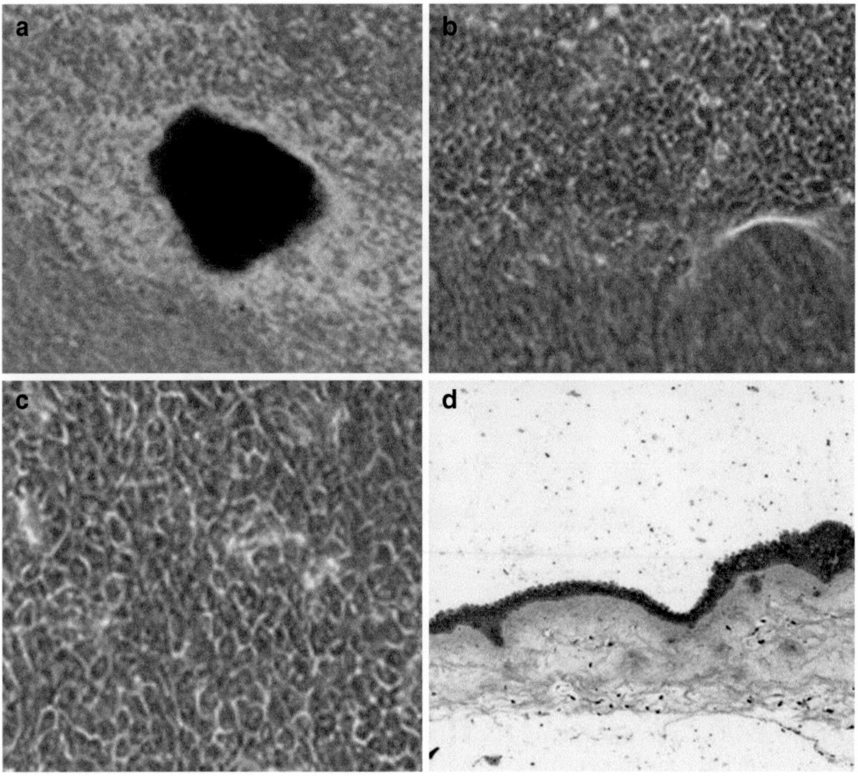

Fig. 18.1 Phase contrast light microscopic pictures of human LESCs cultivated on dHAM. (**a**) Picture at low magnification (32×) on third day showing expansion of LESCs from the edge of the explant. (**b**) Cultured limbal epithelial cells at higher magnification (310×) showing migration of limbal epithelial peripherally outward. (**c**) Picture at 320× magnification showing formation of monolayer with a typical honeycomb-like structure and hexagonal morphology of the cells. (**d**) Hematoxylin and eosin staining showing formation of multilayer of cultivated limbal epithelial cells at low magnification

seems to inhibit inflammation and provide a supportive niche for the transplanted LEST cells. In 2012, Sangwan VS (Sangwan et al. 2012) described this surgical technique. In this procedure, a small 2 × 2 mm strip was removed from the fellow eye and chopped into pieces. Then, the tiny pieces were seeded on the amniotic membrane (AM)-covered cornea. Complete reconstruction with epithelialized, avascular, and stable corneal surface was observed after 6 weeks in all 6 recipient eye.

4. *Corneal Limbal Epithelial Transplant (CLET)*: The cells used for cultured limbal epithelial transplantation (CLET) are obtained from a relatively small biopsy of limbal tissue. This is grown on a denuded amniotic membrane (Fig. 18.1) which is used as a cell substrate to facilitate transfer of the cells from culture to recipient cornea. Several materials such as fibrin gels (Han et al. 2002; Rama et al. 2001; Talbot et al. 2006), collagen (Dravida et al. 2008; McIntosh Ambrose et al. 2009; Takezawa et al. 2004), keratin films (Borrelli et al. 2013; Feng et al. 2014), silk fibroin films (Bray et al. 2011), chitosan hydrogels (Grolik et al. 2012),

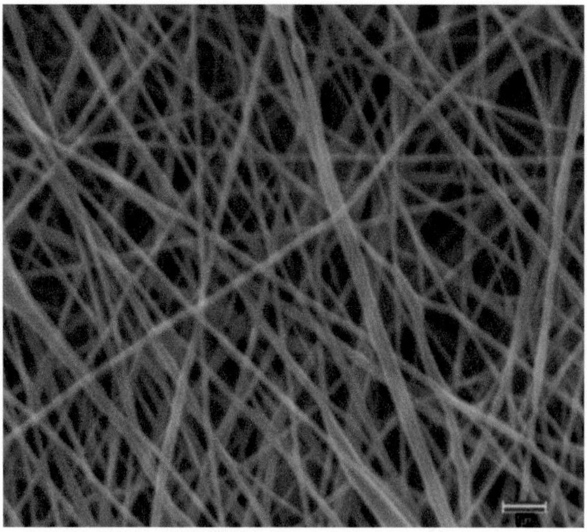

Fig. 18.2 Architecture of electrospun PCL nanofiber scaffold as seen under a scanning electron microscope at 25,000× magnification. The average fiber diameter of nanofibers was 132 ± 42 nm. Scale bar measures 1 μm

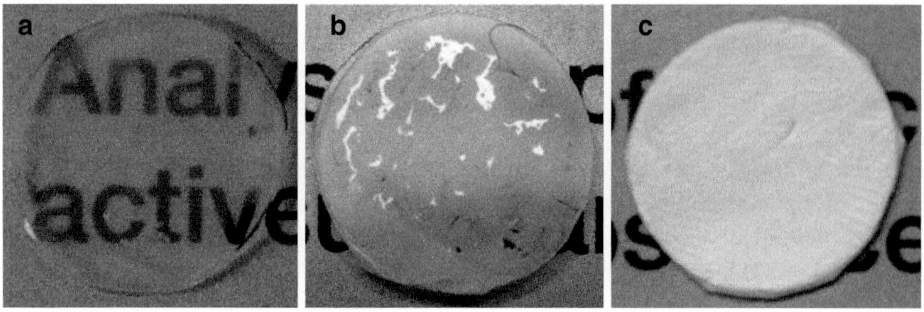

Fig. 18.3 Optical transparency of PCL nanofiber membranes and HAM. (**a**) Wet HAM showing transparency through which the printed text can be easily read. (**b**) Wet PCL membrane showing translucency through which the printed text is slightly visible. (**c**) Dry PCL membrane showing complete opacity and the text underneath cannot be read through it

siloxane–hydrogel contact lens (Di Girolamo et al. 2007), polystyrene, and nanofiber scaffold (Sharma et al. 2011a) (Figs. 18.2 and 18.3) have been tested as scaffolds. All of these material have been found to support the growth of LEST cells in vivo, but only human amniotic membrane and fibrin gels have been investigated in clinical studies with positive outcomes (Fig. 18.2).

Due to the high risk of rejection associated with allografts, ex vivo expansion of limbal epithelial stem cells is a preferable solution for bilateral LSCD.

CLET may also have a reduced risk of allograft rejection compared with direct tissue transfer because antigen-presenting macrophages do not survive the process of ex vivo culture. Limbal epithelial stem cells (LESCs) transplantation has been clinically recognized of therapeutic value in hereditary conditions such as aniridia (Gomes et al. 2005) and in acquired diseases characterized by LESC deficiency, such as SJS, chemical or thermal injury, chronic limbitis, limbal surgery, and contact lens keratopathy (Tsubota et al. 1999). Successful transplants of cultured autologous

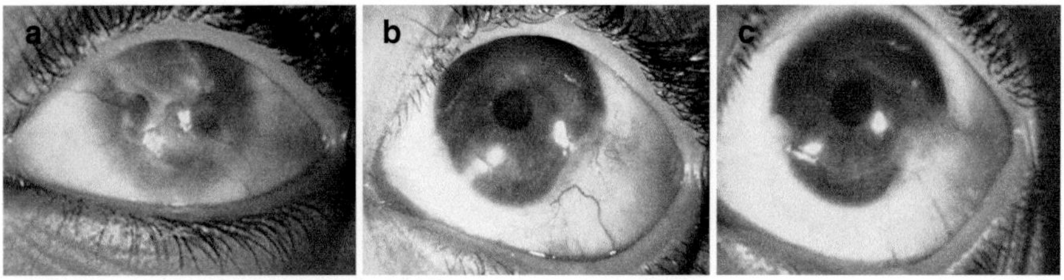

Fig. 18.4 Representative case of patient no. 8, a 10-year-old girl who suffered from lime injury. Patient underwent autologous ex vivo cultured LSCT. (**a**) Preoperative clinical appearance of ocular surface with 360° of conjunctivalization, corneal haze, and VA finger counting close to the face (FCCF). (**b**) Three-month postoperative clinical appearance with improved VA 3/60 and ocular surface. (**c**) 24-month postoperative appearance with stable VA 3/60 and ocular surface

limbal epithelium in patients with unilateral limbal stem cell deficiency have been achieved (Sharma et al. 2011b) (Fig. 18.4).

18.1.2 Oral Mucosal Epithelium

Apart from limbus tissue-derived SC, oral mucosal tissue has also been tested as an alternative stem cell source. The safety and efficiency of oral mucosal epithelium base transplantation have been evaluated clinically. Several groups from Japan demonstrated that cultured oral mucosal epithelium can be used to reconstruct the corneal epithelium in animal models as well as patients with LSCD due to chemical injury and SJS (Nakamura et al. 2011; Sen et al. 2011).

1. *Cultured oral mucosa stem cell transplant (COMET)*: It is closely related to LSCT. It has also been used for LSCD treatment. Cultured oral mucosal epithelial transplantation (COMET) has several potential advantages. There are no risk of immune-mediated rejection, and, in the absence of autoimmune disease, immunosuppression is not required. Published outcomes for COMET show that a stable corneal surface is achieved in up to 100 % of eyes at 1 year, 100 % at 14 months, 67 % at 20 months, and 92 % at 4 years. Visual acuity was better than pretreatment levels in 90 % of eyes at 1 year, 100 % at 14 months, and 67 % at 20 months, and 53 % remained improved for 4 years following surgery (Figs. 18.5 and 18.6).

18.1.3 Bone Marrow-Derived Stem Cells

Some studies have suggested that bone marrow-derived stem cells might be implicated in promoting corneal wound healing in vivo and in retinal disease (Ma et al. 2006; Otani et al. 2004; Ye et al. 2008; Kumar et al. 2012). Briefly, cultured human BM-MSCs on amniotic membrane were transplanted into chemically burned rat corneas achieving the same results in corneal epithelialization and vision acuity as achieved by same procedure using LESCs (Ma et al. 2006; Ye et al. 2008).

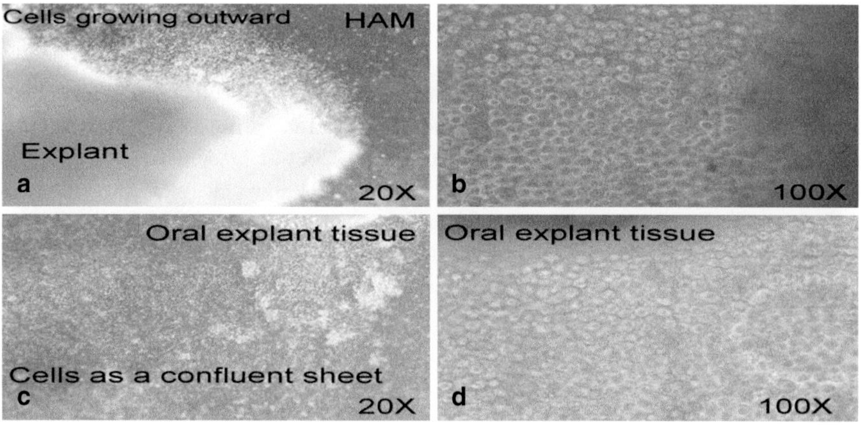

Fig. 18.5 (**a**, **b**) Morphologic findings of OMEC growing on HAM for 2–3 days. Magnification: (**a**) 20×; (**b**) 100× (**c**, **d**) OMEC as a confluent sheet on HAM (after 1–2 weeks). Magnification: (**c**) 20×; (**d**) 100×

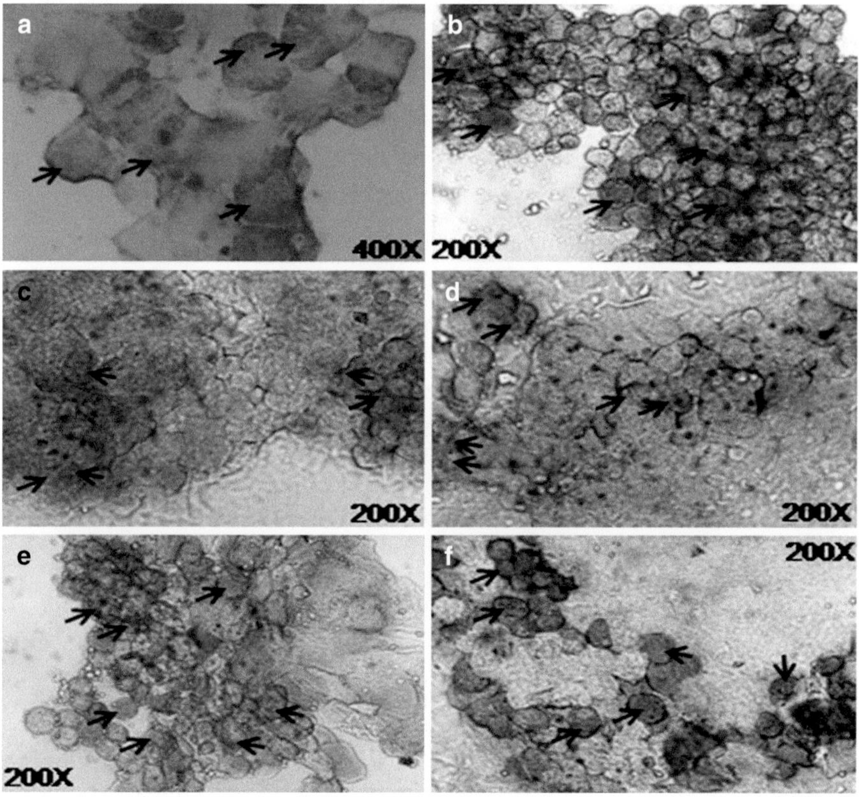

Fig. 18.6 Expression of various marker proteins as assessed by immunocytochemistry in cultivated OMEC for 1–2 weeks. (**a**) Expression of cytokeratin K3/K12; magnification, 400×. (**b**) Expression of connexin 43; magnification, 200×. (**c**) Expression of p63; magnification, 200×. (**d**) Expression of −1 integrin (CD29); magnification, 200×. (**e**) Expression of p75; magnification, 200×. (**f**) Expression of MUC1; magnification, 200×

18.1.4 Hair Follicle Bulge Cells

Hair follicle bulge is an essential niche for keratinocyte stem cells (KSCs), and hair follicle stem cells have been found to successfully trans-differentiate into corneal epithelial-like cells (Ohyama 2007; Ohyama et al. 2006; Blazejewska et al. 2009). In preclinical studies, isolated autologous hair follicle bulge cells were expanded on a fibrin carrier in vitro and then transferred into the mice with LSCD. It contributes to the reconstruction of corneal epithelium by crossing the lineage boundaries and terminally differentiating into corneal epithelial-like cells.

18.1.5 Bioengineered Cornea

In vitro tissue engineering is an approach where healthy mammalian cells are used with a supporting matrix to produce a composite implant. Before the tissue can be assembled from specific cells and be ready for implantation, a series of highly orchestrated events in the correct sequential order must take place. To ensure reliable large-scale production of a durable and easily stored implant, the following criteria should be met:

- Source of healthy self-renewing cells
- Bioactive scaffolds with correct chemical/physical properties to promote cell

  Differentiation/integration and tissue formation
- In vitro conditions that mimic the in vivo environment
- Non-immunogenic: biocompatible

Several materials such as human amniotic membrane (Sharma et al. 2011a), fibrin gels (Han et al. 2002; Rama et al. 2001; Talbot et al. 2006), collagen (Dravida et al. 2008; McIntosh Ambrose et al. 2009; Takezawa et al. 2004), keratin films (Borrelli et al. 2013; Feng et al. 2014), silk fibroin films (Bray et al. 2011), chitosan hydrogels (Grolik et al. 2012), siloxane–hydrogel contact lens (Di Girolamo et al. 2007), polystyrene (Takezawa et al. 2004), and nanofiber scaffold (Kuno and Fujii 2011; Sharma et al. 2011a) have been tested as scaffolds. All of these materials have been found to support the growth of LEST cells in vitro.

18.1.6 New Frontiers

1. *Induced pluripotent stem cells (iPSCs)*: Patient-specific *iPSCs* represent an excellent tool for modeling ocular disease and therapy. This disease-specific iPSCs generation is based on the work of Nobel laureate Prof. Shinya Yamanaka who showed in 2006 that the introduction of four specific genes encoding transcription factors (Oct3/4, Sox2, Klf4, and c-Myc) with a retroviral system could convert adult cells into pluripotent stem cells. These can be generated from adult somatic cells, thus avoiding the ethical considerations involved with

using embryonic stem cells. Human iPS-derived RPE (iPS-RPE) cells have been developed, and restoration of RPE phagocytic function has been observed (Carr et al. 2009; Jin et al. 2005).Recently, a pilot study in Japan has been undertaken to treat age-related macular degeneration using iPSC. This was led by Masayo Takahashi, Laboratory for Retinal Regeneration, RIKEN Center for Developmental Biology, and has been conducted in collaboration with the Institute for Biomedical Research and Innovation.

2. *Embryonic stem cells: Steven D Schwartz et al. conducted a clinical trial using ESC*. Two prospective phase 1/2 studies were done to assess the primary endpoints safety and tolerability of subretinal transplantation of hESC-derived retinal pigment epithelium in nine patients with Stargardt's macular dystrophy and nine with atrophic age-related macular degeneration. The study reported the medium-term to long-term safety, graft survival, and possible biological activity of cells derived from human embryonic stem cells (hESC) when transplanted into patients (Schwartz et al. 2012).

18.2 Conclusion

Stem cells from a wide variety of sources are being considered, both from inside the eye (limbal and retinal stem cells) and outside the eye (embryonic, induced pluripotent stem cells or iPS cells, bone marrow, and neural stem cells). The road to finding a stem cell therapy for eye diseases is paved with many challenges that will take time to overcome. But the wealth of information generated from labs around the globe is converging to help with the transition from basic research to the clinic. Currently, to enhance the stem cell expansion and transplantation efficiency, research is being focused on optimizing the culture conditions; exploring novel scaffolds supporting stem cell proliferation , maintenance, and differentiation; and evaluating the therapeutic potential of different kinds of autologous stem cells.

However, several different barriers still remain. The characteristics and anatomical structure of the limbal stem cell niche are still obscure, and the specific markers for limbal stem cell remain uncertain. Besides, the molecular networks responsible for modulation of stem cell biobehaviors are unclear. More work needs to be done to address these important concerns and make stem cell-based therapy for treating eye disorder more successful.

References

Arpitha P, Prajna NV, Srinivasan M, Muthukkaruppan V. High expression of p63 combined with a large N/C ratio defines a subset of human limbal epithelial cells: implications on epithelial stem cells. Invest Ophthalmol Vis Sci. 2005;46:3631–6.

Banin E, Obolensky A, Idelson M, Hemo I, Reinhardtz E, Pikarsky E. Retinal incorporation and differentiation of neural precursors derived from human embryonic stem cells. Stem Cells. 2006;24(2):246–57.

Blazejewska EA, Schlotzer-Schrehardt U, Zenkel M, Bachmann B, Chankiewitz E, Jacobi C. Corneal limbal microenvironment can induce transdifferentiation of hair follicle stem cells into corneal epithelial-like cells. Stem Cells. 2009;27(3):642–52.

Borrelli M, Reichl S, Feng Y, Schargus M, Schrader S, Geerling G. In vitro characterization and ex vivo surgical evaluation of human hair keratin films in ocular surface reconstruction after sterilization processing. J Mater Sci Mater Med. 2013;24(1):221–30.

Bray LJ, George KA, Ainscough SL, Hutmacher DW, Chirila TV, Harkin DG. Human corneal epithelial equivalents constructed on Bombyx mori silk fibroin membranes. Biomaterials. 2011;32(22):5086–91.

Budak MT, Alpdogan OS, Zhou M, Lavker RM, Akinci MA, Wolosin JM. Ocular surface epithelia contain ABCG2-dependent side population cells exhibiting features associated with stem cells. J Cell Sci. 2005;118:1715–24.

Carr AJ, Vugler AA, Hikita ST, Lawrence JM, Gias C, Chen LL. Protective effects of human iPS-derived retinal pigment epithelium cell transplantation in the retinal dystrophic rat. PLoS One. 2009;4:e8152.

Cotsarelis G, Cheng SZ, Dong G, Sun TT, Lavker RM. Existence of slow-cycling limbal epithelial basal cells that can be preferentially stimulated to proliferate: implications on epithelial stem cells. Cell. 1989;57(2):201–9.

De Paiva CS, Chen Z, Corrales RM, Pflugfelder SC, Li DQ. ABCG2 transporter identifies a population of clonogenic human limbal epithelial cells. Stem Cells. 2005;23(1):63–73.

Di Girolamo N, Chui J, Wakefield D, Coroneo MT. Cultured human ocular surface epithelium on therapeutic contact lenses. Br J Ophthalmol. 2007;91:459–64.

Di Iorio E, Barbaro V, Ruzza A, Ponzin D, Pellegrini G, De Luca M. Isoforms of DeltaNp63 and the migration of ocular limbal cells in human corneal regeneration. Proc Natl Acad Sci U S A. 2005;102(27):9523–8.

Dravida S, Gaddipati S, Griffith M, Merrett K, Lakshmi Madhira S, Sangwan VS. A biomimetic scaffold for culturing limbal stem cells: a promising alternative for clinical transplantation. J Tissue Eng Regen Med. 2008;2(5):263–71.

Feng Y, Borrelli M, Meyer-Ter-Vehn T, Reichl S, Schrader S, Geerling G. Epithelial wound healing on keratin film, amniotic membrane and polystyrene in vitro. Curr Eye Res. 2014;39(6):561–70.

Goldberg MF, Bron AJ. Limbal palisades of Vogt. Trans Am Ophthalmol Soc. 1982;80:155–71.

Grolik M, Szczubialka K, Wowra B, Dobrowolski D, Orzechowska-Wylęgała B, Wylęgała E. Hydrogel membranes based on genipin-cross-linked chitosan blends for corneal epithelium tissue engineering. J Mater Sci Mater Med. 2012;23(8):1991–2000.

Han B, Schwab IR, Madsen TK, Isseroff RR. A fibrin-based bioengineered ocular surface with human corneal epithelial stem cells. Cornea. 2002;21(5):505–10.

Hirano M, Yamamoto A, Yoshimura N, Tokunaga T, Motohashi T, Ishizaki K. Generation of structures formed by lens and retinal cells differentiating from embryonic stem cells. Dev Dyn. 2003;228(4):664–71.

Huang T, Wang Y, Zhang H, Gao H, Hu A. Limbal allografting from living related donors to treat partial limbal deficiency secondary to ocular chemical burns. Arch Ophthalmol. 2011;129(10):1267–73.

Jin M, Li S, Moghrabi WN, Sun H, Travis GH. Rpe65 is the retinoid isomerase in bovine retinal pigment epithelium. Cell. 2005;122(3):449–59.

Kenyon KR, Tseng SC. Limbal autograft transplantation for ocular surface disorders. Ophthalmology. 1989;96(5):709–22.

Kumar A, Mohnaraj SN, Mochi TB, Mohanty S, Seth T, Azad R. Assessment of central retinal function after autologous bone marrow derived intravitreal stem cell injection in patients with retinitis pigmentosa using multifocal ERG: a pilot study. World J Retina Vitreous. 2012;2(1):5–13.

Kuno N, Fujii S. Ocular drug delivery systems for the posterior segment: A review. Retina Today (May/June) 2012;54–9.

Lagali N, Eden U, Utheim TP, Chen X, Riise R, Dellby A, Fagerholm P. In vivo morphology of the limbal palisades of Vogt correlates with progressive stem cell deficiency in aniridia-related keratopathy. Invest Ophthalmol Vis Sci. 2013;54:5333–42.

Lam DS, Young AL, Leung AT, Fan DS, Wong AK. Limbal stem cell allografting from related live donors for corneal surface reconstruction. Ophthalmology. 2000;107(7):411–2.

Ma Y, Xu Y, Xiao Z, Yang W, Zhang C, Song E. Reconstruction of chemically burned rat corneal surface by bone marrow-derived human mesenchymal stem cells. Stem Cells. 2006;24:315–21.

McIntosh Ambrose W, Salahuddin A, So S, Ng S, Ponce Márquez S, Takezawa T. Collagen Vitrigel membranes for the in vitro reconstruction of separate corneal epithelial, stromal, and endothelial cell layers. J Biomed Mater Res B Appl Biomater. 2009;90(2):818–31.

Meallet MA, Espana EM, Grueterich M, Ti SE, Goto E, Tseng SC. Amniotic membrane transplantation with conjunctival limbal autograft for total limbal stem cell deficiency. Ophthalmology. 2003;110(8):1585–92.

Mittal V, Sangwan VS, Fernandes M, Thomas R. Survival analysis of conjunctival limbal grafts and amniotic membrane transplantation in eyes with total limbal stem cell deficiency. Am J Ophthalmol. 2006;141:599–600.

Nakamura T, Takeda K, Inatomi T. Long-term results of autologous cultivated oral mucosal epithelial transplantation in the scar phase of severe ocular surface disorders. Br J Ophthalmol. 2011;95:942–6.

Ohyama M. Hair follicle bulge: a fascinating reservoir of epithelial stem cells. J Dermatol Sci. 2007;46:81–9.

Ohyama M, Terunuma A, Tock CL, Radonovich MF, Pise-Masison CA, Hopping SB. Characterization and isolation of stem cell-enriched human hair follicle bulge cells. J Clin Invest. 2006;116(1):249–60.

Otani A, Dorrell MI, Kinder K, Moreno SK, Nusinowitz S, Banin E, Heckenlively J. Rescue of retinal degeneration by intravitreally injected adult bone marrow-derived lineage-negative hematopoietic stem cells. J Clin Invest. 2004;114(6):765–74.

Pellegrini G, Golisano O, Paterna P, Lambiase A, Bonini S, Rama P. Location and clonal analysis of stem cells and their differentiated progeny in the human ocular surface. J Cell Biol. 1999;145(4):769–82.

Rama P, Bonini S, Lambiase A, Golisano O, Paterna P, De Luca M. Autologous fibrin-cultured limbal stem cells permanently restore the corneal surface of patients with total limbal stem cell deficiency. Transplantation. 2001;72(9):1478–85.

Rao SK, Rajagopal R, Sitalakshmi G, Padmanabhan P. Limbal allografting from related live donors for corneal surface reconstruction. Ophthalmology. 1999;106:822–8.

Sangwan VS, Basu S, MacNeil S, Balasubramanian D. Simple limbal epithelial transplantation (SLET): a novel surgical technique for the treatment of unilateral limbal stem cell deficiency. Br J Ophthalmol. 2012;96:931–4.

Schermer A, Galvin S, Sun TT. Differentiation-related expression of a major 64K corneal keratin in vivo and in culture suggests limbal location of corneal epithelial stem cells. J Cell Biol. 1986;103(1):49–62.

Schwartz SD, Hubschman JP, Heilwell G, Franco-Cardenas V, Pan CK, Ostrick RM. Embryonic stem cell trials for macular degeneration: a preliminary report. Lancet. 2012;379(25):713–20.

Sen S, Sharma S, Gupta A, Gupta N, Singh N, Roychoudhury A. Molecular characterization of explant cultured human oral mucosal epithelial cells. Invest Ophthalmol Vis Sci IOVS. 2011;52(13):9548–54.

Shanmuganathan VA, Foster T, Kulkarni BB, Hopkinson A, Gray T, Powe DG, Lowe J, Dua HS. Morphological characteristics of the limbal epithelial crypt. Br J Ophthalmol. 2007;91(4):514–9.

Sharma S, Mohanty S, Gupta D, Jassal M, Agrawal AK, Tandon R. Cellular response of limbal epithelial cells on electrospun poly-ε- caprolactone nanofibrous scaffolds for ocular surface bioengineering: a preliminary in vitro study. Mol Vis. 2011a;17:2898–910.

Sharma S, Tandon R, Mohanty S, Sharma N, Vanathi M, Sen S. Culture of corneal limbal epithelial stem cells: experience from benchtop to bedside in a tertiary care hospital in India. Cornea. 2011b;30:1223–32.

Takezawa T, Ozaki K, Nitani A, Takabayashi C, Shimo-Oka T. Collagen vitrigel: a novel scaffold that can facilitate a three-dimensional culture for reconstructing organoids. Cell Transplant. 2004;13(4):463–73.

Talbot M, Carrier P, Giasson CJ, Deschambeault A, Guérin SL, Auger FA. Autologous transplantation of rabbit limbal epithelia cultured on fibrin gels for ocular surface reconstruction. Mol Vis. 2006;12:65–75.

Tsubota K, Satake Y, Kaido M, Shinozaki N, Shimmura S, Bissen-Miyajima H. Treatment of severe ocular surface disorders with corneal epithelial stem cell transplantation. N Engl J Med. 1999;340:1697–703.

Ye J, Lee SK, Kook KH, Yoa K. Bone marrow-derived progenitor cells promote corneal wound healing following alkali injury. Graefes Arch Clin Exp Ophthalmol. 2008;246(2):217–22.

Chapter 19
Drug Delivery Systems for Ocular Use

Jayabalan Nirmal and Gaurav K. Jain

Abstract Various static and dynamic ocular barriers in conjunction with membrane transporters pose a significant challenge for ocular drug therapy. These challenges present unique opportunities for understanding the barriers and overcoming it using novel/innovative drug delivery systems. Recently in response to advent of potent and versatile therapeutic agents, the diversity of conventional ocular formulations has gradually evolved, extending well beyond simple solutions, suspensions and ointments. The field includes a variety of innovative carriers that have shown the capacity to encapsulate wide variety of drugs and macromolecules and maintain extended drug effect in targeted tissues. Vesicular carriers, polymeric and lipid nanoparticles, dendrimers, nanoplexes, nanoemulsions, cubosomes, nanoassemblies, nanomicelles and various hybrid hydrogels as well as drug delivery enhancement devices have been widely explored to overcome various hurdles. This chapter presents an overview about the importance of understanding the blood ocular barriers for developing strategies for appropriate drug delivery systems and applications of innovative carriers for ocular delivery of drugs or macromolecules.

J. Nirmal, PhD (✉)
School of Materials Science & Engineering, NTU-Northwestern Nanomedicine Institute@NTU, Nanyang Technological University, Singapore, Singapore
e-mail: nirmaljayabalan@gmail.com

G.K. Jain, PhD
Department of Pharmaceutics, Faculty of Pharmacy, Jamia Hamdard (Hamdard University), New Delhi, India

T. Velpandian (ed.), *Pharmacology of Ocular Therapeutics*,
DOI 10.1007/978-3-319-25498-2_19

19.1 Sympathetic Understanding of Physiological Constraints

Jayabalan Nirmal, PhD

19.1.1 Blood–Ocular Barriers

The eye is a well-equipped sense organ which detects light from the environment and sends signal to the brain. It equipped itself with various anatomical and physiological barriers (Fig. 19.1). Being an anatomically privileged organ, it

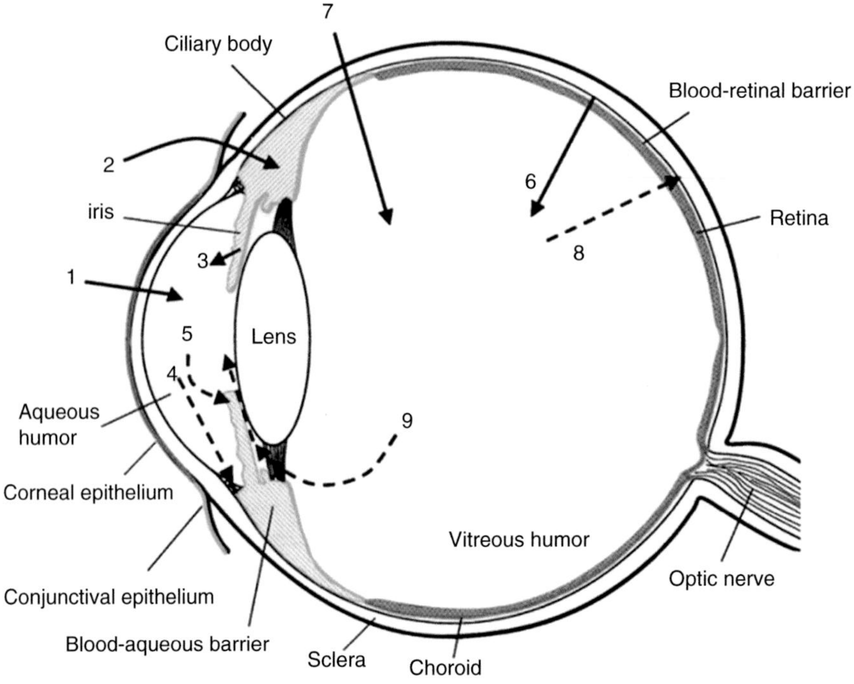

Fig. 19.1 Anatomy of the eye and the biological barriers of the eye (tight barriers are indicated in red, others in green; route of elimination). The main pathway for drugs to enter the anterior chamber is via the cornea (Lee and Robinson 1979). Some large and hydrophilic drugs prefer the conjunctival and scleral route and then diffuse into the ciliary body (Maurice and Mishima 1984). After systemic administration, small compounds can diffuse from the iris blood vessels into the anterior chamber (Young and Heath 2000). From the anterior chamber, the drugs are removed either by aqueous humor outflow (Barar et al. 2008) or by venous blood flow after diffusing across the iris surface (Klyce and Crosson 1985). After systemic administration, drugs must pass across the retinal pigment epithelium or the retinal capillary endothelium to reach the retina and vitreous humor (Sasaki et al. 1999). Alternatively, drugs can be administered by intravitreal injection (Huang et al. 1983). Drugs are eliminated from the vitreous via the blood–retinal barrier (Huang et al. 1989) or via diffusion into the anterior chamber (Dartt 2002) (Reproduced with permission from Hornof et al. 2005)

poses unique challenges to pharmaceutical scientists to deliver therapeutics inside the eye. In the battle of drugs to cross the ocular barriers, drugs often fail or perform poor in the battle. Unfortunately due to these barriers, access for the therapeutic drugs are difficult; hence, the clinical success is very limited. At the cellular level, the corneal epithelium, retinal endothelial cells, and retinal pigmented epithelium all contain tight intercellular junctions prevent the paracellular movement of small hydrophilic compounds. Drug distribution also restricted by anatomical features including blood supply which normally restricts penetration from superficial sites. Physiological (e.g., metabolism and membrane receptors/transporters) are other factors determining effective concentration within the eye. The various ocular barriers are the cornea, conjunctiva, blood aqueous barrier (BAB), and blood–retinal barrier (BRB). These are the fundamental barriers which protect the eye from xenobiotics, hence determining the ocular pharmacokinetics of the therapeutics.

19.1.1.1 Corneal Barrier

The topical ocular route of administration is preferred for many classes of drugs due to ease of access and patient compliance when treating diseases of the anterior segment. The topically applied drugs are rapidly eliminated from the precorneal area. In the precorneal area, solution drainage, tear dilution, tear turnover, tear fluid-enabled lacrimal drainage, and the conjunctival absorption allow only a small fraction of the drug to be absorbed into the eye (Lee and Robinson 1979; Maurice and Mishima 1984). The cornea (transparent tissue) is a front part of the eye, and it can be called as a window of the eye is considered as a major pathway for topical drugs. It provides an important mechanical and chemical barrier, which limits the access of exogenous substances into the eye and protects the intraocular tissues. The cornea is made up of five layers: corneal epithelium, basement membrane, Bowman's layer, stroma, Descemet's membrane, and endothelium (Fig. 19.2) (Young and Heath 2000; Barar et al. 2008). The corneal epithelium constitutes flattened superficial cells, wing cells, and columnar basal cells. The superficial cells are in close contact with one another via desmosomes, and these cells are surrounded by annular tight junctions–zonulae occludentes (Klyce and Crosson 1985; Sasaki et al. 1999). The tight junctions of the corneal epithelium are the rate-limiting barrier for hydrophilic drug permeation, whereas lipophilic drugs have comparatively higher permeability. The stroma and endothelium offer little resistance as compare to epithelium for transcorneal permeation (Huang et al. 1983, 1989). The stroma constitutes 85–90 % of the total corneal mass and is mainly composed of hydrated collagen. Stroma's hydrophilic nature exhibit a diffusional barrier to highly lipophilic drugs (Huang et al. 1983). The innermost layer of cornea–corneal endothelial monolayer conserves an effective barrier between the stroma and aqueous humor.

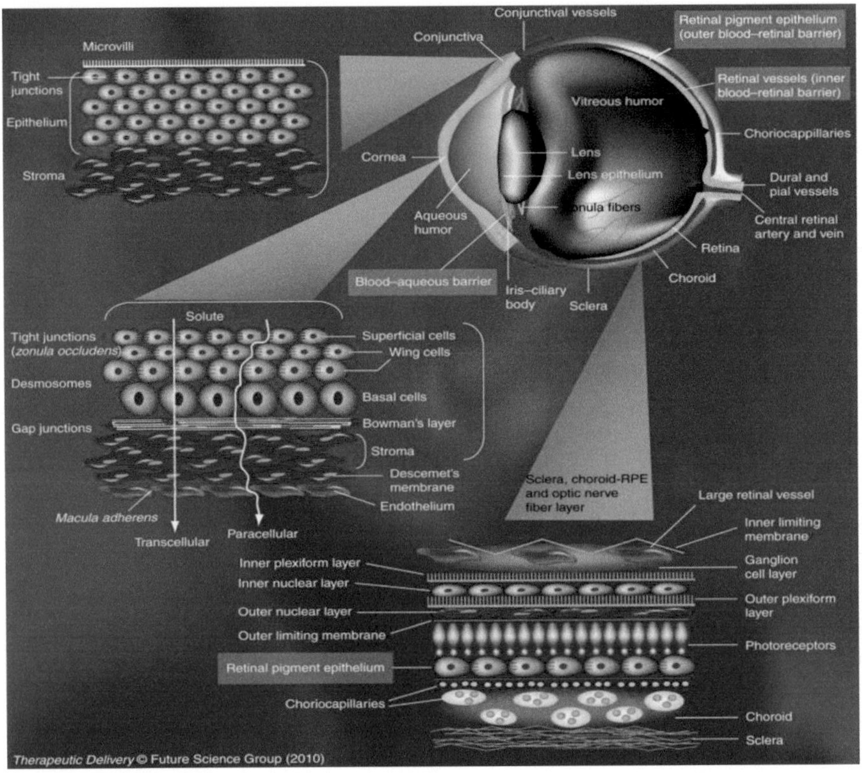

Fig. 19.2 Drug permeability barriers (Reproduced with permission from Kompella et al. 2010)

19.1.1.2 Conjunctival Barrier

Topical drugs reach various ocular structures through corneal and/or the non-corneal conjunctival (non-corneal) pathways (Fig. 19.1). The conjunctiva's greater surface area (17 times larger than human cornea) and relatively weaker epithelium provides opportunity for better topical absorption of drugs. It covers anterior one-third of the eye ball. The conjunctiva consists of an outer epithelium and beneath that lies the stroma. Microvilli cover the epithelium, and they are composed of 5–15 layers of stratified epithelium. Tight junctions connect the adjacent epithelial cells on the apical side due to which it exerts the intercellular drug permeability barrier. The stromal layer which attaches itself to the sclera has nerves, lymphatics, and blood vessels (Dartt 2002).

The palpebral conjunctiva lines the inner surface of the eyelids and bulbar conjunctiva which covers the anterior surface of the sclera. The bulbar conjunctiva represents the first barrier for the non-corneal permeation of topically applied drugs. Conjunctival route is favored for hydrophilic and large polar molecules bypassing anterior segment and having direct access to posterior segment tissues (Hosoya et al. 2005). The drugs can cross the conjunctiva through paracellular or transcellular routes. Also the drugs which are substrates of the influx transporters are reported to have been transported using the transporters (Zhang et al. 2006;

Garrett et al. 2008). However, the transporter-mediated transport in conjunctiva has not been explored much. The pore diameter and pore density was reported to be 2 and 16 times more in conjunctival epithelium than corneal epithelium of rabbits. This also could be the reason for higher drug permeability than cornea (Hamalainen et al. 1997). Another important thing to consider is the conjunctival blood vessels; a significant amount of topical and subconjunctivally injected drugs will be lost to the conjunctival blood circulation (Chang and Lee 1987; Urtti and Salminen 1993). Further details about cellular and metabolic functions various parts of the eye are explained in detail in the Chapter of Ocular Biochemistry (Chap. 5).

19.1.1.3 Blood–Aqueous Barrier (BAB)

The BAB is located at the anterior portion of the eye, and the access of drugs to the aqueous humor of the anterior and posterior chambers is restricted by the BAB (Figs. 19.1 and 19.2). The BAB executes its barrier functions by the presence of nonpigmented cell layer of the ciliary epithelium, posterior iridial epithelium, and endothelium of the iridial blood vessels. These structures are reported to have leaky tight junctions as compared to BRB (Cunha-Vaz 1979). The BAB regulates the solute exchange between the blood and the intraocular fluids – hence limits the entry of plasma albumin/drugs into aqueous humor (discussed in detail in Chap. No.3). However, some pathological conditions like inflammation could disrupt this barrier and allow the improved entry of drugs (Urtti 2006).

19.1.1.4 Blood–Retinal Barrier (BRB)

BRB at the posterior segment of the eye consists of inner BRB (iBRB) and outer BRB (oBRB) (Figs. 19.1 and 19.2). The iBRB and oBRB constitute endothelial membrane of the retinal blood vessels and retinal pigment epithelium (RPE). The cellular tight junctions "zonula occludens" seal off the spaces between the RPE cells (Cunha-Vaz 1976). Both the inner and outer BRB offer significant restriction to the permeability of drugs (discussed in detail in Chap. 3). The diffusion (permeability) of drugs across BRB is determined by its lipid solubility. BRB due to its specific permeability characteristics provide its potential role in the pathophysiology and posterior therapeutics of diabetic retinopathy (DR), age-related macular degeneration (ARMD), and diabetic macular edema (DME) (Cunha-Vaz 1976; Mannermaa et al. 2006). It separates blood from neural retina. The oBRB being a tight ion-transporting barrier restricts paracellular transport of polar solutes from the choroidal side. The iBRB offers significant resistance to systemic penetration of drugs. A drug should possess optimum membrane partition characteristics or should be a substrate for one of the membrane uptake transporters present on the iBRB or oBRB to cross BRB (Cunha-Vaz 1976; Nirmal et al. 2012, 2013a, b). Both BAB and BRB contain epithelium and endothelium with tight junctions that restrict the entry of drugs through paracellular route (Cunha-Vaz 1979; Rizzolo et al. 2011).

19.1.2 Various Routes of Ocular Drug Delivery

To achieve a therapeutic success for various ocular diseases, various possible routes of drug delivery are being used (Fig. 19.1). However, the selection of administration route mainly depends on the targeted site of action. Conventionally, topical, intravitreal, systemic (oral and intravenous), and recently periocular routes are used. To treat the anterior segment of the eye, mostly topical route is used, whereas for posterior segment, intravitreal and periocular routes are used. Systemic route has been used traditionally for treating both anterior and posterior segment (Urtti 2006). Ocular pharmacokinetics of drugs administered through various routes are explained in Chap. 3.

19.1.2.1 Topical Drug Delivery

The most patient compliant and the conventional route is topical delivery into the cul-de-sac using eye drop. In humans, the contact time of the eye drop in the precorneal area is very less (less than 5 min), and it also activates lacrimation and tear turnover which dilutes the drug concentration (Hughes et al. 2005). Hence, less than 1 % reaches the aqueous humor (Lee and Robinson 1986; Mikkelson et al. 1973). During this short time, the drugs which are small ionic and hydrophilic enters the anterior chamber through the pores (60 A°) of the corneal epithelium (Lee 1990). In case of lipophilic drugs, the drug remains in the epithelium due to its lipid solubility and release to the stroma and then to the anterior chamber (Sieg and Robinson 1976). The drug reaches its maximum concentration at 20–30 min in aqueous humor. From there, it gets distributed to the iris and the ciliary body (Maurice and Mishima 1984; Urtti et al. 1990). The elimination from aqueous humor is through the aqueous turnover, Schlemm's canal, and the anterior uveal venous blood flow (Maurice and Mishima 1984). These mechanisms render the overall half-life of topical eye drops in the anterior chamber in around 1 h (Urtti 2006). Hence, a topical delivery requires frequent administration with high concentration. There is a real need for the topical delivery system which could release the drug for extended period without frequent administration.

19.1.2.2 Systemic Drug Delivery (Oral and Intravenous)

For oral drugs, the ocular bioavailability is determined by the plasma concentration it reaches after the intestinal absorption. The intraocular penetration determined by the drugs' physiochemical and transporters susceptibility at ocular barriers (Nirmal et al. 2012, 2013a, b; Velpandian 2010). Both BAB and BRB restrict the entry of systemic drugs. The systemic drugs enter the anterior segment by penetrating the leaky vessels of the ciliary body and diffuse through the iris to aqueous humor (Cunha-Vaz 1979). In the posterior segment, the drugs which could reach choroid will be cleared by choriocapillaris (densely packed network) – luckily, it has numerous fenestrations in the endothelium which offers less resistance. However, the further movement into vitreous is restricted by RPE except for the compounds with extreme lipophilic nature. Additionally, the functional transporter systems present in the RPE and retinal vessels efflux the drugs out from vitreous to plasma (vitreous elimination) which renders the short half-life of the drugs in vitreous. As a result, most of the compounds with good pharmacological activity reaches poorly inside the eye, hence requiring high systemic concentration which provides unwanted side effects and poor therapeutic success. Hence, systemic drug delivery systems with specific targeting are highly needed, without which only a fraction can reach after oral or intravenous administration (Urtti 2006; Nirmal et al. 2013b).

19.1.2.3 Intravitreal Drug Delivery

To overcome the BRB and achieve the required therapeutic concentration inside the vitreous chamber, direct vitreal administration is a more straightforward approach. In many posterior segment diseases like DR, ARMD, and DME, vitreous administration is still the mainstay of treatment (Hughes et al. 2005). However, the intravitreal administration has its own disadvantages like frequent administration, hemorrhage, retinal detachment, and endophthalmitis (Jay and Shockley 1988; Daily et al. 1973). The drug gets eliminated from vitreous through both the anterior and posterior segment. The anterior elimination occurs by diffusion from vitreous to posterior chamber and elimination via aqueous turnover and uveal blood flow (Maurice and Mishima 1984). Recently, it has been revealed that the cationic drugs predominantly undergo anterior elimination using organic cation transporters (Nirmal et al. 2012). The posterior segment elimination occurs due to permeation across BRB through passive permeability or by active efflux transporters (Maurice and Mishima 1984; Senthilkumari et al. 2009; Hosoya et al. 2009). Hence, large or hydrophilic molecules tend to have longer vitreal half-life. In the vitreous, the mobility of large molecules is restricted, especially the positively charged; however, the small drugs could diffuse rapidly (Pitkanen et al. 2003). The influence of compromised BRB in various disease conditions in altering the vitreal drug pharmacokinetics needs further studies and serious consideration. The drug delivery system like injectable implants which could deliver the drugs for prolonged period of time holds the promise for intravitreal therapeutics.

19.1.2.4 Periocular Drug Delivery Systems

Periocular denotes the periphery of the eye or surrounding region of the eye. Periocular drug delivery could be achieved via subconjunctival, sub-Tenon, peribulbar, posterior juxtrascleral, and retrobulbar spaces (Ranta and Urtti 2006). The sclera due to its large surface area provides potential advantage for periocular drug delivery. Periocular drugs could reach posterior segment through the anterior chamber route, systemic circulation route, and direct penetration route (Eljarrat-Binstock et al. 2010). Periocular drug delivery systems need to overcome the episclera, sclera, choroid, Bruch's membrane, and RPE before reaching the vitreous humor or the retina (Kim et al. 2007; Ghate et al. 2007). This could be the longest and most problematic route to reach vitreous and retina due to the presence of static barrier and dynamic clearance mechanisms (Ghate and Edelhauser 2006). Potential capabilities of new novel drug delivery systems could provide a new importance to this route for treating various posterior segment diseases. However, detail studies are still needed to understand the pharmacokinetics of the periocular drug delivery systems from various periocular spaces before questioning its future.

19.1.3 Importance of Understanding Blood–Ocular Barriers to Overcome It Using Drug Delivery Approaches

The clinical success of ophthalmic therapeutics was reported to be approximately 14 % (Kola and Landis 2004). Ophthalmic drugs are one among the various areas have very limited clinical success as compare to other therapeutic areas. This scenario could be due to: (i) no/very few ocular-specific drugs are being developed and (ii) lack of sufficient understanding of blood–ocular barriers to overcome it using appropriate drug delivery systems. The ocular barriers exert its property through (i) regulated diffusion through the paracellular spaces, (ii) transcellular facilitated diffusion, (iii) transcellular active transport, (iv) transcytosis, and (v) metabolic processing (Rizzolo et al. 2011). The contribution of each of these pathways in the drug transport across ocular barriers is not clear. However, the transport of majority of the drug molecules/solutes through various ocular epitheliums occurs by either through the cells (transcellular) or between the cell (paracellular) routes. Generally, hydrophilic drugs have less penetration across various ocular epithelium; hence, they require some active uptake process/transporter for their penetration or transport through paracellular route (Mannermaa et al. 2006; Hughes et al. 2005; Ueda et al. 2000). The size and charge of the intercellular spaces determines the transport of drugs through the paracellular route. The paracellular permeability is limited by four types of cell–cell junctions which include tight junctions (TJ), adherens junctions, gap junctions, and desmosomes in vertebrates. In 1963, the tight junction or zonula occludens was discovered by Farquhar and Palade (1963). The TJs are formed just beneath the apical surface in epithelial cells (to seal neighboring cells) to determine transport of solutes like water, ions, drugs, and other molecules (Farquhar and Palade 1963). The drug/molecule with radii up to 15 A° can cross through the tight junctions. The cells attain the mechanical stability by zonula adherens and desmosomes. Electrical and metabolic coupling are ensured by gap junctions (Simon and Goodenough 1998).

The lipophilic drugs cross the epithelium due to their lipid solubility in the cell membrane lipids. Drugs with specialized transport process utilize the transcellular route (Ho and Kim 2005). The drug interaction with the cell is influenced by both drug and cell characteristics. The transcellular transport mechanisms include passive diffusion, facilitated diffusion, and receptor-mediated endocytosis. These mechanisms are implemented by the cells using the membrane proteins (transporters or receptors). The membrane transporters (so-called drug transporters) are the militants located across the eye. Many of the ocular drugs are substrates of these transporter proteins. It is also very clear that these transporters share a substantial percentage in the ocular pharmacokinetics and disposition of drugs (Mannermaa et al. 2006). Hence, there is a potential opportunity for the drug delivery systems to target the drug transporters to optimize the ocular bioavailability of therapeutics.

Drug transporters could enhance or prevent the entry of drugs across blood–ocular barriers. Based on these characteristics, transporters are divided into uptake (influx) or export (efflux) of the drugs which are their substrates – hence, it could be an opportunity or barrier for drug delivery. Apart from the physicochemical characteristics of the drugs (molecular size, lipophilicity, and the pKa), these transporters determine the transport of the drugs across various ocular barriers. The various ocular barriers are known to express several of these transporters at both apical and basolateral surfaces (Nirmal et al. 2012, 2013a, b; Zhang et al. 2008; Vadlapatla et al. 2014). However, the percentage contribution of various factors is not very clear yet and needs further studies. The transporters could also provide mechanistic details of treatment failure, individual response to the treatment, and adverse drug reaction (Tamai and Tsuji 2000).

The two major superfamilies ATP-binding cassette (ABC) and solute carrier (SLC) transporters consist of 400 membrane transporters (International Transporter Consortium et al. 2010; Schlessinger et al. 2013). Efflux and influx transporters belong to the ABC and SLC superfamily. The various transporters' localization in ocular tissues is reported in (Zhang et al. 2008; Vadlapatla et al. 2014). Efflux transporters reduce intracellular concentration of drugs by expelling it out of the cell, and it operates as a unidirectional transporters. Till now 48 ABC transporters belonging to seven different classes (ABCAABCG) have been identified (Hediger et al. 2004; Vadlapatla et al. 2014). Among them P-glycoprotein (P-gp/MDR1), multidrug-resistant proteins (MRPs), and breast cancer-resistant protein (BCRP) are considered important. Influx transporters help to transport nutrients, peptides, ions, peptides, metabolites, other endogenous amines, and exogenous molecules. In human genome, 386 SLC transporters belonging to 43 different families (SLC1-SLC43) have been identified. Among them organic cation transporters (OCT/OCTN), organic anion transporters (OAT/OATP), peptide transporter (PEPT), monocarboxylate transporters (MCTs), amino acid transporters, and sodium-dependent multivitamin transporter (SMVT) (Vadlapatla et al. 2014).

Transporter-targeted drug delivery could become a clinically significant drug delivery approach (Duvvuri et al. 2004). P-gp and MRPs were the most explored transporters in the eye. Mitra group have demonstrated the importance of inhibiting P-gp and MRPs to improve the ocular bioavailability of various clinically important drugs (Vadlapatla et al. 2014). Several transporters or receptors for nutrients and endogenous compounds are expressed in the cornea, conjunctiva, and RPE representing opportunities for ocular delivery of drugs. For example, corneal permeability of antiviral drugs such as acyclovir and ganciclovir is improved when converted into their L-valyl esters which could be due to targeting dipeptide transporters in the cornea (Anand and Mitra 2002). Evidence suggests that the presence of peptide transporters (PEPT1 and PEPT2) in the cornea is involved in the absorptive mechanism for their drug substrates after topical dosing to the cornea (Zhang et al. 2008). Few of the studies have also reported the utilization of BRB for enhanced nonviral gene transfer, utilizing transporters like folate and vitamin C transporters/receptors located in the RPE (Lee and Huang 1996; Guo and Lee 1999). An oligopeptide transport system is involved in the transport of a model dipeptide after systemic administration across ocular barriers (Atluri et al. 2004).

Carrier-mediated transport process for brimonidine in the RPE has been demonstrated in bovine RPE-choroid explants and polarized human adult retinal pigment epithelial cells (ARPE-19), suggesting its role in modulating the movement of brimonidine into and out of the eye (Zhang et al. 2006). Organic cation drug absorption could be greatly enhanced by targeting OCT in the cornea and BRB (Nirmal et al. 2012, 2013a, b). Transporter-mediated drug penetration present at iBRB would confer great advantage over passive diffusion due to the tight barrier of the retinal endothelium. Therefore, it is important to design and select optimal drug candidates by taking into account the fact that drugs should be recognized by influx transporters, while efflux transporters at the iBRB be avoided (Hosoya et al. 2009). To effectively implement the current drug delivery strategies, it is critical to understand the distribution and functional importance of the various transporters which are exerting the barrier properties of the eye. Also the varied expression of the influx and efflux transporters in disease conditions needs careful consideration during design of drug delivery systems (Vadlapatla et al. 2014). It might be the key to successful topical, periocular, intravitreal, and systemic drug delivery to the ocular structures.

19.1.4 *Importance of Ocular-Specific Novel Drug Delivery for Overcoming Blood–Ocular Barriers for Providing Optimum Therapeutics*

Several experimental studies in in vitro and in vivo models promise the possibility of successful therapeutic effect. However, clinical trials could not show the similar beneficial effect due to subtherapeutic concentrations of the drug in the eye (Velpandian 2010). Figure 19.3 shows the existing problem of the ocular drugs and the potential strategies to overcome it.

Few of the classical examples discussed below could show the compelling need for the ocular-specific drugs/novel drug delivery systems to overcome blood–ocular barriers and to provide optimum therapeutics for various sight-threatening diseases.

19.1.4.1 Challenges and Potential Opportunities for siRNA Ocular Delivery

Any gene that is responsible for a disease is susceptible to suppression by RNA interference (RNAi) (Guo et al. 2010). Through evolution, it has been a conserved posttranscriptional pathway (Fire et al. 1998). Specific siRNA will be able to target and cleaves the complementary messenger RNA (mRNA), hence inhibits the protein synthesis (gene silencing) through RNAi pathway (Ketting et al. 2001). The synthetically produced siRNA has promising future in the biomedical applications for various diseases. Especially for the eye being a secluded organ, the application of siRNA has great advantage to provide therapeutic activity without unwanted side effects (Guzman-Aranguez et al. 2013). Because of these potential benefits, currently several siRNA therapeutics

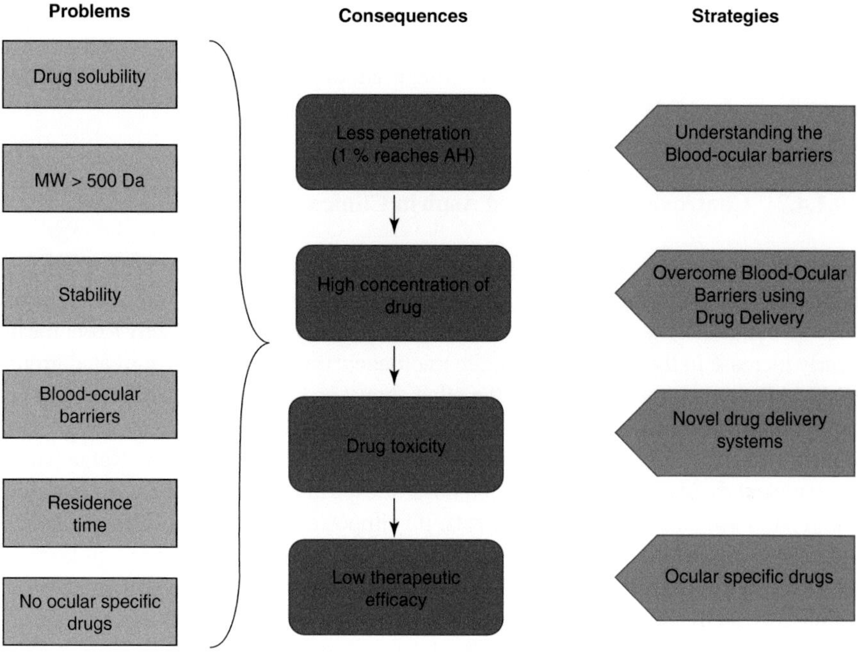

Fig. 19.3 Intricacies with the existing ocular therapeutics

are being tested at various clinical phase trials by pharmaceutical companies for age-related macular degeneration, diabetic macular edema, and glaucoma (Thakur et al. 2012). However, the clinical studies for bevasiranib and siRNA-027 are terminated or have been completed without significant positive results because of possible failure to meet its key efficacy against inhibiting VEGF or VEGFR1 and possible stimulation of Toll-like receptors 3 (TLR3) (Guzman-Aranguez et al. 2013; Kaiser et al. 2010). Important lessons can be learned from these studies and it is clear that siRNA needs to overcome several barriers to have a successful therapeutic effect. siRNAs electrostatically repel negatively charged cell membrane due to its negative charges from phosphate groups hence cannot cross the membrane and reach cytoplasm. Once it reaches the cytoplasm, it has to escape the endosomes or lysosomes. It also has short half-life in the physiological conditions, poor specificity and tissue uptake, cellular toxicity, and off-target effects (Reischl and Zimmer 2009). Another important issue to consider is that siRNA half-life needs to be at least three times (at the site of action) the half-life of targeted protein for silencing. The rapidly dividing cells and active clearance mechanism of the eye decrease the siRNA half-life hence compels the need for multiple dosing which leads to patient incompliance (Bartlett and Davis 2006).

Drug delivery systems like liposomes, polyplexes, polymers, self-penetrating peptides, and dendrimers could overcome the above said problems to provide optimum siRNA therapeutics in the eye (Thakur et al. 2012). Cells can uptake these nanocarriers through multiple pathways including endocytosis, micropinocytosis, and phagocytosis (Zuhorn et al. 2002). Using these nanocarriers, the siRNA can be delivered to specific cellular compartment and also can escape the endosome/lysosome degradation. For example, polyethylenimine (PEI) is a cationic polymer in which the siRNA could be conjugated (PEI-siRNA delivery system) to deliver sufficient payload inside the cytoplasm through endocytosis and also can escape the endosomes due to its high buffering capability (Boussif et al. 1995).

19.1.4.2 Controversial Results of Aspirin Clinical Trials

Aspirin's anti-inflammatory property and its effect on DR already has been studied in clinical trials and animal studies. However, prospective clinical trials in humans showed contradictory conclusions, with one study showing a significantly lower mean yearly increase in the number of definite microaneurysms in the aspirin-treated group (DAMAD Study Group 1989), and the other shows no benefit (or harm) of aspirin on the retinopathy (Early Treatment Diabetic Retinopathy Research Group 1991). The aspirin's failure to inhibit retinopathy in the Early Treatment Diabetic Retinopathy Research study gives us a clue that the dose of aspirin reached the eye was not high enough to have anti-inflammatory effects. It is important to note that all these studies are carried out using oral aspirin therapy (Tang and Kern 2011). The lesson learned from this study compels the need for the sufficient concentration of aspirin required at retina to treat DR. Recent prospective, randomized study using another NSAID, sulindac shows that the salicylates can inhibit development and progression of DR if anti-inflammatory dose is delivered (Hattori et al. 2007). These clinical studies show the need for the ocular drug delivery systems for aspirin to treat DR. The novel drug delivery systems (e.g., nanoparticles) can deliver aspirin to the vitreous compartment in a sustained manner with offered protection from metabolizing enzymes, avoiding cellular toxicity and specific cell uptake using surface modifications or decorations.

19.1.4.3 Partial Protective Effect of *Erigeron breviscapus* (vant.) Hand. Mazz in Clinical Trial

Velpandian (2010) described BRB as closed gateways. The inability of the active ingredients to cross closed gates could be a possible reason for the failure of randomized, double-blind, clinical trial while commenting on Chinese traditional herb *Erigeron breviscapus* (vant.) Hand. Mazz for glaucoma (Velpandian 2010). This commentary also compels the need for the ocular delivery systems to deliver therapeutics to overcome ocular barriers for optimum therapeutics.

19.1.4.4 Limited Success of Calcium Dobesilate

Calcium dobesilate (CDO) was developed more than four decades ago for treating DR and chronic venous insufficiency (Zhang et al. 2015). Recently, a meta-analysis study by Zhang et al. (2015) concluded the efficacy of CDO to treat DR. However, despite its multiple modes of action, clinical studies failed to show the significant efficacy to treat clinically significant macular edema (CSME) (Feghhi et al. 2014; Haritoglou et al. 2009). It gave a mixed signal to use CDO for posterior segment diseases. Considering its multiple actions and hypothesizing the lack of ocular penetration of CDO, our group (Velpandian et al. 2009) developed an ocular-specific eye drops and evaluated its pharmacological efficacy against various cataract models. The study reported sufficient transcorneal penetration after single topical administration of CDO eye drops and also significant effect of CDO in vivo cataract model (Velpandian et al. 2009). Pedro Cuevas et al., even though in a different disease condition, reconfirmed the need for ocular-specific drug delivery by demonstrating the significant effect of CDO eye drop to treat primary pterygium. The report also suggested that the failed efficacy of calcium dobesilate in CSME could be due to its unstable nature and lack of ocular penetration after oral administration (Cuevas et al. 2012).

19.1.5 Conclusion

The major goal in providing optimum therapeutics to the eye is to circumvent the various blood–ocular barriers. Even though new ocular drugs have been developed, still effective concentration could not be reached at site of action due to these ocular barriers. Various drug delivery systems have been developed to increase the ocular bioavailability of ophthalmic drugs after topical instillation. But an ideal topical drug delivery is not yet available. Drugs administered systemically also have poor access to retina and vitreous humor. It is also recognized that drug transporter activity is an essential component for ocular barrier function. Transporter-targeted systemic delivery could be an ideal drug delivery system; however, extensive research is needed to establish the functional importance of these transporters to utilize for the drug delivery systems. Although intravitreal administration overcomes both these barriers, it is also associated with several other problems. Therefore, a smart way of drug delivery is required at this stage to treat various sight-threatening diseases.

19.2 Innovative Drug Delivery Systems

Gaurav K. Jain, PhD

19.2.1 Introduction

Ocular drug delivery remains a challenging task due to restrictive barrier functionalities of the eye structure. Structural variation of each layer of ocular tissue can pose a significant barrier following drug administration by any route, i.e., topical, systemic, periocular, and intravitreal. Topical instillation as an eye drop formulation is the most widely preferred noninvasive route of ocular drug administration and accounts for ~90 % of the marketed ophthalmic formulations. Nonetheless, the ocular bioavailability is very low (<5 %) with topical eye drop administration (Khar et al. 2010; Patel et al. 2013; Chaurasia et al. 2015; Reimondez-Troitiño et al. 2015). Static and dynamic ocular barriers impede transport and efficacy of various topically administered medications. Furthermore, it is difficult to achieve therapeutic drug concentration to the back of the eye, viz., vitreous, retina, and choroid, following topical eye drops instillation (Nagarwal et al. 2009; Jain et al. 2012). In addition, physicochemical properties of the drug also have an impact on limiting the ocular drug bioavailability. Tight barriers and layers of alternating polarity make the tear film and cornea an important barrier to most low-molecular-weight hydrophilic and lipophilic drugs. Delivery of high-molecular-weight compounds such as nucleic acids, proteins, peptides, Fab fragments, growth factors, and genetic material, which are gaining increased attention in the ophthalmic field, is also challenging (Khar et al. 2010). Indeed, these compounds are rapidly degraded by extracellular enzymes, and their entry, either by a paracellular or by a transcellular route, is totally restricted. Since most drugs poorly penetrate the cornea, fulminating diseases of the posterior segment are required to be treated with either systemic administration or through intravitreal or periocular injections/implants. Therapy with systemic administration requires large doses due to strong blood–ocular tissue barrier, making it an impractical approach. Though direct injections through intravitreal and periocular route appear to be a promising approach to attain high drug concentrations at the back of the eye, these routes are very invasive requiring skilled administration and are associated with a high degree of risk, such as development of retinal detachment and endophthalmitis (Lee et al. 2010).

Clearly, there is a strong case in favor of formulating ocular delivery systems by focusing on improved ocular bioavailability and extended drug effect in targeted tissues. In particular, the improved ocular bioavailability could be achieved by (i) increasing residence time of carrier on the ocular surface, (ii) enhancing corneal penetration, (iii) prolonged release of drug, and (iv) targeting of drug to intraocular tissues. Advances in development of ocular delivery system is continuing and, with the better understanding of physiology and barriers of the eye, has gathered momentum in recent years. Innovative delivery systems that can efficiently target the diseased ocular tissues generate effective and prolonged drug effective concentrations for treating both anterior and posterior segment disorders are emerging (Fig. 19.4).

Conventional approach to prolong precorneal residence or to improve corneal permeation of topical eye drop formulation is through the addition of viscosity and permeation enhancers. Viscosity enhancers such as hydroxy methyl cellulose, hydroxy ethyl cellulose, sodium carboxymethyl cellulose, and hydroxypropyl methylcellulose improve contact time of drug with the ocular mucosa but suffer from the disadvantage of poor ocular penetration (Patel et al. 2013). Permeation enhancers improve corneal uptake by modifying the corneal integrity. Examples of permeation enhancers investigated for improving ocular delivery include benzalkonium chloride, polyoxyethylene glycol ethers, ethylenediaminetetraacetic acid sodium salt, sodium taurocholate, saponins, and Cremophor EL. However, local toxicity has been observed with the use of permeation enhancers (Patel et al. 2013). To circumvent the problems associated with these delivery systems, emulsions and suspensions have been developed.

These formulations improve both solubility and bioavailability of drug and hold a strong marketplace. Nevertheless, these conventional formulations, because of their micron-size particle range, are associated with stability issues and various side effects such as ocular irritation, redness, inflammation, and vision interference

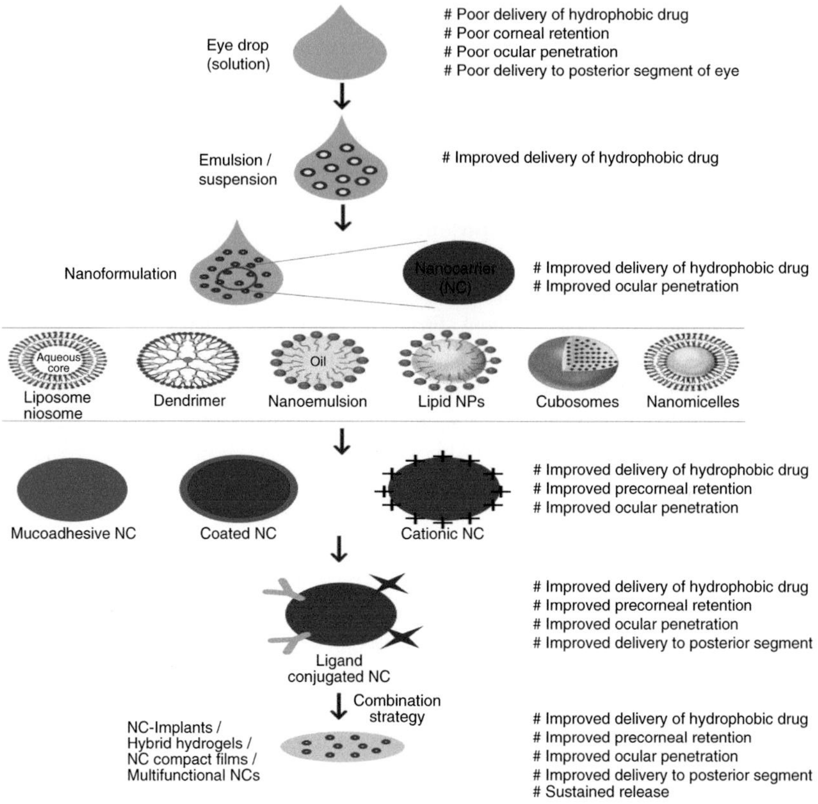

Fig. 19.4 Development stages and attributes of innovative ocular drug delivery systems

(Patel et al. 2013). In addition, coarse particles do not prevail corneal and conjunctival epithelial barriers of the eye. Attempts to overcome the problems associated with conventional formulations resulted in the development of innovative carriers and technologies that have shown the capacity to (i) encapsulate wide variety of drugs, including biomacromolecules, (ii) reduce the degradation of labile drugs, (iii) increase the precorneal residence time, (iv) improve the corneal penetration, and (v) maintain extended drug effect in targeted tissues. Innovative drug delivery systems such as nanoparticles, nanoplexes, micro- and nanoemulsions, liposomes, niosomes, cubosomes, lipid nanoparticles, nanomicelles, dendrimers, hybrid hydrogels, implants, and drug delivery enhancement devices possess combination of these properties to attain optimum drug levels in desired ocular tissue. Although there are many potential improvements in the field of ocular drug delivery resulting in burgeoning development of innovative ocular drug delivery systems (Fig. 19.4), advancement of these innovative carriers is continuing to allow them to undergo rapid internalization, to enhance target recognition, to sustain the release of encapsulated drug, to enhance gene transfection, and to achieve optimum drug concentration at target site. Such emerging drug delivery technologies have the potential to maintain and/or improve therapeutic indices of active agents. In this section, we provide an overview on the success achieved until now using a number of innovative drug delivery systems for the delivery of drug to ocular tissues.

19.2.2 Innovative Drug Delivery Systems

19.2.2.1 Vesicular Carriers: Liposomes and Niosomes

Vesicular carriers are lamellar structures made up of amphiphilic molecules surrounded by an aqueous compartment. From the early 1980s, vesicular carriers, particularly liposomes and niosomes, have gained wide attention by researchers for their use as ocular drug delivery carriers (Stratford et al. 1983; Kaur et al. 2004). Liposomes are biocompatible and biodegradable vesicles comprising of an aqueous volume surrounded by a phospholipid bilayer (Agarwal et al. 2014). Niosomes are structurally similar to liposomes; however, bilayers are made up of nonionic surfactant instead of phospholipids (Moghassemi and Hadjizadeh 2014). Vesicular carriers are useful for the delivery of both hydrophilic and hydrophobic drugs which are encapsulated in the core or bilayer, respectively. These carriers have been widely explored to overcome the problems of conventional ocular therapy. Vesicles can vary in size from nanometers to micrometers, can be uni- or multilamellar, and can vary considerably in size, surface charge, lipid composition, and fluidity of the bilayers. Drug encapsulation by these carriers results in improved pharmacokinetics, stability, precorneal residence time, and transcorneal permeation. Because of their unique features, liposomes and niosomes are a promising means of delivering ocular drugs for the treatment of both anterior and posterior segment eye disorders. Topical bioavailability can be improved by maximizing corneal drug absorption, minimizing precorneal drug loss, and continuous delivery of ophthalmic drugs to the ocular tissues. When applied topically, vesicles can attach to the hydrophobic corneal epithelium (Schaeffer and Krohn 1982). Effect of vesicle type, charge, and size on precorneal retention and transcorneal permeation is well investigated and generally follows the order of (+)SUV > (+)MLV = (−)SUV > SUV > MLV > free drug. It has been shown that positively charged vesicles composed of cationic lipids such as stearylamine, didodecyldimethylammonium bromide, and 1,2-dioleyl-3-trimethyl ammonium propane have higher binding affinity to the corneal surface than neutral or negatively charged vesicles (Velpandian et al. 1999; Law et al. 2000; Hathout et al. 2007). Several experiments using animal models have shown that cationic liposome-entrapped drugs have improved ocular bioavailability compared to their free drug counterparts. Cationic vesicles also exert adjuvant immunity when they are used as a delivery system for protein vaccines and DNA (Yan et al. 2007). Moreover, the performance of liposomes and niosomes can be further improved by their surface modification. Surface modification of vesicles with carbopol, chitosan, and its derivative, N-trimethyl chitosan, not only improve the physicochemical stability but also prolong precorneal retention and enhance bioavailability over uncoated counterparts and drug solutions (Li et al. 2009; Mehanna et al. 2010; Abdelbary 2011; Li et al. 2012). In a recent study, coating of liposome with mucoadhesive silk fibroin has shown to improve cellular uptake and therapeutic efficacy (Dong et al. 2015). Liposomes incorporated into hydrogels or soft contact lenses or complexed with either chitosan nanoparticle or noisome has been used to improve precorneal retention and to extend optimal ocular pharmacodynamics over a prolonged period (Nagarsenker et al. 1999).

Topical administration for posterior segment delivery is the greatest challenge and opportunity of ocular liposomal drug delivery. It has been shown that liposomal drug can reach the neural retina and ganglion cells after topical administration (Masuda et al. 1996; Davis et al. 2014). Liposome formulation variables might be used to tune the delivery properties to the ocular tissues. It is very unlikely that large-sized liposomes could permeate in the tight corneal barrier. Blood vessel-mediated liposomal delivery to the posterior segment can be achieved only if the liposomes are able to distribute to the ocular tissues. For this purpose, the size of the liposomes is critically important due to the limited size of choroidal and conjunctival fenestrations. Hironaka et al. demonstrated that liposomes with a size of 105–125 nm reach the retina (Hironaka et al. 2009). In another study, size-dependent distribution of liposomes to different posterior segment tissues was seen. Liposomes with the diameter less than 80 nm produced by microfluidization permeated to the retinal pigment epithelium, whereas liposomes with the diameter of 100 nm or more were distributed to the choroidal endothelium (Lajunen et al. 2014). However, active targeting using transferring or phospholipid-binding protein annexin A5 was shown to be necessary for liposome retention to the target tissue (Hironaka et al. 2009; Davis et al. 2014). Direct intravitreal injection of liposomes is a more definitive method of posterior segment drug delivery than topical administration, but it is more invasive and associated with greater risks of infection and bleeding. Despite some advantages that make vesicular carrier a potentially useful system for ocular drug delivery, the utility of these carriers may be limited by a short shelf life, limited drug loading, difficulty associated with thorough sterilization, and long-term side effects. Additionally, vesicles may not be able to release the entire payload of active drug relative to a free solution form. Therefore, all these factors should be taken into account while developing vesicular formulation for ophthalmic application.

19.2.2.2 Polymeric Nanoparticles

Nanoparticles (NPs) are colloidal carriers with a size range of 10–1000 nm. For ocular delivery, nanoparticles are generally composed of proteins, natural or synthetic polymers such as gelatin, modified starch, albumin, sodium alginate, chitosan, hyaluronic acid, carbopol, poly (lactic-co-glycolic acid) (PLGA), poly-ε-caprolactone (PCL), Eudragit® (RS100 and RL100), and poly-(butylcyanoacrylate) (PBCA). Drug-loaded NPs can be nanospheres or nanocapsules. In nanospheres, drug is uniformly distributed throughout polymeric matrix, while in nanocapsules, drug is enclosed inside the polymeric shell. NPs were considered to offer the possibility of a more facile delivery and transport across tissues, and consequently their potential for delivery to both anterior and posterior ocular tissues started to be studied (Khar et al. 2010; Jain et al. 2012). In 1986, an early attempt to use NPs was done with PBCA NPs loaded with highly lipophilic drug, progesterone (Li et al. 1986). After topical application to rabbit eyes, a decreased progesterone concentration in tissues, compared to control solutions, was observed attributed to greater affinity of progesterone for the NP polymer. The lesson learned from these experiments was that it is important to optimize the physicochemical relations between the polymers and drug to obtain an efficient carrier. Later, Juberias et al., used PECL nanocapsules loaded with 1 % cyclosporine (CsA) in a rat model of corneal transplantation rejection. By using PECL nanocapsules, toxic effects of CsA were avoided along with improved ocular penetration; however, corneal graft rejection was not prevented by the CsA-loaded PECL NPs (Juberías et al. 1998). The failure was not considered to be a consequence of negative interactions between the polymer and the drug. Improved formulations using polymers with known biocompatibility and biodegradability, such as PLGA, were developed later and shown to be more effective than commercial formulations (Vega et al. 2006; Garg et al. 2014). Recently, NPs with mucoadhesive properties have been developed to improve precorneal residence time. NPs prepared from chitosan, hyaluronic acid, carbopol, and sodium alginate are commonly employed to improve precorneal residence time of nanoparticles (Kao et al. 2006; Motwani et al. 2008; Ibrahim et al. 2010; Contreras-Ruiz et al. 2010; Ameeduzzafar et al. 2014; Chhonker et al. 2015).

Out of these, chitosan NPs or chitosan-coated NPs are most widely explored for improving precorneal residence. Chitosan is a natural polysaccharide with interesting features, such as biocompatibility and biodegradability, mucoadhesiveness, and the ability to transiently enhance the permeability of ocular barriers. Chitosan NPs are able to interact with the ocular surface and get through the corneal and conjunctival epithelium without causing toxicity. Several studies using chitosan NPs, chitosan/carbopol NPs, chitosan/lecithin NPs, and chitosan/alginate NPs have demonstrated improved pharmacokinetics and pharmacodynamic activity of encapsulated drugs (Motwani et al. 2008). The surface characteristics of the nanocarriers also have an influence on the interaction with the ocular surface structures. For instance, chitosan-coated PECL NPs enter the corneal epithelium in vivo more efficiently than uncoated PECL or polyethylene glycol-coated PECL NPs (de Campos et al. 2003). The transport pathways by which NPs penetrate the ocular surface tissues are of great interest. For NPs composed of hydrophobic polymers such as PECL or PLGA, uptake via transcellular route has been proposed, whereas for NPs composed of hydrophilic polymers such as chitosan, paracellular route has been proposed. These results moved us to explore different biomaterial combinations intended specifically for the ocular surface tissues. Consequently, we joined PLGA and chitosan to form a new matrix-based nanosystem that we termed "nanoplex" (Jain et al. 2010a, b, 2011; Warsi et al. 2014). The theoretical advantages of these nanoplexes are encapsulation of both hydrophilic and hydrophobic drugs, better control over drug release, prolonged corneal retention, and penetration (Jain et al. 2010a, b). We tested nanoplex formulation, showing their potential for ocular administration. In an in vivo study using rabbit eye, we investigated the interaction of nanoplexes with ocular mucosa. Confocal microscopy of the cornea revealed both paracellular and transcellular uptake of the nanoplex. The uptake mechanism postulated was adsorptive-mediated endocytosis and opening of tight junctions between epithelial cells. Results demonstrated prolonged precorneal retention of nanoplexes. Further, these carriers were found to be well tolerated (Jain et al. 2011).

NPs have also been lucratively employed as an alternative strategy for prolonged drug delivery to the posterior segment ocular tissues. For posterior segment delivery, disposition of NPs depends on the size and surface property. Following periocular administration into Sprague–Dawley rats, NPs in the range of 200–2000 nm were retained at the site of administration for at least 2 months. On the other hand, NPs with size 20 nm were cleared rapidly from periocular tissues (Amrite and Kompella 2005; Amrite et al. 2008). Therefore, it can be concluded that for transscleral drug delivery to the back of the eye, NPs with low clearance by blood and lymphatic circulations and slow drug release are suitable delivery carriers. Following intravitreal injection, NPs migrate through the retinal layers and tend to accumulate in the RPE cells. Following single intravitreal injection, the PLA NPs were retained in rat RPE tissues up to 4 months, suggesting great potential for achieving steady and continuous delivery to the back of the eye using NPs. In another study using PLGA NPs, authors concluded that NPs provide sustained delivery of dexamethasone for the treatment of posterior segment eye diseases (Pan et al. 2015). The surface property of nanoparticles is a key factor affecting their distribution from vitreous humor to retinal layers following intravitreal injection. Koo et al. found that polyethyleneimine/glycol chitosan NPs and human serum albumin/glycol chitosan NPs easily penetrated the vitreal barrier and reached at the inner limiting membrane but could not penetrate to the deeper retinal layers. On the other hand, negatively charged human serum albumin/hyaluronic acid NPs could penetrate the whole retina structures and reach the outer retinal layers such as the photoreceptor layer and RPE which was attributed to interaction between anionic surface and Müller cells (Koo et al. 2012). Therefore, the anionic NPs could be promising drug delivery carrier for the treatment of choroid and retinal disorders. Additionally, molecules such as folate and hyaluronic acid have been proposed as a targeting strategy. Specifically, folate-decorated NPs have shown increased uptake in retinal pigment epithelium cells in vitro (Suen et al. 2013). On the other side, the inclusion of hyaluronan into chitosan NPs was explored as a strategy to target the CD44 receptors expressed by epithelial corneal and conjunctival cells (Contreras-Ruiz et al. 2011). Few other reports highlighted the importance of polymeric NPs to deliver drug and genes to the retina more specifically to the RPE cells (de la Fuente et al. 2008; Khar et al. 2010). More recently, novel pentablock copolymeric NPs have been developed using biodegradable polyglycolic acid, polyethylene glycol, polylactic acid, and polycaprolactone polymers. Results indicated that pentablock polymeric NPs can serve a platform for sustained delivery of therapeutic proteins in the treatment of posterior segment diseases (Patel et al. 2014).

19.2.2.3 Dendrimers

Dendrimers are globular, nanostructured polymers (~1–100 nm), which have received significant attention as ocular drug delivery systems, due to their well-defined size, tailorable structure, and potentially favorable ocular biodistribution. Dendrimers have tree-like branched architecture formed by repetitive branched molecules surrounding a central core allowing them to act as efficient carriers for nucleic acids and water insoluble drugs. Because of their electrophoretic, dimensional length scaling and other biomimetic properties, similar to globular proteins, dendrimers display good ocular tolerance. The large number of surface functional groups on dendrimers can lead to multivalent interactions, with a potential for mucoadhesive properties that could lead to a reduction in tear washing and dilution and improved precorneal residence. The most commonly used dendrimers in ocular delivery are poly-(amidoamine) (PAMAM), polypropylenimines (PPI), and phosphorus dendrimers (Yavuz et al. 2013). Although the mechanisms of interaction of the dendrimers with the ocular mucosa have not been fully disclosed, it has been reported that anionic high-generation PAMAM dendrimers can act as permeability enhancers and they are mainly internalized by caveolin-mediated process, whereas neutral and cationic low-generation dendrimers promote higher permeability and are endocytosed by clathrin-mediated pathway (Perumal et al. 2008; Spataro et al. 2010; Durairaj et al. 2010; Kambhampati and Kannan 2013). Various research groups have shown enhanced bioavailability of pilocarpine (Vandamme and Brobeck 2005), tropicamide (Vandamme and Brobeck 2005), puerarin (Yao et al. 2010), brimonidine (Holden et al. 2012), and timolol maleate (Holden et al. 2012) after topical application of PAMAM dendrimer formulation. Phosphorus dendrimers are reported to be beneficial in the delivery of carteolol to aqueous humor (Spataro et al. 2010). Dendrimer glucosamine and dendrimer glucosamine 6-sulfate conjugates have shown to have synergistic immunomodulatory and antiangiogenic effect (Shaunak et al. 2004).

There are promising studies reported in the recent literature on the use of dendrimers for the delivery of drugs to the back of the eye. In vivo experiments demonstrated that following subconjunctival administration, carboplatin-loaded PAMAM dendrimer nanoparticles not only crossed the sclera but were also retained for an extended period of time in the tumor vasculature, providing a sustained treatment effect (Kang et al. 2009). In another study, hydroxyl-terminated fourth-generation PAMAM dendrimers have been reported for targeted delivery of fluocinolone acetonide for retinal neuroinflammation (Lezzi et al. 2012). Animal studies revealed selective localization and prolonged retention (~35 days) of PAMAM dendrimers within activated outer retinal microglia after intravitreal injection. Dendrimer-based approach was used for antivascular endothelial growth factor oligonucleotide (VEGF-ODN) delivery and successfully tested in a rat model to treat choroidal neovascularization (Marano et al. 2005). The results indicated that dendrimer/ODN-1 complexes significantly suppressed VEGF expression in cell level studies around 40–60 %. Examinations of injected rat eyes also showed that no significant toxicity and damage were caused by the complex injections (Marano et al. 2005). Porphyrin-based dendrimers have also been explored as photosensitizers for treatment of retinal tumors and degenerative disorders of the eye (Nishiyama et al. 2003, 2009). Targeting to retinal tumor is achieved via conjugation with Concanavalin A, mannose-specific ligand protein. Dendrimer porphyrin-encapsulated polymeric micelles and phthalocyanine core-based dendrimer photosensitizers were used for photodynamic therapy as well as drug delivery.

19.2.2.4 Micro-/Nanoemulsions

Microemulsions or nanoemulsions are dispersions of water and oil that require surfactant and cosurfactant to stabilize the interfacial area. These emulsified systems have nanosized globules (<1.0 μm) in the dispersed phase and are transparent and thermodynamically stable. Oil-in-water nanoemulsions were proposed for topical ocular delivery during early 1990s (Alany et al. 2006). The surfactants used to stabilize these systems have been found to play a critical role in their interaction with the ocular surface. For example, it has been observed that the use of cationic surfactants prolong the drug residence time on the ocular surface due to the electrostatic interactions with the corneal epithelia and, consequently, its bioavailability and therapeutic efficacy. On the other hand, the use of nonionic surfactants may lead to an opening of the tight junctions and also to an inhibition of the activity of the glycoprotein P (P-gp) on the epithelial cells; both effects result in an enhancement of the corneal transport of the drug (Jiao 2008). Apart from this, nanoemulsions can also interact with the lipid layer of the tear film, remaining in the conjunctival sac for longer times and consequently acting as a drug depot (Alany et al. 2006). Furthermore, the low surface tension of microemulsions also guarantees a good spreading effect on the cornea and mixing with the precorneal film constituents, thus possibly improving the contact between the drug and the corneal epithelium. Studies have also shown that some pilocarpine-based microemulsions delay the activity of the drug in such a way that twice daily instillations of these systems were equivalent to four instillations of conventional eye drops (Ince et al. 2015). Recently, emulsions with lipid additives such as phospholipid, lecithin, stearylamine, oleylamine, and medium-chain triglycerides were evaluated as carrier system for better ocular performance and bioavailability. Our group is also working on the preparation of cationic lipid-based emulsions for the delivery of drugs to posterior segment of the eye. More recently, Garg et al. has hypothesized the potential of cationic nanoemulsion for the delivery of tacrolimus for the management of uveitis (Garg et al. 2013).

19.2.2.5 Lipid Nanoparticles: SLN and NLC

Lipid NPs received considerable attention over the past few years among the most popular drug delivery systems for ophthalmic application. Solid lipid nanoparticles (SLN) and nanostructured lipid carriers (NLC), regarded as the first and second generation of lipid nanoparticles, respectively, have emerged as promising carriers for ocular delivery of various drug moieties due to their ability to prolong the residence time of dosage forms, reduce systemic absorption and administration frequency, and enhance bioavailability of drugs (Gan et al. 2013; Puglia et al. 2015). SLNs were developed in a manner analogous to o/w nanoemulsions, by replacing the oil phase of the nanoemulsion by a lipid that is solid at room temperature. As drug delivery devices, SLN show great promise for ocular administration, due to their better biocompatibility, modified drug release kinetics, avoidance of organic solvents during production process, and feasibility of large-scale production. As novel generation of nanoparticles, NLC consist of a mixture of biocompatible lipids (solid and liquid), surfactants, and drugs, resulting in a structure with more crystal imperfections favorable to accommodate drugs. NLC combine the advantages of SLN and overcome limitations, such as poor long-term stability, low drug loading capacity, and possibility of drug expulsion. Enhanced ocular bioavailability, prolonged release, increased precorneal retention, and enhanced corneal permeation of various ocular drugs have been reported after encapsulation of these drugs in either SLN or NLC (Gan et al. 2013; Puglia et al. 2015).

Many efforts have been made in modification of SLN and NLC to prolong the retention of drug on the corneal surface. New strategy reports the development of positively charged SLN since the slightly anionic characteristic of the ocular mucosa contributes to particle adhesion onto the ocular surface increasing drug residence time (Başaran et al. 2010). In another study, a thiolated nonionic surfactant, cysteine–polyethylene glycol–stearate (Cys–PEG–SA), was developed to modify the NLC (Shen et al. 2010). Such modified thiolated NLC has PEG moiety and free thiol group that facilitate the interpenetration and in situ cross-linking between the thiolated NLC and the mucus gel layer, which resulted in the enhanced mucoadhesion of thiolated NLC to the eye surface. After application into rabbit eyes, thiolated NLC demonstrated extended preocular residence time (up to 6 h), resulting in not only a higher precorneal concentration of cyclosporine than with the unmodified NLC ($P<0.05$) but also a higher level of cyclosporine in the anterior chamber (Shen et al. 2010). Electrostatic interactions between the negatively charged mucus and the cationic polymer can be exploited to provide an effective means of improving drug bioavailability. Chitosan oligosaccharide-coated NLC increased the transcorneal penetration to 2.4 times than that of uncoated NLC. Cytotoxicity studies of SLNs and NLCs performed in various cell lines showed that these systems are well tolerated and nonirritant to the eye tissues (Luo et al. 2011). The critical point to the cytotoxicity of the NLCs seems to be the nature of the surfactants used in the formulation, and therefore, the nonionic surfactants should be selected, as they cause lower toxicity to the eye tissues. Despite that the drug plays the most important role in therapy, the selection of suitable lipids, surfactant, appropriate size, narrow size distribution, and high encapsulation efficiency are of great importance, as they are crucial for the performance of the SLN and NLCs.

19.2.2.6 Cubosomes

Cubosomes are self-assembled nanostructured particles with bicontinuous aqueous and aliphatic domains formed with amphiphilic lipid molecules. The surfactant assembles to form a tightly packed structure resembling a honeycomb with an ability to accommodate hydrophilic, hydrophobic, and amphiphilic molecules. The microstructure of cubosomes is similar to that of biological membranes. This enables the lipid carriers to fuse with the lipid bilayers of the corneal epithelial cells. Once these lipid layers become integrated, cubosomes become a drug reservoir, releasing the drug through their unique bicontinuous cubic phase (Lakshmi et al. 2014). The basic building block of the bicontinuous cubic phase is the lipid bilayer, which is often based on glyceryl monostearate (GMS), Poloxamer 407, and Peceol. A dexamethasone (DEX) cubosome system was prepared by fragmenting a cubic crystalline phase of GMS and water in the presence of Poloxamer 407 (Gan et al. 2010). Preocular retention studies revealed that the retention of cubosomes was significantly longer than that of solution and carbopol gels. In vivo aqueous humor pharmacokinetics indicated a 1.8-fold increase in $AUC_0 \rightarrow_4$ h of DEX administered in cubosomes relative to that of DEX eye drops, showing about an eightfold increase over DEX suspension (Gan et al. 2010). Cubosomal formulation of flurbiprofen showed enhanced ocular bioavailability compared to eye drop formulation (Han et al. 2010). Based on their excellent colloidal stability, high internal surface area, sustained release properties, and low-irritant potential, cubosomes might be a promising system for effective ocular drug delivery.

19.2.2.7 Core–Shell Nanoassemblies

Core–shell nanoassemblies are nanostructures composed of a lipid shell and a defined core thus combining the advantages of lipid vesicles and colloidal cores. These nanoassemblies have excellent mechanical stability, high drug loading capacity, and sustained drug release behavior. Diebold et al. prepared core–shell structured liposome-chitosan nanoparticle complexes. These nanoassemblies were identified inside IOBA-NHC cells after 15 min and inside primary cultures of conjunctival epithelial cells after 30 min. It was proposed that the nanoassemblies might travel through the mucous layer of the tear film and deliver drug molecules to the corneal and conjunctival cells via the bionic action of the outer lipid membrane (Diebold et al. 2007).

19.2.2.8 Nanomicelles

Nanomicelles consist of amphiphilic molecules (surfactants or block copolymers) that self-assemble in aqueous media to form organized supramolecular structures. During micellization, the hydrophobic segments associate to form the core region, whereas the hydrophilic segments form hydrophilic shell of micelles. Micelles of various sizes (10–1000 nm) and shapes can be prepared depending on the molecular weights of the core and corona-forming blocks and can be tailored to have unique properties with respect to delivery requirements, such as to prolong the stability of micelles in eye fluid, to enhance residence time at cornea, and to modify the drug release profiles. Currently, tremendous interest is being shown toward development of nanomicellar formulation-based technology for ocular drug delivery. The reasons may be attributed to their small size, ease of preparation, high drug encapsulation capability, and hydrophilic nanomicellar corona-generating aqueous solution. In addition, nanomicellar formulation can enhance the ocular bioavailability of the encapsulated drug. Researchers have utilized both polymeric and surfactant-based nanomicellar approach for topical delivery of small molecules as well as genes to the anterior segment of the eye. For instance, nanomicellar formulation prepared from copolymers such as N-isopropylacrylamide, methoxy poly(ethylene glycol)-hexyl-substituted poly(lactides), Pluronic F127, and polyhydroxyethyl aspartamide and have been reported to improve ocular bioavailability of ketorolac (Gupta et al. 2000), cyclosporin A (Kuwano et al. 2002), pilocarpine (Pepić et al. 2004), and dexamethasone (Rafie et al. 2010), respectively. Recently, Pepic et al. have demonstrated the application of chitosan micellar system as a novel eye drop formulation. Addition of mucoadhesive chitosan to Pluronic F127 micelles resulted in enhanced intraocular dexamethasone absorption and nearly 2.4-fold increase in bioavailability, which was attributed to permeability enhancement property of both pluronic and chitosan (Pepić et al. 2010). Improved drug solubility in the nanomicelle core is long known, but their utilization to deliver drugs to posterior target tissue in the eye has recently been pursued and is still emerging. Highly hydrophobic drugs, such as voclosporin, rapamycin, and dexamethasone, could be efficiently delivered to retina and choroid after topical administration through mixed nanomicelles made up of vitamin E TPGS and octoxynol-40 (Velagaleti et al. 2010). Delivery to posterior segment through the aqueous pores of conjunctival/scleral (non-corneal) pathway has been postulated for extremely small-sized and hydrophilic nanomicelles. In addition, the hydrophilic corona prevents drug wash out into systemic circulation. Minimal/no drug accumulation in the nontarget ocular tissues and systemic circulation support this assumption. Further, after reaching the basolateral side, EPR effect is observed which helps in selective accumulation of micelles to the targeted tissues. Minimal/no drug accumulation in the nontarget ocular tissues and systemic circulation indicate avoidance of drug-induced side effects such as increased intraocular pressure or cataract formation (Cholkar et al. 2012). Proper selection of surfactant/polymers and formulation techniques can produce nanomicelles which could be utilized to deliver drugs, proteins, and nucleic acid to both anterior and posterior ocular tissues noninvasively in therapeutic levels. Emerging nanomicellar topical drop approach, in the near future, may replace the patient noncompliant route of drug administration to posterior ocular tissues such as intravitreal and periocular injections to the globe.

19.2.2.9 Inserts and Implants

Soft contact lenses, punctual plugs, cul-de-sac inserts (Ocusert, Lacrisert, Ocufit), and episcleral inserts (LX201) have been explored for sustained and prolonged drug release for anterior segment of the eye. However, for posterior delivery, intraocular implants are designed to be placed intravitreally by making incision through minor surgery at pars plana. Though implantation is an invasive procedure, these devices are gaining interest due to their associated advantages such as prolonged and targeted drug release. In addition, these devices help in circumventing complications associated with systemic dosages and multiple intraocular injections

(Bourges et al. 2006; Jain et al. 2012; Morrison and Khutoryanskiy 2014). Ocular implants are available as nonbiodegradable and biodegradable drug-releasing devices. Nonbiodegradable implants offer long-lasting release by achieving near zero-order release kinetics. Polymers such as ethylene vinyl acetate (EVA), polyvinyl alcohol (PVA), and polysulfone capillary fiber (PCF) are being employed for fabricating nonbiodegradable implants. Retisert® (Jaffe et al. 2005) and Vitrasert® (Dhillon et al. 1998) are the examples of marketed nonbiodegradable implants used for the treatment of chronic uveitis and AIDS-associated cytomegalovirus retinitis, respectively. Recently, biodegradable implants are gaining much attention because these implants are not required to be surgically removed which signify a distinctive advantage over the nonbiodegradable implants (Lee et al. 2010). Polylactic acid (PLA), polyglycolic acid (PGA), PLGA, and polycaprolactones are the most commonly used polymers for the fabrication of biodegradable implants (Bourges et al. 2006). Examples of biodegradable implants for ocular delivery include Surodex™ (Kodama et al. 2003) and Ozurdex® (Totan et al. 2015), which are designed for the sustained delivery of dexamethasone for the treatment of intraocular inflammation and macular edema, respectively. These implants, however, are associated with local complications such as scarring, pain, and infection at the incision site. A novel approach to overcome the disadvantages of presently used vitreous implant is the use of injectable particulate system. Icon Bioscience, Inc. (Sunnyvale, CA, USA) has developed Verisome™ drug delivery platform technology. The Verisome™ is a translucent liquid made up of benzyl benzoate, which forms gel when injected to ocular tissue resulting in sustained drug release (Noriyuki et al. 2011). Intravitreally injected PLGA microspheres (REETAC) have been found to be safe and well tolerated by the retina (Cardillo et al. 2006). Cortiject® (NOVA63035, Novagali Pharma S.A.) is an oily emulsion for sustained release of target tissue-activated, dexamethasone palmitate, following intravitreal injection (Noriyuki et al. 2011). Such phase-transition systems and particulate formulations offer advantages of implants without having complications associated with implants.

19.2.2.10 Hybrid Hydrogels

A diverse range of hybrid hydrogels have been developed with varying types of nanocarriers embedded in a bulk hydrogel framework. Five main approaches have been used: (1) hydrogel formation in a nanocarrier suspension, (2) physically embedding the nanocarrier into hydrogel matrix after gelation, (3) reactive nanocarrier formation within a preformed gel, and (4) cross-linking using nanocarrier to form hydrogels, and (5) gel formation using nanocarrier, polymers, and distinct gelator molecules. The approach chosen will be, in part, determined by the final application of hybrid hydrogel (Thoniyot et al. 2015). Recently, hyaluronic acid-based composite hydrogels incorporating liposomes have been evaluated as ocular carriers (Widjaja et al. 2014). In vitro release study shows longer sustained release of latanoprost from composite hydrogels as compared to liposomes or hydrogels alone indicating additional resistance to drug diffusion because of the incorporation of liposomes inside the hydrogels. These hybrid hydrogels, with controlled degradation properties and sustained release, could serve as potential drug delivery systems for many ocular diseases.

19.2.2.11 Nanoparticle Compact Films

NP-loaded contact lenses have been developed to provide longer residence time of the loaded drug in the tear film; however, these lenses suffer from disadvantages including loss of loaded drug, poor tolerance, and chances of ocular irritation and corneal ulceration (Fazly Bazzaz et al. 2014; Phan et al. 2014). A better and safer way would be to disperse the NPs in a thin film of a polymer like chitosan, gellan, or HPMC for placing in the lower cul-de-sac (El-Sousi et al. 2013). The film impregnated with NPs is prepared by dispersing NPs in the polymer solution which is then allowed to dry. Drug can also be added to polymer solution to provide the loading dose. The films, after placement in the cul-de-sac, will imbibe the tear, the process of biodegradation of NPs proceeds, and the NPs will slowly release their drug content into the surrounding tear film, thus providing a continuous release of the loaded drug over extended period. NP compacts can be designed to release one or more pharmacologically active agents over an extended period of time, such as for more than 1 week and up to 1 year or more.

19.2.2.12 Encapsulated Cell Technology

Encapsulated cell technology (ECT) is a cell-based device that can be used to deliver large-molecular-weight compounds to the eye. ECT developed by Neurotech Pharmaceuticals, Inc. (Lincoln, RI, USA) contains human RPE cells, genetically modified to secrete recombinant human ciliary neurotrophic factor, packaged in a hollow tube of semipermeable membrane that allows the outward diffusion of CNTF and the inward diffusion of nutrients necessary to support the cell survival (Kauper et al. 2012). The device is surgically implanted in the vitreous through a tiny scleral incision anchored through a titanium loop at one end of the device. The results of the phase I clinical trial for the use of this device for retinal pigmentation are successful, and the device was well tolerated for 6 months postimplantation. Clinical application of ECT in dry or wet ARMD is under investigation (Tao 2006).

19.2.2.13 Photonic Crystals

The optical properties of porous Si have been extensively investigated. Porous Si is a biocompatible and bioresorbable material that has also been investigated for in vivo drug delivery and biomedical application. Recently, Cheng et al. explored the potential of microparticulate porous Si photonic crystals capable of acting as a self-reporting ocular drug delivery system (Cheng et al. 2008). From the results, it was evident that hydrosilylated or oxidized porous Si particles have long vitreous lifetimes and can be safely injected into rabbit vitreous humor without any apparent toxicity. This suggests that it is plausible for porous Si particles to be used as a long-lasting intravitreal drug delivery vehicle. The drug can be housed in the porous matrix by either encapsulation or by covalent or electrostatic interactions, and the drug would be slowly released as the particles degrade (Anglin et al. 2004; Cheng et al. 2008). Furthermore, the optical spectrum of the photonic crystal could be utilized to monitor drug release through the transparent optical medium of the eye using a simple CCD spectrometer device that would allow noninvasive method to monitor drug release. Nevertheless, further studies to characterize the drug loading, intravitreal release profiles, and noninvasive remote monitoring of drug release are needed to determine the viability of the approach for effective patient treatment.

19.2.2.14 Transporter-Targeted Prodrugs

Recently, transporter-targeted prodrugs were developed following the identification of various influx and efflux transporters on ocular tissues (Barot et al. 2012; Cholkar et al. 2013). Transporter-targeted prodrugs have the potential of improving ocular absorption of poorly permeating parent drug. One of the example of such technology is the utilization of amino acid transporters (ATB(0,+)) on corneal surface, primarily responsible for uptake of neutral and cationic amino acids. Various amino acids such as aspartate, gamma glutamate, phenylalanine, and valine have been covalently coupled to the acyclovir (Katragadda et al. 2008) and ganciclovir (Patel et al. 2005) to form prodrugs that are recognized by ATB(0,+). Prodrugs are recognized by the membrane transporters as substrates resulting in their translocation across the epithelia and consequently significantly enhanced ocular bioavailability. Recently, glucose prodrugs (Dalpiaz et al. 2007) and lipid prodrugs (Vadlapudi et al. 2012; Cholkar et al. 2014) have been used to enhance delivery of drug to posterior segment. More recently, prodrugs have been encapsulated into nanocarriers to attain dual advantage of targeted delivery and sustained drug release resulting in significantly improved drug delivery (Jwala et al. 2011; Vadlapudi et al. 2014). Recently, our group is exploring the effect of various polymers, used in drug delivery, on transporters in the eye. This would facilitate development of transporter-targeted nanocarriers.

19.2.2.15 Drug Penetration Enhancement Devices

Microneedles

Microneedle-based technique is an emerging and minimally invasive mode of drug delivery to ocular tissues. Microneedle insertion into target tissues creates temporary micro pathways resulting in enhanced drug transport with minimum damage. They are custom designed to penetrate only hundreds of microns into the sclera, so that damage to deeper ocular tissues may be avoided. Injection into the suprachoroidal space using a microneedle offers a simple and minimally invasive way to target the delivery of drugs or carrier system to the choroid and retina (Jiang et al. 2007, 2011; Donnelly et al. 2010). In a study, Jiang et al. demonstrated that microneedles were able to infuse approximately 10–35 μL of fluid into tissues. Further, microparticles and nanoparticles were also delivered into the sclera by microneedles; however, the former were delivered only in the presence of collagenase spreading enzymes and hyaluronidase (Jiang et al. 2009). Nevertheless, the application of microneedles to ocular tissues such as the cornea or sclera is extremely challenging due to the round surface and lack of a supporting pressure that is required for insertion. To overcome this problem, recently, a microneedle pen system having a single microneedle with a spring-loaded microneedle applicator has been designed. The fabricated microneedle pen could deliver drugs to target sites in a more localized and minimally invasive manner than hypodermic needles could (Song et al. 2015).

Iontophoresis

Iontophoresis is a noninvasive technique, to deliver drug to the posterior segment of the eye, in which a small electric current is applied to enhance transscleral penetration of ionized drug (Myles et al. 2005). The sclera appears to be a cation-permselective membrane, supporting a net negative charge at physiological pH, supporting iontophoretic drug delivery. Significant transscleral delivery of timolol, dexamethasone phosphate, and vancomycin was achieved by iontophoresis (Gungor et al. 2010; Nicoli et al. 2009). The experimental results suggest that iontophoretic fluxes are proportional to the applied current, at least for the tested small anionic and cationic drugs. The results from the vancomycin experiments suggest that for the delivery of macromolecule, the driving concentration and the applied current need to be judiciously chosen. Another limitation of transscleral iontophoresis is the fast clearance of the drug from the eye to the systemic circulation such as through episcleral vessels and conjunctival lymphatic system, leading to the requirement of repeated iontophoresis administration. Recently, a micellar carrier system has been designed, which could be able to deliver by iontophoretic transport and provide sustained release of encapsulated drug (Chopra et al. 2012). Despite this, future studies are required to fully evaluate the safety of the nanocarriers for transscleral iontophoretic delivery.

Ultrasonication

The treatment of glaucoma and ultrasonic drug delivery are the two main areas of research and potential clinical applications of high-intensity focused ultrasound (Aptel and Lafon 2012). For the treatment of glaucoma, the specific advantage of ultrasound is that the energy can be focused through the sclera which is an optically opaque strongly light-scattering medium. Thus, ultrasound is a possible method for partial coagulation of the ciliary body, an anatomical structure responsible for the production of the liquid filling the eye, hence, reducing intraocular pressure. Locally applied ultrasound has also been proposed as a way to modulate transscleral barriers for delivering macromolecular therapeutics to posterior segment of the eye (Suen et al. 2013). Ultrasonication was found to be potentially safe and effective physical approach for drug delivery to the back of the eye. A study by Murugappan et al. showed that 50-ms ultrasonication can increase the transscleral penetration by two- to threefold without morphological changes on the sonicated sclera (Murugappan and Zhou 2014). Despite the fact that experimental studies seem to confirm the potential benefit of ultrasound ocular drug delivery, there is still a lack of clinical evidence.

19.2.3 Conclusion

Ophthalmology is currently emerging out with many exciting technologies for improving drug delivery for potential clinical application. However, as new pharmacotherapies continue to be developed for ocular disorders, innovative drug delivery systems will be required, with preference for noninvasive methods. The potential for the growth of drug delivery systems is limitless, and extended drug effect in ocular tissues by means of targeting transporters or receptors in the eye using ligands, advances in nanotechnology, and use of hybrid or combinational drug delivery systems will remain in the forefront of innovative and novel ophthalmic drug delivery systems.

References

Abdelbary G. Ocular ciprofloxacin hydrochloride mucoadhesive chitosan-coated liposomes. Pharm Dev Technol. 2011;16(1):44–56.

Agarwal R, Iezhitsa I, Agarwal P, Abdul Nasir NA, Razali N, Alyautdin R, Ismail NM. Liposomes in topical ophthalmic drug delivery: an update. Drug Deliv. 2014;12:1–17.

Alany RG, Rades T, Nicoll J, Tucker IG, Davies NM. W/O microemulsions for ocular delivery: evaluation of ocular irritation and precorneal retention. J Control Release. 2006;111:145–52.

Ameeduzzafar, Ali J, Bhatnagar A, Kumar N, Ali A. Chitosan nanoparticles amplify the ocular hypotensive effect of cateolol in rabbits. Int J Biol Macromol. 2014;65:479–91.

Amrite AC, Kompella UB. Size-dependent disposition of nanoparticles and microparticles following subconjunctival administration. J Pharm Pharmacol. 2005;57(12):1555–63.

Amrite AC, Edelhauser HF, Singh SR, Kompella UB. Effect of circulation on the disposition and ocular tissue distribution of 20 nm nanoparticles after periocular administration. Mol Vis. 2008;14:150–60.

Anand BS, Mitra AK. Mechanism of corneal permeation of L-valyl ester of acyclovir: targeting the oligopeptide transporter on the rabbit cornea. Pharm Res. 2002;19:1194–202.

Anglin EJ, Schwartz MP, Ng VP, Perelman LA, Sailor MJ. Engineering the chemistry and nanostructure of porous silicon Fabry-Pérot films for loading and release of a steroid. Langmuir. 2004;20(25):11264–9.

Aptel F, Lafon C. Therapeutic applications of ultrasound in ophthalmology. Int J Hyperthermia. 2012;28(4):405–18.

Atluri H, Anand BS, Patel J, Mitra AK. Mechanism of a model dipeptide transport across blood-ocular barriers following systemic administration. Exp Eye Res. 2004;78:815–22.

Barar J, Javadzadeh AR, Omidi Y. Ocular novel drug delivery: impacts of membranes and barriers. Expert Opin Drug Deliv. 2008;5:567–81.

Barot M, Bagui M, Gokulgandhi MR, Mitra AK. Prodrug strategies in ocular drug delivery. Med Chem. 2012;8(4):753–68.

Bartlett DW, Davis ME. Insights into the kinetics of siRNA-mediated gene silencing from live-cell and live-animal bioluminescent imaging. Nucleic Acids Res. 2006;34:322–33.

Başaran E, Demirel M, Sirmagül B, Yazan Y. Cyclosporine-A incorporated cationic solid lipid nanoparticles for ocular delivery. J Microencapsul. 2010;27(1):37–47.

Bourges JL, Bloquel C, Thomas A, Froussart F, Bochot A, Azan F, Gurny R, BenEzra D, Behar-Cohen F. Intraocular implants for extended drug delivery: therapeutic applications. Adv Drug Deliv Rev. 2006;58(11):1182–202.

Boussif O, Lezoualc'h F, Zanta MA, Mergny MD, Scherman D, et al. A versatile vector for gene and oligonucleotide transfer into cells in culture and in vivo: polyethylenimine. Proc Natl Acad Sci U S A. 1995;92:7297–301.

Cardillo JA, Souza-Filho AA, Oliveira AG. Intravitreal bioerudivel sustained-release triamcinolone microspheres system (RETAAC). Preliminary report of its potential usefulness for the treatment of diabetic macular edema. Arch Soc Esp Oftalmol. 2006;81:675–82.

Chang SC, Lee VH. Nasal and conjunctival contributions to the systemic absorption of topical timolol in the pigmented rabbit: implications in the design of strategies to maximize the ratio of ocular to systemic absorption. J Ocul Pharmacol. 1987;3:159–69.

Chaurasia SS, Lim RR, Lakshminarayanan R, Mohan RR. Nanomedicine approaches for corneal diseases. J Funct Biomater. 2015;6(2):277–98.

Cheng L, Anglin E, Cunin F, Kim D, Sailor MJ, Falkenstein I, Tammewar A, Freeman WR. Intravitreal properties of porous silicon photonic crystals a potential self-reporting intraocular drug-delivery vehicle. Br J Ophthalmol. 2008;92(5):705–11.

Chhonker YS, Prasad YD, Chandasana H, Vishvkarma A, Mitra K, Shukla PK, Bhatta RS. Amphotericin-B entrapped lecithin/chitosan nanoparticles for prolonged ocular application. Int J Biol Macromol. 2015;72:1451–8.

Cholkar K, Patel A, Vadlapudi AD, Mitra AK. Novel nanomicellar formulation approaches for anterior and posterior segment ocular drug delivery. Recent Pat Nanomed. 2012;2(2):82–95.

Cholkar K, Patel SP, Vadlapudi AD, Mitra AK. Novel strategies for anterior segment ocular drug delivery. J Ocul Pharmacol Ther. 2013;29(2):106–23.

Cholkar K, Trinh HM, Vadlapudi AD, Mitra AK. Synthesis and characterization of ganciclovir Long chain lipid prodrugs. Adv Ophthalmol Vis Syst. 2014;1(2):00007.

Chopra P, Hao J, Li SK. Sustained release micellar carrier systems for iontophoretic transport of dexamethasone across human sclera. J Control Release. 2012;160(1):96–104.

Contreras-Ruiz L, de la Fuente M, García-Vázquez C, Sáez V, Seijo B, Alonso MJ, Calonge M, Diebold Y. Ocular tolerance to a topical formulation of hyaluronic acid and chitosan-based nanoparticles. Cornea. 2010;29(5):550–8.

Contreras-Ruiz L, de la Fuente M, Párraga JE, López-García A, Fernández I, Seijo B, Sánchez A, Calonge M, Diebold Y. Intracellular trafficking of hyaluronic acid-chitosan oligomer-based nanoparticles in cultured human ocular surface cells. Mol Vis. 2011;17:279–90.

Cuevas P, Outeirino LA, Angulo J, Gimenez-Gallego G. Topical dobesilate eye drops for ophthalmic primary pterygium. BMJ Case Rep. 2012; pii: bcr1220115449.

Cunha-Vaz JG. The blood-retinal barriers. Doc Ophthalmol. 1976;41:287–327.

Cunha-Vaz J. The blood-ocular barriers. Surv Ophthalmol. 1979;23:279–96.

Daily MJ, Peyman GA, Fishman G. Intravitreal injection of methicillin for treatment of endophthalmitis. Am J Ophthalmol. 1973;76:343–50.

Dalpiaz A, Filosa R, de Caprariis P, Conte G, Bortolotti F, Biondi C, Scatturin A, Prasad PD, Pavan B. Molecular mechanism involved in the transport of a prodrug dopamine glycosyl conjugate. Int J Pharm. 2007;336(1):133–9.

DAMAD Study Group. Effect of aspirin alone and aspirin plus dipyridamole in early diabetic retinopathy: a multicenter randomized controlled clinical trial. Diabetes. 1989;38:491–8.

Dartt DA. Regulation of mucin and fluid secretion by conjunctival epithelial cells. Prog Retin Eye Res. 2002;21:555–76.

Davis BM, Normando EM, Guo L, Turner LA, Nizari S, O'Shea P, Moss SE, Somavarapu S, Cordeiro MF. Topical delivery of Avastin to the posterior segment of the eye in vivo using annexin A5-associated liposomes. Small. 2014;10(8):1575–84.

De Campos AM, Sánchez A, Gref R, Calvo P, Alonso MJ. The effect of a PEG versus a chitosan coating on the interaction of drug colloidal carriers with the ocular mucosa. Eur J Pharm Sci. 2003;20:73–81.

De la Fuente M, Seijo B, Alonso MJ. Novel hyaluronic acid-chitosan nanoparticles for ocular gene therapy. Invest Ophthalmol Vis Sci. 2008;49(5):2016–24.

Dhillon B, Kamal A, Leen C. Intravitreal sustained-release ganciclovir implantation to control cytomegalovirus retinitis in AIDS. Int J Std Aids. 1998;9(4):2227–30.

Diebold Y, Jarrín M, Sáez V, Carvalho EL, Orea M, Calonge M, Seijo B, Alonso MJ. Ocular drug delivery by liposome-chitosan nanoparticle complexes (LCS-NP). Biomaterials. 2007;28(8):1553–64.

Dong Y, Dong P, Huang D, Mei L, Xia Y, Wang Z, Pan X, Li G, Wu C. Fabrication and characterization of silk fibroin-coated liposomes for ocular drug delivery. Eur J Pharm Biopharm. 2015;91:82–90.

Donnelly RF, Raj Singh TR, Woolfson AD. Microneedle-based drug delivery systems: microfabrication, drug delivery, and safety. Drug Deliv. 2010;17(4):187–207.

Durairaj C, Kadam RS, Chandler JW, Hutcherson SL, Kompella UB. Nanosized dendritic polyguanidilyated translocators for enhanced solubility, permeability and delivery of gatifloxacin. Invest Ophthalmol Vis Sci. 2010;51(11):5804–16.

Duvvuri S, Majumdar S, Mitra AK. Role of metabolism in ocular drug delivery. Curr Drug Metab. 2004;5:507–15.

Early Treatment of Diabetic Retinopathy Research Group: effects of aspirin treatment on diabetic retinopathy. Ophthalmology. 1991;98(5 Suppl):757–65.

Eljarrat-Binstock E, Pe'er J, Domb AJ. New techniques for drug delivery to the posterior eye segment. Pharm Res. 2010;27:530–43.

El-Sousi S, Nácher A, Mura C, Catalán-Latorre A, Merino V, Merino-Sanjuán M, Díez-Sales O. Hydroxypropylmethylcellulose films for the ophthalmic delivery of diclofenac sodium. J Pharm Pharmacol. 2013;65(2):193–200.

Farquhar MG, Palade GE. Junctional complexes in various epithelia. J Cell Biol. 1963;17:375–412.

Fazly Bazzaz BS, Khameneh B, Jalili-Behabadi MM, Malaekeh-Nikouei B, Mohajeri SA. Preparation, characterization and antimicrobial study of a hydrogel (soft contact lens) material impregnated with silver nanoparticles. Cont Lens Anterior Eye. 2014;37(3):149–52.

Feghhi M, Farrahi F, Abbaspour M, Takhtaeian A. Effect of adding oral calcium dobesilate to laser photocoagulation on the macular thickness in patients with diabetic macular edema: a randomized clinical trial. Adv Pharm Bull. 2014;4:375–8.

Fire A, Xu S, Montgomery MK, Kostas SA, Driver SE, Mello CC. Potent and specific genetic interference by double-stranded RNA in Caenorhabditis elegans. Nature. 1998;391(6669):806–11.

Gan L, Han S, Shen J, Zhu J, Zhu C, Zhang X, Gan Y. Self-assembled liquid crystalline nanoparticles as a novel ophthalmic delivery system for dexamethasone: improving preocular retention and ocular bioavailability. Int J Pharm. 2010;396(1–2):179–87.

Gan L, Wang J, Jiang M, Bartlett H, Ouyang D, Eperjesi F, Liu J, Gan Y. Recent advances in topical ophthalmic drug delivery with lipid-based nanocarriers. Drug Discov Today. 2013;18(5–6):290–7.

Garg V, Jain GK, Nirmal J, Kohli K. Topical tacrolimus nanoemulsion, a promising therapeutic approach for uveitis. Med Hypotheses. 2013;81(5):901–4.

Garg V, Jain GK, Jayabalan N, Warsi MH, Ahmad FJ, Khar RK. Development of poly lactide-co-glycolide nanodispersions for enhanced ocular delivery of moxifloxacin. Sci Adv Mater. 2014;6(5):990–9.

Garrett Q, Xu S, Simmons PA, Vehige J, Flanagan JL, et al. Expression and localization of carnitine/organic cation transporter OCTN1 and OCTN2 in ocular epithelium. Invest Ophthalmol Vis Sci. 2008;49:4844–9.

Ghate D, Edelhauser HF. Ocular drug delivery. Expert Opin Drug Deliv. 2006;3:275–87.

Ghate D, Brooks W, McCarey BE, Edelhauser HF. Pharmacokinetics of intraocular drug delivery by periocular injections using ocular fluorophotometry. Invest Ophthalmol Vis Sci. 2007;48:2230–7.

Gungor S, Delgado-Charro MB, Ruiz-Perez B, Schubert W, Isom P, Moslemy P, Patane MA, Guy RH. Trans-scleral iontophoretic delivery of low molecular weight therapeutics. J Control Release. 2010;147:225–31.

Guo W, Lee RL. Receptor-targeted gene delivery via folate-conjugated polyethylenimine. AAPS PharmSci. 1999;1:E19.
Guo J, Fisher KA, Darcy R, Cryan JF, O'Driscoll C. Therapeutic targeting in the silent era: advances in non-viral siRNA delivery. Mol Biosyst. 2010;6:1143–61.
Gupta AK, Madan S, Majumdar DK, Maitra A. Ketorolac entrapped in polymeric micelles: preparation, characterisation and ocular anti-inflammatory studies. Int J Pharm. 2000;209:1–14.
Guzman-Aranguez A, Loma P, Pintor J. Small-interfering RNAs (siRNAs) as a promising tool for ocular therapy. Br J Pharmacol. 2013;170:730–47.
Hamalainen KM, Kananen K, Auriola S, Kontturi K, Urtti A. Characterization of paracellular and aqueous penetration routes in cornea, conjunctiva, and sclera. Invest Ophthalmol Vis Sci. 1997;38:627–34.
Han S, Shen JQ, Gan Y, Geng HM, Zhang XX, Zhu CL, Gan L. Novel vehicle based on cubosomes for ophthalmic delivery of flurbiprofen with low irritancy and high bioavailability. Acta Pharmacol Sin. 2010;31(8):990–8.
Haritoglou C, Gerss J, Sauerland C, Kampik A, Ulbig MW, et al. Effect of calcium dobesilate on occurrence of diabetic macular oedema (CALDIRET study): randomised, double-blind, placebo-controlled, multicentre trial. Lancet. 2009;373:1364–71.
Hathout RM, Mansour S, Mortada ND, Guinedi AS. Liposomes as an ocular delivery system for acetazolamide: in vitro and in vivo studies. AAPS PharmSciTech. 2007;8(1):1.
Hattori Y, Hashizume K, Nakajima K, Nishimura Y, Naka M, et al. The effect of long-term treatment with sulindac on the progression of diabetic retinopathy. Curr Med Res Opin. 2007;23:1913–7.
Hediger MA, Romero MF, Peng JB, Rolfs A, Takanaga H, et al. The ABCs of solute carriers: physiological, pathological and therapeutic implications of human membrane transport proteins Introduction. Pflugers Arch. 2004;447:465–8.
Hironaka K, Inokuchi Y, Tozuka Y, Shimazawa M, Hara H, Takeuchi H. Design and evaluation of a liposomal delivery system targeting the posterior segment of the eye. J Control Release. 2009;136(3):247–53.
Ho RH, Kim RB. Transporters and drug therapy: implications for drug disposition and disease. Clin Pharmacol Ther. 2005;78:260–77.
Holden CA, Tyagi P, Thakur A, et al. Polyamidoamine dendrimer hydrogel for enhanced delivery of antiglaucoma drugs. Nanomedicine. 2012;8(5):776–83.
Hornof M, Toropainen E, Urtti A. Cell culture models of the ocular barriers. Eur J Pharm Biopharm. 2005;60(2):207–25.
Hosoya K, Lee VH, Kim KJ. Roles of the conjunctiva in ocular drug delivery: a review of conjunctival transport mechanisms and their regulation. Eur J Pharm Biopharm. 2005;60:227–40.
Hosoya K, Makihara A, Tsujikawa Y, Yoneyama D, Mori S, et al. Roles of inner blood-retinal barrier organic anion transporter 3 in the vitreous/retina-to-blood efflux transport of p-aminohippuric acid, benzylpenicillin, and 6-mercaptopurine. J Pharmacol Exp Ther. 2009;329:87–93.
Huang HS, Schoenwald RD, Lach JL. Corneal penetration behavior of beta-blocking agents II: assessment of barrier contributions. J Pharm Sci. 1983;72:1272–9.
Huang AJ, Tseng SC, Kenyon KR. Paracellular permeability of corneal and conjunctival epithelia. Invest Ophthalmol Vis Sci. 1989;30:684–9.
Hughes PM, Olejnik O, Chang-Lin JE, Wilson CG. Topical and systemic drug delivery to the posterior segments. Adv Drug Deliv Rev. 2005;57:2010–32.
Ibrahim HK, El-Leithy IS, Makky AA. Mucoadhesive nanoparticles as carrier systems for prolonged ocular delivery of gatifloxacin/prednisolone bitherapy. Mol Pharm. 2010;7(2):576–85.
Ince I, Karasulu E, Ates H, Yavasoglu A, Kirilmaz L. A novel pilocarpine microemulsion as an ocular delivery system: in vitro and in vivo studies. J Clin Exp Ophthalmol. 2015;6:408.
International Transporter Consortium, Giacomini KM, Huang SM, Tweedie DJ, Benet LZ, et al. Membrane transporters in drug development. Nat Rev Drug Discov. 2010;9:215–36.
Jaffe GJ, McCallum RM, Branchaud B, Skalak C, Butuner Z, Ashton P. Long-term follow-up results of a pilot trial of a fluocinolone acetonide implant to treat posterior uveitis. Ophthalmology. 2005;112(7):1192–8.
Jain GK, Jain N, Pathan SA, Akhter S, Ahmad N, Jain N, Talegaonkar S. Mechanistic study of hydrolytic erosion and drug release behaviour of PLGA nanoparticles: influence of chitosan. Polym Degrad Stab. 2010a;95(12):2360–6.

Jain GK, Jain N, Pathan SA, Akhter S, Talegaonkar S, Chander P, Khar RK, Ahmad FJ. Ultra high-pressure liquid chromatographic assay of moxifloxacin in rabbit aqueous humor after topical instillation of moxifloxacin nanoparticles. J Pharm Biomed Anal. 2010b;52(1):110–3.
Jain GK, Pathan SA, Akhter S, Jayabalan N, Talegaonkar S, Khar RK, Ahmad FJ. Microscopic and spectroscopic evaluation of novel PLGA-chitosan Nanoplexes as an ocular delivery system. Colloids Surf B Biointerfaces. 2011;82(2):397–403.
Jain GK, Warsi MH, Nirmal J, Garg V, Pathan SA, Ahmad FJ, Khar RK. Therapeutic stratagems for vascular degenerative disorders of the posterior eye. Drug Discov Today. 2012;17(13–14):748–59.
Jay WM, Shockley RK. Toxicity and pharmacokinetics of cefepime (BMY-28142) following intravitreal injection in pigmented rabbit eyes. J Ocul Pharmacol. 1988;4:345–9.
Jiang J, Gill HS, Ghate D, McCarey BE, Patel SR, Edelhauser HF, Prausnitz MR. Coated microneedles for drug delivery to the eye. Invest Ophthalmol Vis Sci. 2007;48(9):4038–43.
Jiang J, Moore JS, Edelhauser HF, Prausnitz MR. Intrascleral drug delivery to the eye using hollow microneedles. Pharm Res. 2009;26(2):395–403.
Jiao J. Polyoxyethylated nonionic surfactants and their applications in topical ocular drug delivery. Adv Drug Deliv Rev. 2008;60:1663–73.
Juberías JR, Calonge M, Gómez S, López MI, Calvo P, Herreras JM, Alonso MJ. Efficacy of topical cyclosporine-loaded nanocapsules on keratoplasty rejection model in the rat. Curr Eye Res. 1998;17:39–46.
Jwala J, Boddu SHS, Shah S, Sirimulla S, Pal D, Ashim K. Ocular sustained release nanoparticles containing stereoisomeric dipeptide prodrugs of acyclovir. J Ocul Pharmacol Ther. 2011;27(2):163–72.
Kaiser PK, Symons RC, Shah SM, Quinlan EJ, Tabandeh H, et al. RNAi-based treatment for neovascular age-related macular degeneration by Sirna-027. Am J Ophthalmol. 2010;150:33–9 e32.
Kambhampati SP, Kannan RM. Dendrimer nanoparticles for ocular drug delivery. J Ocul Pharmacol Ther. 2013;29(2):151–65.
Kang SJ, Durairaj C, Kompella UB, O'Brien JM, Grossniklaus HE. Subconjunctival nanoparticle carboplatin in the treatment of murine retinoblastoma. Arc Ophthal. 2009;127(8):1043–7.
Kao HJ, Lin HR, Lo YL, Yu SP. Characterization of pilocarpine-loaded chitosan/carbopol nanoparticles. J Pharmacokinet Pharmacodyn. 2006;58:179–86.
Katragadda S, Jain R, Kwatra D, Hariharan S, Mitra AK. Pharmacokinetics of amino acid ester prodrugs of acyclovir after oral administration: interaction with the transporters on Caco-2 cells. Int J Pharm. 2008;362(1–2):93–101.
Kauper K, McGovern C, Sherman S, Heatherton P, Rapoza R, Stabila P, Dean B, Lee A, Borges S, Bouchard B, Tao W. Two-year intraocular delivery of ciliary neurotrophic factor by encapsulated cell technology implants in patients with chronic retinal degenerative diseases. Invest Ophthalmol Vis Sci. 2012;53(12):7484–91.
Kaur IP, Garg A, Singla AK, Aggarwal D. Vesicular systems in ocular drug delivery: an overview. Int J Pharm. 2004;269(1):1–14.
Ketting RF, Fischer SE, Bernstein E, Sijen T, Hannon GJ, et al. Dicer functions in RNA interference and in synthesis of small RNA involved in developmental timing in C. elegans. Genes Dev. 2001;15:2654–9.
Khar RK, Jain GK, Warsi MH, Mallick N, Akhter S, Pathan SA, Ahmad FJ. Nano-vectors for the ocular delivery of nucleic acid-based therapeutics. Indian J Pharm Sci. 2010;72:675–88.
Kim SH, Galban CJ, Lutz RJ, Dedrick RL, Csaky KG, et al. Assessment of subconjunctival and intrascleral drug delivery to the posterior segment using dynamic contrast-enhanced magnetic resonance imaging. Invest Ophthalmol Vis Sci. 2007;48:808–14.
Klyce SD, Crosson CE. Transport processes across the rabbit corneal epithelium: a review. Curr Eye Res. 1985;4:323–31.
Kodama M, Numaga J, Yoshida A, Kaburaki T, Oshika T, Fujino Y, Wu GS, Rao NA, Kawashima H. Effects of a new dexamethasone-delivery system (Surodex) on experimental intraocular inflammation models. Graefes Arch Clin Exp Ophthalmol. 2003;241(11):927–33.
Kola I, Landis J. Can the pharmaceutical industry reduce attrition rates? Nat Rev Drug Discov. 2004;3:711–5.
Kompella UB, Kadam RS, Lee VHL. Recent advances in ophthalmic drug delivery. Ther Deliv. 2010;1(3):435–56.

Koo H, Moon H, Han H, Na JH, Huh MS, Park JH, Woo SJ, Park KH, Kwon IC, Kim K, Kim H. The movement of self-assembled amphiphilic polymeric nanoparticles in the vitreous and retina after intravitreal injection. Biomaterials. 2012;33:3485–93.

Kuwano M, Ibuki H, Morikawa N, Ota A, Kawashima Y. Cyclosporine A formulation affects its ocular distribution in rabbits. Pharm Res. 2002;19:108–11.

Lajunen T, Hisazumi K, Kanazawa T, Okada H, Seta Y, Yliperttula M, Urtti A, Takashima Y. Topical drug delivery to retinal pigment epithelium with microfluidizer produced small liposomes. Eur J Pharm Sci. 2014;62:23–32.

Lakshmi NM, Yalavarthi PR, Vadlamudi HC, Thanniru J, Yaga G, KH. Cubosomes as targeted drug delivery systems – a biopharmaceutical approach. Curr Drug Discov Technol. 2014;11(3):181–8.

Law SL, Huang KJ, Chiang CH. Acyclovir-containing liposomes for potential ocular delivery. Corneal penetration and absorption. J Control Release. 2000;63(1–2):135–40.

Lee VHL. Mechanisms and facilitation of corneal drug penetration. J Controlled Release. 1990;11:79–90.

Lee RJ, Huang L. Folate-targeted, anionic liposome-entrapped polylysine-condensed DNA for tumor cell-specific gene transfer. J Biol Chem. 1996;271:8481–7.

Lee VH, Robinson JR. Mechanistic and quantitative evaluation of precorneal pilocarpine disposition in albino rabbits. J Pharm Sci. 1979;68:673–84.

Lee VH, Robinson JR. Topical ocular drug delivery: recent developments and future challenges. J Ocul Pharmacol. 1986;2:67–108.

Lee SS, Hughes P, Ross AD, Robinson MR. Biodegradable implants for sustained drug release in the eye. Pharm Res. 2010;27(10):2043–53.

Lezzi R, Guru BR, Glybina IV, Mishra MK, Kennedy A, Kannan RM. Dendrimer-based targeted intravitreal therapy for sustained attenuation of neuroinflammation in retinal degeneration. Biomaterials. 2012;33(3):979–88.

Li VH, Wood RW, Kreuter J, Harmia T, Robinson JR. Ocular drug delivery of progesterone using nanoparticles. J Microencapsul. 1986;3:213–8.

Li N, Zhuang C, Wang M, Sun X, Nie S, Pan W. Liposome coated with low molecular weight chitosan and its potential use in ocular drug delivery. Int J Pharm. 2009;379(1):131–8.

Li N, Zhuang CY, Wang M, Sui CG, Pan WS. Low molecular weight chitosan-coated liposomes for ocular drug delivery: in vitro and in vivo studies. Drug Deliv. 2012;19(1):28–35.

Luo Q, Zhao J, Zhang X, Pan W. Nanostructured lipid carrier (NLC) coated with Chitosan Oligosaccharides and its potential use in ocular drug delivery system. Int J Pharm. 2011;403(1–2):185–91.

Mannermaa E, Vellonen KS, Urtti A. Drug transport in corneal epithelium and blood-retina barrier: emerging role of transporters in ocular pharmacokinetics. Adv Drug Deliv Rev. 2006;58:1136–63.

Marano RJ, Toth I, Wimmer N, Brankov M, Rakoczy PE. Dendrimer delivery of an anti-VEGF oligonucleotide into the eye: a long-term study into inhibition of laser-induced CNV, distribution, uptake and toxicity. Gene Ther. 2005;12(21):1544–50.

Masuda I, Matsuo T, Yasuda T, Matsuo N. Gene transfer with liposomes to the intraocular tissues by different routes of administration. Invest Ophthalmol Vis Sci. 1996;37(9):1914–20.

Maurice DM, Mishima S. Ocular pharmacokinetics. In: Sears ML, editor. Pharmacology of the eye: handbook of experimental pharmacology. Berlin: Springer; 1984. p. 19–116.

Mehanna MM, Elmaradny HA, Samaha MW. Mucoadhesive liposomes as ocular delivery system: physical, microbiological, and in vivo assessment. Drug Dev Ind Pharm. 2010;36(1):108–18.

Mikkelson TJ, Chrai SS, Robinson JR. Altered bioavailability of drugs in the eye due to drug-protein interaction. J Pharm Sci. 1973;62:1648–53.

Moghassemi S, Hadjizadeh AJ. Nano-niosomes as nanoscale drug delivery systems: an illustrated review. Control Release. 2014;10(185):22–36. doi:10.1016/j.jconrel.2014.04.015.

Morrison PW, Khutoryanskiy VV. Advances in ophthalmic drug delivery. Ther Deliv. 2014;5(12):1297–315.

Motwani SK, Chopra S, Talegaonkar S, Kohli K, Ahmad FJ, Khar RK. Chitosan-sodium alginate nanoparticles as submicroscopic reservoirs for ocular delivery: formulation, optimisation and in vitro characterization. Eur J Pharm Biopharm. 2008;68:513–25.

Murugappan SK, Zhou Y. Transsclera drug delivery by pulsed High-Intensity Focused Ultrasound (HIFU): an ex vivo study. Curr Eye Res. 2014;7:1–9.
Myles ME, Neumann DM, Hill JM. Recent progress in ocular drug delivery for posterior segment disease: emphasis on transscleral iontophoresis. Adv Drug Deliv Rev. 2005;57:2063–79.
Nagarsenker MS, Londhe VY, Nadkarni GD. Preparation and evaluation of liposomal formulations of tropicamide for ocular delivery. Int J Pharm. 1999;190:63–71.
Nagarwal RC, Kant S, Singh PN, Maiti P, Pandit JK. Polymeric nanoparticulate system: a potential approach for ocular drug delivery. J Control Release. 2009;136(1):2–13.
Nicoli S, Ferrari G, Quarta M, Macaluso C, Santi P. In vitro transscleral iontophoresis of high molecular weight neutral compounds. Eur J Pharm Sci. 2009;36:486–92.
Nirmal J, Velpandian T, Singh SB, Biswas NR, Azad R, et al. Evaluation of the functional importance of organic cation transporters on the ocular disposition of its intravitreally injected substrate in rabbits. Curr Eye Res. 2012;37:1127–35.
Nirmal J, Singh SB, Biswas NR, Thavaraj V, Azad RV, et al. Potential pharmacokinetic role of organic cation transporters in modulating the transcorneal penetration of its substrates administered topically. Eye (Lond). 2013a;27:1196–203.
Nirmal J, Sirohiwal A, Singh SB, Biswas NR, Thavaraj V, et al. Role of organic cation transporters in the ocular disposition of its intravenously injected substrate in rabbits: implications for ocular drug therapy. Exp Eye Res. 2013b;116:27–35.
Nishiyama N, Stapert HR, Zhang GD, et al. Light-harvesting ionic dendrimer porphyrins as new photosensitizers for photodynamic therapy. Bioconj Chem. 2003;14(1):58–66.
Nishiyama N, Morimoto Y, Jang WD, Kataoka K. Design and development of dendrimer photosensitizer-incorporated polymeric micelles for enhanced photodynamic therapy. Adv Drug Del Rev. 2009;61(4):327–38.
Pan Q, Xu Q, Boylan NJ, Lamb NW, Emmert DG, Yang JC, Tang L, Heflin T, Alwadani S, Eberhart CG, Stark WJ, Hanes J. Corticosteroid-loaded biodegradable nanoparticles for prevention of corneal allograft rejection in rats. J Control Release. 2015;201:32–40.
Patel K, Trivedi S, Luo S, Zhu X, Pal D, Kern ER, Mitra AK. Synthesis, physicochemical properties and antiviral activities of ester prodrugs of ganciclovir. Int J Pharm. 2005;305:75–89.
Patel SR, Lin AS, Edelhauser HF, Prausnitz MR. Suprachoroidal drug delivery to the back of the eye using hollow microneedles. Pharm Res. 2011;28(1):166–76.
Patel A, Cholkar K, Agrahari V, Mitra AK. Ocular drug delivery systems: an overview. World J Pharmacol. 2013;2(2):47–64.
Patel SP, Vaishya R, Yang X, Pal D, Mitra AK. Novel thermosensitive pentablock copolymers for sustained delivery of proteins in the treatment of posterior segment diseases. Protein Pept Lett. 2014;21(11):1185–200.
Pepić I, Jalsenjak N, Jalsenjak I. Micellar solutions of triblock copolymer surfactants with pilocarpine. Int J Pharm. 2004;272:57–64.
Pepić I, Hafner A, Lovrić J, Pirkić B, Filipović-Grcić J. A nonionic surfactant/chitosan micelle system in an innovative eye drop formulation. J Pharm Sci. 2010;99(10):4317–25.
Perumal OP, Inapagolla R, Kannan S, Kannan RM. The effect of surface functionality on cellular trafficking of dendrimers. Biomaterials. 2008;29(24–25):3469–76.
Phan CM, Subbaraman L, Liu S, Gu F, Jones L. In vitro uptake and release of natamycin Dex-b-PLA nanoparticles from model contact lens materials. J Biomater Sci Polym Ed. 2014;25(1):18–31.
Pitkanen L, Ruponen M, Nieminen J, Urtti A. Vitreous is a barrier in nonviral gene transfer by cationic lipids and polymers. Pharm Res. 2003;20:576–83.
Puglia C, Offerta A, Carbone C, Bonina F, Pignatello R, Puglisi G. Lipid Nanocarriers (LNC) and their applications in ocular drug delivery. Curr Med Chem. 2015;22(13):1589–602.
Rafie F, Javadzadeh Y, Javadzadeh AR, Ghavidel LA, Jafari B, Moogooee M. In vivo evaluation of novel nanoparticles containing dexamethasone for ocular drug delivery on rabbit eye. Curr Eye Res. 2010;35:1081–9.
Ranta VP, Urtti A. Transscleral drug delivery to the posterior eye: prospects of pharmacokinetic modeling. Adv Drug Deliv Rev. 2006;58:1164–81.
Reimondez-Troitiño S, Csaba N, Alonso MJ, de la Fuente M. Nanotherapies for the treatment of ocular diseases. Eur J Pharm Biopharm. 2015. doi:10.1016/j.ejpb.2015.02.019.

Reischl D, Zimmer A. Drug delivery of siRNA therapeutics: potentials and limits of nanosystems. Nanomedicine. 2009;5:8–20.

Rizzolo LJ, Peng S, Luo Y, Xiao W. Integration of tight junctions and claudins with the barrier functions of the retinal pigment epithelium. Prog Retin Eye Res. 2011;30:296–323.

Sasaki H, Yamamura K, Mukai T, Nishida K, Nakamura J, et al. Enhancement of ocular drug penetration. Crit Rev Ther Drug Carrier Syst. 1999;16:85–146.

Schaeffer H, Krohn D. Liposomes in topical drug delivery. Invest Ophthalmol Vis Sci. 1982;22:220–7.

Schlessinger A, Khuri N, Giacomini KM, Sali A. Molecular modeling and ligand docking for solute carrier (SLC) transporters. Curr Top Med Chem. 2013;13:843–56.

Senthilkumari S, Velpandian T, Biswas NR, Bhatnagar A, Mittal G, et al. Evidencing the modulation of P-glycoprotein at blood-ocular barriers using gamma scintigraphy. Curr Eye Res. 2009;34:73–7.

Shaunak S, Thomas S, Gianasi E, et al. Polyvalent dendrimer glucosamine conjugates prevent scar tissue formation. Nat Biotech. 2004;22(8):977–84.

Shen J, Deng Y, Jin X, Ping Q, Su Z, Li L. Thiolated nanostructured lipid carriers as a potential ocular drug delivery system for cyclosporine A: improving in vivo ocular distribution. Int J Pharm. 2010;402(1–2):248–53.

Sieg JW, Robinson JR. Mechanistic studies on transcorneal permeation of pilocarpine. J Pharm Sci. 1976;65:1816–22.

Simon AM, Goodenough DA. Diverse functions of vertebrate gap junctions. Trends Cell Biol. 1998;8:477–83.

Song HB, Lee KJ, Seo IH, Lee JY, Lee SM, Kim JH, Kim JH, Ryu W. Impact insertion of transfer-molded microneedle for localized and minimally invasive ocular drug delivery. J Control Release. 2015;209:272–9.

Spataro GG, Malecaze F, Turrin C-O. Designing dendrimers for ocular drug delivery. Eur J Med Chem. 2010;45(1):326–34.

Stratford RE, Yang DC, Redell MA, Lee VHL. Effects of topically applied liposomes on disposition of epinephrine and inulin in the albino rabbit eye. Int J Pharm. 1983;13:263–72.

Suen WL, Chau Y. Specific uptake of folate-decorated triamcinolone-encapsulating nanoparticles by retinal pigment epithelium cells enhances and prolongs antiangiogenic activity. J Control Release. 2013;167(1):21–8.

Suen WL, Wong HS, Yu Y, Lau LC, Lo AC, Chau Y. Ultrasound-mediated transscleral delivery of macromolecules to the posterior segment of rabbit eye in vivo. Invest Ophthalmol Vis Sci. 2013;54(6):4358–65.

Tamai I, Tsuji A. Transporter-mediated permeation of drugs across the blood-brain barrier. J Pharm Sci. 2000;89:1371–88.

Tang J, Kern TS. Inflammation in diabetic retinopathy. Prog Retin Eye Res. 2011;30:343–58.

Tao W. Application of encapsulated cell technology for retinal degenerative diseases. Expert Opin Biol Ther. 2006;6(7):717–26.

Thakur A, Fitzpatrick S, Zaman A, Kugathasan K, Muirhead B, et al. Strategies for ocular siRNA delivery: potential and limitations of non-viral nanocarriers. J Biol Eng. 2012;6:7.

Thoniyot P, Tan MJ, Karim AA, Young DJ, Loh XJ. Nanoparticle–hydrogel composites: concept, design, and applications of these promising, multi-functional materials. Adv Sci. 2015;2(1–2):1–13.

Totan Y, Güler E, Gürağaç FB. Dexamethasone intravitreal implant for chronic diabetic macular edema resistant to intravitreal bevacizumab treatment. Curr Eye Res. 2015;22:1–7.

Ueda H, Horibe Y, Kim KJ, Lee VH. Functional characterization of organic cation drug transport in the pigmented rabbit conjunctiva. Invest Ophthalmol Vis Sci. 2000;41:870–6.

Urtti A. Challenges and obstacles of ocular pharmacokinetics and drug delivery. Adv Drug Deliv Rev. 2006;58:1131–5.

Urtti A, Salminen L. Minimizing systemic absorption of topically administered ophthalmic drugs. Surv Ophthalmol. 1993;37:435–56.

Urtti A, Pipkin JD, Rork GS, Sendo T, Finne U, et al. Controlled drug delivery devices for experimental ocular studies with timolol. 2. Ocular and systemic absorption in rabbits. Int J Pharm. 1990;61:241–9.

Vadlapatla RK, Vadlapudi AD, Pal D, Mitra AK. Role of membrane transporters and metabolizing enzymes in ocular drug delivery. Curr Drug Metab. 2014;15:680–93.
Vadlapudi AD, Vadlapatla RK, Kwatra D, Earla R, Samanta SK, Pal D, Mitra AK. Targeted lipid based drug conjugates: a novel strategy for drug delivery. Int J Pharm. 2012;434(1–2):315–24.
Vadlapudi AD, Cholkar K, Vadlapatla RK, Mitra AK. Aqueous nanomicellar formulation for topical delivery of biotinylated lipid prodrug of acyclovir: formulation development and ocular biocompatibility. J Ocul Pharmacol Ther. 2014;30(1):49–58.
Vandamme TF, Brobeck L. Poly(amidoamine) dendrimers as ophthalmic vehicles for ocular delivery of pilocarpine nitrate and tropicamide. J Control Release. 2005;102(1):23–38.
Vega E, Egea MA, Valls O, Espina M, García ML. Flurbiprofen loaded biodegradable nanoparticles for ophthalmic administration. J Pharm Sci. 2006;95:2393–405.
Velagaleti PR, Anglade E, Khan JI, Gilger BC, Mitra AK. Topical delivery of hydrophobic drugs using a novel mixed nanomicellar technology to treat diseases of the anterior & posterior segments of the eye. Drug Delivery Technol. 2010;10:42–7.
Velpandian T. Intraocular penetration of antimicrobial agents in ophthalmic infections and drug delivery strategies. Expert Opin Drug Deliv. 2009;6:255–70.
Velpandian T. Closed gateways–can neuroprotectants shield the retina in glaucoma? Drugs R D. 2010;10:93–6.
Velpandian T, Gupta SK, Gupta YK, Biswas NR, Agarwal HC. Ocular drug targeting by liposomes and their corneal interactions. J Microencapsul. 1999;16(2):243–50.
Warsi MH, Anwar M, Garg V, Jain GK, Talegaonkar S, Ahmad FJ, Khar RK. Dorzolamide-loaded PLGA/vitamin E TPGS nanoparticles for glaucoma therapy: pharmacoscintigraphy study and evaluation of extended ocular hypotensive effect in rabbits. Colloids Surf B Biointerfaces. 2014;1(122):423–31.
Widjaja LK, Bora M, Chan PN, Lipik V, Wong TT, Venkatraman SS. Hyaluronic acid-based nanocomposite hydrogels for ocular drug delivery applications. J Biomed Mater Res A. 2014;102(9):3056–65.
Yan W, Chen W, Huang L. Mechanism of adjuvant activity of cationic liposome: phosphorylation of a MAP kinase, ERK and induction of chemokines. Mol Immunol. 2007;44(15):3672–81.
Yao WJ, Sun KX, Mu HJ, et al. Preparation and characterization of puerarin dendrimer complexes as an ocular drug delivery system. Drug Dev Ind Pharm. 2010;36(9):1027–35.
Yavuz B, Pehlivan SB, Unlü N. Dendrimeric systems and their applications in ocular drug delivery. ScientificWorldJournal.2013;2013:1–13.ArticleID732340.http://dx.doi.org/10.1155/2013/732340.
Young B, Heath JW. Wheater's functional histology. Edinburgh: Churchill Livingstone; 2000.
Zhang N, Kannan R, Okamoto CT, Ryan SJ, Lee VH, et al. Characterization of brimonidine transport in retinal pigment epithelium. Invest Ophthalmol Vis Sci. 2006;47:287–94.
Zhang T, Xiang CD, Gale D, Carreiro S, Wu EY, et al. Drug transporter and cytochrome P450 mRNA expression in human ocular barriers: implications for ocular drug disposition. Drug Metab Dispos. 2008;36:1300–7.
Zhang X, Liu W, Wu S, Jin J, Li W, et al. Calcium dobesilate for diabetic retinopathy: a systematic review and meta-analysis. Sci China Life Sci. 2015;58:101–7.
Zuhorn IS, Kalicharan R, Hoekstra D. Lipoplex-mediated transfection of mammalian cells occurs through the cholesterol-dependent clathrin-mediated pathway of endocytosis. J Biol Chem. 2002;277:18021–8.

Chapter 20
Herbal Drugs for Ophthalmic Use

Thirumurthy Velpandian, Aruna Singh, and Rama Jayasundar

Abstract The traditional medicinal systems of various civilizations are well known to use herbal remedies for various ocular conditions. Plant derived compounds came to ocular use in the last century in which cocaine, physostigmine, pilocarpine and atropine are still holding a place in modern ophthalmology practice. The traditional knowledge available at different populations are of current interest among researchers throughout the world for finding new therapeutic modalities for ocular disorders like glaucoma, uveitis, cataract and neovascular conditions etc. This chapter documents the studies exhibiting the usefulness of such attempts to have a place in ocular therapeutics from the alternative systems of medicine.

20.1 Introduction

Herbal medicines have been accepted worldwide with a long recorded history. With an increase in burden of side effects of synthetic drugs and cost, herbal sources are now more focused upon. The ancient Chinese, Greek, Egyptian, and Indian medicinal systems have proved to be a reference for discovery of new therapeutics in various areas including ocular drugs. Century-old plant-derived compounds like pilocarpine, physostigmine, atropine, and cocaine are extensively used in ophthalmic investigations and still holding a value in modern ocular therapy. The understanding of ocular diseases is increasing every day and giving more and more space for therapeutic interventions (Velpandian & Mathur 2010).

T. Velpandian, BPharm, MS(Pharmacol), PhD (✉)
Ocular Pharmacology and Pharmacy, Dr. Rajendra Prasad Centre for Ophthalmic Sciences, All India Institute of Medical Sciences, New Delhi 110 029, India
e-mail: tvelpandian@hotmail.com

A. Singh, MPharm • R. Jayasundar, PhD
Department of NMR, All India Institute of Medical Sciences, New Delhi, India

T. Velpandian (ed.), *Pharmacology of Ocular Therapeutics*,
DOI 10.1007/978-3-319-25498-2_20

20.2 Natural Mucoadhesive Substances

Dry eye is a very common, multifactorial ocular disease especially in dry and hot areas of the world resulting in discomfort, visual disturbance, and tear film instability with potential damage to the ocular surface. Increased osmolarity of the tear film and inflammatory responses on the ocular surface can be regularly observed in dry eye. Ocular lubricants like hydroxypropylmethylcellulose (HPMC), methyl cellulose, polyvinylpyrrolidone, polyethylene glycol, propylene glycol, etc., are the first line of agents used along with or without anti-inflammatory or immunosuppressive drugs if the symptoms are severe and persistent. Methyl cellulose is a methylated derivative of naturally occurring cellulose. A polysaccharide derived from tamarind seeds has shown to be equally effective to HPMC, sodium hyaluronate, and sodium polyacrylate in the form of eyedrops in rabbit model as well as in clinical settings (Burgalassi et al. 1999; Rolando and Valente 2007). Synergistic interactions between hyaluronic acid (HA) and tamarind seed polysaccharide due to its mucoadhesive properties have been demonstrated by means of nuclear magnetic resonance spectroscopy and Ocular Surface Disease Index (OSDI) score in patients (Barabino et al. 2014; Uccello-Barretta et al. 2010). Another polysaccharide, galactomannan from natural gums is recently patented for use in one of the formulations for dry eye (Hong and Meadow 2009). Curcumin (diferuloylmethane) is the main curcuminoid of Indian spice turmeric (Curcuma longa). Several studies, documented the main role of polyphenols and curcumin for the prevention and treatment of many different inflammatory diseases and tumors. In the hyperosmoticity-induced in vitro dry eye model, curcumin has been reported to exhibit anti-inflammatory activity by inhibiting IL-1beta elevation via MAPK pathway in human corneal epithelial cells (Chen et al. 2010). Polyherbal Ayurvedic topical eye drops contain Curcuma longa extract as one of its component had showed anti-inflammatory properties in animal models (Velpandian et al 2013). These studies exhibit the rationale of combining curcuma longa extract in topical Ayurvedic eye drop formulations.

20.3 Antiglaucoma Agents

Glaucoma refers to a group of progressive optic neuropathies characterized by slow and progressive degeneration of retinal ganglion cells (RGCs) and their axons, resulting in reduced visual field sensitivity. With the ever increasing number of people affected by glaucoma, it becomes the major cause of irreversible blindness worldwide (Resnikoff et al. 2004). Increased intraocular pressure is the only proved treatable risk factor, with others like increased glutamate levels, alterations in nitric oxide (NO) metabolism, vascular alterations, and oxidative damage caused by reactive oxygen species are currently under investigation. Elevated IOP is believed to result from an increase in aqueous humor outflow resistance at the level of the trabecular meshwork (TM)/Schlemm's canal. Malfunction of the TM in POAG is associated with the expression of markers of inflammation, cellular senescence, oxidative damage, and decreased cellularity. Current pharmacological treatment of glaucoma lowers IOP by decreasing the rate of aqueous inflow and/or increasing the rate of aqueous outflow via any of the five major classes of drugs (administered as eyedrops) either individually or in combination with drugs from one or more classes. Glaucoma is a group of manifestations therefore, multiple targeting by stabilizing ocular blood flow, restoring the compromised antioxidative defense mechanisms and neuroprotection are the the need of the hour in addition to normalizing of IOP (Gupta et al. 2008). The interest in research of herbal drugs has paved the path for many new avenues of treatment that include agents improving blood flow, restoring antioxidant mechanisms, and halting further loss of neurons with an added advantage of low side effects (Ritch 2005; Kathleen Head 2001). Among the IOP-lowering herbals, the aqueous seed extract of *Foeniculum vulgare* (*mishreyaa* in Ayurveda) exhibited reduction of intraocular pressure (IOP) in normotensive rabbits at 0.3, 0.6, and 1.2 % (w/v) concentrations. The extract at the concentration of 0.6 % showed optimum effect in acute, chronic and steroid induced experimental models of glaucoma (Agarwal et al. 2008).

Lycium barbarum, known as Fructus Lycii or wolfberry, is reported in traditional Chinese medicine (TCM) for antiaging effects. Various studies have reported potential neuroprotective effects of *Lycium barbarum* polysaccharides (LBPs) and other small molecules such as betaine, cerebroside, beta-sitosterol, p-coumaric acid, and various vitamins on neurons in the CNS (Song et al. 1995; Ho et al. 2007, 2009). The bioactive component of LBP showed neuroprotective effects on retinal ganglion cells (RGCs) and blood-retinal barrier (BRB), evidenced by less loss of RGCs and prevention of IgG leakage. At molecular level, LBP has been reported to act by down regulating the expressions of RAGE, ET-1, AGE, Aβ in retina and arresting their signaling pathways leading to cause vascular damage and neuronal degeneration in the model of acute ocular hypertension (Mi et al. 2012).

Ginkgo biloba is another important herb mentioned in traditional Chinese medicine for several biological actions which combine to make it a potentially important agent in the treatment of glaucoma. Possessing properties like, improving central/peripheral blood flow, reduction of vasospasm, decrease in serum viscosity, anti-apoptotic, antioxidant, inhibition of platelet activating factor and excitotoxicity make this plant a suitable candidate for anti-glaucoma therapy. (Ritch 2000). Ginkgolide B, a terpenoid from *Gingko biloba* extract, promotes axonal growth of retinal ganglion cells by anti-apoptosis in vitro (Wang et al. 2012). Effect of topical *Ginkgo biloba* extract (GBE) was seen on steroid-induced changes in the trabecular meshwork and intraocular pressure. This study showed that GBE, a nontoxic, herbal compound, significantly suppressed steroid-induced IOP elevation in rabbits, and reported to prevent the adverse effects of dexamethasone on trabecular meshwork cells. Therefore, it could be a therapeutic agent or dietary supplement to prevent steroid-induced ocular hypertension (Jia et al. 2008). The extract is also reported to improve visual field damage in patients with normotensive glaucoma (Quaranta et al. 2014; Shim et al. 2012). Oral aqueous saffron extract seems to exert an ocular hypotensive effect in primary open-angle glaucoma along with its antioxidant properties and can be used as adjunct therapy (Jabbarpoor Bonyadi et al. 2014).

The triterpene forskolin from the plant *Coleus forskohlii* (*Parna Yavaani*) is one of the most useful herbs described in Ayurveda and stimulates the enzyme adenylate cyclase (Caprioli et al. 1984). Adenylate cyclase then stimulates the ciliary epithelium to produce cyclic adenosine monophosphate (cAMP), which in turn decreases IOP by decreasing aqueous humor inflow. A dose-dependent decrease in IOP of normal rabbits was found, when 1 % of solution was applied topically (Zeng et al. 1995; Li et al. 2000). The results are also reproduced on healthy volunteers in different clinical settings, although the efficacy in glaucoma patients is yet to be established (Meyer et al. 1987; Brubaker et al. 1987).

The active component of *Cannabis Sativa* (marijuana; *bhangaa* in Ayurveda), delta9-tetrahydrocannabinol (THC)–is reported to be responsible for numerous beneficial effects, including analgesia, appetite stimulation, and nausea reduction, in addition to its psychotropic effects. Interestingly, THC mimics the action of endogenous fatty acid derivatives, referred to as endocannabinoids, and an enzyme – fatty acid amidohydrolase – to metabolize the endoligands. The cannabinoid receptor system (CB1, CB2 receptors) is reported to have endoligands and, as antagonists, agonists in full or partial, and cannabinoids have diverse effects on the ocular fluid dynamics accounting for intraocular pressure (Scholten 2006) and neuroprotection (Yazulla 2008). Another possible mechanism proposed for antiglaucomatous action of cannabinoids is COX-2-dependent upregulation of tissue inhibitor of matrix metalloproteinase-1 (TIMP-1) conferring the antimigratory action. A decreased migration confers a reduced TM cell loss in glaucoma (Ramer and Hinz 2010). Topical semisynthetic derivative of THC, (WIN55212), has been reported to decrease the IOP in rats, monkeys, and human beings with a tolerable side-effect profile (Porcella et al. 2001; Chien et al. 2003; Fischer et al. 2013).

Epigallocatechin gallate (EGCG), a component of green tea, is reported to successfully prevent injury to the retina caused by ischemia/reperfusion (activation of caspases) in rats and white light-induced apoptosis in RGC-5 cell line as well (Zhang et al. 2008). *Salvia miltiorrhiza*, a commonly used herb in Chinese medicine is observed to improve microcirculation of the retinal ganglion cells in rabbits and protect the optic nerve from the damaging effects of increased IOP, with better results when used in conjunction with a medication to lower IOP (Zhu and Cai 1991). Romano et al. (1993) reported the neuroprotective properties of Hong Hua, an extract of safflower, in several experimental models of retinal ischemia.

Resveratrol is a phytoalexin produced naturally by several plants when under attack by pathogens such as bacteria or fungi. Resveratrol is found in the skin of red grapes and is a constituent of red wine. Long-term dietary resveratrol treatment has been reported to protect retinal ganglion cell (RGC) dendrite loss after optic nerve injury and altered the resolution of the unfolded protein response in mice model (Lindsey et al. 2015) . It has also been reported to significantly delay the RGC loss in the experimental model of glaucoma (Pirhan et al. 2015). Resveratrol treatment effectively prevented increased production of intracellular reactive oxygen species (iROS) and inflammatory markers (IL1alpha, IL6, IL8, and ELAM-1) and reduced expression of the senescence markers SA-beta-gal and lipofuscin and accumulation of carbonylated proteins. Furthermore, the anti-apoptotic effect of resveratrol is expected to have a potential a role in preventing the TM tissue abnormalities observed in POAG. Red wine polyphenols (e.g., resveratrol) have been shown to exert vasoprotective effects by inhibiting the synthesis of endothelin 1 and proved useful for glaucoma.

There are several other nutrients and botanicals that hold promise in improving circulation to the optic nerve, protecting retinal ganglion cells from oxidative stress, and even lowering IOP including vitamins B12 and C, melatonin, lipoic acid, curcumin, lutein, zeaxanthin, etc. Many of these studies have been performed on normal, healthy eyes. Further investigations into the mechanism of action, possible toxicity, and human clinical trials are warranted before these substances find a place in the arsenal of antiglaucoma drugs.

20.4 Anticataract Agents

Cataract is another most important leading cause of blindness in the world especially in developing countries of Africa and Asia. Extensive research showed that oxidative stress may play an important role in the initiation and progression of a cataract. Generation of reactive oxygen and nitrogen species in the eye tissue has been reported to be one of the most important risk factor for cataract and other age-related eye diseases. The oxidative hypothesis of cataract formation showed that ROS can damage lenticular proteins and fiber cell membranes. ROS can also perturb the homeostasis of the lens by disrupting the water and electrolyte balance and by causing DNA damage and proteolysis, thus leading to loss of lenticular transparency (Bhuyan and Bhuyan 1984; Spector 1995). Cataract is also one of the several complications of long-standing diabetes. Accumulation of advanced glycation end products (AGEs) from nonenzymatic glycation of proteins has been implicated in diabetic cataract (Sisková and Wilhelm 2000).

So far no single drug has been approved to prevent or to delay the progression of cataract. As of now only surgical removal of the lens and substituting it with artificial lenses is the viable option available with ophthalmologists. Therefore, a drug which could slow down the progression of cataract would be expected to reduce the backlog of cataract in developing countries.

There are reports of numerous plant extracts including *Momordica charantia*, *Eugenia jambolana*, *Tinospora cordifolia*, *T. foenum-graecum*, *Ocimum sanctum*, *P. marsupium*, *Murraya koenigii*, *Brassica juncea*, and *Mucuna pruriens* that are shown to have beneficial effect by mitigating diabetes-induced cataract, based on their hypoglycemic and antioxidant properties (Rathi et al. 2002).

Cineraria maritima is a medicinal herb whose aerial parts (leaves and stem) are used in homeopathic preparations for treating ophthalmic conditions such as corneal clouding, opacity, cataract, and conjunctivitis. The ethanolic extract of *C. maritima* exerts an anticataractogenic effect in in vitro and in vivo selenite-induced rat models (Anitha et al. 2011). These effects may be attributed to the plant's ability to reduce the formation of formazan crystals and scavenging ability of hydroxyl, superoxide, and nitric oxide. Alterations in the mRNA and protein expression levels of iNOS are also reported to be prevented in the selenite-challenged, *C. maritima* extract-treated rat lenses (Anitha et al. 2013).

Allium sativum (garlic) is a common cooking spice and has a long history as a folk remedy of several ailments including diabetes. It is known as rasona in Ayurveda and and used extensively for medicinal purpose. Data from animal studies indicating the hypoglycemic effect of garlic in diabetic animals and the preventive effects of garlic on diabetic complications such as cataract have been reported. Intraperitoneal injection of the garlic in rat model appeared to effectively prevent selenite-induced cataract. The action may be attributed to antioxidant, anti-inflammatory, and antiglycative properties of the plant that are also responsible for garlic's role in preventing diabetes progression (Liu et al. 2007; Javadzadeh et al. 2009).

Cinnamon is one of the commonly used spice and medicinal herb of India. It has been reported to have the potential to scavenge dicarbonyls. The fraction of cinnamon enriched in procyanidin B2 inhibited the formation of glycosylated hemoglobin in human blood under *ex vivo* conditions and also demonstrated a delay of diabetic cataract through inhibition of AGE in diabetic rats (Muthenna et al. 2013).

Rosemary (*Rosmarinus officinalis* Linn.) is a common household plant grown in many parts of the world, employed in traditional medicine for its healing properties. Rosemary is a rich source of active antioxidant constituents such as phenolic diterpenes, flavonoids, and phenolic acids. Caffeic acid and its derivative, rosmarinic acid, are the most important bioactive constituents of Rosemary (Nabavi et al. 2015). It increases the production of prostaglandin E2 and reduces the production of leukotriene B4 in human polymorphonuclear leukocytes and inhibits the complement system. It is concluded that rosemary and its constituents especially caffeic acid derivatives such as rosmarinic acid have a therapeutic potential in the treatment or prevention of cataract (al-Sereiti et al. 1999).

There are many other herbal drugs/phytochemicals possessing anticataract activity has been reported in the literature. Lutein, anthocyanins from the seed coat of black soybean, nobiletin and other abundant polymethoxyflavones (PMFs) from citrus peel, curcumin and aminoguanidine, ellagic acid, aqueous extract of *Trigonella foenum-graecum* (*methika* in Ayurveda), saffron (*kunkuma* in Ayurveda), *Ginkgo biloba* extract, *Ocimum sanctum* Linn. (*tulasi* in Ayurveda), and magnolol, from the Chinese herb *Magnolia officinalis*, have been documented to possess anticataract activity in experimental animal models. The protective effect was supported by one or more mechanisms such as restoration of the antioxidant defense system, inhibition of protein insolubilization and inhibition of lipid peroxidation in lens (Manayi et al. 2015; Mok et al. 2014; Miyata et al. 2013; Manikandan et al. 2009; Sakthivel et al. 2008; Gupta et al. 2005, Gupta et al. 2010b; Makri et al. 2013; Lu et al. 2014; Yao et al. 2009).

Gymnema sylvestre (*mesha shrngi* in Ayurveda), one of the constituent herbs of a polyherbal formulation, is reported to protect the lens against sugar-induced cataract by multiple mechanisms (Moghaddam et al. 2005). A polyherbal formulation in Ayurveda called "Chyawanprash" has been reported to decrease the progression of cataract in experimental models (Velpandian et al. 1998). Another polyherbal formulation – Diabecon – is reported to decrease protein carbonyls and prevented the loss of beta(L)-crystallin from rat lens; most of the beneficial effects are mainly due to *Gymnema sylvestre* (Moghaddam et al. 2005).

The role of nutritional supplementation in prevention of onset or progression of cataract is well documented. Those highlighted for possible inclusion are vitamins B and C; carotenoids beta-carotene, lutein, and zeaxanthin; and minerals selenium and zinc. Vitamins B and C have been linked with a reduced risk of cataract, and studies have provided evidence supporting their prevention. Selenium has been linked with a reduced risk of cataract and activates the antioxidant enzyme glutathione peroxidase, protecting cell membranes from oxidative damage whereas zinc acts as an essential component of antioxidant enzymes (Bartlett and Eperjesi 2004). Observational studies and clinical trials showed that with higher intake of phytochemicals such as lutein and zeaxanthein, a lower risk of cataract incidence observed in healthy post menopausal women (Rhone and Basu 2008).

Diabetic complications including neuropathy, nephropathy, cataract, and retinopathy are considerably caused by accumulation of sorbitol, which is produced from glucose by aldose reductase (AR) in polyol pathway. Studies reporting the AR inhibitory activity of aqueous extracts of ayurvedic medicinal plants such as *Withania somnifera*, *Curcuma longa*, *Azadirachta indica* and *Ocimum Sanctum* have been well documented. The extracts possessing a significant anticataract activity in vitro in high glucose environment could be related to their AR inhibitor effect (Halder et al. 2003).

Ellagic acid, 3,3′-di-*O*-methylellagic acid, 3,3′,4-tri-*O*-methylellagic acid, isovitexin, kaempferol 3-*O*-beta-D-glucuronide methyl ester, quercetin 3-*O*-alpha-L-arabinopyranosyl-(1-->6)-beta-D-galactopyranoside, ursolic acid, pomolic acid, tormentic acid, euscaphic acid, euscaphic acid 28-*O*-beta-D-glucopyranoside, and maslinic acid have been isolated from *Duchesnea chrysantha*. These isolated compounds have been subjected to in vitro bioassays to evaluate their inhibitory activity on rat lens aldose reductase and formation of advanced glycation end products (AGEs). It is now established that ellagic acids and associated flavonoids possess moderate inhibitory effects on rat lens AR. Compounds such as isovitexin, kaempferol 3-*O*-beta-D-glucuronide methyl ester, and quercetin 3-*O*-alpha-L-arabinopyranosyl-(1-->6)-beta-D-galactopyranoside have also shown excellent inhibitory activities toward the formation of AGEs (Kim et al. 2008).

Ethyl acetate extract of *Aegle marmelos* (*bilva* in Ayurveda) has pharmacologically active components with a potential to inhibit rat lens AR and consequential decrease in osmotic stress. It has also prevented the loss of antioxidants and contributed to the integrity of α-crystallin's chaperone activity and thereby delayed cataract formation (Sankeshi et al. 2013). Preliminary reports have also indicated a possible inhibitory effect of *Corydalis tuber*, *Buddlejae flos*, *Ganoderma applanatum*, isorhamnetin-3-*O*-beta-D-glucoside from *Salicornia herbacea*, and isoflavones such as tectorigenin, irigenin, and their glucosides from *Belamcanda chinensis* on rat lens AR enzyme system. Luteolin, luteolin-7-*O*-beta-d-glucopyranoside, apigenin, and acacetin-7-*O*-alpha-L-rhamnopyranosyl (6-1)-beta-D-glucopyranoside isolated from *Buddlejae flos* showed the AR inhibitory activity (Matsuda et al. 1995; Jung et al. 2002, 2005; Kubo et al. 1994).

20.5 Anti-angiogenic Compounds

One of the pathological characteristics of proliferative diabetic retinopathy is retinal neovascularization responsible for visual impairment in diabetic patients. The degree of retinopathy is closely associated with the duration of the diabetes. Two types of DR have been identified: (1) non-proliferative or background retinopathy, characterized by increased capillary permeability, edema, hemorrhages, microaneurysms, and exudates, and (2) proliferative retinopathy, characterized by neovascularization extending from the retina to the vitreous, scarring, fibrous tissue causing retinal detachment. Human clinical trials with anti-angiogenic modalities targeting VEGF/VEGFR-2 signaling have shown limited efficacy and occasional toxic side effects. Therefore, screening for potential molecules from herbal resources gained much of interest among several investigators around the world.

Ginkgo biloba has been found, to have potential for the treatment of diabetic retinopathy with improved retinal function as assessed by electroretinogram in experimental animal model. The effect was attributed majorly to ginkgo's antioxidant effects (Doly et al. 1986; Alekseev et al. 2013). Another report from a clinical study showed that oral administration of gingko for 3 months significantly reduced malondialdehyde levels of erythrocyte membranes, decreased fibrinogen levels, promoted erythrocyte deformability, and improved blood viscosity and viscoelasticity. This may facilitate blood perfusion, and may improve retinal capillary blood flow rate in type 2 diabetic patients with retinopathy (Huang et al. 2004).

Vaccinium myrtillus (bilberry) has been used for a wide array of ocular disorders, including diabetic retinopathy. Oral administration of this plant extract has yielded very promising results in preventing or delaying the onset of complications of diabetic retinopathy. Decreased markers of diabetic retinopathy, such as retinal vascular endothelial growth factor (VEGF) expression and degradation of zonula occludens-1, occludin, and claudin-5, were observed after the administration of this extract. The flavonoid (anthocyanoside) contents have been implicated with the connective tissue stabilization, decreased capillary fragility, and antioxidant effects resulted in the therapeutic benefit in DR (Kim et al. 2015). A reduced vascular permeability and incidence of hemorrhage were reported when standardized *Vaccinium* extract (containing 25 % anthocyanosides) was administered (80–160mg, TID) to 31 patients suffering from various retinal pathologies (Scharrer and Ober 1981).

Tetrandrine, isolated from *Stephania tetrandra* S. Moore (root), and related synthetic compounds have been investigated in both in vitro and in vivo experimental models. Tetrandrine and its related synthetic compounds, 6,7-dimethoxy-1-[[4-[4-(6,7-dimethoxy-2-methyl-1,2,3,4-tetrahydroiso quinolinyl)methyl]phenoxy]benzyl]-2-methyl-1,2,3,4-tetrahydroisoquinoline and KS-1-4, showed anti-choroidopathic and anti-retinopathic activity in the diabetic state (Kobayashi et al. 1999). The results for *Stephania tetrandra* S. Moore (root) extracts have been confirmed by other groups in in vitro models (Liang et al. 2002).

Magnolol, a natural product isolated from *Magnolia officinalis*, was evaluated on TGF-beta1 and fibronectin expression in human retinal pigment epithelial cells under diabetic conditions. This study reported that high glucose- or S100b (a specific receptor of advance glycation end products-ligand)-induced TGF-beta1 and fibronectin expression is inhibited by magnolol via the ERK/MAPK/Akt signaling pathway in human retinal pigment epithelial cells (Kim et al. 2007b). Another active compound, honokiol, isolated from Magnolia plants manifested potent anti-angiogenic effect on human retinal microvascular endothelial cells (Vavilala et al. 2014). A mixture of extracts obtained from *Pueraria lobata*, *Magnolia officinalis*, *Glycyrrhiza uralensis*, and *Euphorbia pekinensis* were also found to inhibit vascular endothelial growth factor (VEGF) expression in human retinal pigment epithelial (RPE) cells under diabetic conditions (Kim et al. 2007a). Anti-angiogenic effects of acetyl-11-keto-β-boswellic acid (AKBA), one of the active principles derived from the plant *Boswellia serrata*, employed in Ayurvedic system of medicine was investigated by Lulli et al. (2015) on mouse model. The compound is proposed to inhibit VEGF expression as well as act on VEGF receptor phosphorylation.

20.6 Plant-Derived Compounds for Uveitis

Uveitis is an inflammatory process of the uveal tract, which includes the iris, ciliary body, and choroid. Uveitis is often idiopathic, but it can be triggered by genetic, traumatic, or infectious mechanisms. Many plants have been documented in traditional medicinal systems for their anti-inflammatory properties. Curcumin is one of the foremost phytochemicals studied for its potent anti inflammatory activity. Application of aqueous extracts of *C. longa* or curcumin is reported to suppress vascular and cellular inflammatory responses as measured by low levels of inflammatory cells, proteins, and TNF-α levels in aqueous humor in animal models of uveitis (Gupta et al. 2008; Lal et al. 1999). Nagaki et al. (2001) evaluated the possible inhibitory effects of hot water extract of *Scutellariae radix* (containing baicalein, baicalin, and wogonin) on experimental elevation of aqueous flare in pigmented rabbits. This study reported that hot water extract of *Scutellariae radix* may have an inhibitory effect on experimental anterior uveitis induced by lipopolysaccharide (LPS) in pigmented rabbits. Berberine from *Berberis aristata* (*daaru haridra* in Ayurveda), plant sterol guggulsterone, polyphenols from *Lonicera caerulea* L. and *Aronia* extract, anthocyanins from *Vaccinium myrtillus* L., and *Gingko biloba* have exhibited potent anti-inflammatory activity against endotoxin-induced uveitis in vivo (Kalariya et al. 2010; Jin et al. 2006; Ohgami et al. 2005; Yao et al. 2010). Plant pigments such as, fucoxanthin, lutein, and *Lycium* have been reported to show protection against LPS-induced uveitis; however further investigations elucidating the working mechanism are anticipated. A clinical study evaluated the effect of *Tripterygium wilfordii* polyglycoside (TWP) on serum levels of IL-2 and tumor necrosis factor alpha (TNF-alpha) in patients of acute anterior uveitis. TWP has been reported to markedly suppress both parameters in patients and showed a possibility of using it for the treatment of acute anterior uveitis (Huang et al. 2002).

20.7 Ocular Side Effects of Herbal Drugs

Plants are the inexhaustible source for bioactive compounds, however, their therapeutics utility need to be rationalized based on their mechanism of action (Table 20.1). There are plethora of documents reporting the useful pharmacological activities of medicinal herbs and other botanicals; however, few attempts have been made to document the side effects of herbal therapy (Fraunfelder 2004; Ishtiaq et al. 2007). Recently, reports revealing the ocular side effects of herbal medicines and nutritional supplements have come into fore. The problem is further compounded by usage of herbal medications by patients without the knowledge of the treating physician. Current data does not support the use of antioxidants or herbal medications in the prevention or treatment of cataract, glaucoma, or diabetic retinopathy (Wilkinson and Fraunfelder 2011). Usage of canthaxanthin, chamomile, *datura, Echinacea purpurea*, *Ginkgo biloba*, licorice, niacin, and vitamin A are reported to be associated with clinically significant ocular side effects and is advocated to be used with caution. Consequently, plant-based drugs are now under scrutiny so as to enable a judicious selection of plants for ocular diseases (Fraunfelder 2005). A rational utilization of herbal constituents would be highly beneficial, whereas "herbal drugs are lacking side effects" stands unenforceable.

Table 20.1 Medicinal plants reported to be effective in various ocular conditions

S. no.	Ocular condition	Herbs reported to have beneficial effect
1	Dry eye	Natural polymer (gum) from tamarind seed, curcumin
2.	Glaucoma	*Foeniculum vulgare*, *Lycium barbarum*, *Gingko biloba*, *Coleus forskohlii*, *Cannabis sativa*, lutein, zeaxanthin, green tea, resveratrol, curcumin, safflower
3.	Cataract	*Cineraria maritime*, *Momordica charantia*, *Eugenia jambolana*, *Tinospora cordifolia*, *T. foenum-graecum*, *Ocimum sanctum*, *P. marsupium*, *Murraya koenigii*, *Brassica juncea*, *Mucuna pruriens*, *Coleus forskohlii*, *Rosmarinus officinalis*, *Allium sativum*, *Ocimum sanctum*, *Gymnema sylvestre*, *Buddlejae flos*, cinnamon, lutein, nobiletin, *Withania somnifera*, *Aegle marmelos*, *Duchesnea chrysantha*
4.	Anti-angiogenic	*Gingko biloba*, *Vaccinium myrtillus*, *Stephania tetrandra*, *Magnolia officinalis*, *Dendrobium chrysotoxum*, *Boswellia serrata*
5.	Uveitis	Curcumin, *Scutellariae radix*, *Tripterygium wilfordii*, *Vaccinium myrtillus*, *Berberis aristata*, *Lonicera caerulea*, fucoxanthin, lutein, *Lycium*

20.8 Polyherbal Formulations and Methods from Alternative Systems of Medicine for Ocular Therapeutics

Complementary and alternative medicine (CAM) embrace tremendous therapeutic potential, attracting more research groups and governing authorities to conduct critical analysis of the formulations and variety of approaches (acupuncture, homeopathy, massage, reflexology, Reiki healing, etc.) which are differing markedly from conventional modern biomedicine. Unlike the research in modern medicine where the specific efficacy of active component of formulation or therapy is taken as parameter to determine the effectiveness often discounting synergistic effects. CAM treatments are to be evaluated as a whole, rather than splitting up into parts and investigating separately (Fønnebø et al. 2007). A number of clinical trials are now being conducted with traditional medicine therapies in ocular disorders. Sharma et al. (1992) reported rapid absorption of retinal hemorrhages in 24 patients suffering from diabetes and hypertension when treated with indigenous ayurvedic formulation and *Saptamrita Lauha*. The beneficial effect was attributed to the flavonoid-like properties of one of the ingredients of this natural product (Sharma et al. 1992). Clinical trials have successfully proved the usefulness of Ayurvedic treatment and herbal formulations in different eye allergies such as conjunctivitis (Das et al. 1995; Dhiman et al. 2010; Bhardwaj and Tanwar 2011). The percentage level of efficacy of *Triyushnadi Anjana*, mentioned in literature of the *Shalakya Netra Roga Chikitsa* for inflammatory conditions of eyes, was found to be better than sodium cromoglycate 2 % eyedrops. Another clinical study evaluated the comparative efficacy of ayurvedic *Bilvadi Yoga* (a formulation for conjunctivitis) as *Ashchyotana* (eyedrops prepared by traditional method) and eyedrops. *Ashchyotana* formulation is a time-consuming procedure, but it is more effective than the eyedrops depicting the importance of method of administration of Ayurvedic formulations in governing its efficacy (Udani et al. 2012). Unani medicine also mentions treatment for conjunctivitis and other inflammatory conditions. Qatoor Ramad (QR) is an ophthalmic formulation of Unani medicine reputed for its beneficial effects in the inflammatory conditions of the eyes as evident from a comparative double-blind randomized placebo-controlled clinical trial conducted in 70 patients suffering from different types of conjunctivitis, as reported by Siddiqui et al. (2002). Ayurvedic proprietary formulations such as Ophthacare and Itone eyedrops have been reported to be beneficial for various ocular conditions like dry eye, inflammatory, and angiogenesis (Biswas et al. 2001; Velpandian et al. 2013). Clinical study of ayurvedic formulations *Shatavaryaadi Churna* (orally) and *Go-Ghrita Netra Tarpana* (topically), when evaluated in 30 patients of computer vision syndrome, led to a significant improvement in the ocular symptoms such as blurred vision, headache, redness, dry eye, and slow refocusing (Dhiman et al. 2012).

Refractive errors of eyes can be correlated with *Timira* mentioned in Ayurvedic literature. Several clinical trials have been conducted with formulations and other non-pharmacological methods used in Ayurveda for treatment of refractive disorders specially myopia (Gupta et al. 2010a, b; Poonam 2011; Gopinathan et al. 2012). The clinical studies have shown effectiveness in reduction of the dioptric power and improvement in visual acuity of patients. Although there is a mention of the mechanism of action of therapy, the correlation of this mechanism with the modern medicine remains poorly explained. Also there is a need to conduct these studies on a larger scale, with longer duration, to scientifically validate the effectiveness.

Hu et al. (2014) reported a clinical study of traditional Chinese medicine compound Sheng-Jin-Run-Zao-Yang-Xue granules on 240 patients of primary Sjögren's syndrome, exhibiting advantages over Western medicine in terms of fewer side effects and improved patient conditions including dry eyes. Chang et al. submitted a scientific report on clinical evaluation of Chi-Ju-Di-Huang-Wan, a Chinese herbal medicine, as an alternative for dry eye treatment. The herb is an effective stabilizer of tear film and decreases the abnormality of corneal epithelium (Chang and So 2008). Others have reported a composite herbal recipe known as Huoxue-Huayu, used in traditional Chinese medicine for invigoration of blood circulation and reduction of blood stasis, for patients with retinal vein occlusion (Deng et al. 1995; Peng et al. 2009). Diabetic retinopathy is one of the major complications of advanced diabetes. Qiming granules, a traditional patent medicine, has gained wide clinical application in China and has been widely used in clinical settings for alleviating symptoms of diabetic retinopathy (Luo et al. 2009). The main active constituents of the formulation include astragalosides, astragalus polysaccharides, puerarin, and catalpol from *Radix* species. This formulation improved blood rheology, enhanced insulin receptor sensitivity, inhibited protein glycosylation, regulated lipid metabolism and reduced blood sugar levels. There are other formulations in Chinese herbal medicine which are reported to improve retinal cone activity of patients of retinitis pigmentosa, even in those with advanced retinal degeneration as confirmed by flicker response of electroretinogram (Wu and Tang 1996).

Traditional Japanese herbal (Kampo) formulas are approved as ethical drugs and are in clinical practice for many years. Numerous investigators have reported

Japanese herbal medicines as efficacious treatment for several human diseases. Oral Orengedoku-to and Kakkon-to are shown to inhibit postoperative uveitis symptoms (aqueous flare) in humans. Oral Gosha-jinki-gan improved ocular surface disorders in patients with type 1 diabetes mellitus, while oral Hachimi-jio-gan increased retinal blood flow. Topical glycyrrhizinate improved allergic conjunctivitis in humans, and oral crocetin is reported to improve eyestrain in humans (Hayasaka et al. 2012).

The research and clinical trials in traditional medicinal systems followed pharmacological research methods used for modern medicine until now. But now it is well understood by researchers that research strategies and methodologies employed and developed by clinical pharmacologists to evaluate efficacy and eventual effectiveness of a drug yield a "gap" between the results of randomized controlled trials showing little or no effect and the widespread use and reports of beneficial outcomes of traditional medicinal systems (Launsø and Gannik 2000). Researchers and government authorities have initiated harmonizing and quality improvement of clinical research in traditional medicinal systems. The Consolidated Standards of Reporting Trials (CONSORT) offers a minimum set of recommendations and guidelines for reporting randomized clinical trials on herbal products (Altman et al. 2001; Gagnier et al. 2006). Specifically concerned with clinical trials of Ayurvedic interventions, a standard framework for developing clinical ethnic protocols and subsequent reporting was formulated by Narahari et al. (2008).

20.9 Conclusion

Natural products are the most consistently successful source of drug leads. Despite the fact, their use in drug discovery has fallen out of favor. Less than 10 % of the world's biodiversity has been tested for biological activity, whereas many more useful natural lead compounds are awaiting discovery. The challenge is how to access this natural chemical diversity and use them as reservoir for finding new chemical entities for several ocular disorders. In modern science, the technique for the isolation, analysis, and identification of plant-derived new chemical entities has been renovated to make them simple, fast, cost effective, and efficient. All these advances have enabled to develop data libraries and chemical libraries from various classes of phytochemicals such as nucleosides, anthocyanosides, flavonoids, polyketides, and taxanes. These libraries can now be screened efficiently against an increasing number of ever more challenging molecular assay targets, leading to generation of more appropriate lead compounds. The chemical diversity derived from natural products will be increasingly relevant to the future of drug discovery including novel ocular therapeutics. Apart from allopathic medicine and isolated compound of herbal origin, alternative and complimentary systems of medicines offer ethnic and time-tested formulations and methods for ocular therapeutics. A systematic evaluation and inclusion of such systems would be of help in conditions where definite therapeutic strategies are so far not achieved.

References

Agarwal R, Gupta SK, Agrawal SS, Srivastava S, Saxena R. Oculohypotensive effects of foeniculum vulgare in experimental models of glaucoma. Indian J Physiol Pharmacol. 2008;52(1):77–83.

Alekseev IB, Kochergin SA, Vorob'eva IV, Mikhaleva LG. On some pathogenic features of diabetic retinopathy in type II diabetes mellitus and the role of antioxidants and Ginkgo biloba. Vestn Oftalmol. 2013;129(3):89–93.

al-Sereiti MR, Abu-Amer KM, Sen P. Pharmacology of rosemary (Rosmarinus officinalis Linn.) and its therapeutic potentials. Indian Exp J Biol. 1999;37(2):124–30.

Altman DG, Schulz KF, Moher D, Egger M, Davidoff F, Elbourne D, Gøtzsche PC, Lang T, CONSORT Group (Consolidated Standards of Reporting Trials). The revised CONSORT statement for reporting randomized trials: explanation and elaboration. Ann Intern Med. 2001; 134(8):663–94.

Anitha TS, Annadurai T, Thomas PA, Geraldine P. Prevention of selenite-induced cataractogenesis by an ethanolic extract of Cineraria maritima: an experimental evaluation of the traditional eye medication. Biol Trace Elem Res. 2011;143(1):425–36.

Anitha TS, Muralidharan AR, Annadurai T, Christdas Jesudasan AN, Thomas PA, Geraldine P. Putative free radical-scavenging activity of an extract of Cineraria maritima in preventing selenite-induced cataractogenesis in Wistar rat pups. Mol Vis. 2013;19:2551–60.

Barabino S, Rolando M, Nardi M, Bonini S, Aragona P, Traverso CE. The effect of an artificial tear combining hyaluronic acid and tamarind seeds polysaccharide in patients with moderate dry eye syndrome: a new treatment for dry eye. Eur J Ophthalmol. 2014;24(2):173–8.

Bartlett H, Eperjesi F. An ideal ocular nutritional supplement? Ophthalmic Physiol Opt. 2004; 24(4):339–49.

Bhardwaj A, Tanwar M. Effect of rasanjana madhu ashchyotana in netra abhishyanda (mucopurulent conjunctivitis). Ayu. 2011;32(3):365–9.

Bhuyan KC, Bhuyan DK. Molecular mechanism of cataractogenesis: III. Toxic metabolites of oxygen as initiators of lipid peroxidation and cataract. Curr Eye Res. 1984;3(1):67–81.

Biswas NR, Gupta SK, Das GK, Kumar N, Mongre PK, Haldar D, Beri S. Evaluation of Ophthacare eye drops – a herbal formulation in the management of various ophthalmic disorders. Phytother Res. 2001;15(7):618–20.

Brubaker RF, Carlson KH, Kullerstrand LJ, McLaren JW. Topical forskolin (colforsin) and aqueous flow in humans. Arch Ophthalmol. 1987;105(5):637–41.

Burgalassi S, Panichi L, Chetoni P, Saettone MF, Boldrini E. Development of a simple dry eye model in the albino rabbit and evaluation of some tear substitutes. Ophthalmic Res. 1999;31(3):229–35.

Caprioli J, Sears M, Bausher L, et al. Forskolin lowers intraocular pressure by reducing aqueous inflow. Invest Ophthalmol Vis Sci. 1984;25(3):268–77.

Chang RC, So KF. Use of anti-aging herbal medicine, Lycium barbarum, against aging-associated diseases. What do we know so far? Cell Mol Neurobiol. 2008;28(5):643–52.

Chen M, Hu DN, Pan Z, Lu CW, Xue CY, Aass I. Curcumin protects against hyperosmoticity-induced IL-1beta elevation in human corneal epithelial cell via MAPK pathways. Exp Eye Res. 2010;90(3):437–43.

Chien FY, Wang RF, Mittag TW, Podos SM. Effect of WIN 55212–2, a cannabinoid receptor agonist, on aqueous humor dynamics in monkeys. Arch Ophthalmol. 2003;121(1):87–90.

Das GK, Pandey RM, Biswas NR. Comparative double masked randomised placebo controlled clinical trial of a herbal eye drop preparation in trachoma and conjunctivitis. J Indian Med Assoc. 1995;93(10): 383–4.

Deng Y, Wang M, Duan J. The modality of huoxue-huayu in treatment of retinal vein occlusion. Yan Ke Xue Bao. 1995;11(1):57–60.

Dhiman KS, Sharma G, Singh S. A clinical study to assess the efficacy of Triyushnadi Anjana in Kaphaja Abhishyanda with special reference to vernal keratoconjunctivitis. Ayu. 2010; 31(4):466–72.

Dhiman KS, Ahuja DK, Sharma SK. Clinical efficacy of Ayurvedic management in computer vision syndrome: a pilot study. Ayu. 2012;33(3):391–5.

Doly M, Droy-Lefaix MT, Bonhomme B, Braquet P. Effect of Ginkgo biloba extract on the electrophysiology of the isolated retina from a diabetic rat. Presse Med. 1986;15(31): 1480–3.

Fischer KM, Ward DA, Hendrix DV. Effects of a topically applied 2% delta-9-tetrahydrocannabinol ophthalmic solution on intraocular pressure and aqueous humor flow rate in clinically normal dogs. Am J Vet Res. 2013;74(2):275–80.

Fønnebø V, Grimsgaard S, Walach H, Ritenbaugh C, Norheim AJ, MacPherson H, Lewith G, Launsø L, Koithan M, Falkenberg T, Boon H, Aickin M. Researching complementary and alternative treatments – the gatekeepers are not at home. BMC Med Res Methodol. 2007;7:7.

Fraunfelder FW. Ocular side effects from herbal medicines and nutritional supplements. Am J Ophthalmol. 2004;138(4):639–47.

Fraunfelder FW. Ocular side effects associated with dietary supplements and herbal medicines. Drugs Today (Barc). 2005;41(8):537–45.

Gagnier JJ, Boon H, Rochon P, Moher D, Barnes J, Bombardier C, CONSORT Group. Reporting randomized, controlled trials of herbal interventions: an elaborated CONSORT statement. Ann Intern Med. 2006;144(5):364–7.

Gopinathan G, Dhiman KS, Manjusha R. A clinical study to evaluate the efficacy of Trataka Yoga Kriya and eye exercises (non-pharmocological methods) in the management of Timira (Ammetropia and Presbyopia). Ayu. 2012;33(4):543–6.

Gupta SK, Srivastava S, Trivedi D, Joshi S, Halder N. Ocimum sanctum modulates selenite-induced cataractogenic changes and prevents rat lens opacification. Curr Eye Res. 2005; 30(7):583–91.

Gupta SK, Niranjan DG, Agrawal SS, Srivastava S, Saxena R. Recent advances in pharmacotherapy of glaucoma. Indian J Pharmacol. 2008; 40(5):197–208.

Gupta DP, Rajagopala M, Dhiman KS. A clinical study on Akshitarpana and combination of Akshitarpana with Nasya therapy in Timira with special reference to myopia. Ayu. 2010; 31(4):473–7.

Gupta SK, Kalaiselvan V, Srivastava S, Saxena R, Agrawal SS. Trigonella foenum-graecum (Fenugreek) protects against selenite-induced oxidative stress in experimental cataractogenesis. Biol Trace Elem Res. 2010;136(3):258–68.

Halder N, Joshi S, Gupta SK. Lens aldose reductase inhibiting potential of some indigenous plants. J Ethnopharmacol. 2003;86(1):113–6.

Hayasaka S, Kodama T, Ohira A. Traditional Japanese herbal (kampo) medicines and treatment of ocular diseases: a review. Am J Chin Med. 2012;40(5):887–904.

Ho YS, Yu MS, Lai CS, So KF, Yuen WH, Chang RC. Characterizing the neuroprotective effects of alkaline extract of Lycium barbarum on beta-amyloid peptide neurotoxicity. Brain Res. 2007;1158:123–34.

Ho YS, Yu MS, Yik SY, So KF, Yuen WH, Chang RC. Polysaccharides from wolfberry antagonizes glutamate excitotoxicity in rat cortical neurons. Cell Mol Neurobiol. 2009;29(8):1233–44.

Hong BS, Meadows DL. Methods and compositions for treating dry eye. US patent 20090131303 A1. 2009.

Hu W, Qian X, Guo F, Zhang M, Lyu C, Tao J, Gao Z, Zhou Z. Traditional Chinese medicine compound Sheng Jin Run Zao Yang Xue granules for treatment of primary Sjögren's syndrome: a randomized, double-blind, placebo-controlled clinical trial. Chin Med J (Engl). 2014;127(15):2721–6.

Huang QS, Zhang ZL, Liu YM. Effect of Tripterygium wilfordii polyglycoside on serum IL-2 and TNF-alpha in patients with acute anterior Uveitis. Zhongguo Zhong Xi Yi Jie He Za Zhi. 2002;22(6):432–4.

Huang SY, Jeng C, Kao SC, Yu JJ, Liu DZ. Improved haemorrheological properties by Ginkgo biloba extract (Egb 761) in type 2 diabetes mellitus complicated with retinopathy. Clin Nutr. 2004;23(4):615–21.

Ishtiaq M, Hanif W, Khan MA, Ashraf M, Butt AM. An ethnomedicinal survey and documentation of important medicinal folklore food phytonims of flora of Samahni valley, (Azad Kashmir) Pakistan. Pak J Biol Sci. 2007;10(13):2241–56.

Jabbarpoor Bonyadi MH, Yazdani S, Saadat S. The ocular hypotensive effect of saffron extract in primary open angle glaucoma: a pilot study. BMC Complement Altern Med. 2014;14:399.

Javadzadeh A, Ghorbanihaghjo A, Arami S, Rashtchizadeh N, Mesgari M, Rafeey M, Omidi Y. Prevention of selenite-induced cataractogenesis in Wistar albino rats by aqueous extract of garlic. J Ocul Pharmacol Ther. 2009;25(5):395–400.

Jia LY, Sun L, Fan DS, Lam DS, Pang CP, Yam GH. (DEX)-induced ocular hypertension. Arch Ophthalmol. 2008;126(12):1700–6.

Jin XH, Ohgami K, Shiratori K, Suzuki Y, Koyama Y, Yoshida K, Ilieva I, Tanaka T, Onoe K, Ohno S. Effects of blue honeysuckle (Lonicera caerulea L.) extract on lipopolysaccharide-induced inflammation in vitro and in vivo. Exp Eye Res. 2006;82(5):860–7.

Jung SH, Lee YS, Lee S, Lim SS, Kim YS, Shin KH. Isoflavonoids from the rhizomes of Belamcanda chinensis and their effects on aldose reductase and sorbitol accumulation in streptozotocin induced diabetic rat tissues. Arch Pharm Res. 2002;25(3):306–12.

Jung SH, Lee YS, Shim SH, Lee S, Shin KH, Kim JS, Kim YS, Kang SS. Inhibitory effects of Ganoderma applanatum on rat lens aldose reductase and sorbitol accumulation in streptozotocin-induced diabetic rat tissues. Phytother Res. 2005;19(6):477–80.

Kalariya NM, Shoeb M, Reddy AB, Zhang M, van Kuijk FJ, Ramana KV. Prevention of endotoxin-induced uveitis in rats by plant sterol guggulsterone. Invest Ophthalmol Vis Sci. 2010; 51(10):5105–13.

Kathleen Head ND. Natural therapies for ocular disorders part two: cataracts and glaucoma. Altern Med Rev. 2001;6(2):141–66.

Kim YS, Jung DH, Kim NH, Lee YM, Jang DS, Song GY, Kim JS. KIOM-79 inhibits high glucose or AGEs-induced VEGF expression in human retinal pigment epithelial cells. J Ethnopharmacol. 2007a;112(1):166–72.

Kim YS, Jung DH, Kim NH, Lee YM, Kim JS. Effect of magnolol on TGF-beta1 and fibronectin expression in human retinal pigment epithelial cells under diabetic conditions. Eur J Pharmacol. 2007b;562(1–2):12–9.

Kim JM, Jang DS, Lee YM, Yoo JL, Kim YS, Kim JH, Kim JS. Aldose-reductase- and protein-glycation-inhibitory principles from the whole plant of Duchesnea chrysantha. Chem Biodivers. 2008;5(2):352–6.

Kim J, Kim CS, Lee YM, Sohn E, Jo K, Kim JS. Vaccinium myrtillus extract prevents or delays the onset of diabetes—induced blood-retinal barrier breakdown. Int J Food Sci Nutr. 2015;66(2): 236–42.

Kobayashi S, Kimura I, Fukuta M, Kontani H, Inaba K, Niwa M, Mita S, Kimura M. Inhibitory effects of tetrandrine and related synthetic compounds on angiogenesis in streptozotocin-diabetic rodents. Biol Pharm Bull. 1999;22(4):360–5.

Kubo M, Matsuda H, Tokuoka K, Kobayashi Y, Ma S, Tanaka T. Studies of anti-cataract drugs from natural sources. I. Effects of a methanolic extract and the alkaloidal components from Corydalis tuber on in vitro aldose reductase activity. Biol Pharm Bull. 1994;17(3):458–9.

Lal B, Kapoor AK, Asthana OP. Efficacy of curcumin in the management of chronic anterior uveitis. Phytother Res. 1999;13(4):318–22.

Launsø L, Gannik DE. The need for revision of medical research designs. In: Gannik DE, Launsø L, editors. Disease knowledge and society. Copenhagen: Forlaget Samfunds Litteratur; 2000.

Li X, Nie L, Yang W, Chen Z, Wang X, Luo L. Suppressing effect of isoforskolin and forskolin on ocular hypertension in rabbits. Zhonghua Yan Ke Za Zhi. 2000;36(4):292–4.

Liang XC, Hagino N, Guo SS, Tsutsumi T, Kobayashi S. Therapeutic efficacy of Stephania tetrandra S. Moore for treatment of neovascularization of retinal capillary (retinopathy) in diabetes – in vitro study. Phytomedicine. 2002;9(5):377–84.

Lindsey JD, Duong-Polk KX, Hammond D, Leung CK, Weinreb RN. Protection of injured retinal ganglion cell dendrites and unfolded protein response resolution after long-term dietary resveratrol. Neurobiol Aging. 2015;36(5):1969–81.

Liu CT, Sheen LY, Lii CK. Does garlic have a role as an antidiabetic agent? Mol Nutr Food Res. 2007;51(11):1353–64.

Lu Q, Yang T, Zhang M, Du L, Liu L, Zhang N, Guo H, Zhang F, Hu G, Yin X. Preventative effects of Ginkgo biloba extract (EGb761) on high glucose-cultured opacity of rat lens. Phytother Res. 2014;28(5):767–73.

Lulli M, Cammalleri M, Fornaciari I, Casini G, Dal Monte M. Acetyl-11-keto-β-boswellic acid reduces retinal angiogenesis in a mouse model of oxygen-induced retinopathy. Exp Eye Res. 2015;135:67–80.

Luo XX, Duan JG, Liao PZ, Wu L, Yu YG, Qiu B, Wang YL, Li YM, Yin ZQ, Liu XL, Yao K. Effect of qiming granule on retinal blood circulation of diabetic retinopathy: a multicenter clinical trial. Chin J Integr Med. 2009;15(5):384–8.

Makri OE, Ferlemi AV, Lamari FN, Georgakopoulos CD. Saffron administration prevents selenite-induced cataractogenesis. Mol Vis. 2013;19:1188–97.

Manayi A, Abdollahi M, Raman T, Nabavi SF, Habtemariam S, Daglia M, Nabavi SM. Lutein and cataract: from bench to bedside. Crit Rev Biotechnol. 2015;4:1–11.

Manikandan R, Thiagarajan R, Beulaja S, Chindhu S, Mariammal K, Sudhandiran G, Arumugam M. Anti-cataractogenic effect of curcumin and aminoguanidine against selenium-induced oxidative stress in the eye lens of Wistar rat pups: an in vitro study using isolated lens. Chem Biol Interact. 2009;181(2):202–9.

Matsuda H, Cai H, Kubo M, Tosa H, Iinuma M. Study on anti-cataract drugs from natural sources II. Effects of buddlejae flos on in vitro aldose reductase activity. Biol Pharm Bull. 1995; 18(3):463–6.

Meyer BH, Stulting AA, Müller FO, Luus HG, Badian M. The effects of forskolin eye drops on intra-ocular pressure. S Afr Med J. 1987;71(9):570–1.

Mi X-S, Feng Q, Lo ACY, et al. Protection of retinal Ganglion cells and retinal vasculature by Lycium barbarum polysaccharides in a mouse model of acute ocular hypertension. Barnes S, ed. PLoS One. 2012;7(10):e45469. doi:10.1371/journal.pone.0045469.

Miyata Y, Oshitari T, Okuyama Y, Shimada A, Takahashi H, Natsugari H, Kosano H. Polymethoxyflavones as agents that prevent formation of cataract: nobiletin congeners show potent growth inhibitory effects in human lens epithelial cells. Bioorg Med Chem Lett. 2013;23(1):183–7.

Moghaddam MS, Kumar PA, Reddy GB, Ghole VS. Effect of Diabecon on sugar-induced lens opacity in organ culture: mechanism of action. J Ethnopharmacol. 2005;97(2):397–403.

Mok JW, Chang DJ, Joo CK. Antiapoptotic effects of anthocyanin from the seed coat of black soybean against oxidative damage of human lens epithelial cell induced by H_2O_2. Curr Eye Res. 2014;39(11):1090–8.

Muthenna P, Raghu G, Akileshwari C, Sinha SN, Suryanarayana P, Reddy GB. Inhibition of protein glycation by procyanidin-B2 enriched fraction of cinnamon: delay of diabetic cataract in rats. IUBMB Life. 2013;65(11):941–50.

Nabavi SM, Nabavi SF, Tenore GC, Daglia M, Tundis R, Loizzo MR. The cellular protective effects of rosmarinic acid: from bench to bedside. Curr Neurovasc Res. 2015;12(1): 98–105.

Nagaki Y, Hayasaka S, Kadoi C, Nakamura N, Hayasaka Y. Effects of scutellariae radix extract and its components (baicalein, baicalin, and wogonin) on the experimental elevation of aqueous flare in pigmented rabbits. Jpn J Ophthalmol. 2001;45(3):216–20.

Narahari SR, Ryan TJ, Aggithaya MG, Bose KS, Prasanna KS. Evidence-based approaches for the Ayurvedic traditional herbal formulations: toward an Ayurvedic CONSORT model. J Altern Complement Med. 2008;14:769–76.

Ohgami K, Ilieva I, Shiratori K, Koyama Y, Jin XH, Yoshida K, Kase S, Kitaichi N, Suzuki Y, Tanaka T, Ohno S. Anti-inflammatory effects of Aronia extract on rat endotoxin-induced uveitis. Invest Ophthalmol Vis Sci. 2005;46(1):275–81.

Peng QH, Yao XL, Zeng ZC, Su RB, Wei YP. Effects of Huoxue Tongmai Lishui method on fundus fluorescein angiography of non-ischemic retinal vein occlusion: a randomized controlled trial. Zhong Xi Yi Jie He Xue Bao. 2009;7(11):1035–41.

Pirhan D, Yüksel N, Emre E, Cengiz A, Kürşat Yıldız D. Riluzole- and resveratrol-induced delay of retinal Ganglion cell death in an experimental model of glaucoma. Curr Eye Res. 2015:1–11.

Poonam, Vaghela DB, Shukla VJ. A clinical study on the role of Akshi Tarpana with Jeevantyadi Ghrita in Timira (Myopia). Ayu. 2011;32(4):540–5.

Porcella A, Maxia C, Gessa GL, Pani L. The synthetic cannabinoid WIN55212-2 decreases the intraocular pressure in human glaucoma resistant to conventional therapies. Eur J Neurosci. 2001;13(2):409–12.

Quaranta L, Riva I, Floriani I. Ginkgo biloba extract improves visual field damage in some patients affected by normal-tension glaucoma. Invest Ophthalmol Vis Sci. 2014;55(4):2417.

Ramer R, Hinz B. Cyclooxygenase-2 and tissue inhibitor of matrix metalloproteinases-1 confer the antimigratory effect of cannabinoids on human trabecular meshwork cells. Biochem Pharmacol. 2010;80(6):846–57.

Rathi SS, Grover JK, Vats V, Biswas NR. Prevention of experimental diabetic cataract by Indian ayurvedic plant extracts. Phytother Res. 2002;16(8):774–7.

Resnikoff S, Pascolini D, Etya'ale D, Kocur I, Pararajasegaram R, Pokharel GP, Mariotti SP. Global data on visual impairment in the year 2002. Bull World Health Organ. 2004;82(11):844–51.

Rhone M, Basu A. Phytochemicals and age-related eye diseases. Nutr Rev. 2008;66(8):465–72.

Ritch R. Potential role for Ginkgo biloba extract in the treatment of glaucoma. Med Hypotheses. 2000;54(2):221–35.

Ritch R. Complementary therapy for the treatment of glaucoma: a perspective. Ophthalmol Clin North Am. 2005;18(4):597–609.

Rolando M, Valente C. Establishing the tolerability and performance of tamarind seed polysaccharide (TSP) in treating dry eye syndrome: results of a clinical study. BMC Ophthalmol. 2007;7(5).

Romano C, Price M, Bai HY, Olney JW. Neuroprotectants in Honghua: glucose attenuates retinal ischemic damage. Invest Ophthalmol Vis Sci. 1993;34(1):72–80.

Sakthivel M, Elanchezhian R, Ramesh E, Isai M, Jesudasan CN, Thomas PA, Geraldine P. Prevention of selenite-induced cataractogenesis in Wistar rats by the polyphenol, ellagic acid. Exp Eye Res. 2008;86(2): 251–9.

Sankeshi V, Kumar PA, Naik RR, Sridhar G, Kumar MP, Gopal VV, Raju TN. Inhibition of aldose reductase by Aegle marmelos and its protective role in diabetic cataract. J Ethnopharmacol. 2013;149(1):215–21.

Scharrer A, Ober M. Anthocyanosides in the treatment of retinopathies. Klin Monatsbl Augenheilkd. 1981;178:386–9.

Scholten WK. The mechanism of action of cannabis and cannabinoids. Ned Tijdschr Geneeskd. 2006;150(3):128–31.

Sharma KR, Bhatia RP, Kumar V. Role of the indigenous drug saptamrita lauha in hemorrhagic retinopathies. Ann Ophthalmol. 1992;24(1):5–8.

Shim SH, Kim JM, Choi CY, Kim CY, Park KH. Ginkgo biloba extract and bilberry anthocyanins improve visual function in patients with normal tension glaucoma. J Med Food. 2012; 9:818–23.

Siddiqui TA, Zafar S, Iqbal N. Comparative double-blind randomized placebo-controlled clinical trial of a herbal eye drop formulation (Qatoor Ramad) of Unani medicine in conjunctivitis. J Ethnopharmacol. 2002;83(1–2):13–7.

Sisková A, Wilhelm J. Role of nonenzymatic glycation and oxidative stress on the development of complicated diabetic cataracts. Cesk Fysiol. 2000;49(1):16–21.

Song Y, Wei G, Li C, Lu N. Effect of Lycium barbarum polysaccharides on cerebral ischemia and reperfusion in mice. J Ningxia Med Coll. 1995;17:12–4.

Spector A. Oxidative stress-induced cataract: mechanism of action. FASEB J. 1995;9(12): 1173–82.

Uccello-Barretta G, Nazzi S, Zambito Y, Di Colo G, Balzano F, Sansò M. Synergistic interaction between TS-polysaccharide and hyaluronic acid: implications in the formulation of eye drops. Int J Pharm. 2010;395(1–2):122–31.

Udani J, Vaghela DB, Rajagopala M, Matalia PD. A comparative study of Bilvadi Yoga Ashchyotana and eye drops in Vataja Abhishyanda (Simple Allergic Conjunctivitis). Ayu. 2012;33(1):97–101.

Vavilala DT, Ponnaluri VK, Kanjilal D, Mukherji M. Evaluation of anti-HIF and anti-angiogenic properties of honokiol for the treatment of ocular neovascular diseases. PLoS One. 2014;9(11): e113717.

Velpandian T, Mathur P, Sengupta S, Gupta SK. Preventive effect of chyvanprash against steroid induced cataract in the developing chick embryo. Phytother Res. 1998;12(5):320–3.

Velpandian T, Gupta P, Ravi AK, Sharma HP, Biswas NR. Evaluation of pharmacological activities and assessment of intraocular penetration of an ayurvedic polyherbal eye drop (Itone™) in experimental models. BMC Complement Altern Med. 2013;13:1. doi:10.1186/1472-6882-13-1.

Velpandian T & Mathur R. Potential therapeutic entities from plants for various ocular disorders (In) Recent Advances in Herbal Drug Research and Therapy Ed. Ray and Gulati, IK International Publishing House, New Delhi, 2010, pp. 449–59.

Wang ZY, Mo XF, Jiang XH, Rong XF, Miao HM. Ginkgolide B promotes axonal growth of retina ganglion cells by anti-apoptosis in vitro. Sheng Li Xue Bao. 2012;64(4):417–24.

Wilkinson JT, Fraunfelder FW. Use of herbal medicines and nutritional supplements in ocular disorders: an evidence-based review. Drugs. 2011;71(18):2421–34.

Wu XW, Tang YZ. Study on treatment of retinitis pigmentosa with traditional Chinese medicine by Flicker electroretinogram. Zhongguo Zhong Xi Yi Jie He Za Zhi. 1996;16(6):336–9.

Yao K, Zhang L, Ye PP, Tang XJ, Zhang YD. Protective effect of magnolol against hydrogen peroxide-induced oxidative stress in human lens epithelial cells. Am J Chin Med. 2009; 37(4):785–96.

Yao N, Lan F, He RR, Kurihara H. Protective effects of bilberry (Vaccinium myrtillus L.) extract against endotoxin-induced uveitis in mice. J Agric Food Chem. 2010;58(8):4731–6.

Yazulla S. Endocannabinoids in the retina: from marijuana to neuroprotection. Prog Retin Eye Res. 2008;27(5):501–26.

Zeng S, Shen B, Wen L, et al. Experimental studies of the effect of forskolin on the lowering of intraocular pressure. Yan Ke Xue Bao. 1995;11(3):173–6.

Zhang B, Rusciano D, Osborne NN. Orally administered epigallocatechin gallate attenuates retinal neuronal death in vivo and light-induced apoptosis in vitro. Brain Res. 2008;1198:141–52.

Zhu MD, Cai FY. The effect of Inj. Salviae Miltiorrhizae Co. on the retrograde axoplasmic transport in the optic nerve of rabbits with chronic IOP elevation. Chung Hua Yen Ko Tsa Chih. 1991;27(3):174–8.

Printed in the United States
By Bookmasters